# Atlas of Toxicological Pathology

Chirukandath Gopinath
Vasanthi Mowat

# Atlas of Toxicological Pathology

Springer

Chirukandath Gopinath
Consultant in Toxicology and Pathology
Cambridgeshire
UK

Vasanthi Mowat
Huntingdon Life Sciences
Cambridgeshire
UK

ISBN 978-1-4939-6197-9 ISBN 978-1-62703-998-7 (eBook)
DOI 10.1007/978-1-62703-998-7
Springer New York Heidelberg Dordrecht London


Softcover reprint of the hardcover 1st edition 2014


Printed on acid-free paper

Humana Press is a brand of Springer
Springer is part of Springer Science+Business Media (www.springer.com)

# Preface

This colour atlas follows in the footsteps of the *Atlas of Experimental Toxicological Pathology*, edited and authored by Gopinath, Prentice, and Lewis and published by MTP Press Ltd, Lancaster, UK, in 1987. This atlas is still widely used and is recognised as one of the standard reference texts in this field. This latest version is an update with numerous new illustrations that the authors have collected over the years, and with references and information pertaining to recently developed drug classes, including biologics.

The field of toxicological pathology has expanded vastly, and although several excellent textbooks on toxicological pathology have been published over the past two decades, the authors still feel that this atlas has a significant role to play and will be useful for practising toxicological pathologists of all levels of experience.

Toxicological pathology is a subspeciality of pathology and is a comparatively young profession, dealing mainly with the pathology of laboratory animals used in toxicity studies. As such, it includes a variety of animal species that are used in this field. Different strains of rats, mice, beagle dogs and nonhuman primates form the bulk of animals used in safety assessment studies. Rabbits, hamsters, mini-pigs, guinea pigs, and chickens form a smaller proportion of these studies. Less commonly, domestic animals including goats, sheep, and cattle are also used in these studies. This makes veterinarians, by virtue of their training, ideally suited as candidates for toxicological pathologists.

Toxicity studies are generally driven by protocols designed by various governmental regulatory bodies, mainly from Europe, the USA and Japan. These studies are carried out to assess potential toxicity of the test substances. The test articles may be novel pharmaceuticals, agrochemicals or chemical entities, and include biologics such as vaccines and antibodies.

Toxicity studies are designed with one or more control groups and a few incremental dose levels of the test substance that are selected to represent multiples of the potential exposure levels in humans. The high doses are chosen to induce toxicity in target organs, and lower doses are used to determine no effect levels and no adverse effect levels where possible. With pharmaceuticals, these studies provide information on potential risk during human use and also on side effects during therapy. With chemicals and agrochemicals, these provide data on potential human hazard due to either industrial or environmental exposure. Exposure through either the food chain or the water supply, due to contamination of the environment by use on crops or soil, are also causes for concern.

Toxicity studies are carried out by different routes of administration that mimic expected routes of human exposure. These include dietary, oral, inhalation and parenteral administration. Parenteral routes include subcutaneous, dermal, intradermal or intravenous (bolus or continuous infusion) administration. The duration of the studies varies according to the intended use of the test substance and may vary from a single dose to a few days to lifelong exposure. The aim of all toxicity studies is to assess the potential risk of the test substance to man when in use.

Pathology is an integral part of these studies at termination, as all animals are subject to autopsies and tissue preservation followed by histopathological evaluation and reporting. A full list of organs/tissues is routinely processed from control animals and some or all treated groups, according to the study protocol and using standard operating procedures. By comparing the results between treated and control groups, the pathologist identifies treatment-related changes and target organs. A sound knowledge of the background pathology of the strain/species of the animals used and of the induced lesions associated with different compound classes is essential for accurate evaluation and interpretation of these studies. This atlas includes a few common spontaneous lesions, but the illustrations are primarily of induced lesions, mostly of a nonneoplastic nature. A few examples of induced rodent tumours from carcinogenicity studies are included. The atlas is organised into different chapters based on systemic pathology. Each chapter has illustrations with legends that briefly identify the changes and a text that explains the changes with references wherever possible. Most of the illustrations are recently sourced from the authors' own collections. A small number that have been used from the previous atlas are acknowledged. The atlas includes some rare examples of unique lesions found during toxicity studies over many years.

It is hoped that the atlas will be useful as a bench reference for practising pathologists and will also be used as a reference text by other experts from related fields.

Cambridgeshire, UK Chirukandath Gopinath
Cambridgeshire, UK Vasanthi Mowat

# Acknowledgement

We are very grateful to Huntingdon Life Sciences for the wealth of experience we have gained here and for the opportunity to publish this atlas.

We have followed the general pattern/theme of a previous atlas on a similar topic, and we are thankful to D.E. Prentice and D.J. Lewis (editors/authors of *Atlas of Experimental Toxicological Pathology*) for their general approval and encouragement for the present book and their permission to reuse some of the photographs.

We are indebted to many people who have helped us in the preparation of this atlas, especially the pathology group at HLS. In particular, we would like to acknowledge David Bell, Dianne Creasy, James Cartwright, and Andrew Pilling for variously helping with photography, providing photographs, and reviewing sections of the manuscript.

Lastly, we thank our partners and children for their unfailing understanding and patience during the preparation of this atlas. Without their support, this project would not have been possible.

# Contents


**1 The Cardiovascular System** . . . 1
- 1.1 Heart . . . 1
  - 1.1.1 Introduction . . . 1
- 1.2 Vascular Changes . . . 13
- References . . . 18

**2 The Respiratory System** . . . 19
- 2.1 Introduction . . . 19
- 2.2 Nasal Turbinates . . . 20
- 2.3 Pharynx . . . 26
- 2.4 Larynx . . . 27
- 2.5 Trachea/Tracheal Bifurcation . . . 29
- 2.6 Bronchi/Bronchioles . . . 30
- 2.7 Terminal Bronchioles/Alveolar Ducts . . . 33
- 2.8 Lungs . . . 35
- References . . . 44

**3 The Liver** . . . 47
- 3.1 Introduction . . . 47
- 3.2 Hydropic Degeneration . . . 48
- 3.3 Fatty Change (Steatosis) . . . 49
- 3.4 Necrosis . . . 51
- 3.5 Apoptosis . . . 54
- 3.6 Nuclear Changes . . . 55
- 3.7 Intracytoplasmic Inclusions . . . 56
- 3.8 Pigments . . . 57
- 3.9 Mineralisation . . . 59
- 3.10 Hepatocellular Hypertrophy . . . 59
- 3.11 Hyperplasia . . . 62
  - 3.11.1 Regenerative Hyperplasia . . . 62
  - 3.11.2 Diffuse Nodular Hyperplasia . . . 63
- 3.12 Foci of Cellular Alteration . . . 64
- 3.13 Bile Duct Hyperplasia . . . 66
- 3.14 Oval Cell Proliferation . . . 67
- 3.15 Cholangiofibrosis . . . 68
- 3.16 ItoCell Prominence or Hyperplasia . . . 69
- 3.17 Cirrhosis . . . 71
- 3.18 Neoplasia . . . 72
  - 3.18.1 Cholangiocarcinomas . . . 73
- 3.19 Gall Bladder . . . 74
- References . . . 75

**4 The Alimentary System and Pancreas** ... 77
4.1 The Oral Cavity ... 77
4.1.1 Teeth ... 79
4.2 Salivary Glands ... 81
4.3 Oesophagus ... 82
4.4 Stomach ... 84
4.4.1 The Rodent Forestomach ... 84
4.4.2 The Glandular Stomach ... 85
4.5 Small Intestines ... 90
4.6 Large Intestines ... 95
4.7 The Exocrine Pancreas ... 99
References ... 105

**5 The Urinary System** ... 109
5.1 Kidney ... 109
5.1.1 Introduction ... 109
5.1.2 Glomerular Changes ... 110
5.1.3 Tubular Changes ... 112
5.1.4 Papilla ... 120
5.1.5 Vascular Changes ... 123
5.1.6 Tumours ... 125
5.2 Urinary Bladder ... 126
References ... 128

**6 The Male Reproductive System** ... 131
6.1 Testes ... 132
6.2 Epididymis ... 140
6.3 Accessory Sex Glands ... 142
6.3.1 Seminal Vesicles/Prostate ... 142
References ... 145

**7 The Female Reproductive System** ... 149
7.1 Introduction ... 149
7.2 Ovaries ... 149
7.2.1 Ovarian Tumours ... 154
7.3 Uterus ... 155
7.3.1 Uterine Tumours ... 159
7.4 Vagina and Cervix ... 161
7.4.1 Vaginal and Cervical Tumours ... 161
7.5 Mammary Gland ... 163
References ... 167

**8 The Endocrine System** ... 169
8.1 Introduction ... 169
8.2 Adrenal Glands ... 169
8.2.1 Lesions of the Adrenal Cortex ... 170
8.2.2 Lesions of the Adrenal Medulla ... 175
8.3 Thyroid Gland ... 178
8.3.1 Induced Changes in the Thyroid Gland ... 178
8.4 Parathyroid Gland ... 186
8.5 Pancreatic Islets ... 187
8.6 Pituitary Gland ... 190
References ... 194

**9 The Lymphoid System** 197
9.1 Introduction 197
9.2 Thymus 199
9.3 Lymph Nodes 201
9.4 Spleen 205
9.5 Bone Marrow 209
9.6 Neoplasms 212
References 213

**10 The Nervous System** 215
10.1 Introduction 215
10.2 Neuronopathy 216
10.3 Axonopathy 218
10.4 Myelinopathy 220
10.5 Gliopathies 222
10.6 Other Changes 223
10.6.1 Choroid Plexus Vacuolation 225
10.6.2 CNS Tumours 225
References 226

**11 The Musculoskeletal System and Skin** 229
11.1 Muscle 229
11.2 Bones 235
11.3 Joints 241
11.4 Skin and Adipose Tissue 242
11.4.1 Skin 242
11.4.2 Adipose Tissue 248
References 250

**12 The Eye and Ear** 253
12.1 The Eye 253
12.1.1 Cornea 254
12.1.2 Retina 259
12.1.3 Uveal Tract 264
12.1.4 Lens 265
12.1.5 Harderian Glands 267
12.1.6 Lacrimal and Meibomian Glands 268
12.2 The Ear 270
12.2.1 Zymbal's Gland 271
References 272

**Index** 275

# 1 The Cardiovascular System

Induced myocardial lesions such as myocardial degeneration/necrosis, haemorrhage, and fibrosis are described with illustrations. The mechanisms underlying myocardial injuries are discussed. Changes occurring as a result of exaggerated pharmacological actions and those occurring because of direct toxicity are included. Other changes discussed include myocardial hypertrophy, coronary and myocardial vascular lesions, and changes to the valves and pericardium. Lesions affecting peripheral vessels are also described. Drug-induced vascular injury, inflammatory and degenerative changes affecting vessel walls, thrombosis, mineralisation, and atherosclerosis are illustrated.

## 1.1 Heart

### 1.1.1 Introduction

Spontaneous cardiovascular injury is somewhat rare in routine toxicity studies. However, cardioactive drugs target the heart quite regularly in toxicity studies. Several good reviews of drug-induced cardiac lesions exist [1–4]. Many cardioactive drugs and some chemicals and metals are known to produce myocardial injuries. Myocardial toxicity induced by cytotoxic agents usually produces widespread and multifocal lesions, and pharmacologically mediated changes are mostly focal with specific anatomical locations, leaving large areas of the myocardium unaffected [1, 5]. Routine screening can sometimes miss lesions in the myocardium owing to restricted sampling. Accurate detailed dissection techniques and sampling are essential to avoid missing vital information/lesions [6]. The myocardium on rare occasions reveals lesions that are secondary to renal failure, stress, or certain central nervous system lesions. Functional tests employed do not always correlate with pathologic changes in the myocardium in toxicity studies. The use of biomarkers, notably troponins, is valuable in monitoring myocardial lesions [7, 8]. An integrated approach evaluating a number of cardiovascular parameters allows detection of minimal early changes and thorough characterisation of any lesions [9].

Induced myocardial lesions are summarised as:

- Myocardial degeneration/necrosis
- Myocardial vacuolation
- Myocardial haemorrhage
- Myocardial pigmentation
- Myocardial calcification
- Myocardial hypertrophy
- Valvular changes
- Myocardial vascular changes
- Pericarditis

Catecholamines and a few other cardioactive agents produce myocardial injuries through exaggerated pharmacological responses. Myocardial fibres are excessively

C. Gopinath, V. Mowat, *Atlas of Toxicological Pathology*,
DOI 10.1007/978-1-62703-998-7_1, © Springer Science+Business Media New York 2014

stimulated, resulting in increased energy and oxygen demand. Functional stimulation causes transmembrane calcium influx, which enhances muscle activity. Vasodilation results in a localised drop in coronary blood pressure, reduced perfusion time, perturbation of transmural blood flow, and development of subendothelial steal phenomenon and set up reflex tachycardia. All these in turn contribute to local ischaemia leading to myocardial degeneration and necrosis in the most vulnerable sites, such as subendocardial foci in papillary muscles and left ventricles. It is interesting to note that cardiostimulants (resulting in tachycardia) and cardioinhibitors (causing extreme bradycardia) can both induce similar myocardial lesions owing to local ischaemia at very high doses (personal observation). Dogs appear to be more susceptible than rodents to cardiotoxicity.

Histologically, small foci or groups of myocardial fibres show swelling, increased eosinophilia of the sarcoplasm, and loss of striation (Figs. 1.1 and 1.2). Frequently this is accompanied by increased granularity, fragmentation, and development of contraction bands. Affected fibres reveal transverse bands that are condensed contractile materials (Fig. 1.3). Preparation artefacts can also reveal focal myocardial fibres with increased eosinophilia (Fig. 1.4). The degenerating fibres occasionally show intracytoplasmic

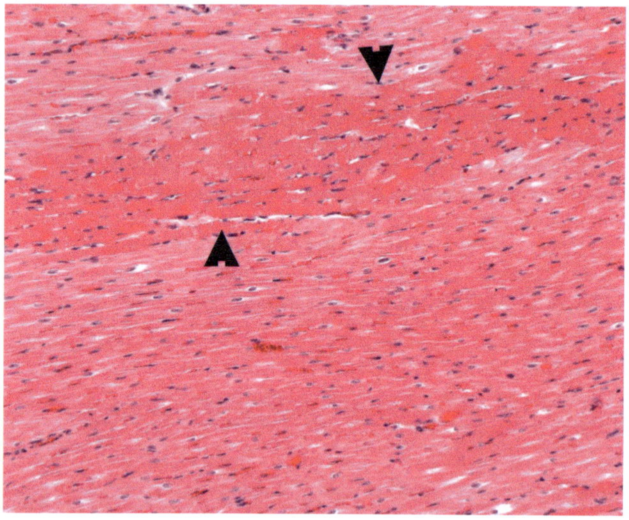

**Figure 1-1.** Myocardial degeneration, left ventricle, in a dog treated with a cardioactive agent. Affected fibres (*arrowheads*) appear more eosinophilic with loss of striations. Haematoxylin and eosin (H&E).

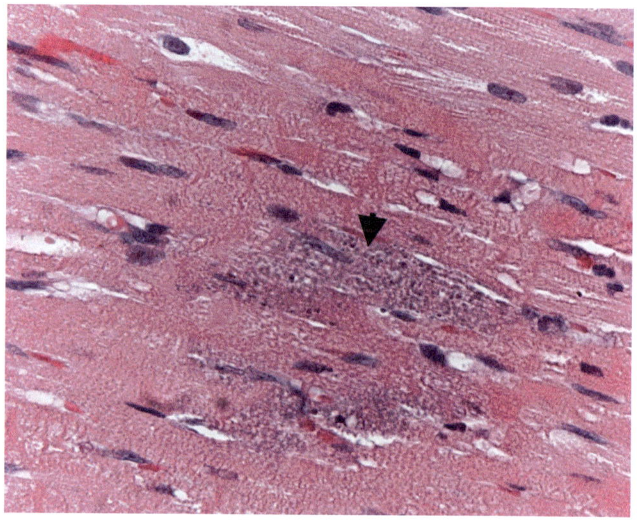

**Figure 1-2.** Myocardial degeneration and calcification, left ventricle, in a dog treated with a cardioactive agent. Affected fibres reveal increased eosinophilia and contraction bands. A few fibres reveal basophilic granular intracytoplasmic deposits (*arrowhead*) representing calcium. H&E.

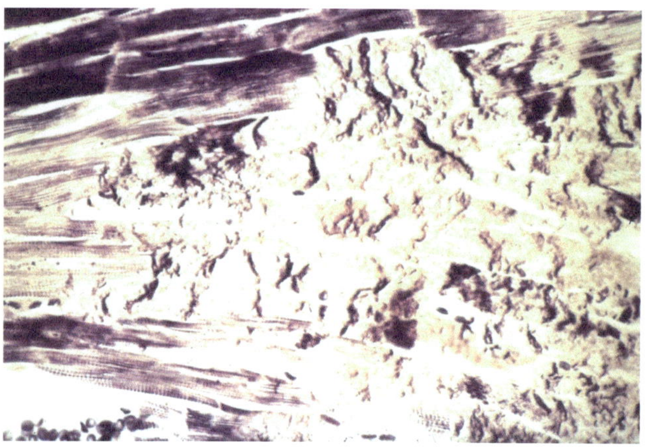

**Figure 1-3.** Myocardial necrosis, left ventricle, in a dog treated with isoprenaline. Affected fibres show loss of staining (striations), but show several contraction bands. Phosphotungstic acid haematoxylin (PTAH).

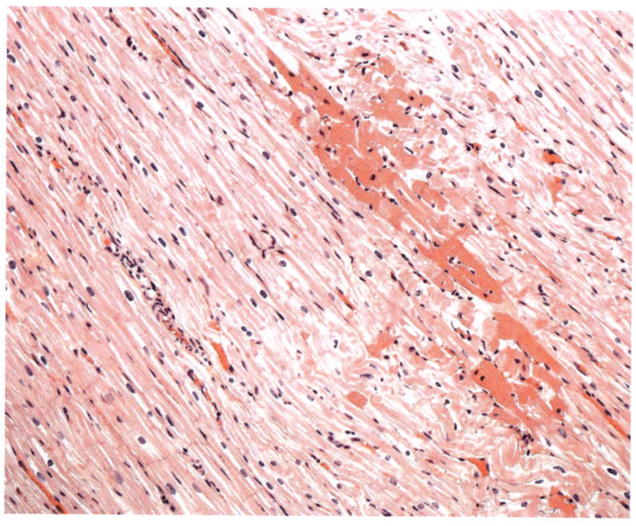

**Figure 1-4.** Eosinophilic shrunken myocardial fibres, untreated dog heart, represent a preparation artefact. H&E.

granular basophilic calcium deposits (Figs. 1.5 and 1.6). The fibres undergo vacuolation, lysis, and nuclear changes including loss of fibres (Fig. 1.7). Initially a minimal inflammatory response (with notable absence of neutrophil infiltration) is followed by a more marked histiocytic infiltration and, later still, a fibroblastic response (Figs. 1.8 and 1.9). Phosphotungstic acid haematoxylin (PTAH) staining is useful in demarcating degenerative/necrotic lesions in the myocardium (Fig. 1.10). In the early stages (acute), heart-specific enzymes like transaminases, lactate dehydrogenases, creatine phosphokinase, and other cardiac biomarkers such as troponins show elevations in serum, along with changes in the electrocardiogram (ECG) during

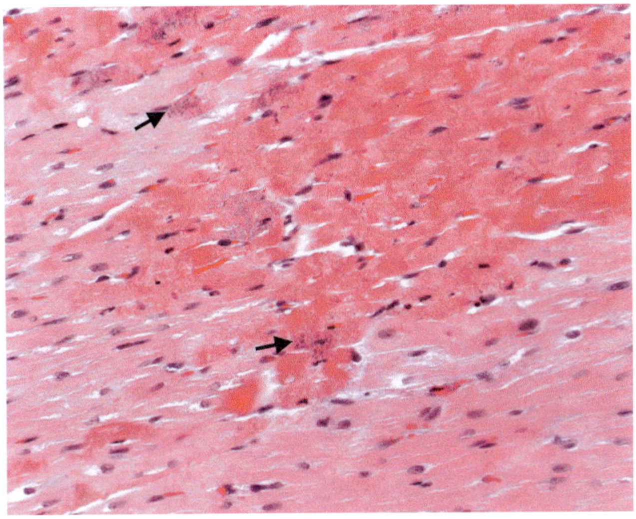

**Figure 1-5.** Myocardial calcification, left ventricle, in a dog treated with a cardioactive agent. Basophilic intracytoplasmic deposits (*arrows*) represent calcium within degenerating (eosinophilic) fibres. H&E.

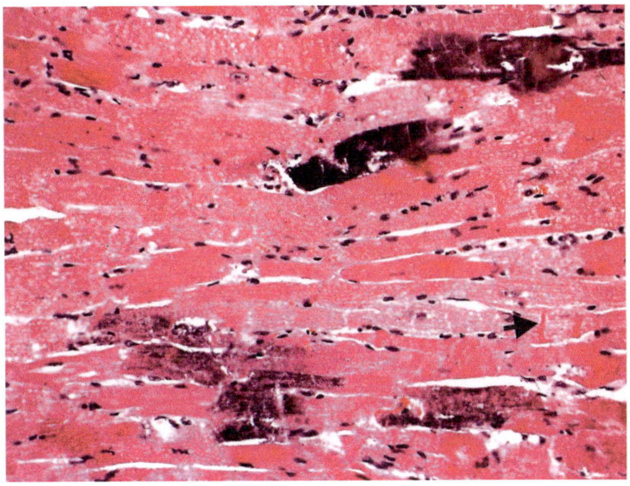

**Figure 1-6.** Myocardial degeneration and calcification, left ventricle, in a dog treated with a cardioactive agent. Dark basophilic deposits of calcium in the degenerating fibres also show occasional contraction bands (*arrow*). H&E.

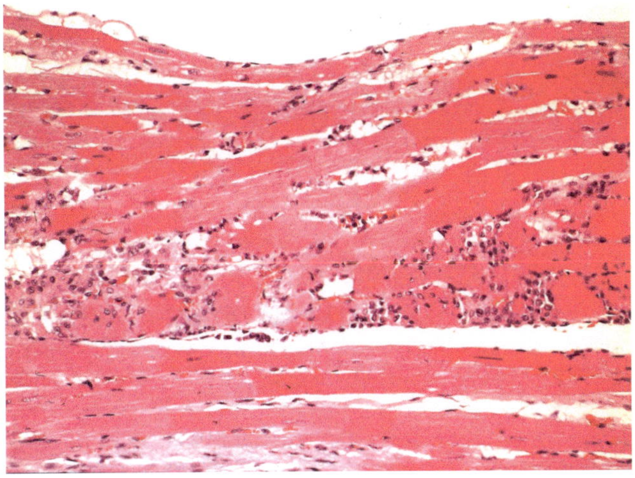

**Figure 1-7.** Subendocardial myocardial necrosis and vacuolation, left ventricle, in a dog treated with a cardioactive agent reveal vacuolation, minimal inflammatory response, and loss of fibres. H&E.

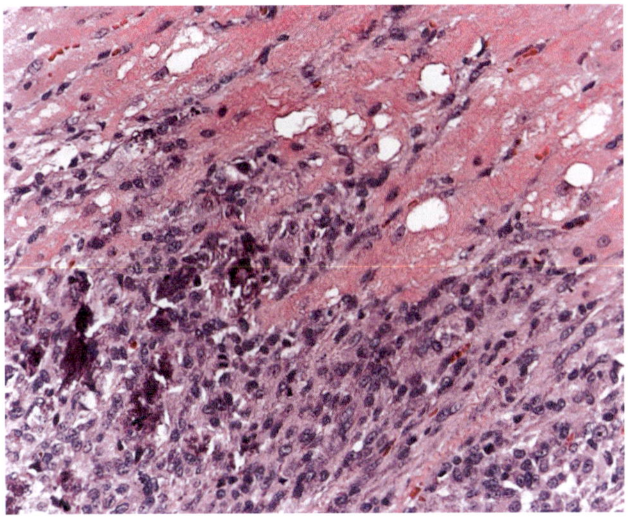

**Figure 1-8.** Myocardial necrosis, left ventricle, in a dog treated with a cardioactive agent. Extensive fibrohistiocytic response is present. Adjacent fibres show vacuolation and focal calcification. H&E.

the ischaemic stages. In the later stages these are not very helpful in animal studies because levels decline to baseline soon after acute injury [10, 11]. In addition to myocardial necrosis, a number of β-adrenergic stimulants and antihypertensive vasodilators produce subendocardial and intramyocardial haemorrhage (Figs. 1.11 and 1.12). The areas of haemorrhage are frequently accompanied by pigmented macrophages, inflammation, and fibrosis (Fig. 1.13). Areas of fibrosis are a common sequel to myocardial necrosis (Fig. 1.14). Cardioactive drugs in dogs can result in endocardial haemorrhage, inflammation, and fibroblastic proliferation (Figs. 1.15 and 1.16). Haemorrhagic cardiomyopathy in male mice has been induced by a reverse transcriptase inhibitor and was found to be secondary to an induced vitamin K deficiency [12].

Digitoxin and theobromine and antihypertensive agents like minoxidil all can produce vascular lesions, haemorrhage, and myocardial necrosis (Fig. 1.17). These agents induce changes in the right ventricle and

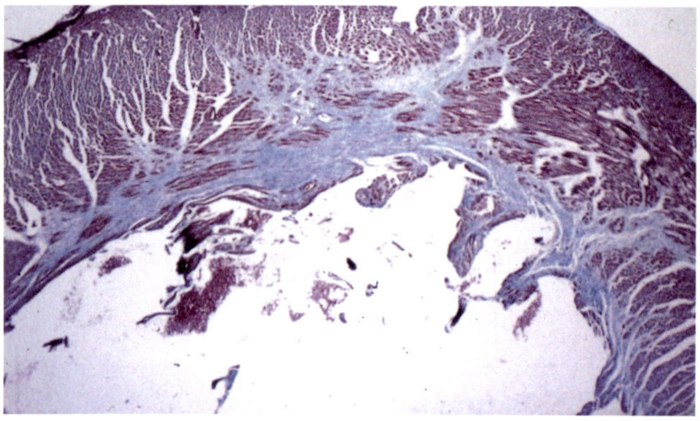

**Figure 1-9.** Myocardial fibrosis, left ventricle, in a dog treated with a cardioactive agent. Fibroblast proliferation replaces injured myocardial fibres. Trichrome.

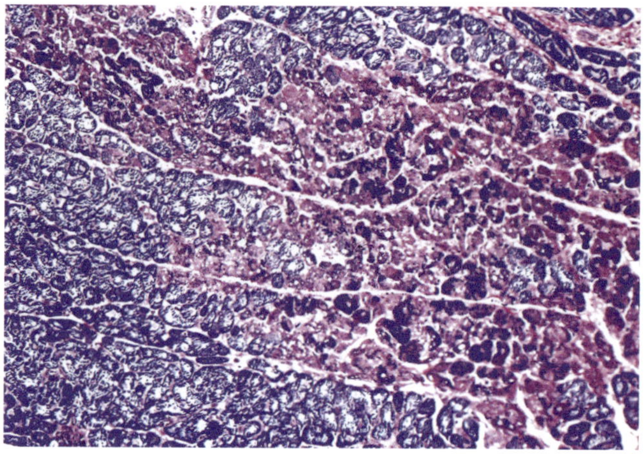

**Figure 1-10.** Early myocardial degeneration/necrosis, left ventricle, in a dog treated with isoprenaline. Loss of cytoplasmic staining clearly demarcates the lesion. PTAH.

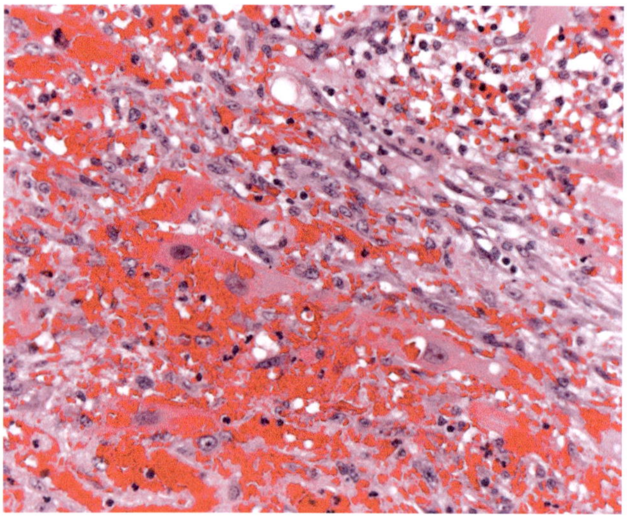

**Figure 1-11.** Myocardial necrosis and haemorrhage, interventricular septum in a monkey treated with a cardioactive agent. Myocardial necrosis, interstitial haemorrhage, fibroblasts, and inflammation are present. H&E.

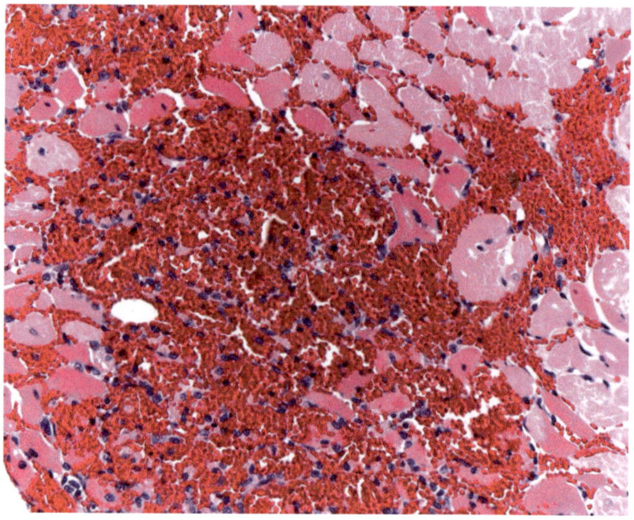

**Figure 1-12.** Myocardial haemorrhage, left ventricle, in a monkey treated with an antithrombotic agent. Extensive haemorrhage and adjacent fibres are necrotic. H&E.

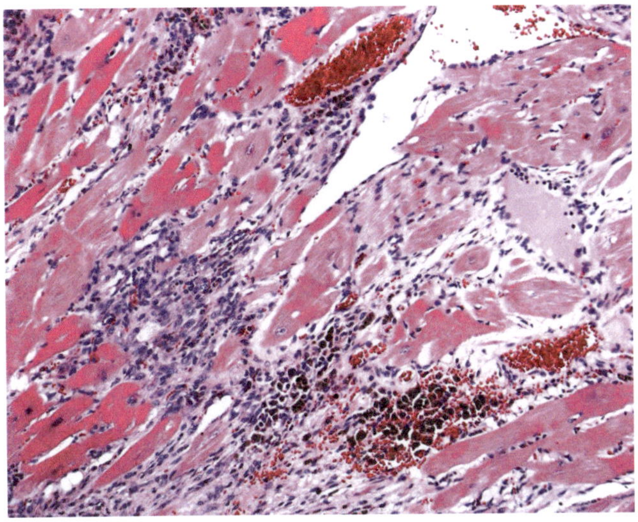

**Figure 1-13.** Myocardial fibrosis and pigmentation, interventricular septum, in a monkey treated with an antithrombotic agent, reveal areas of fibrosis, haemorrhage, and dark brown pigment. H&E.

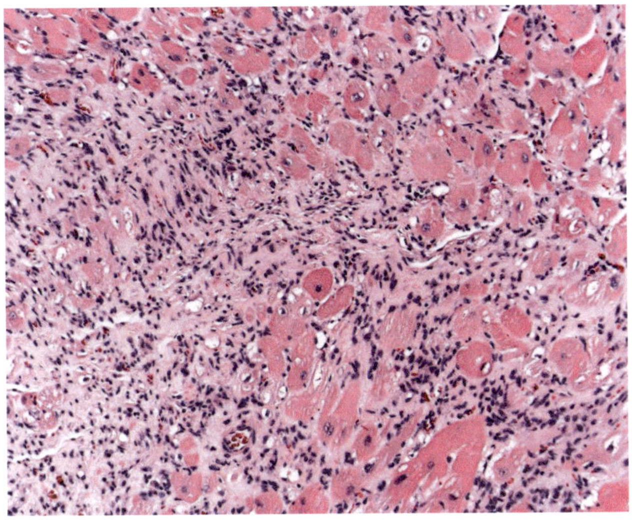

**Figure 1-14.** Myocardial fibrosis, left ventricle, in a rat treated with a cardioactive agent. Areas of myocardium are replaced by fibrosis. H&E.

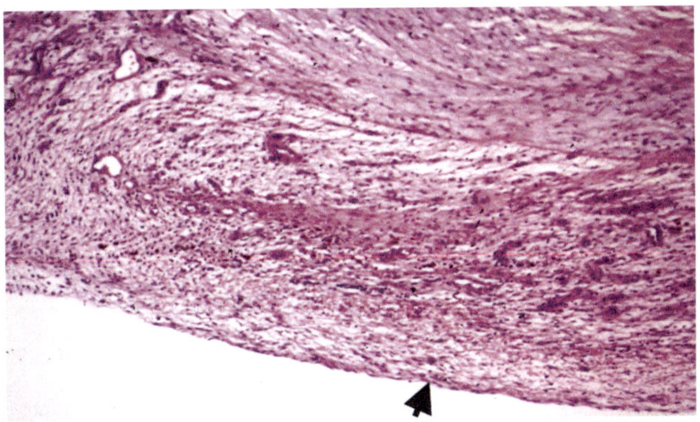

**Figure 1-15.** Endocardial inflammation, left ventricle, in a dog treated with a cardioactive agent. Endocardium is thickened (*arrow*) and reveals inflammation and early fibroblastic proliferation. H&E.

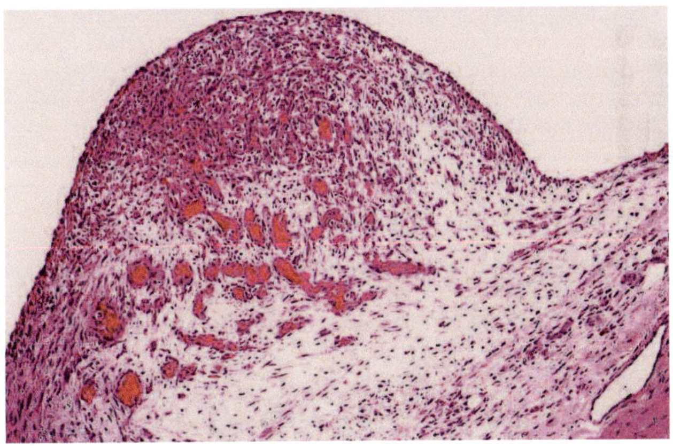

**Figure 1-16.** Endocardial inflammation, left ventricle, in a dog treated with a cardioactive agent reveals inflammation, neovascularisation, and fibroblastic proliferation. H&E.

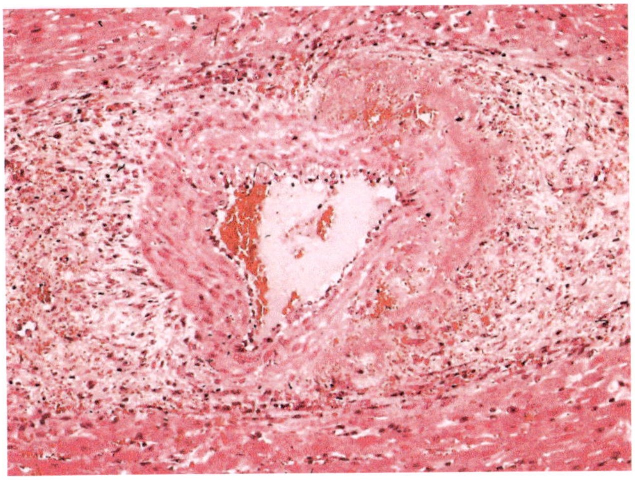

**Figure 1-17.** Vascular injury, intramyocardial artery, left ventricle, in a dog treated with a vasoactive agent. The artery shows intramural necrosis and haemorrhage and perivascular inflammation, haemorrhage, and fibrosis. H&E.

left ventricles associated with arteritis of the intramural arteries [13]. The affected arteries show medial haemorrhage, fibrinoid necrosis, and inflammation of the media and adventitia [14]. This may progress to thickening of the tunica media and fibrosis and inflammation of the tunica adventitia (Figs. 1.18 and 1.19). Tyrosine kinase receptor inhibitors are associated with myocardial degeneration in the ventricular walls, apex, and interventricular septum when administered to rats (Figs. 1.20 and 1.21) [15]. With the tyrosine kinase inhibitor imatinib, severity of cardiotoxic changes is influenced by arterial blood pressure [16]. Chronic inflammation of the heart base, major blood vessels, and valves has been induced in mice by a phosphodiesterase-4 (PDE-4) inhibitor [17].

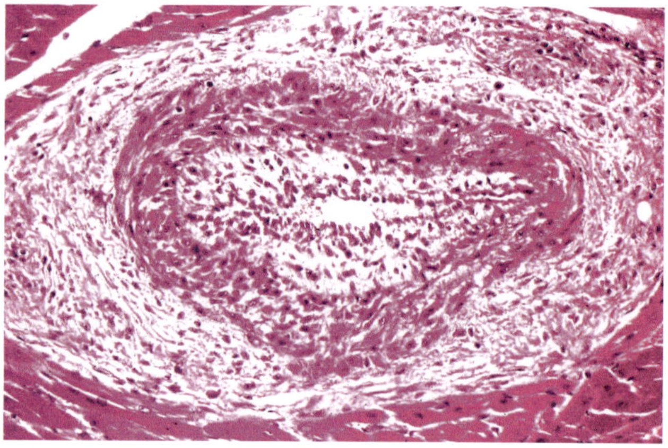

**Figure 1-18.** Arterial hypertrophy, intramyocardial artery, left ventricle, in a dog treated with a cardioactive agent. Thickening of tunica media, inflammation, and periarteritis are present. H&E (With kind permission from Springer Science + Business Media B.V [1]).

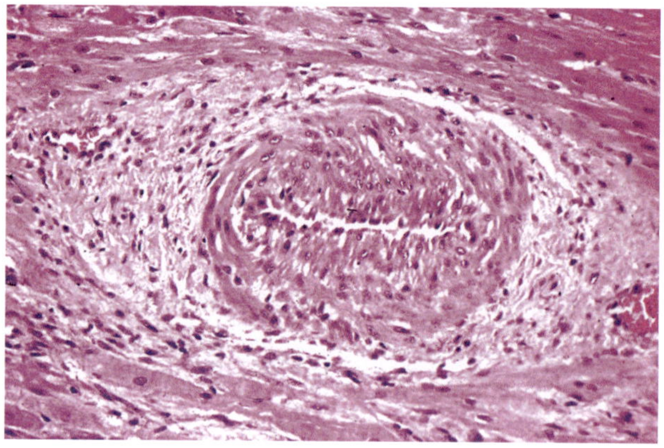

**Figure 1-19.** Arterial hypertrophy, intramyocardial artery, left ventricle, in a dog treated with a cardioactive agent. Smooth muscle hyperplasia of tunica media and periarterial fibrosis are present. H&E (With kind permission from Springer Science + Business Media B.V [1]).

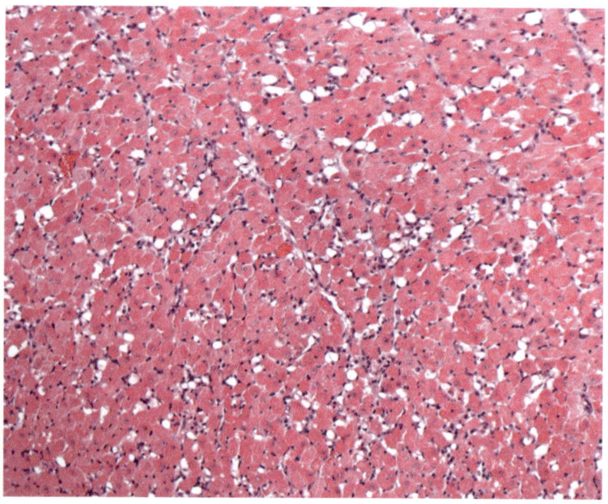

**Figure 1-20.** Myocardial degeneration, multifocal, interventricular septum, in a rat, shows widespread involvement. H&E.

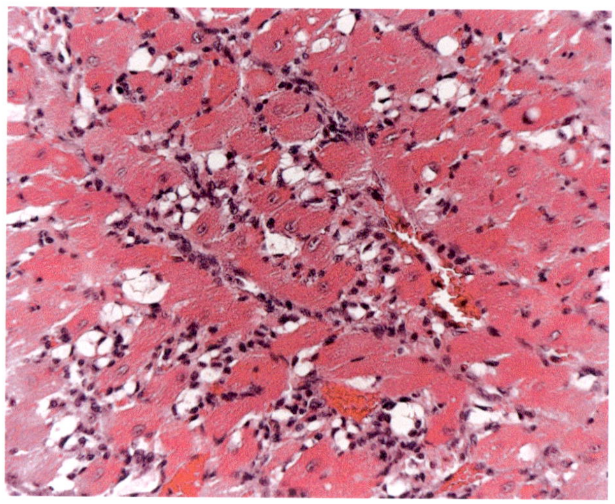

**Figure 1-21.** Myocardial degeneration, widespread involvement, affecting different areas of myocardium suggests cardiotoxicity. H&E.

Prolonged administration of β-stimulants and other cardioactive agents to rats results in an increase in incidence and severity of spontaneous chronic cardiomyopathy in older rodents, mainly affecting the left ventricle (Figs. 1.22 and 1.23). Therefore, it is important to record severity grades in such studies. In advanced cases marked fibrosis and cardiac dilation occur. Sometimes cartilaginous metaplasia of chordae tendineae and valves develops (Figs. 1.24 and 1.25).

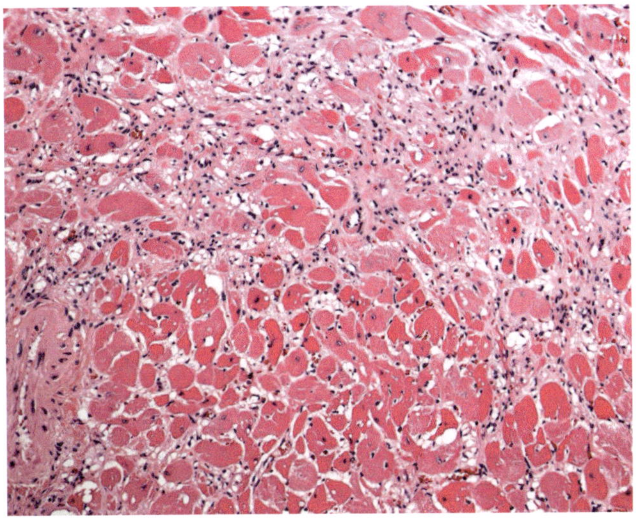

**Figure 1-22.** Cardiomyopathy, left ventricle, in a rat from a chronic toxicity study with a cardioactive agent. Myocardial degeneration, fibre loss, and fibrosis are present. H&E.

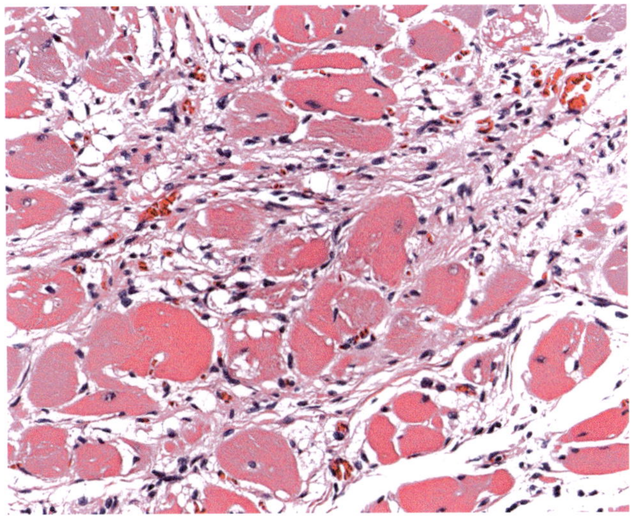

**Figure 1-23.** Cardiomyopathy, left ventricle, in a rat. Note concurrent appearance of active degeneration/necrosis and fibrous replacement. H&E.

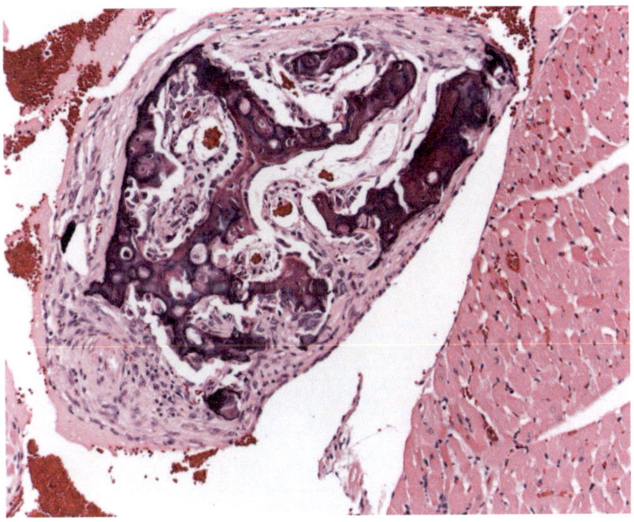

**Figure 1-24.** Extensive cartilaginous metaplasia, papillary muscle, left ventricle, in a rat from a chronic study with a cardioactive agent. H&E.

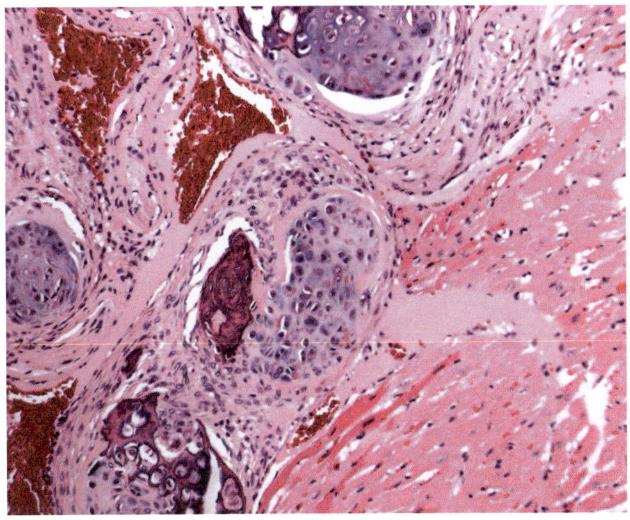

**Figure 1-25.** Myocardial fibrosis and cartilaginous metaplasia, left ventricle, in a rat with advanced cardiomyopathy. H&E.

Histamine induces multifocal myocardial necrosis of the right ventricle in rabbits. Cobalt salts induce myocardial necrosis and calcification in piglets, affecting mainly the atria. Protein deficiency exaggerates myocardial injury by cobalt; the affected myocardium shows macrophage infiltration, fibrosis, and oedema. Gossypol produces multifocal myocardial vacuolation and necrosis in experimental animals including monkeys (Figs. 1.26 and 1.27) [1, 18]. In pigs gossypol produces ventricular dilation and congestive heart failure. Cyclophosphamide induces haemorrhagic myocardial necrosis in monkeys and dogs. Ionophores like monensin are associated with myocardial vacuolation and necrosis in experimental animals (Figs. 1.28 and 1.29). Rodenticides, fluoroacetates, and 5-fluorouracil are capable of producing multifocal myocardial necrosis [19].

Anthracycline antibiotics like Adriamycin, daunomycin, and doxorubicin induce multifocal myocardial vacuolation, hyalinisation, and loss of fibres [19, 20]. The vacuolation is due to distension of endoplasmic reticulum and t-tubules. Lesions can be associated with fibrosis, oedema, and often cardiac dilation. Adriamycin is cardiotoxic to several species of experimental animals and humans [21]. Rodents are slow to develop Adriamycin-induced toxicity.

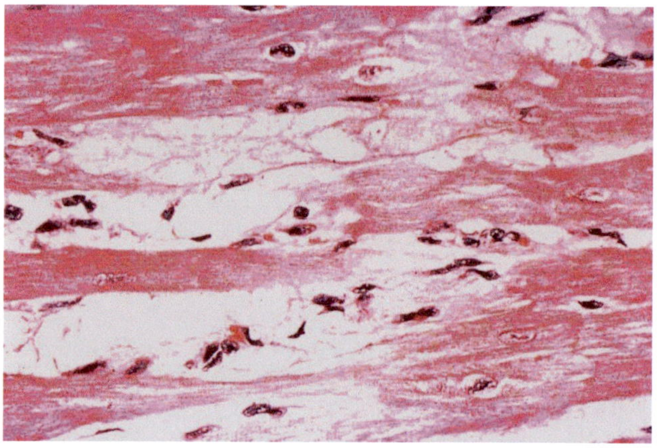

**Figure 1-26.** Myocardial vacuolation, interventricular septum, in a dog treated with an anticancer agent. Swelling, vacuolation of myocardial fibres, and minimal inflammatory cell infiltration are noted. H&E.

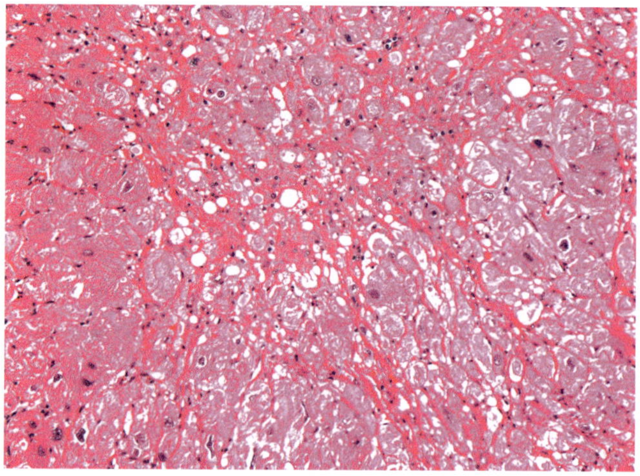

**Figure 1-27.** Myocardial vacuolation and fibrosis, interventricular septum, in a cynomolgus monkey. Similar lesions at low incidences have been noted in untreated monkeys. H&E.

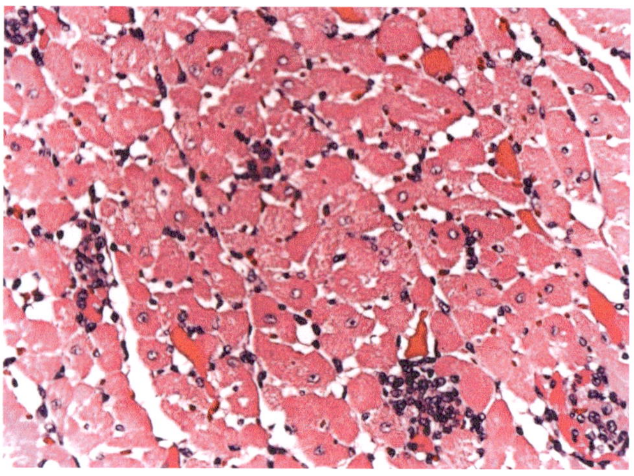

**Figure 1-28.** Myocardial necrosis, multifocal, right ventricle, in a rat treated with an industrial chemical. Necrotic fibres associated with inflammation are present. H&E.

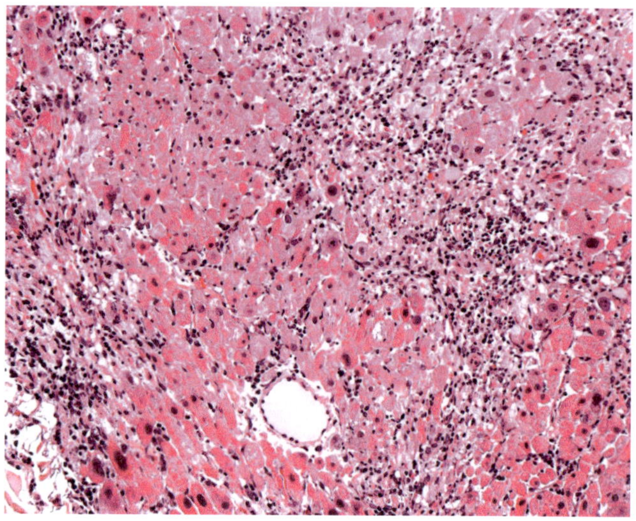

**Figure 1-29.** Myocardial necrosis, multifocal, interventricular septum, in a monkey treated with a novel pharmaceutical. Areas of necrosis and inflammation are noted. H&E.

Fatty degeneration and myocytolysis are induced in rats given high doses of brominated vegetable oils [1]. Glucocorticoids when given to rats result in lipid accumulation and myocardial degeneration. Cardiac muscles can develop phospholipidosis, manifesting as vacuolation (confirmed as phospholipidosis by electron microscopy), when exposed to agents like chloroquine. Administration of a food pigment, Brown FK, to rats results in lipofuscin-like pigment deposition along with focal necrosis. Hypervitaminosis D causes metastatic calcification of the myocardium and myocardial arteries and aorta (Figs. 1.30 and 1.31). Hypothyroidism and diabetes mellitus can cause fat accumulation in the myocardium. Allylamine also causes fatty degeneration and myocardial necrosis [22].

Right atrial damage including fibrosis, haemorrhage, and inflammation occurs in treatment with minoxidil and hydralazine [1, 19]. Digitoxin also causes haemorrhagic lesions in the right atrium (Fig. 1.32). Subendocardial haemorrhage is seen in dogs with renal failure and uraemia.

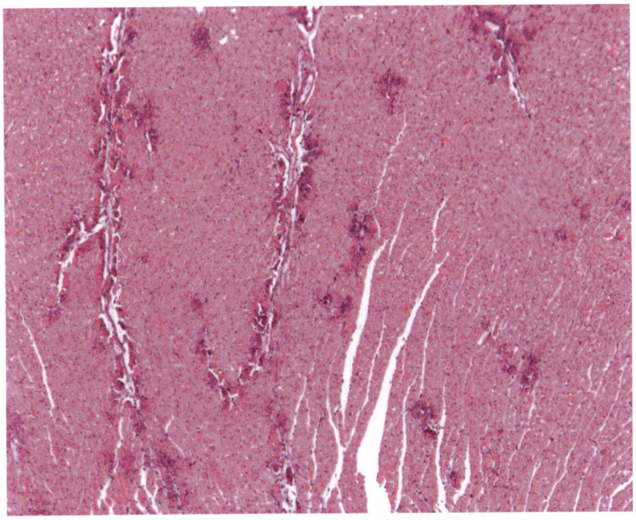

**Figure 1-30.** Myocardial calcification, multifocal, right ventricle, in a rat treated with a vitamin D analogue. Multifocal deposits of calcium, mostly adjacent to vessels, are present. H&E.

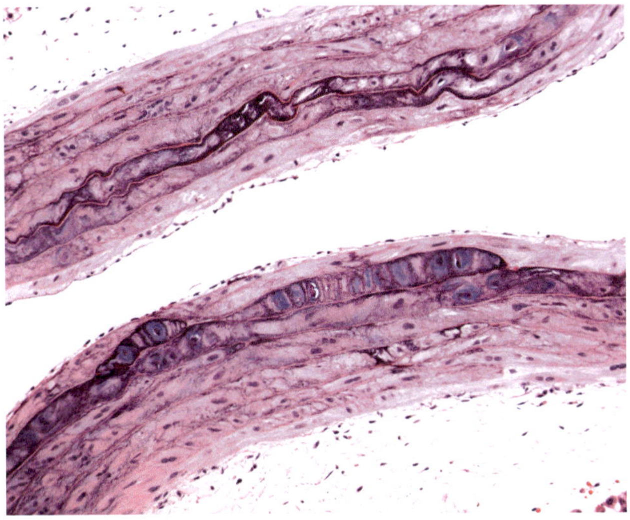

**Figure 1-31.** Calcification and cartilaginous metaplasia, aorta, in a rat from a chronic toxicity study with a vitamin D analogue. Elastic fibres in aortic wall reveal mineralisation along with cartilaginous metaplasia. H&E.

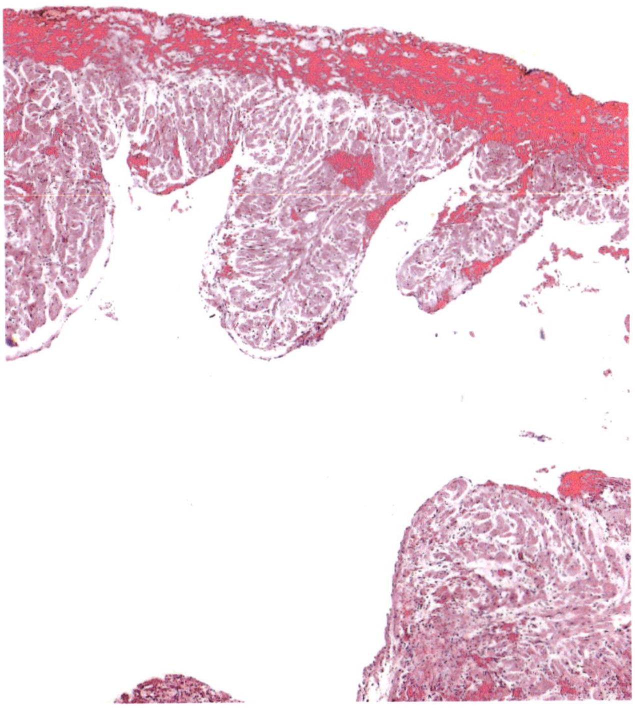

**Figure 1-32.** Myocardial haemorrhage, right atrium, in a monkey treated with a novel pharmaceutical. H&E.

Myocardial hypertrophy can be induced in response to mechanical, haemodynamic, hormonal, and physiological stimulation. Systemic hypertension produces left ventricular hypertrophy. Hypertrophy can also be physiological, as seen in athletes and racehorses, owing to increased exercise and in females during pregnancy. Chronic exposure to catecholamines and administration of thyroxine, growth hormone, testosterone, and anabolic steroids cause myocardial hypertrophy. Oxfenicine produces an increase in heart weight in dogs and rats [23]. Troglitazone causes myocardial hypertrophy in rodents but not in monkeys [24]. Some other related antidiabetic agents are known to result in myocardial hypertrophy in monkeys. Myocardial hypertrophy can be localised, affecting only a few fibres as seen in areas adjacent to chronic myocardial lesions, or it can affect the entire chamber(s). Certain calcium channel blockers given to dogs cause myocardial hypertrophy. The affected fibres appear larger and broader with large vesicular nuclei (Fig. 1.33). A growth hormone analogue resulted in visible enlargement of the heart in rats (hypertrophy) without producing any frank microscopic changes in the myocardium (Fig. 1.34). Arsenic, when given to mice in the drinking water, produces hypertension and left ventricular concentric hypertrophy [25].

Endothelin antagonists can induce arteritis of coronary arteries with thrombosis. Pericarditis, vasculitis, and myocarditis have been induced in dogs by an immunomodulator. Muramyl peptide given to dogs induces pericarditis and myocarditis (Fig. 1.35). Epicarditis has been induced by a sweetener in dogs. Treatment of dogs with certain immunostimulants has produced vasculitis, with endothelial proliferation and thrombosis with associated myocardial necrosis (Fig. 1.36). In later stages the thrombi cause occlusion and undergo recanalisation (Figs. 1.37–1.39) [1].

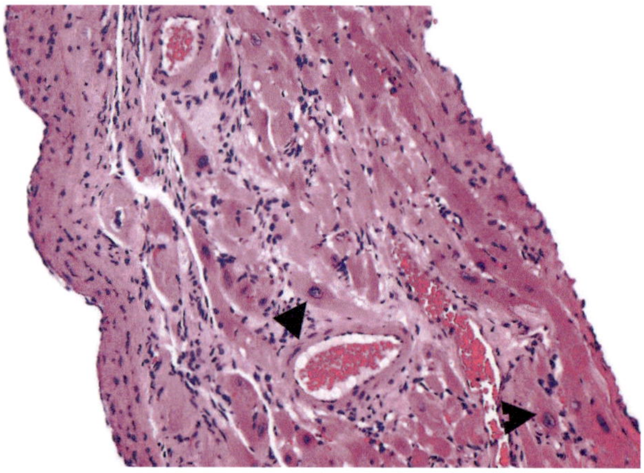

**Figure 1-33.** Myocardial hypertrophy, focal, right ventricle, in a monkey. Affected fibres (*arrowheads*) are larger with large open nuclei. There is some interstitial fibrosis. H&E.

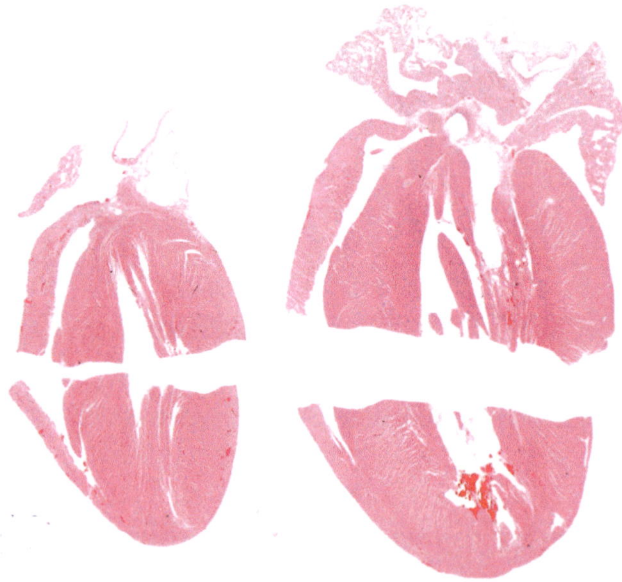

**Figure 1-34.** Myocardial hypertrophy, left ventricle, on a rat, with no change in histological appearance of individual fibres. H&E.

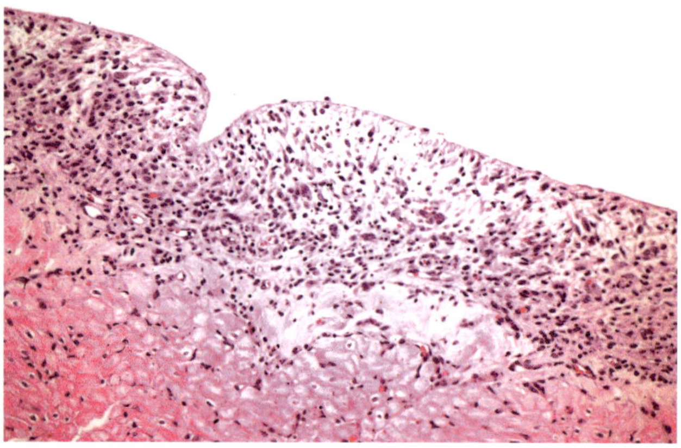

**Figure 1-35.** Epicarditis, left ventricle, in a dog treated with an immunomodulator. Inflammation and oedema of epicardium are present. H&E.

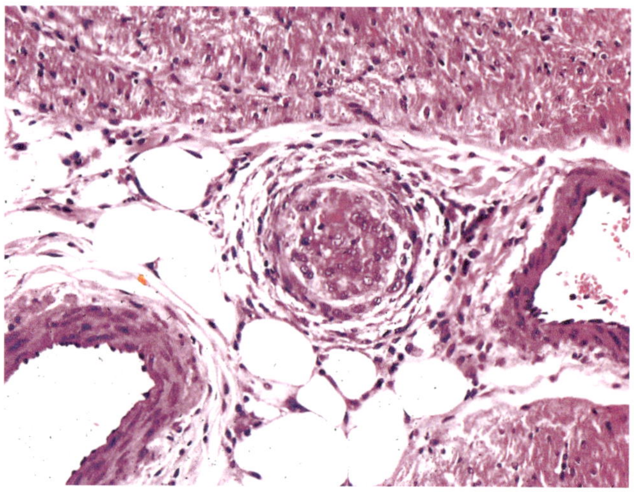

**Figure 1-36.** Vasculitis, myocardium, of a dog treated with an immunostimulant. Note the intimal proliferation and thrombosis. H&E.

Arteritis and periarteritis of the extramural coronary artery have been recorded in dogs treated with certain immunomodulators. Coronary arterial inflammation was noted in mice treated with an immunomodulator (Fig. 1.40). These lesions in the dog can sometimes be difficult to differentiate from those seen spontaneously in laboratory beagles. Valvular inflammation and stromal proliferation of atrioventricular valves have been noticed in dogs treated with a variety of agents including immunomodulators, biologicals, and certain cardioactive agents (Figs. 1.41 and 1.42) [26–28]. Fat necrosis of epicardial adipose tissue has been seen in dogs treated with novel glucocorticoids (Fig. 1.43) [1]. Atrial thrombosis is sometimes associated with prolonged cases of cardiomyopathy in rodents (Fig. 1.44). Complications in infusion studies can sometimes lead to the development of valvular endocarditis (Fig. 1.45).

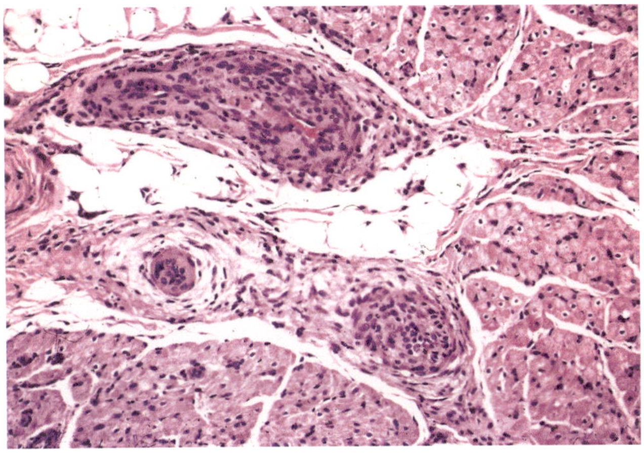

**FIGURE 1-37.** Vasculitis and intimal proliferation, coronary artery, in a dog treated with an immunostimulant. Note the luminal occlusion. H&E (With kind permission from Springer Science + Business Media B.V [1]).

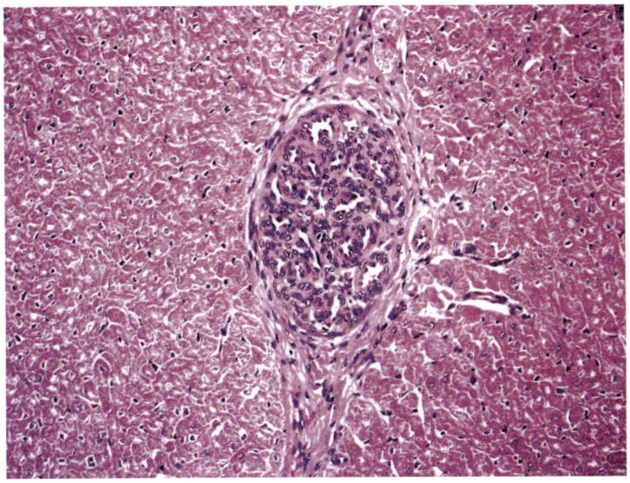

**FIGURE 1-38.** Vascular occlusion and recanalisation, myocardial arteries, left ventricle, in a dog treated with an immunostimulant. H&E.

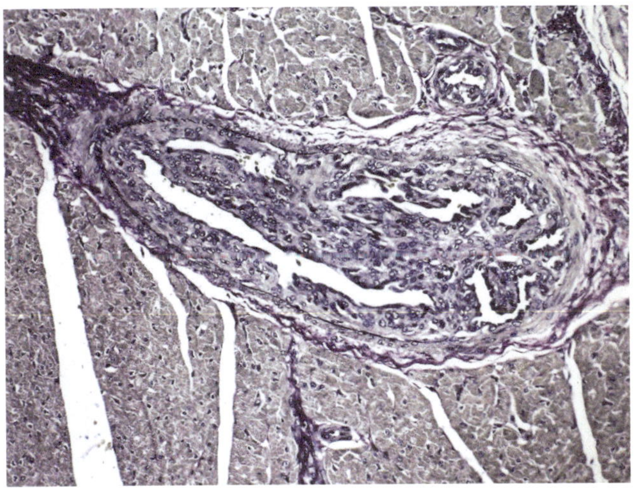

**FIGURE 1-39.** Occlusion, myocardial arteries, in a dog treated with an immunostimulant. Note the distinct recanalisation. Elastic van Gieson (With kind permission from Springer Science + Business Media B.V [1]).

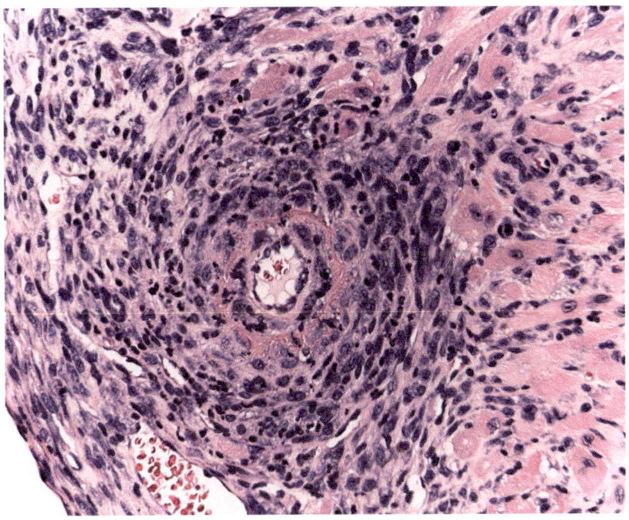

**FIGURE 1-40.** Coronary arteritis in a dog treated with an immunomodulator. Note inflammation and necrosis of arterial wall, periarterial inflammation, and fibrosis. H&E.

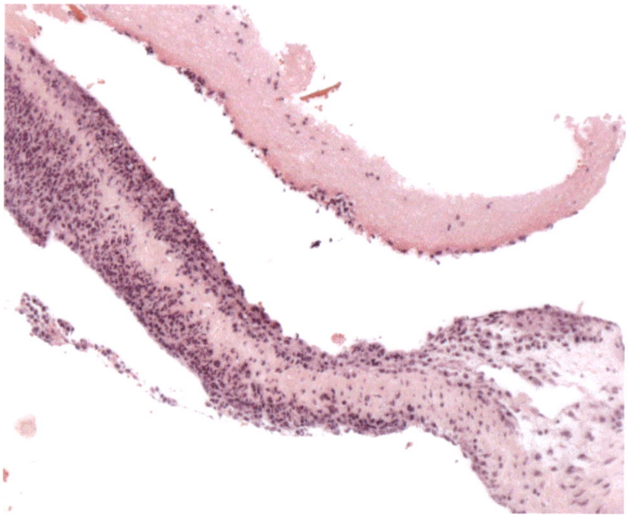

**Figure 1-41.** Valvular inflammation in a dog treated with an immunomodulator. Note the thickening and inflammatory cell infiltration. H&E.

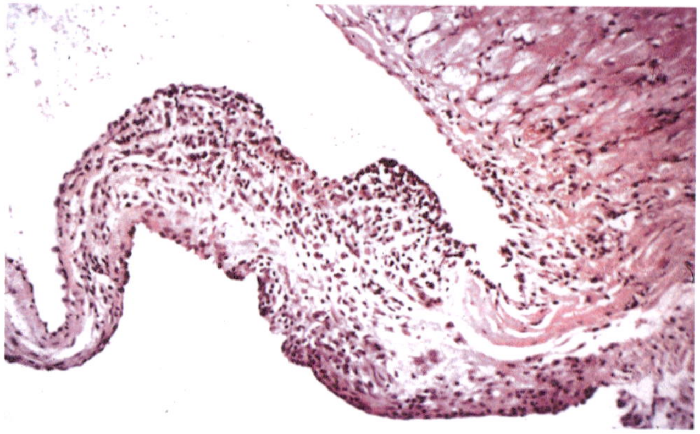

**Figure 1-42.** Valvular inflammation in a dog treated with an immunomodulator. There is stromal increase and inflammatory cell infiltration causing increased thickness. H&E.

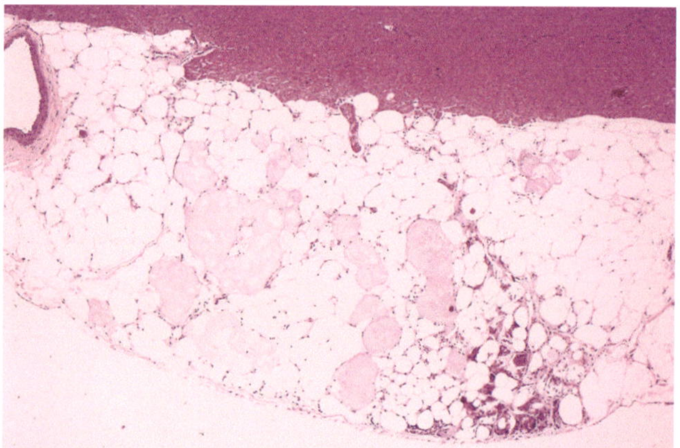

**Figure 1-43.** Fat necrosis, epicardial fat, in a dog treated with a glucocorticoid agent. H&E (With kind permission from Springer Science + Business Media B.V [1]).

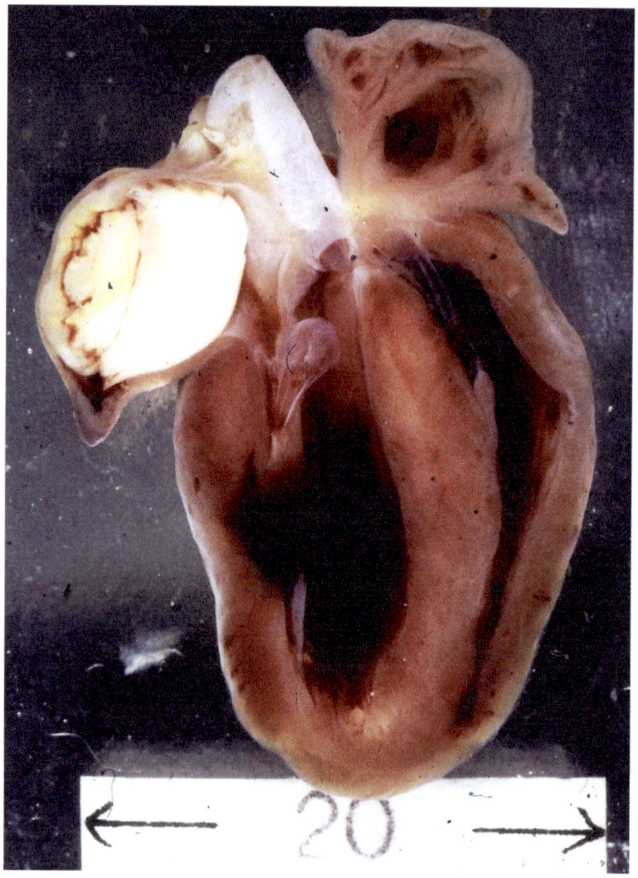


**Figure 1-44.** Atrial thrombosis in a rat from a chronic toxicity study.

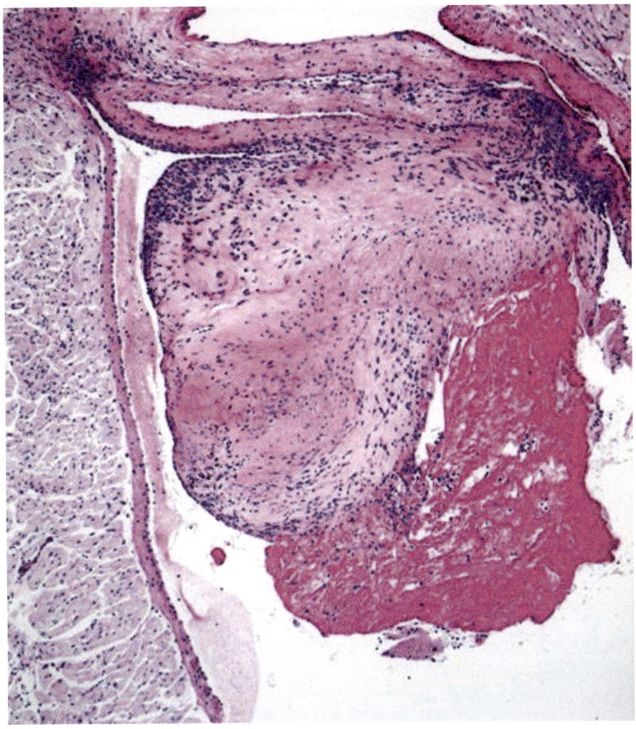

**Figure 1-45.** Valvular endocarditis, aortic valve, in a dog from an infusion study. The valve is thickened and inflamed and shows thrombosis. H&E.

## 1.2 Vascular Changes

In addition to the cardiac vessels, peripheral vessels can also become targets in toxicity studies, albeit rarely. Mercury salts induce a vasculopathy in pigs, resulting in degeneration of arteries in meninges, oesophagus, and stomach [29]. The affected arteries show thickening of all layers of the artery, fibrinoid degeneration of the tunica media, and narrowing of the lumen. Monocrotaline, a pyrrolizidine alkaloid, induces occlusive arteritis with thrombosis in the lungs of treated monkeys and rats. Certain immunostimulants have induced necrotising arteritis with extensive inflammation of the periarterial connective tissue in dogs (Fig. 1.46). This type of vasculitis can occur spontaneously in dogs and rodents.

β-Aminopropionitrile causes intramural damage to arteries, with haemorrhage, and can progress to aneurysms in rats [30]. Ergotamine toxicity affects peripheral arteries causing medial degeneration and intimal proliferation. Drug-induced vascular injury (DIVI) in toxicology studies is a frequent problem with several drugs; their mechanisms and extrapolative significance to human safety are poorly understood. Vasodilating antihypertensive agents and PDE inhibitors cause degeneration of the tunica media along with necrosis, inflammation, and haemorrhage, affecting small to medium-sized arteries in experimental animals (Figs. 1.47 and 1.48) [31–36]. The exact location of DIVI is not always predictable, although it frequently affects mesenteric vessels. It is important to note and report the location of affected vessels. Ionotropic vasodilators produce a plexiform vasculopathy in mesenteric vessels (Figs. 1.49 and 1.50) [34]. The affected vessels show intramural vascular channel formation. Thrombosis is often seen with higher incidences in chronic intravenous studies, as a result of direct local effects (Figs. 1.51 and 1.52). Varying degrees of intimal and mural injuries and responses are frequently seen in the vessels of animals used in chronic infusion studies (Fig. 1.53). A novel biotechnological product resulted in adherence of macrophages to the vascular endothelium in the lungs in rats in our laboratories.

Hypervitaminosis D results in widespread and extensive mineralisation of the tunica media of arteries and aorta, sometimes resulting in cartilaginous metaplasia (Fig. 1.54).

Experimental atherosclerosis can be induced in several species. Hyperlipidaemic diets, homocystine, carbon disulphide, and carbon monoxide exposure are known to influence development of atherosclerosis by causing injury to endothelium in experimental animals [1, 37]. Diets rich in cholesterol alone induced atherosclerotic lesions of the coronary arteries, aorta,

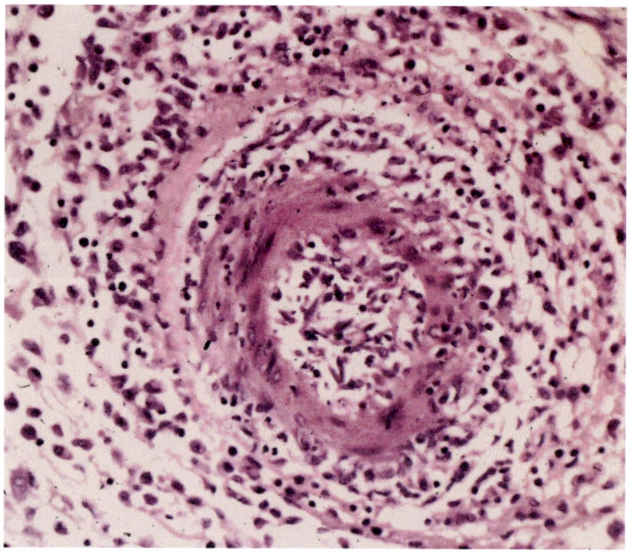

**Figure 1-46.** Arteritis, coronary artery, in a dog treated with an immunomodulator. Inflammatory cell infiltration of the arterial wall and periarterial connective tissue are noted. H&E.

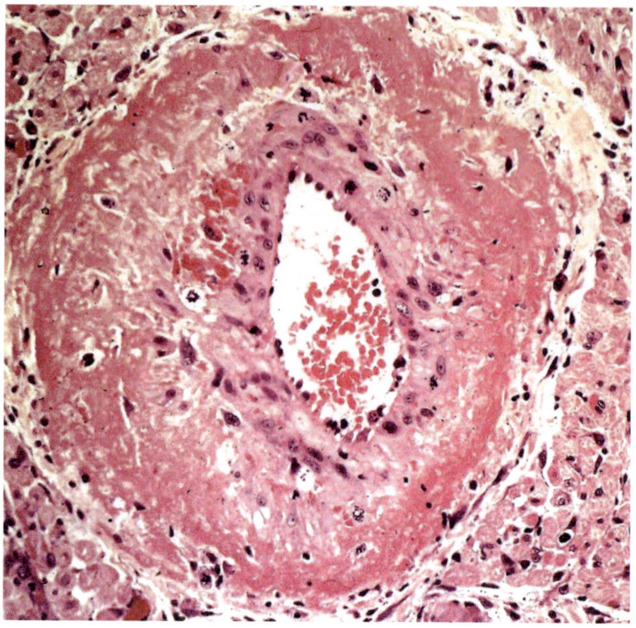

**Figure 1-47.** Vascular injury, artery, in a dog treated with a phosphodiesterase (PDE) inhibitor. Tunica media reveal necrosis and haemorrhage. H&E.

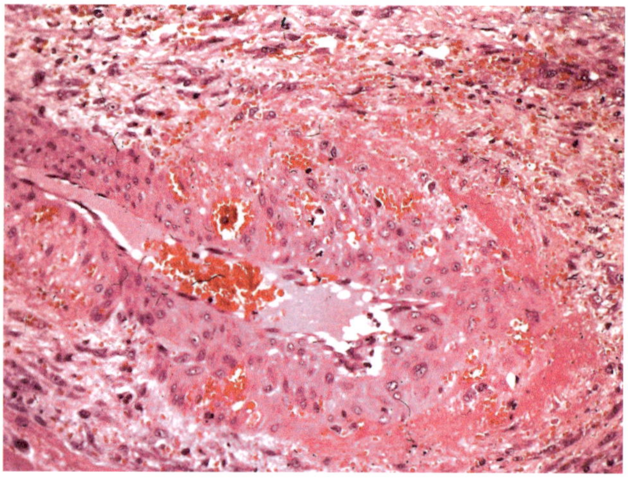

**Figure 1-48.** Drug-induced vascular injury, artery, in a dog treated with an antihypertensive agent. Arterial wall reveals necrosis, haemorrhage and periarterial inflammation, haemorrhage, and fibroblastic proliferation. H&E.

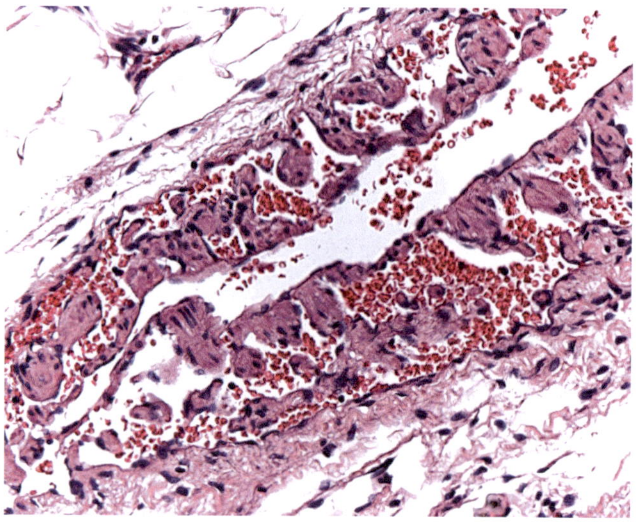

**Figure 1-49.** Plexiform vasculopathy, mesenteric vessels, in a rat treated with an ionotropic agent. Vessel shows intramural vascular channel formation. H&E.

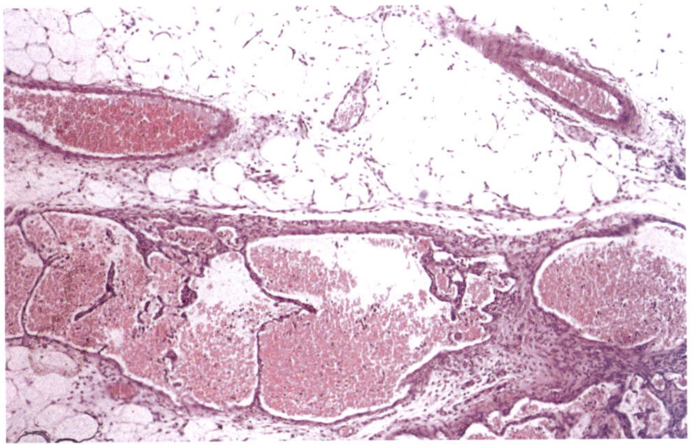

**Figure 1-50.** Plexiform vasculopathy in a rat. Note the large vascular channels within the mesenteric vessel wall. H&E.

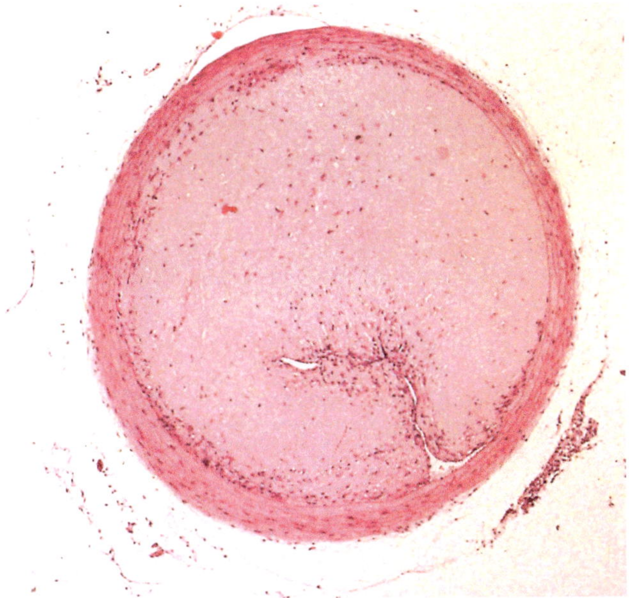

**Figure 1-51.** Occluding thrombus in a subcutaneous vein at the site of injection. H&E.

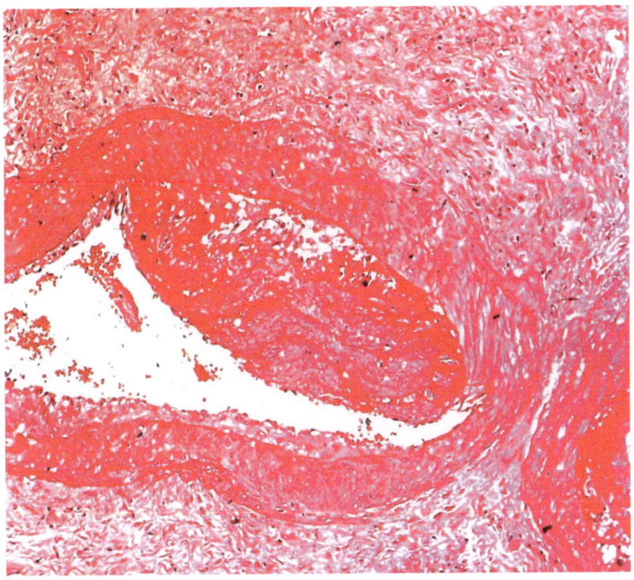

**Figure 1-52.** Thrombosis at the site of injection in a dog. H&E.

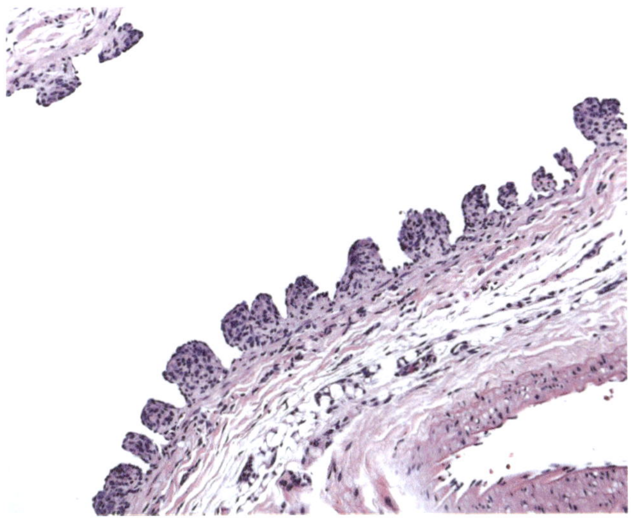

**Figure 1-53.** Intimal proliferation, multifocal, subcutaneous vessel, in a dog from an infusion study. H&E.

and peripheral vessels in monkeys in our laboratories (Fig. 1.55) [1]. The affected arteries appear thickened, opaque creamy white, and tortuous on the cardiac surface (Fig. 1.56). The affected arteries reveal plaques containing lipoid and mucoid substances along with tissue components such as myofibres, fibroblasts, and macrophages. The plaques are frequently located subendothelially and project into the lumen, causing varying degrees of stenosis (Figs. 1.57 and 1.58). The affected areas show amorphous matrix containing lipid, cholesterol clefts, mucoglycoproteins, calcification, collagen mixed with fibroblasts, smooth muscle cells,

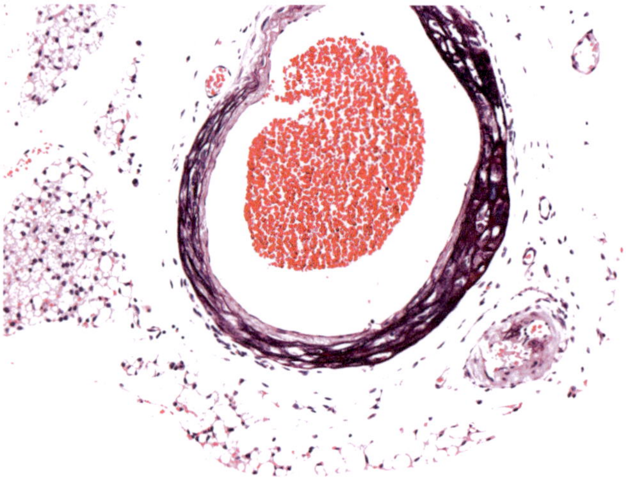

**Figure 1-54.** Mineralisation and cartilaginous metaplasia, visceral artery, in a rat from a chronic toxicity study with vitamin D analogue. H&E.

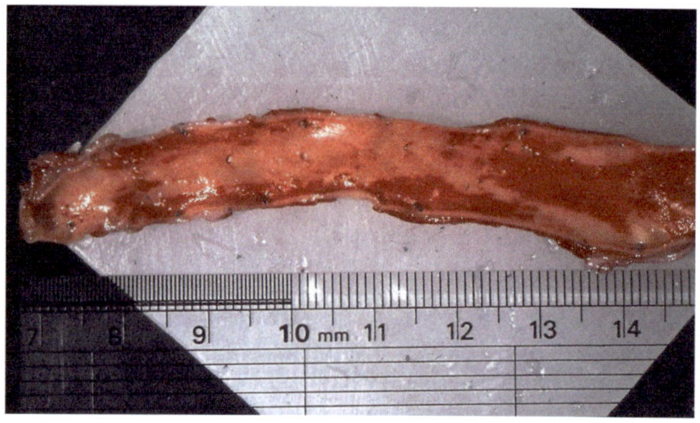

**Figure 1-55.** Fatty streaks, abdominal aorta, in a monkey. Many raised reddish plaques are seen on the intimal surface. Oil red O (ORO).

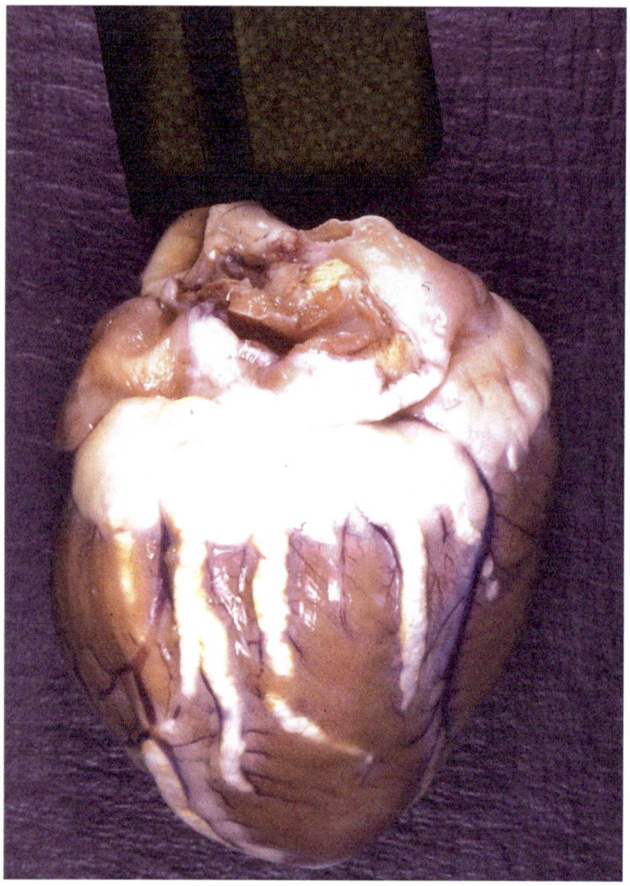

**Figure 1-56.** Atherosclerosis, coronary arteries, in a monkey. Creamy white coronary arteries appear nodular and thickened.

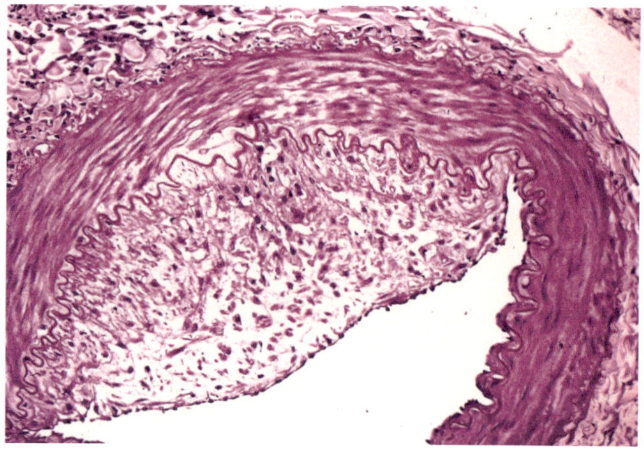

**Figure 1-57.** Intimal plaque, renal artery, in a monkey. An intimal plaque is present over the internal elastic lamina. H&E (With kind permission from Springer Science + Business Media B.V [1]).

and macrophages. The lesion can extend to involve the tunica media. In extreme cases the lesion can affect all layers. Lymphoid foci were noticed in the tunica adventitia in occasional cases. Ulceration and thrombosis were not recorded in any of the monkeys with atherosclerosis of the coronary arteries.

Vasculitis, mainly affecting medium-sized to small arteries of different organs and tissues, is noted in animals treated with certain PDE-4 inhibitors and other agents (Figs. 1.59 and 1.60). Focal arterial hypertrophy of pulmonary arterioles was seen in rats treated with an industrial chemical (Fig. 1.61).

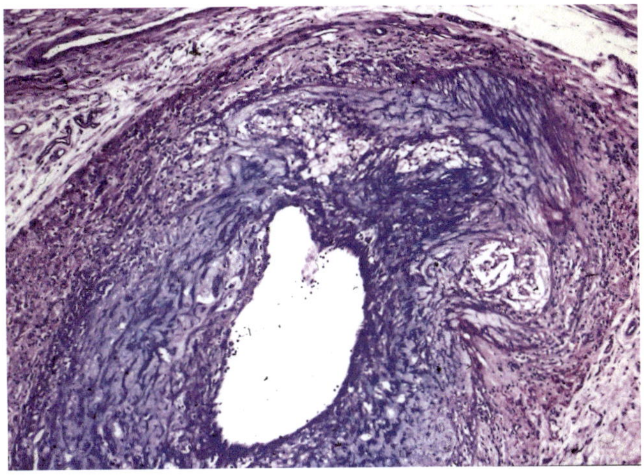

**Figure 1-58.** Atherosclerotic plaque, coronary artery, in a monkey. Narrowing of the lumen is caused by the plaque with accumulation of mucopolysaccharide in the matrix. Periodic acid–Schiff (PAS)/Alcian blue (With kind permission from Springer Science + Business Media B.V [1]).

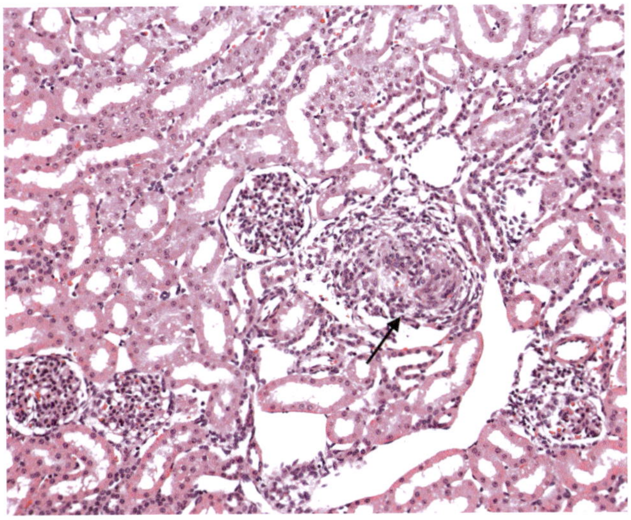

**Figure 1-59.** Vasculitis, kidney, in a rat treated with a PDE-4 inhibitor shows intramural and perivascular inflammation (*arrow*). H&E.

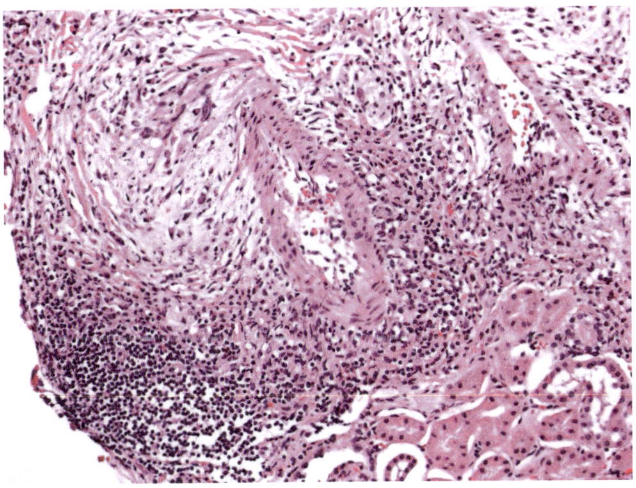

**Figure 1-60.** Vasculitis in a monkey treated with an immunomodulator. Inflammation of the vessel wall and extensive periarteriolar inflammation and fibroblastic proliferation are seen. H&E.

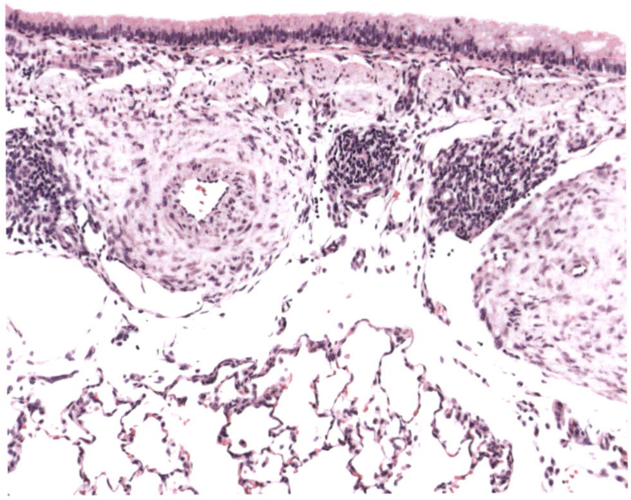

**Figure 1-61.** Arteriolar hypertrophy, lung, in a rat treated with an industrial chemical. Affected artery shows thickening of the wall and narrowing of the lumen. H&E.

## References


1. Gopinath C, Prentice DE, Lewis DJ. The cardiovascular system. In: Atlas of experimental toxicological pathology. Boston: MTP Press Limited; 1987. p. 11–22.
2. Greaves P. Patterns of drug-induced cardiovascular pathology in the beagle dog: relevance for humans. Exp Toxicol Pathol. 1998;50:283–93.
3. Greaves P. Patterns of cardiovascular pathology induced by diverse cardioactive drugs. Toxicol Lett. 2000;112–113: 547–52.
4. Jokinen MP, Lieuallen WG, Boyle MC, Johnson CL, Malarkey DE, Nyska A. Morphologic aspects of rodent cardiotoxicity in a retrospective evaluation of national toxicology program studies. Toxicol Pathol. 2011;39:850–60.
5. Glaister JR. Cardiovascular system. In: Glaister JR, editor. Principles of toxicological pathology. London: Taylor & Francis; 1986. p. 116.
6. Keenan CM, Vidal JD. Standard morphologic evaluation of the heart in the laboratory dog and monkey. Toxicol Pathol. 2006;34:67–74.
7. Herman E, Knapton A, Rosen E, Zhang J, Estis J, Agee SJ, et al. Baseline serum cardiac troponin I concentrations in Sprague–Dawley, spontaneous hypertensive, Wistar, Wistar-Kyoto, and Fisher rats as determined with an ultrasensitive immunoassay 2. Toxicol Pathol. 2011;39:653–63.
8. Walker DB. Serum chemical biomarkers of cardiac injury for nonclinical safety testing. Toxicol Pathol. 2006;34:94–104.
9. Casartelli A, Lanzoni A, Comelli R, Crivellente F, Defazio R, Dorigatti R, et al. A novel and integrated approach for the identification and characterization of drug-induced cardiac toxicity in the dog. Toxicol Pathol. 2011;39:361–71.
10. Balazs T, Earl FL, Bierbower GW, Weinberger MA. The cardiotoxic effects of pressurized aerosol isoproterenol in the dog. Toxicol Appl Pharmacol. 1973;26:407–17.
11. Gopinath C, Thuring J, Zayed I. Isoprenaline-induced myocardial necrosis in dogs. Br J Exp Pathol. 1978;59:148–57.
12. De JS, Verbeeck J, Vinken P, Lammens L, Starckx S, Lachau-Durand S, et al. Hemorrhagic cardiomyopathy in male mice treated with an NNRTI: the role of vitamin K. Toxicol Pathol. 2008;36:321–9.
13. Teske RH, Bishop SP, Righter HF, Detweiler DK. Subacute digoxin toxicosis in the beagle dog. Toxicol Appl Pharmacol. 1976;35:283–301.
14. Gans JH, Korson R, Cater MR, Ackerly CC. Effects of short-term and long-term theobromine administration to male dogs. Toxicol Appl Pharmacol. 1980;53:481–96.
15. Aguirre SA, Heyen JR, Collette III W, Bobrowski W, Blasi ER. Cardiovascular effects in rats following exposure to a receptor tyrosine kinase inhibitor. Toxicol Pathol. 2010;38:416–28.
16. Herman EH, Knapton A, Rosen E, Thompson K, Rosenzweig B, Estis J, et al. A multifaceted evaluation of imatinib-induced cardiotoxicity in the rat. Toxicol Pathol. 2011;39:1091–106.
17. Losco PE, Poulet FM, Kaminska-McNamara GZ, Klein MF. Myocardial and reproductive system toxicity of SCH 351591, a selective phosphodiesterase-4 inhibitor, in CD-1 mice. Toxicol Pathol. 2010;38:568–82.
18. Smith HA. The pathology of gossypol poisoning. Am J Pathol. 1957;33:353–65.
19. Van Vleet JF, Ferrans VJ. Myocardial diseases of animals. Am J Pathol. 1986;124:98–178.
20. Jaenke RS. An anthracycline antibiotic-induced cardiomyopathy in rabbits. Lab Invest. 1974;30:292–304.
21. Billingham ME, Mason JW, Bristow MR, Daniels JR. Anthracycline cardiomyopathy monitored by morphologic changes. Cancer Treat Rep. 1978;62:865–72.
22. Boor PJ, Moslen MT, Reynolds ES. Allylamine cardiotoxicity: I. Sequence of pathologic events. Toxicol Appl Pharmacol. 1979;50:581–92.
23. Greaves P, Martin J, Michel MC, Mompon P. Cardiac hypertrophy in the dog and rat induced by oxfenicine, an agent which modifies muscle metabolism. Arch Toxicol. 1984;7: 488–93.
24. Breider MA, Gough AW, Haskins JR, Sobocinski G, de la Iglesia FA. Troglitazone-induced heart and adipose tissue cell proliferation in mice. Toxicol Pathol. 1999;27:545–52.
25. Sanchez-Soria P, Broka D, Monks SL, Camenisch TD. Chronic low-level arsenite exposure through drinking water increases blood pressure and promotes concentric left ventricular hypertrophy in female mice. Toxicol Pathol. 2012;40:504–12.
26. Donnelly KB. Cardiac valvular pathology: comparative pathology and animal models of acquired cardiac valvular diseases. Toxicol Pathol. 2008;36:204–17.
27. Anderton MJ, Mellor HR, Bell A, Sadler C, Pass M, Powell S, et al. Induction of heart valve lesions by small-molecule ALK5 inhibitors. Toxicol Pathol. 2011;39:916–24.
28. Elangbam CS. Drug-induced valvulopathy: an update. Toxicol Pathol. 2010;38:837–48.
29. Tryphonas L, Nielsen NO. Pathology of chronic alkylmercurial poisoning in swine. Am J Vet Res. 1973;34:379–92.
30. Balazs T, Hanig JP, Herman EH. Toxic responses of the cardiovascular system. In: Klaassen CD, Amdur MO, Doull J, editors. Toxicology. New York: Macmillan; 1986. p. 387.
31. Joseph EC, Rees JA, Dayan AD. Mesenteric arteriopathy in the rat induced by phosphodiesterase III inhibitors: an investigation of morphological, ultrastructural, and hemodynamic changes. Toxicol Pathol. 1996;24:436–50.
32. Joseph EC, Jones HB, Kerns WD. Characterization of coronary arterial lesions in the dog following administration of SK&F 95654, a phosphodiesterase III inhibitor. Toxicol Pathol. 1996;24: 429–35.
33. Joseph EC. Arterial lesions induced by phosphodiesterase III (PDE III) inhibitors and DA(1) agonists. Toxicol Lett. 2000;112–13: 537–46.
34. Westwood FR, Iswaran TJ, Greaves P. Pathologic changes in blood vessels following administration of an inotropic vasodilator (ICI 153,110) to the rat. Fundam Appl Toxicol. 1990;14: 797–809.
35. Weaver JL, Zhang J, Knapton A, Miller T, Espandiari P, Smith R, et al. Early events in vascular injury in the rat induced by the phosphodiesterase IV inhibitor SCH 351591. Toxicol Pathol. 2010;38:738–44.
36. Zhang J, Snyder RD, Herman EH, Knapton A, Honchel R, Miller T, et al. Histopathology of vascular injury in Sprague–Dawley rats treated with phosphodiesterase IV inhibitor SCH 351591 or SCH 534385. Toxicol Pathol. 2008;36:827–39.
37. Wronska-Nofer T, Szendzikowski S, Laurman W. The effect of carbon disulphide and atherogenic diet on the development of atherosclerotic changes in rabbits. Atherosclerosis. 1978; 31:33–9.

# 2 The Respiratory System

Induced lesions of the respiratory tract are described on an organ-by-organ basis with illustrations. Both nonneoplastic and neoplastic changes of the various regions are covered. Examples of test articles causing different lesions are provided. Lesions of the upper respiratory tract in inhalation safety studies are described in some detail, with particular reference to their significance. The mechanisms of toxicity in the various regions of the tract are discussed briefly, along with their relationship to the pathogenesis of these changes. The relevance of certain mechanical and physiological features to the development of these lesions also is mentioned.

## 2.1 Introduction

The respiratory tract was recognised several decades ago as a major target for toxicity due to airborne pollutants. The increasing numbers of people affected by neoplastic and nonneoplastic pathologic conditions of the respiratory tract have made it a major area for research and for the targeting of therapeutic agents.

Inhalation toxicology initially gained importance as a technique to study the effects of environmental airborne pollutants on the respiratory tract, primarily for pulmonary changes. Compounds tested included cigarette smoke, toxic gases such as sulphur dioxide, occupationally inhaled chemicals and particles, solvents, dyes, and particles such as carbon, silica, and asbestos. The increasingly wide range of household products sold as aerosols, such as polishes, cleaning agents, hairsprays, and deodorants, also required safety evaluation to assess potential for damage to the respiratory tract.

More recently, a wide range of therapies including biologics has been developed for treating respiratory conditions via the inhalation route, notably antiasthmatics, treatments for chronic obstructive pulmonary disease and cystic fibrosis, and anti-allergics.

The structure and metabolic function of different areas of the respiratory tract have a bearing on the distribution and severity of induced toxicologic lesions [1, 2]. Several mechanical factors also cause or influence toxicity in studies of this type [3–5]. The size and shape of particles, particle density, and molecular weight are just a few of the factors that can determine the regions of the respiratory tract that may be affected and the nature and extent of their toxicity [6]. Recognition of these variables has initiated considerable interest in the morphology and physiology of the nasal passages. Inhalation toxicology in safety assessment is now an intensively studied field, with an extensive bibliography describing the range of neoplastic and nonneoplastic changes induced in animal models by different classes of pharmaceuticals and chemicals. In addition, transport of toxicants into the brain via the olfactory nerves is recognised and has aroused considerable interest [7].

Systemic administration of chemicals and pharmaceuticals, such as paraquat, bleomycin, and cyclophosphamide, also may produce changes in the respiratory system. Metabolism of xenobiotics may occur throughout the respiratory tract, such as in the nose, conducting passages, and airways, producing toxic metabolites. Specific types and concentrations of enzymes differ among regions, the site-specific localisation of enzymes accounting, at least partially, for regional susceptibility or resistance to injury. Enzymes in the respiratory tract include cytochromes P450 (CYPs), monooxygenases, dehydrogenases, prostaglandin

C. Gopinath, V. Mowat, *Atlas of Toxicological Pathology*,
DOI 10.1007/978-1-62703-998-7_2, © Springer Science+Business Media New York 2014

G synthetase, and phase II enzymes such as glucuronyl and glutathione transferases that facilitate excretion. Enzyme activity and metabolism are greatest in the olfactory mucosa and Clara cells of the bronchioles because of their high CYP content. Types I and II pneumocytes and endothelial cells have lower levels of activity.

Many agents produce toxicity in the respiratory tract by indirect mechanisms; for example, immunosuppressants may result in pneumonia. Impaired clearance mechanisms, such as impaired macrophage function due to phospholipidosis, predispose to bacterial and fungal infections of the airways and lungs. Immune-mediated pathology due to type I or III hypersensitivity reactions also may occur.

To ensure consistent coverage of all susceptible areas of the respiratory tract in an inhalation study, a standard protocol should be followed for selecting, trimming, and examining respiratory organs. A terminology guide for pathologic changes in the respiratory tract in rodents also has been published recently [8].

## 2.2 Nasal Turbinates

To assess the turbinates thoroughly, three to four levels of the nasal passages should be examined, with the sectioning protocol designed to include squamous, transitional, respiratory, and olfactory epithelia. Sections should also include the different areas of turbinates and the vomeronasal organ [9, 10]. Distribution of lesions in the turbinates depends on various factors, including dose to the affected area, site-specific susceptibility, local metabolism, species, and sex [7, 11–13]. Areas affected may also depend on the physical and chemical nature of the test article [14].

Induced changes seen in the nasal turbinates are as follows:

- Eosinophilic inclusions (globules)
- Inflammation
- Disorganisation/degeneration/atrophy
- Erosion/ulceration
- Regeneration/hyperplasia
- Metaplasia, respiratory or squamous
- Vomeronasal organ—degeneration/necrosis
- Tumours—papillomas/adenomas/adenocarcinomas/squamous cell carcinomas/olfactory epithelial carcinoma
- Neuroendocrine cell tumours

Inhaled substances frequently cause histopathological changes localised to the nasal turbinates, as these are the first point of contact and receive a high concentration of the article. Changes may be caused by direct irritation due to their chemical nature or physical properties, or through toxicity by the test article or one of its metabolites. Arguably the commonest cause of lesions is direct irritation, which is caused by a wide range of chemicals, including formaldehyde and alachlor, and pharmaceuticals including β-agonists, Toll-like receptor agonists, and muscarinic antagonists.

The most rostral regions of the nasal cavity are lined by squamous epithelium, which is relatively resistant. Irritant compounds may induce inflammation, hyperplasia, and keratinisation, with erosion and ulceration seen with more strongly irritant materials (Fig. 2.1). The areas of rodent nasal mucosa that develop lesions most frequently are the transitional, respiratory, and olfactory epithelia lining the caudal third of the nasal and maxillary turbinates [8]. Low-grade irritation often results in minimal changes, such as epithelial eosinophilic inclusions in the respiratory and olfactory epithelium and goblet cell hyperplasia (Figs. 2.2 and 2.3) of the respiratory epithelium. Eosinophilic inclusions also may appear in the

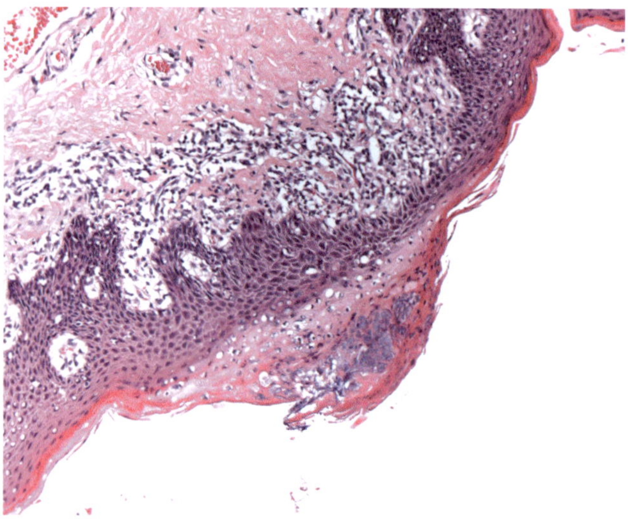

**Figure 2-1.** Focal epithelial erosion of the nasal turbinates in a monkey given an irritant pharmaceutical. Thinning of the squamous epithelium with submucosal lymphocytic infiltration and parakeratosis with nuclear debris and eosinophilic material are seen. Haematoxylin and eosin (H&E).

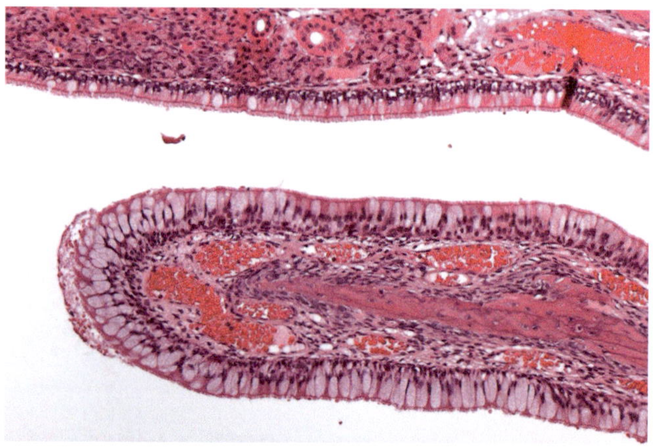

**Figure 2-2.** Goblet cell hyperplasia of the nasal turbinates from a rat given a β-adrenergic agent. The respiratory epithelium lining the turbinates is composed mainly of hypertrophic goblet cells. H&E.

epithelium of the submucosal glands and their ducts (Fig. 2.4). They may be located in any area of the cell, often becoming very large and displacing the nuclei. Ultrastructurally, they appear as membrane-bound ellipsoid bodies containing a homogenous electron-dense matrix. These droplets are negative for polysaccharides on staining by the periodic acid–Schiff (PAS) technique, Alcian blue, and several other stains [15]. They have been induced in rats by a wide range of chemicals and consist of xenobiotic-metabolising enzymes [16].

More marked or prolonged irritancy may result in inflammation, epithelial disorganisation, degeneration, erosion, ulceration, and subsequent regenerative hyperplasia or metaplasia, with several of these changes often being seen simultaneously in studies lasting 4 weeks or longer (Figs. 2.5 and 2.6). Damaged respiratory or transitional epithelium rapidly undergoes repair if the basement membrane is retained, with the development of a thin layer of flattened regenerative cells partially or completely covering the damaged

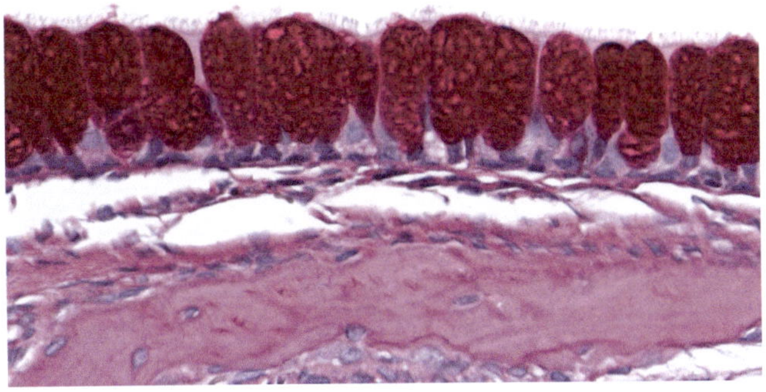

**FIGURE 2-3.** Goblet cell hyperplasia of the nasal turbinates from a rat given a β-adrenergic agent. The hypertrophic mucus-producing cells of the nasopharynx stain strongly positive for neutral mucopolysaccharides. PAS-Haematoxylin staining.

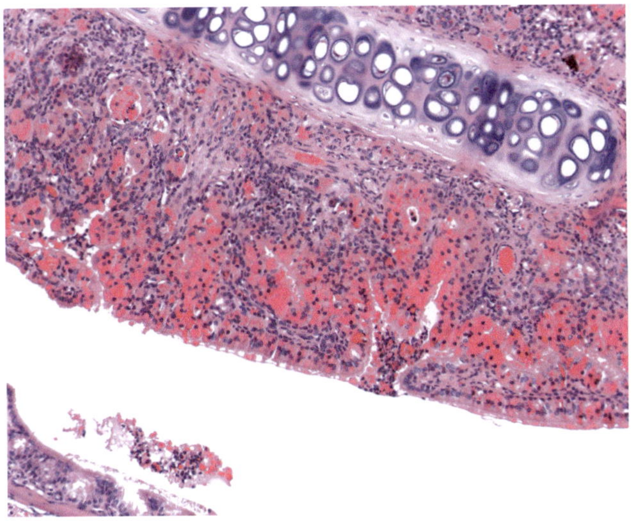

**FIGURE 2-4.** Eosinophilic droplets in the nasal turbinates of a mouse treated with a β-adrenergic agent. The respiratory epithelial cells contain eosinophilic droplets. Also present is marked diffuse hypertrophy of the septal submucosal glands due to distension of acinar and ductal cells with eosinophilic droplets, with mild interstitial inflammation and inflammatory debris in the glands and airways. H&E.

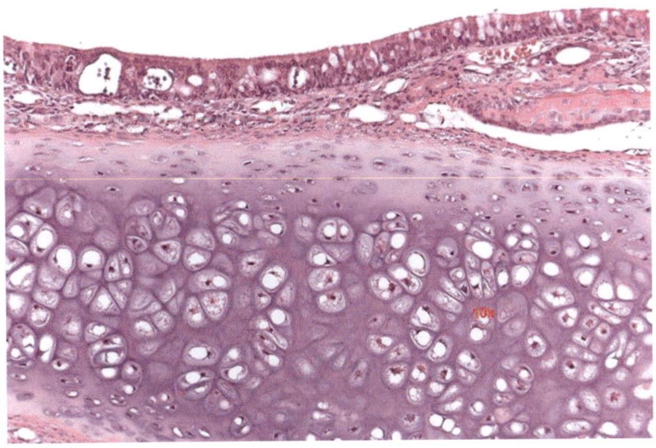

**FIGURE 2-5.** Mild inflammation in the nasal turbinates of a rat given an industrial chemical. Microabscess formation, disorganisation, minimal cell loss, and loss of cilia are present in the septal respiratory epithelium, which is minimally thickened. H&E.

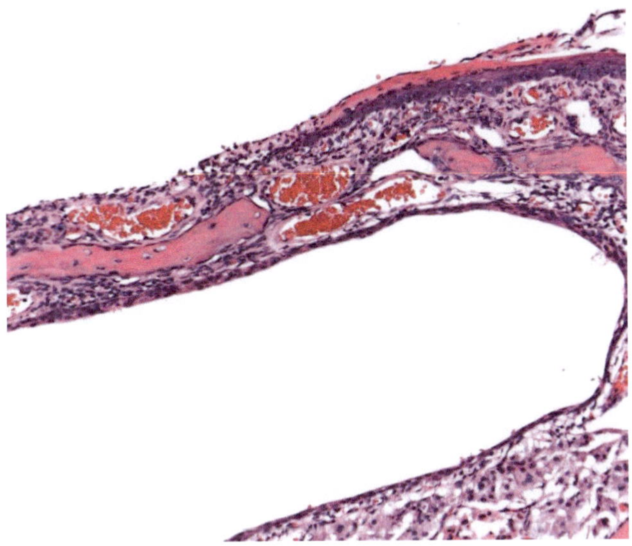

**FIGURE 2-6.** Ulceration and inflammation of the nasal turbinates from a rat given a muscarinic antagonist. The respiratory epithelium shows degeneration, inflammation, ulceration, and localised squamous metaplasia with keratinisation. This combination of changes is seen often with irritant compounds. H&E.

area (Fig. 2.7). The reparative epithelium matures into the original epithelial type or may develop into a more resistant epithelial type, such as respiratory to squamous. True squamous metaplasia, comprising multilayered squamous epithelium with superficial 'umbrella' cells, should be differentiated from the thin layer of flattened epithelial cells seen during early regeneration. Submucosal glands can also undergo inflammation, atrophy, and/or squamous metaplasia as a result of ductal inflammation or blockage (Fig. 2.8).

Ulceration with necrosis of the underlying soft tissues, and sometimes the turbinate bones, also may be induced. Repair results in the development of adhesions, often with fusion of turbinates and subsequent distortion. Marked fibrosis with cartilaginous metaplasia progressing downwards from the dorsal meatus along the septum and extending laterally, involving the turbinates, and partially obliterating the lumen of the nasal cavity has been seen with an industrial chemical (Figs. 2.9 and 2.10).

The vomeronasal organ, or organ of Jacobson, is located at the base of the nasal septum, and is lined laterally by olfactory epithelium and medially by respiratory columnar epithelium. It has important sensory functions in animals. Irritant compounds, such as muscarinics, produce degeneration and necrosis of both epithelial

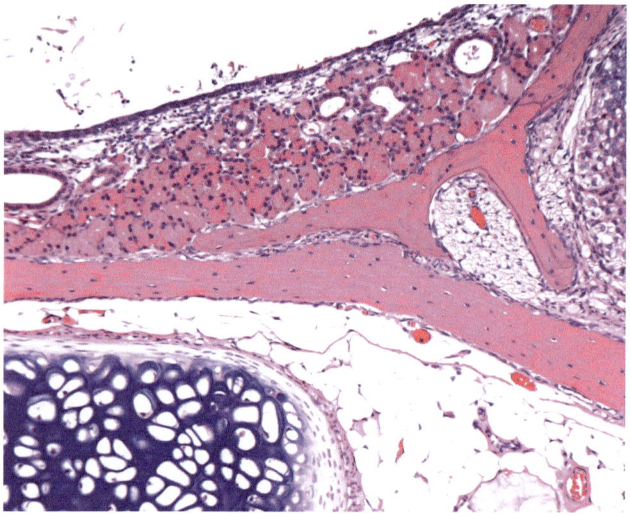

**Figure 2-7.** Regenerating epithelium in the nasal turbinates of a rat given a muscarinic antagonist. A layer of regenerating cuboidal basophilic epithelial cells lines the nasal septum, representing regeneration of the normal respiratory epithelium. Inflammatory cells are present in the lamina propria. H&E.

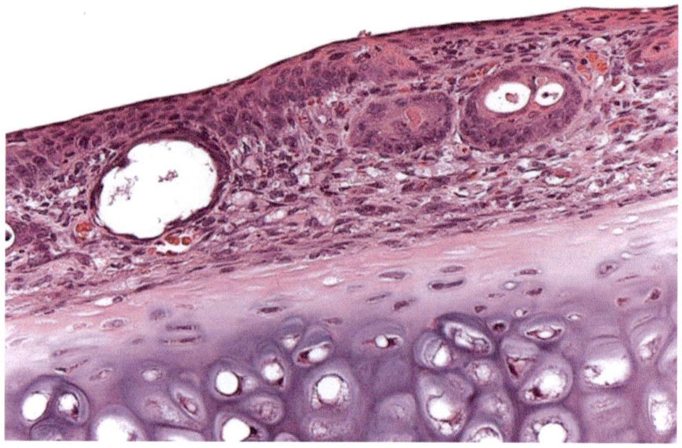

**Figure 2-8.** Squamous metaplasia in the nasal turbinates of a rat given a muscarinic antagonist. Mature squamous epithelium has completely replaced the normal respiratory epithelium of the septum. The submucosal glands and ducts also have undergone squamous metaplasia. H&E.

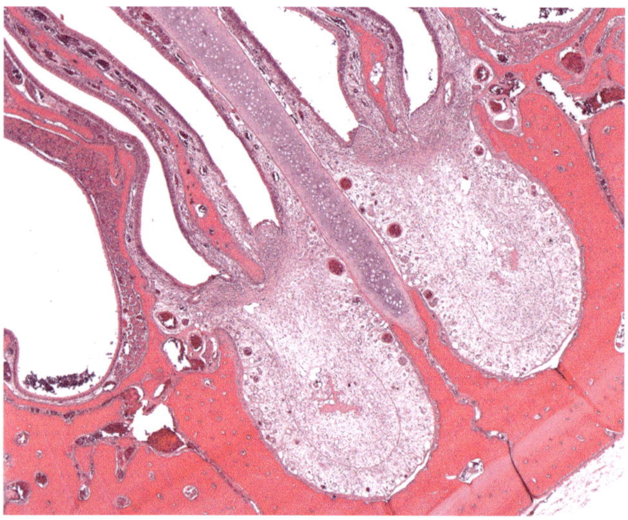

**Figure 2-9.** Severe fibrosis in the nasal cavity of a rat given an inhaled industrial chemical. The normal structures and lumen of the dorsal meatus have been completely replaced by fibrous proliferation. The respiratory epithelium has healed over the fibrotic areas. H&E.

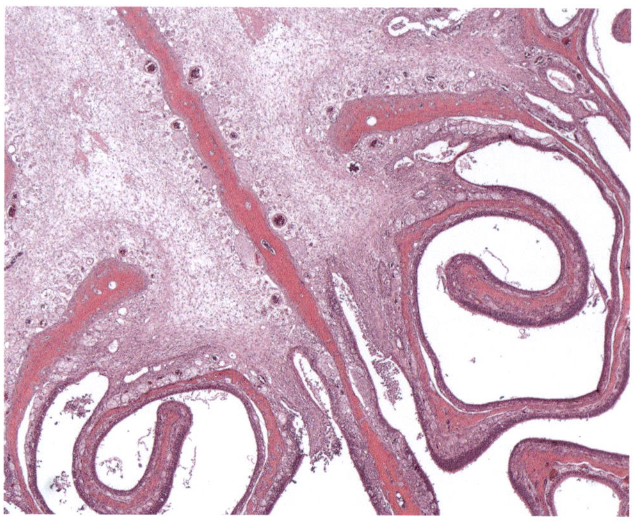

**Figure 2-10.** Fibrosis with early cartilaginous metaplasia in the nasal turbinates of a rat given an inhaled industrial chemical. Fibrosis has partially occluded the nasal cavity, involving the ethmoturbinates. Early cartilaginous differentiation is present in the fibrotic tissue. H&E.

types (Fig. 2.11), with subsequent regeneration of either the original epithelium or squamous metaplasia.

In our experience, changes in the olfactory epithelium due to irritation are most frequently localised to the rostral portion of the dorsal medial meatus of the turbinates, sometimes extending laterally along the dorsal ethmoid turbinates and less frequently along the medial septum. This distribution is similar to that noted by other authors [7, 17]. The ethmoid turbinates often are largely unaffected.

Low-grade irritation may induce eosinophilic droplets in the olfactory epithelium of rodents; however, these are also seen as a spontaneous finding, especially in older animals (Fig. 2.12). More marked induced changes seen in the olfactory epithelium include inflammation, disorganisation, atrophy, apoptosis, degeneration, and necrosis (Fig. 2.13). Olfactory epithelial atrophy, notably in rodents, is frequently associated with atrophy of the underlying nerve bundles and, sometimes, atrophy of the Bowman's glands lying between these bundles (Fig. 2.14). Because of its capacity for regeneration by replication of the basal cell layer, regenerative olfactory epithelial hyperplasia may accompany ongoing degenerative processes. If the insult is prolonged, respiratory or squamous epithelium may replace the olfactory epithelium (Fig. 2.15).

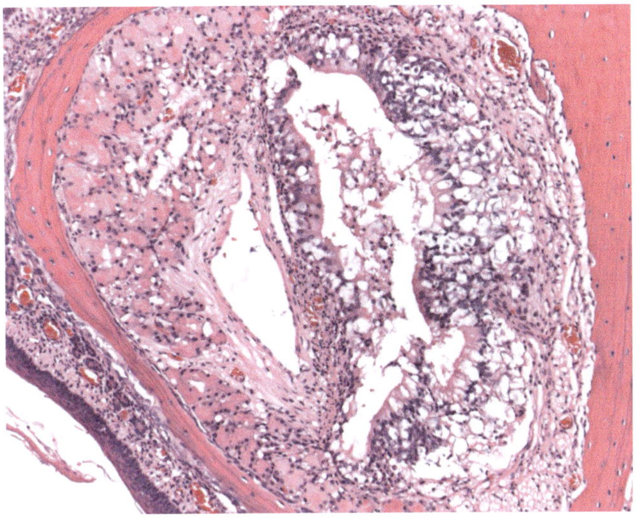

**Figure 2-11.** Necrosis of the vomeronasal organ from a rat given a muscarinic antagonist. Marked degeneration, necrosis, and desquamation of the olfactory and columnar epithelium are present. Inflammatory cells are scattered in the lamina propria, and cellular debris is seen in the lumen. H&E.

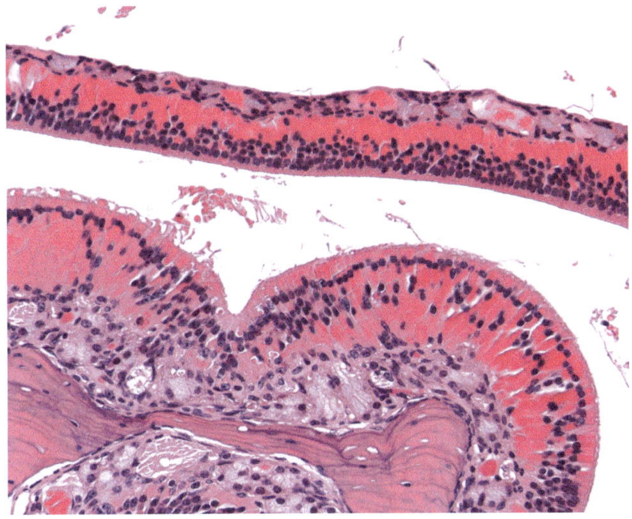

**Figure 2-12.** Eosinophilic droplets in the nasal turbinates of a rat given a β-adrenergic agonist in a long-term study. The olfactory epithelium of the ethmoturbinates is moderately hypertrophic, with loss of architecture. Large eosinophilic droplets have displaced the epithelial nuclei dorsally. H&E.

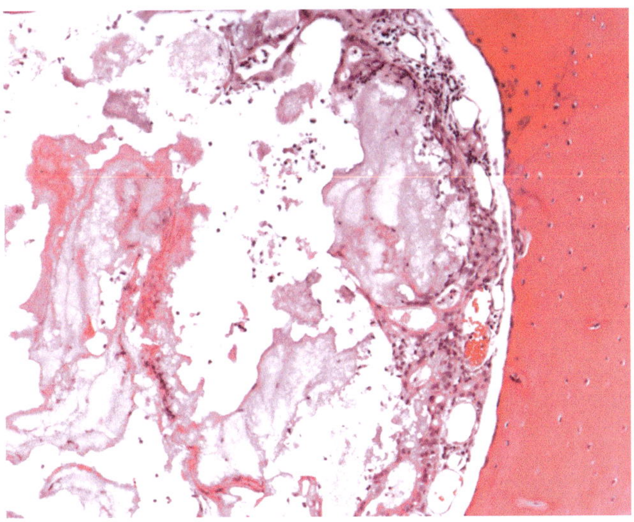

**Figure 2-13.** Degeneration and ulceration of the nasal turbinates in a rat given a biologic. Marked degeneration, erosion, ulceration, and inflammation of the olfactory epithelium are seen at the dorsal meatus, with marked eosinophilic material and cellular debris in the lumen. H&E.

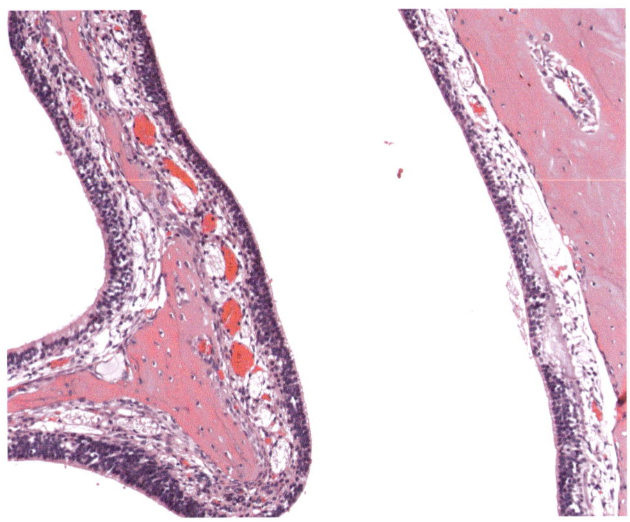

**Figure 2-14.** Atrophy of the nasal turbinates in a rat that received an inhaled industrial chemical. The olfactory epithelium at the dorsal meatus shows moderate atrophy, with almost complete loss of the underlying nerve bundles and Bowman glands. Corpora amylacea are present along the basement membrane. H&E.

In addition, metabolism of inhaled xenobiotics by the olfactory epithelium, because of its high content of mixed function CYP oxidases—and occasionally, metabolism by associated structures, such as Bowman's glands—can generate toxic metabolites. This results in diffuse atrophy, degeneration, and atrophy of the olfactory epithelium, which is most evident on the ethmoid turbinates, where this epithelial type is mostly seen (Fig. 2.16). Depending on the severity and duration of exposure, ongoing regenerative hyperplasia may be present if a population of basal cells is preserved. Olfactory epithelial alterations due to systemic absorption and localised metabolism of the test article also are seen in noninhalation studies, such as with 3-methylindole in mice when administered orally. Local levels of metabolic enzymes within the epithelium govern the distribution of lesions [18]. Methimazole in Long–Evans rats, when administered either orally or intraperitoneally, produces damage to sustentacular and sensory cells while sparing basal cells and the basement membrane [19].

In rodents, lesions of the caudal nasal turbinates also occur in oral gavage studies, as a result of aspiration during dosing or gastric reflux. Findings in the turbinates include proteinaceous fluid or inflammatory exudate in the lumen. Acute necrosis and desquamation of the olfactory epithelium lining the ethmoid turbinates typically are present, sometimes accompanied by inflammatory and degenerative changes of the respiratory epithelium. Changes in the nasopharynx sometimes are present, indicating the pathogenesis of the lesion (Figs. 2.17 and 2.18).

Gastric reflux is a multifactorial phenomenon in rodents, and factors include the animal's size, age, fasting status and the volume administered. Test materials that affect peristalsis or delay gastric emptying, such as antimuscarinics and β-adrenergics, or that display physicochemical properties such as high viscosity, also may predispose to reflux [20].

Tumours of the nasal turbinates have been induced by several classes of compounds administered by systemic or inhalation routes. Nitrosamines cause papillomas and squamous cell carcinomas in rats when given subcutaneously (Fig. 2.19). Dioxane in the drinking water induces papillomas and carcinomas in rats. Formalin administered by inhalation produces squamous cell carcinomas in rats and mice [21]. Olfactory neuroblastomas are rarer but may be induced by genotoxic carcinogens [22] and also by phosphodiesterase (PDE)-4 inhibitors.

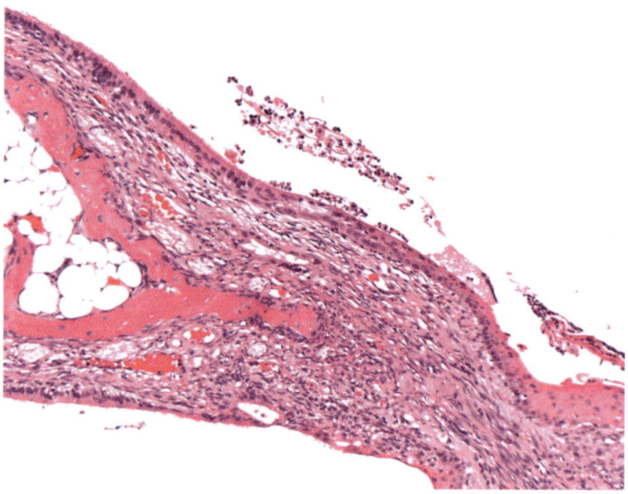

**Figure 2-15.** Respiratory and squamous metaplasia in the nasal turbinates of a rat given a muscarinic antagonist. The olfactory epithelium (*left*) has been partially replaced by a more ciliated cuboidal respiratory epithelium adjacent to it and by squamous epithelium further towards the *right*. Inflammatory cell debris, fibrin, and keratin are present in the lumen. H&E.

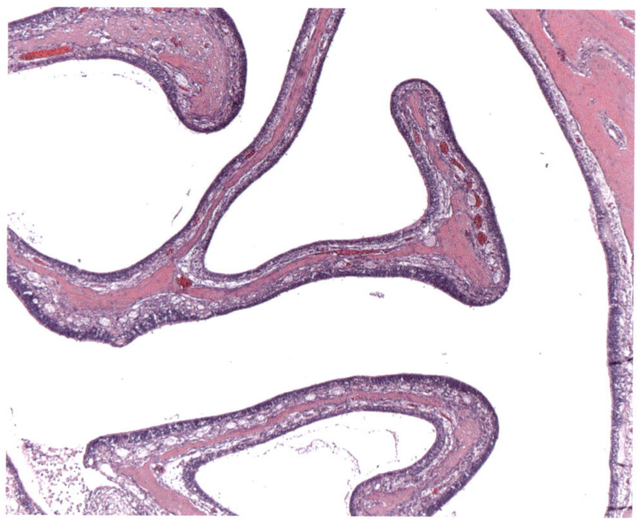

**Figure 2-16.** Diffuse olfactory epithelial atrophy of the nasal turbinates in a rat given an industrial chemical. The olfactory epithelium along the dorsal meatus and turbinates appears unevenly thinner, with cell loss and/or disorganisation in many areas. H&E.

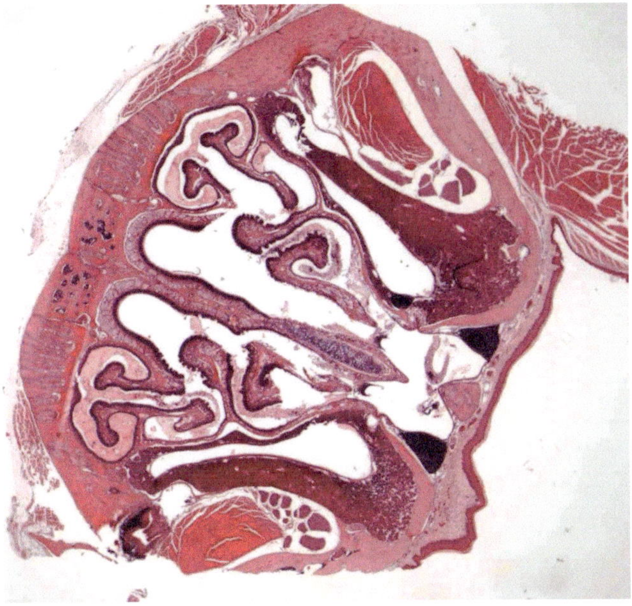

**Figure 2-17.** Reflux-associated changes in the nasal turbinates of a mouse given a pharmaceutical by gavage. Eosinophilic fluid containing inflammatory cells is seen in the dorsolateral aspects of the nasal cavity, between the ethmoid turbinates. Exudate in the nasopharynx indicates the likely pathogenesis. These are the areas often affected in reflux. Volume of dose, increased gastric transit time, and pharmaceutical effects may all be involved in this phenomenon. H&E.

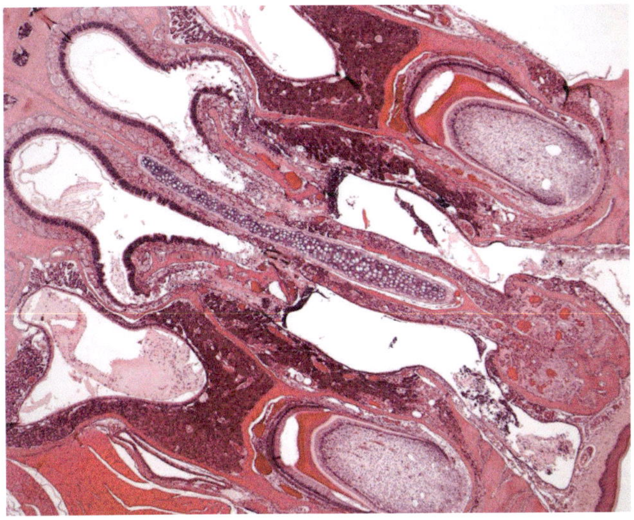

**Figure 2-18.** Reflux-associated changes in the nasal turbinates of a mouse given a pharmaceutical by gavage. Eosinophilic fluid and inflammatory debris are seen in the lumen. Fibrinous adhesions are developing between the lateral walls, turbinates, and middle septum. H&E.

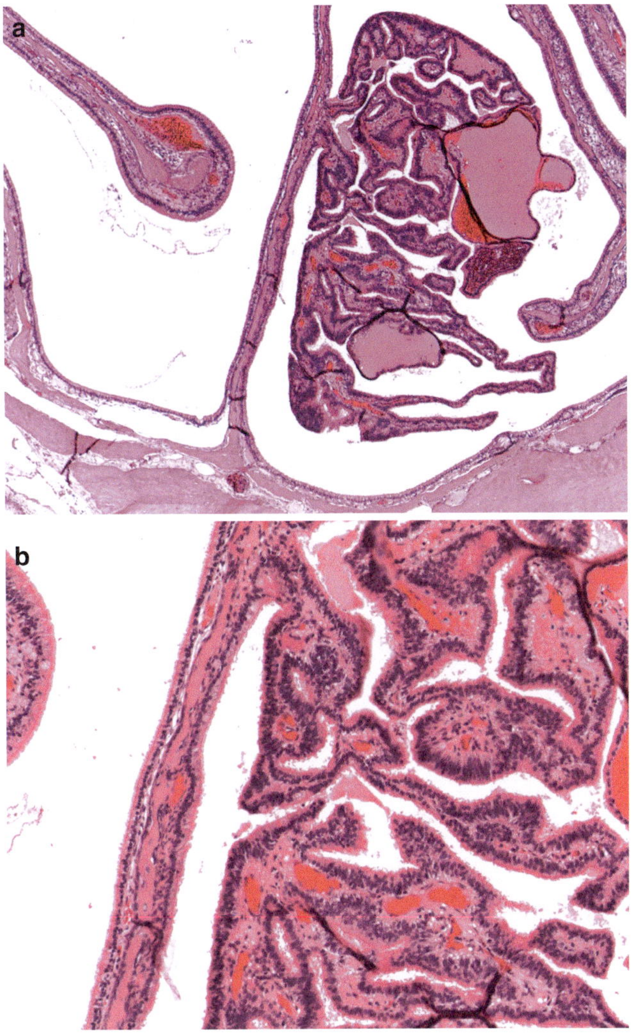

**Figure 2-19.** (**a**, **b**) Papilloma in the nasal turbinates of a mouse. A well-circumscribed papillary proliferation, with a few dilated glandular structures containing eosinophilic fluid, is present between the turbinates. Columnar epithelium covering the papillary projections is well differentiated. H&E.

## 2.3 Pharynx

Although the pharynx and nasopharynx are examined regularly in inhalation studies, induced changes are rare. In dogs and primates, the pharyngeal tonsils and other respiratory-associated lymphoid tissues often reflect stimulatory or depressive effects on the immune system. Inhaled and oral steroids cause immunosuppression and lymphoid depletion. Toll-like receptor inhibitors are associated with germinal centre development because of their immunostimulatory effect (Fig. 2.20).

Eosinophilic droplets in the respiratory epithelium of the pharynx have been recorded with mildly irritant compounds, including neurokinin receptor antagonists. β-adrenergics may cause epithelial degeneration in the pharynx (Fig. 2.21), with the normal respiratory epithelium being replaced by flattened regenerating epithelium.

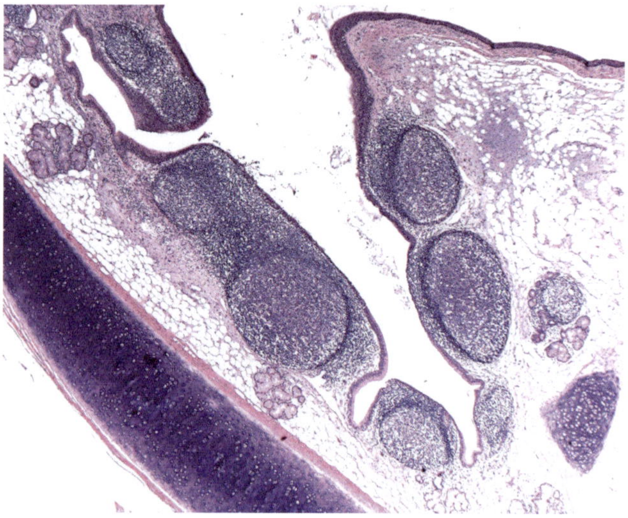

**Figure 2-20.** Lymphoid hyperplasia of the pharynx from a cynomolgus monkey treated with an inhaled immunostimulant. The tonsils display large active germinal centres within the lymphoid follicles. H&E.

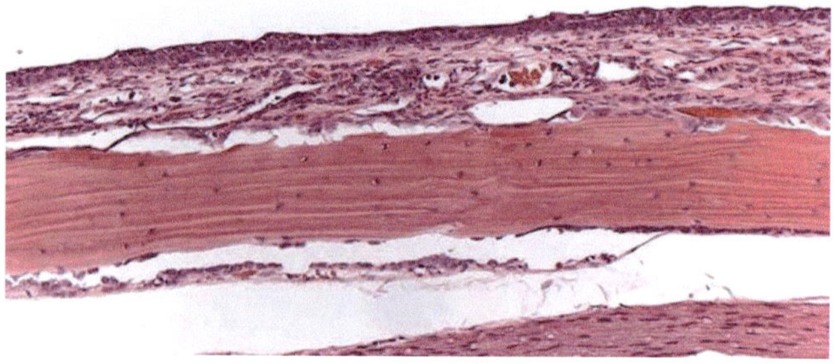

**Figure 2-21.** Regenerating epithelium in the pharynx of a rat given an irritant inhaled compound. The normal ciliated respiratory epithelium has been replaced by flattened regenerating basophilic epithelial cells, with a loss of goblet cells. H&E.

## 2.4 Larynx

The larynx is a well-recognised site of induced toxicity in rodent inhalation studies, in which it is particularly susceptible to even minimal irritant effects. Several schemes for sectioning and examining the rodent larynx are followed in different laboratories, with 3–11 sections generally being examined. It is essential that the predilection sites for toxicologic changes are examined consistently and that the pathologist is familiar with the structure of different areas of the larynx [23–25]. These areas are the inner aspects of the arytenoid cartilage, the laryngeal mucosa rostral and lateral to the ventral pouch, and the ventrolateral region at the base of the epiglottis, which is a transitional zone between the squamous and respiratory epithelium.

Exposure to a range of chemicals and pharmaceuticals is associated with changes in the larynx. Pharmaceuticals include β-adrenergics, p38 inhibitors, muscarinic antagonists, and many other compound classes. Changes seen in the larynx are mostly in the epithelium and are as follows:

- Inflammation, degeneration, and necrosis
- Erosion and ulceration
- Squamous metaplasia
- Cartilage necrosis
- Hyperplasia and neoplasia

The larynx's responses to insult are limited and nonspecific. The most frequently observed change in the rodent is squamous metaplasia, generally seen first in the ventral aspect of the larynx at the base of the epiglottis [23]. This change may manifest as soon as within 3 days of exposure [24]. Often there is little or no inflammatory response associated with this change. Dilation with degeneration and atrophy of the submucosal glands at the base of the epiglottis is seen less commonly. This arises as a result of inflammation and erosion and/or squamous metaplasia of the respiratory epithelium, resulting in the sealing off of the ductal opening and leading to acinar cystic distension and eventually atrophy [24]. Squamous metaplasia of the glands and their ducts also may be a sequel (Fig. 2.22).

If irritation is more marked or prolonged, the lateral aspects of the laryngeal mucosa and the arytenoids also exhibit squamous metaplasia/hyperplasia, sometimes with keratinisation. If recovery is allowed, this finding generally will show partial regression. Squamous metaplasia of the larynx often shows a characteristic lack of progression, even in 2-year studies, and is widely accepted as a rodent-specific adaptive response that is of no relevance to humans [26, 27].

Necrosis of the laryngeal U-shaped cartilage also is associated with low-grade irritation and is thought to be a sequel to initial ulceration of the ventral epithelium, followed by necrosis of the underlying cartilage. The epithelium then regenerates and the larynx presents with intact, often metaplastic, epithelium covering an area of necrotic cartilage. The commonest site for cartilaginous necrosis is at the entrance to the ventral pouch, presumably because of its superficial location here [24]. The cartilage appears as a persistent pink homogenous mass with loss of cell detail, with a noticeable lack of inflammation (Fig. 2.23). More rarely, necrosis of the arytenoid cartilage may occur.

Repair of necrotic cartilage, which may occur depending on the extent of damage, manifests as regenerating cartilage from the intact portion, which appears around, but not within, the necrotic area. The new cartilage appears as foci of basophilic chondrocytes around the margins of the necrotic tissue (Fig. 2.24).

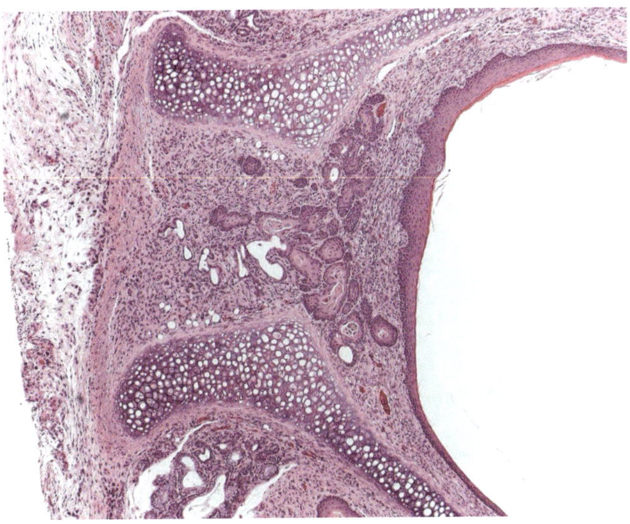

**Figure 2-22.** Squamous metaplasia in the larynx of a rat given an irritant inhaled pharmaceutical. The underlying mucous glands and their ducts also show squamous metaplasia. The submucosa is mildly inflamed, with cellular debris present within the ducts and acini. This site is a common target for irritant compounds in rodent inhalation studies. H&E.

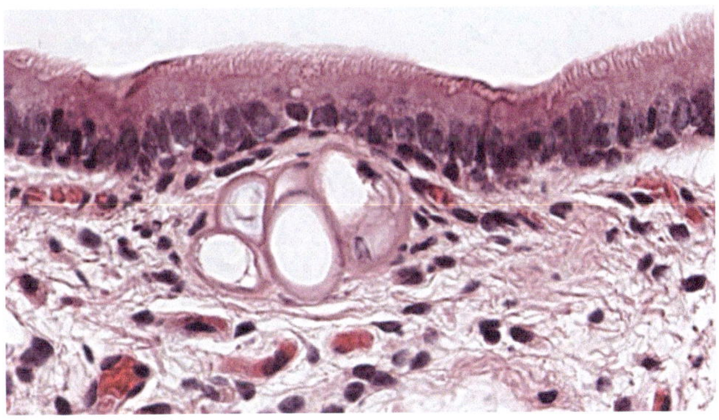

**Figure 2-23.** Necrosis of the U-shaped cartilage in the larynx of a mouse given a β-adrenergic agent. The necrotic cartilage appears as a pink homogenous mass, preserving its outline although cellular detail is lost. Necrotic cartilage persists for a very long period. H&E.

Benign and malignant squamous epithelial neoplasms have been induced in rodent larynges by intratracheal instillation of polycyclic aromatic hydrocarbons.

Induced lesions of the larynx in dogs and monkeys are rare. Irritant compounds sometimes induce varying degrees of inflammatory cell infiltrate and, rarely, erosion and ulceration of the laryngeal epithelium. Occasionally, as a spontaneous finding, focal ulceration with inflammation and necrosis is seen on the vocal folds in dogs, near the junction of the lateral ventricles with the laryngeal lumen. These lesions often are bilateral.

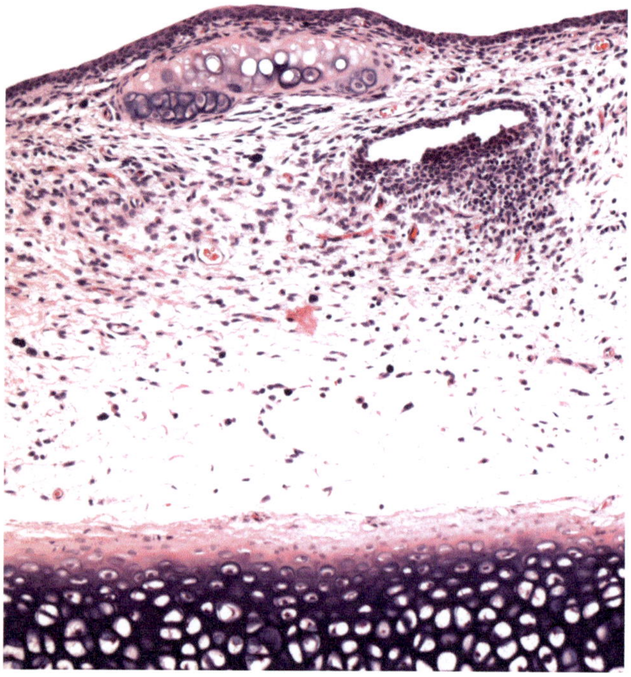

**Figure 2-24.** Cartilage necrosis and regeneration of the larynx from a rat given a muscarinic antagonist. The main portion of the cartilage is pink and necrotic with loss of cellular detail, but some basophilic areas of healthy cartilage are present at the periphery, possibly indicating regeneration. H&E.

## 2.5 Trachea/Tracheal Bifurcation

Treatment-related findings in the upper trachea include the following:

- Loss of cilia with flattening of epithelium
- Epithelial vacuolation
- Inflammation/disorganisation/regeneration
- Degeneration and necrosis
- Erosion and ulceration
- Hyperplasia and neoplasia
- Squamous metaplasia

In reality, however, the trachea rarely displays induced changes. In gavage studies, erosion or degeneration, often with regeneration, of the tracheal epithelium sometimes is seen as the result of small quantities of the test article entering the trachea during the dosing procedure or as a result of reflux. Inflammation with epithelial disorganisation and regeneration has been seen with an inhaled industrial chemical in our laboratory (Fig. 2.25). Vacuolation of the tracheal epithelium is sometimes seen as part of a generalised phospholipidosis.

Unlike the trachea, the carina at the tracheal bifurcation is a common target site for changes in inhalation studies. This is a result of flow dynamics in the upper airways during inhalation, leading to impaction of particles at this site. Changes seen here include loss of cilia; degeneration, disorganisation, and regeneration of the respiratory epithelium at this site; and squamous metaplasia. Loss of cilia appears as a flattening and a basophilic appearance of the epithelial cells at the tip of the carina, with cilia being absent or sparse (Fig. 2.26). Squamous metaplasia is diagnosed when there are several layers of flattened epithelial cells covered by the umbrella cells typical of squamous epithelium (Fig. 2.27). These changes are nonspecific, and their severity depends on the irritancy of the compound, the length of the exposure, the nature of the test article, and other factors. Induced changes are seen with muscarinics, β-adrenergics, and chemicals, including tobacco smoke. Artefactual flattening of the epithelium and erosion are common because of the delicacy of the carina and should be distinguished from genuine induced changes.

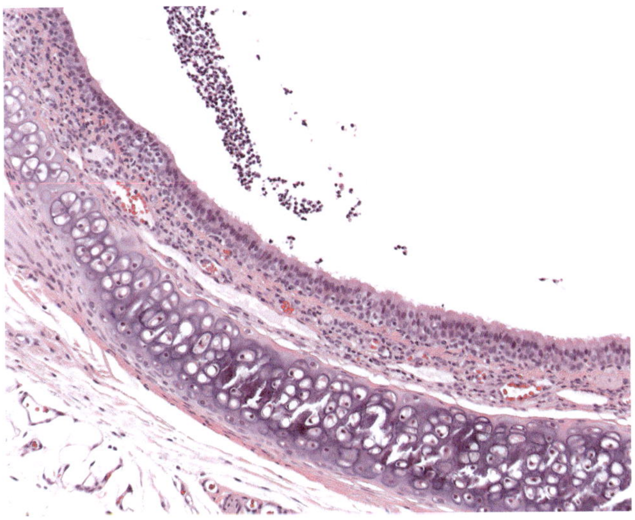

**Figure 2-25.** Inflammation of the trachea from a rat given an industrial chemical by inhalation. The tracheal epithelium is disorganised and mildly hyperplastic, with degenerating cells, inflammation, and focal loss of cilia. Neutrophils are present in the lamina propria and lumen. H&E.

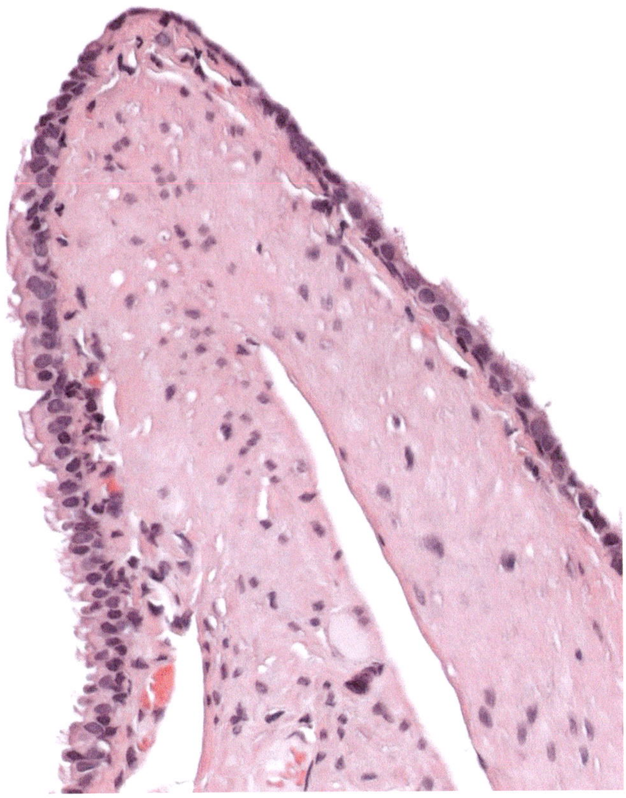

**Figure 2-26.** Loss of cilia in the carina of a rat given an irritant inhaled compound. The tip of the carina shows flattening and basophilia of the epithelial cells, with focal loss of cilia. This is a common site for changes in rodent inhalation studies because of particle impaction at this point. H&E.

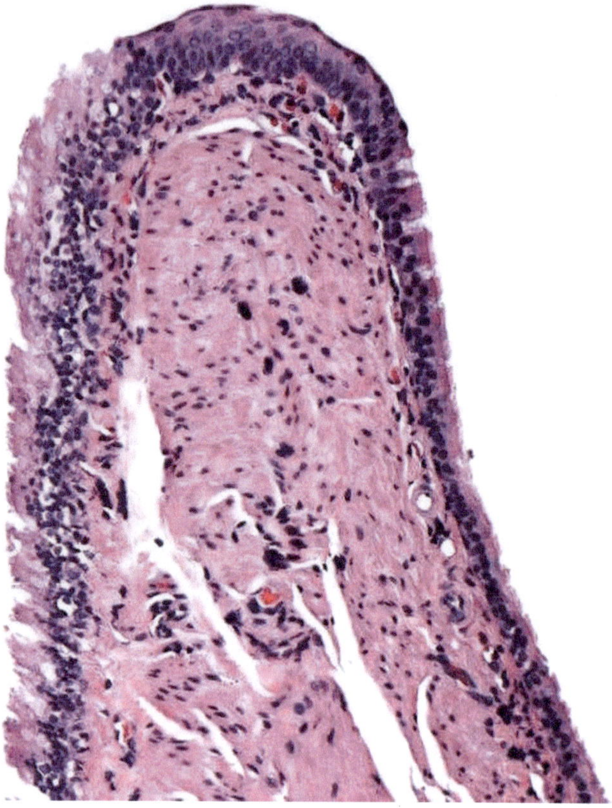

**Figure 2-27.** Squamous metaplasia of the carina from a rat given a muscarinic antagonist. The respiratory epithelium at the tip of the carina has been replaced by stratified squamous epithelium, with characteristic cells. H&E.

## 2.6 Bronchi/Bronchioles

The bronchioles are lined by respiratory epithelium. Epithelial regeneration takes place through the Clara cells, the numbers of which increase with penetration into the lung and are greatest in the terminal bronchioles. Changes in the bronchioles include those typical of respiratory epithelia, along with some more specific changes:

- Clara cells—eosinophilic inclusions
- Mineralisation
- Goblet cell hyperplasia
- Degeneration and necrosis
- Erosion and ulceration
- Hyperplasia and neoplasia
- Squamous metaplasia
- Neuroendocrine cell proliferation

Eosinophilic inclusions may occur as an induced change in the bronchiolar epithelium. Although they also are seen as a background finding, their incidence and severity are exacerbated by a variety of inhaled substances. No widely accepted mechanisms have been described for this change. Large spherical eosinophilic inclusions in the Clara cells are induced by inhaled steroids and steroid receptor agonists (Fig. 2.28). These inclusions have been found to be strongly positive for surfactant protein-D and weakly positive for Clara cell secretory protein [28].

Mineralisation of the bronchiolar epithelium is caused by vitamin D analogues in rats. The bronchiolar epithelial cells and subepithelial collagen contain dark purplish concretions with little or no inflammatory cell reaction (Fig. 2.29).

Low levels of irritation, as seen with gases such as sulphur dioxide, tobacco smoke, and pharmaceuticals, including β-agonists, cause increases in the size and number of mucin-secreting cells, giving the epithelium a hypertrophic appearance (Fig. 2.30). Goblet cells may extend further down the airways than normal, and mucus may accumulate in the airways or alveoli. This finding generally shows complete reversal once the source of irritation is removed. Systemic injections of isoprenaline and pilocarpine also induce changes in goblet cell numbers [29].

A wide range of pharmaceutical classes, chemicals, and gases induce inflammatory and degenerative changes in the bronchiolar epithelium, including tyrosine kinase inhibitors and Toll-like receptor agonists. These changes include peribronchiolar and bronchiolar epithelial inflammation, Clara cell degeneration, and focal or diffuse erosion and ulceration of the bronchiolar epithelium (Fig. 2.31).Varying degrees of inflammatory exudate containing mucus, degenerating inflammatory cells, and other debris sometimes are present in the lumen (Fig. 2.32). Degenerating or ulcerated epithelium may be replaced by regenerating bronchiolar epithelium or may undergo squamous metaplasia (Fig. 2.33).

Neuroendocrine cell hyperplasia occurs spontaneously as a background change in rodents, but physiological conditions such as chronic hyperoxia and pulmonary hypertension cause increases in numbers of neuroendocrine bodies, pulmonary neuroendocrine (PNEC) hyperplasia, or both, in rats. These bodies appear as groups of tightly packed nonciliated cuboidal, oval, columnar, or round cells containing argyrophilic granules, which are positive for corticotropin, calcitonin gene-related peptide (CGRP), and neuron-specific enolase. The cells have round basophilic nuclei and scant cytoplasm, closely resembling lymphocytes, and require immunohistochemical staining for confirmation (Fig. 2.34). Ultrastructurally, dense-core cytoplasmic granules of the amine-precursor update decarboxylase type may be seen. Silica induces hyperplasia of rat alveolar neuroendocrine bodies but not bronchiolar neuroendocrine bodies [30]. Exposure of hamsters to chemical carcinogens such as nitrosamines often leads to marked but reversible PNEC hyperplasia [31].

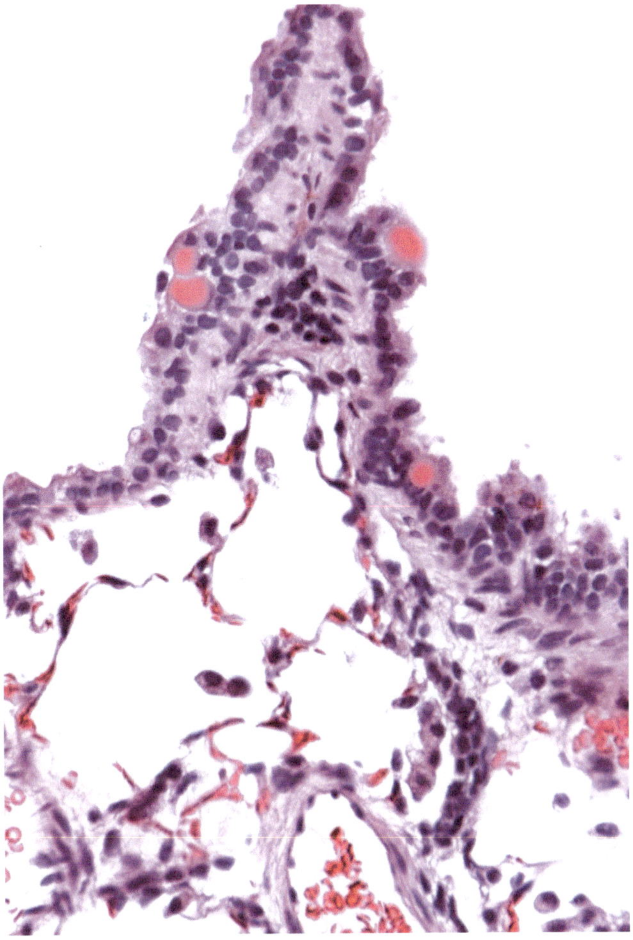

**Figure 2-28.** Eosinophilic inclusions in a bronchiole from a rat treated with a steroid in a long-term study. Large spherical eosinophilic inclusions are present in some of the Clara cells. These inclusions consist of surfactant and secretory proteins. H&E.

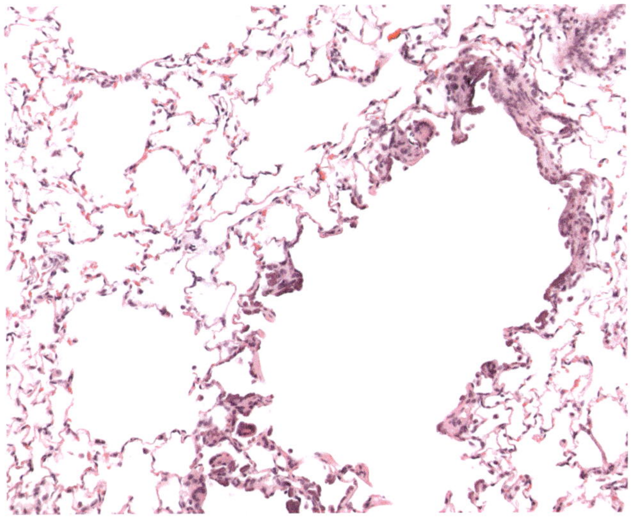

**Figure 2-29.** Mineralisation of the bronchiolar epithelium in a rat given a vitamin D analogue. Dark purplish concretions are seen within the bronchiolar epithelial cells and sometimes within the underlying collagen. H&E.

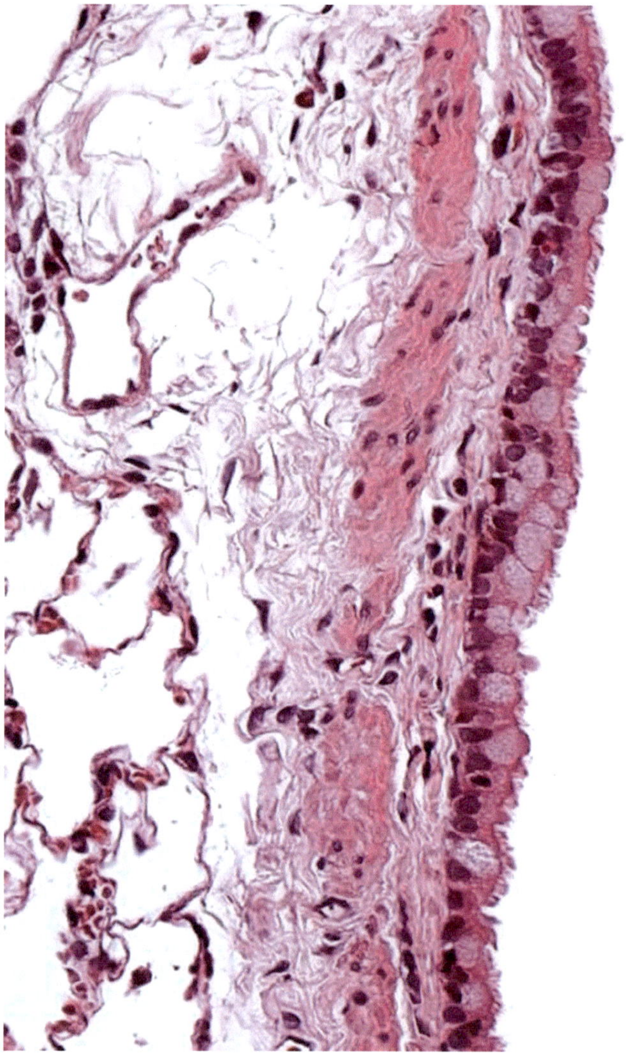

**Figure 2-30.** Goblet cell hypertrophy/hyperplasia of the terminal bronchiole in a rat. This is characterised by an increase in the size and number of goblet cells. The respiratory epithelium consists largely of mucus-producing goblet cells, which have replaced the normal varied epithelial population. H&E.

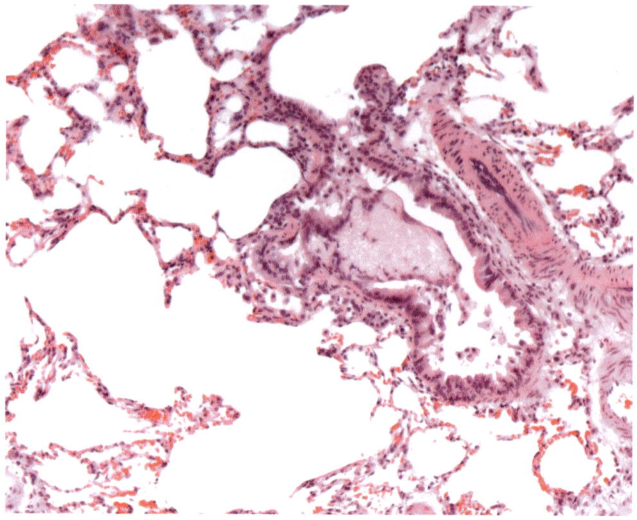

**Figure 2-31.** Focal inflammation of the terminal bronchiole in a rat that received a biologic. Amorphous debris has accumulated beneath and is elevating the bronchiolar epithelium, causing focal erosion. Inflammatory cell debris is present in the bronchiolar lumen. H&E.

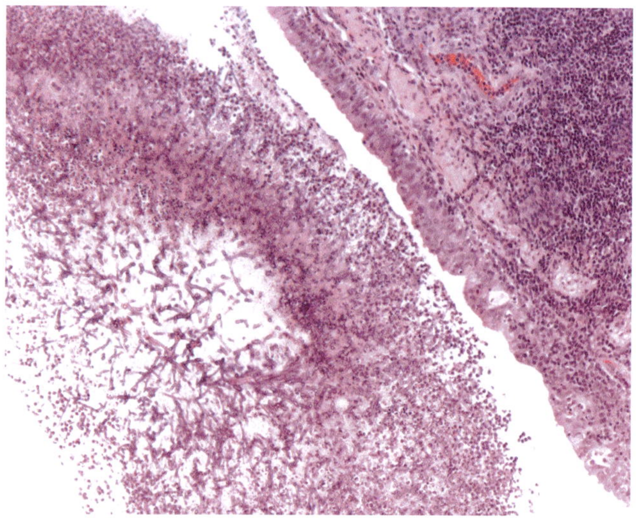

**Figure 2-32.** Inflammation in the bronchiole of a rat given a biologic. Exudate comprising degenerating neutrophils and fibrin is present in the airway, with numerous fungal hyphae evident in the exudate. The broncholar epithelium is mildly inflamed and hyperplastic. H&E.

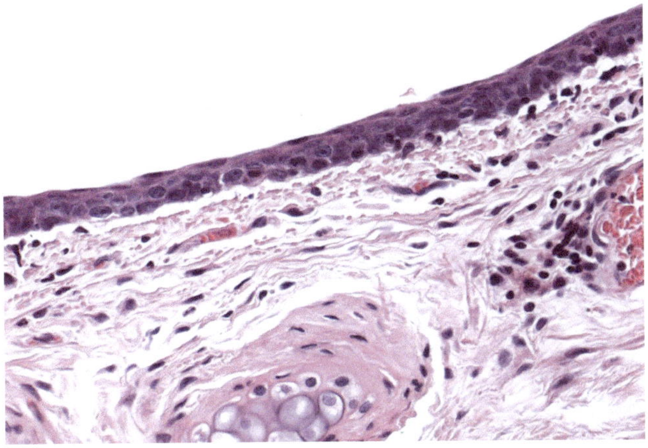

**Figure 2-33.** Squamous metaplasia in the bronchus of a rat given an irritant test article. The normal bronchial epithelium has been replaced by mature stratified squamous epithelium. A few lymphocytes are present in the submucosal tissue associated with the area of squamous metaplasia. H&E.

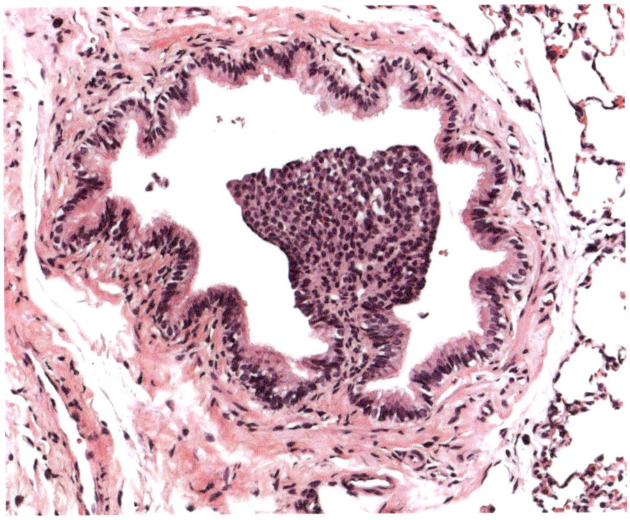

**Figure 2-34.** Neuroendocrine cell hyperplasia in the bronchiole of a rat. A polypoid structure composed of round cells with round dark nuclei and scanty cytoplasm protrudes into the bronchiolar lumen. Immunohistochemistry is necessary to differentiate these from similar-appearing lymphoid aggregates. H&E.

## 2.7 Terminal Bronchioles/Alveolar Ducts

In inhalation studies, induced changes commonly are seen in the terminal bronchioles, where the test material is deposited. The nature of the induced changes depends on several factors including particle size, the nature of the test material, and its pharmacological action. Because this area contains both airways lined by respiratory epithelium and alveoli, toxicologic changes in these regions often involve the cell types of both areas. Changes affecting the terminal bronchioles alone are similar to those described in the previous section. Changes in the alveolar ducts are listed below:

- Increased alveolar macrophages
- Eosinophilic deposits/hyaline membranes
- Epithelialisation/bronchialisation/type II pneumocyte proliferation
- Squamous metaplasia
- Collagenisation/fibroplasia

Oxidant gases (nitrous oxide, oxygen, ozone) tend to affect ciliated cells in the terminal bronchioles more severely, probably because protective mucus is thinner at this site.

Increases in alveolar macrophages reflect an increased nonspecific clearance response to inert inhaled materials (Fig. 2.35). With more reactive compounds, macrophages may coalesce, forming multinucleate cells or granulomas [32].

Deposition of amorphous eosinophilic material, seen lining the alveolar ducts, occurs in treatment with Toll-like receptor agonists and other agents causing alveolar damage (Fig. 2.36).

At the bronchiolar–alveolar junction, ciliated cuboidal cells may proliferate and extend along the alveolar septae, a process known as bronchialisation (Fig. 2.37). This is a protective adaptation. Bronchialisation often is accompanied by thickening of the alveolar septum and sometimes an inflammatory reaction. Squamous metaplasia of the terminal bronchiolar epithelium also may develop as a protective response to inert particles, sometimes becoming quite extensive (Fig. 2.38).

Perivascular and peribronchiolar collagenisation or fibrosis at the junction is associated with a range of compounds, including industrial chemicals and pharmaceuticals such as PDE-4 inhibitors. Morphologically, varying degrees of subepithelial collagen deposition and/or fibrosis are seen in the alveolar ducts and bronchiolar walls (Fig. 2.39).

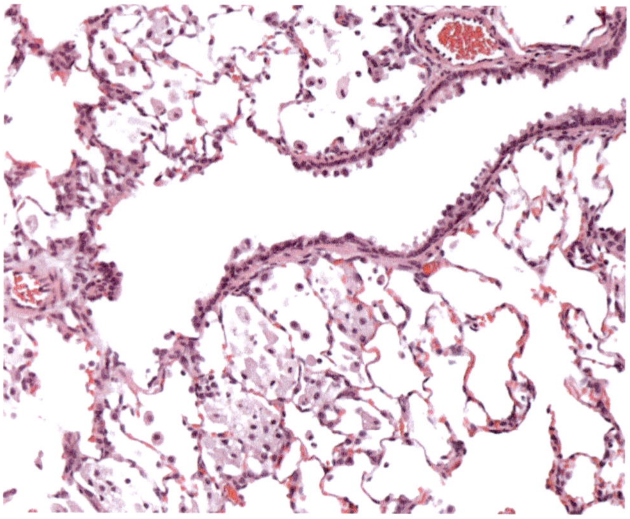

**Figure 2-35.** Foamy macrophage aggregates in the lung of a rat. Foamy macrophages are seen in the alveoli surrounding the terminal bronchiole and alveolar duct. This is a characteristic target site in inhalation studies and indicates an increased clearance response to inert inhaled materials. H&E.

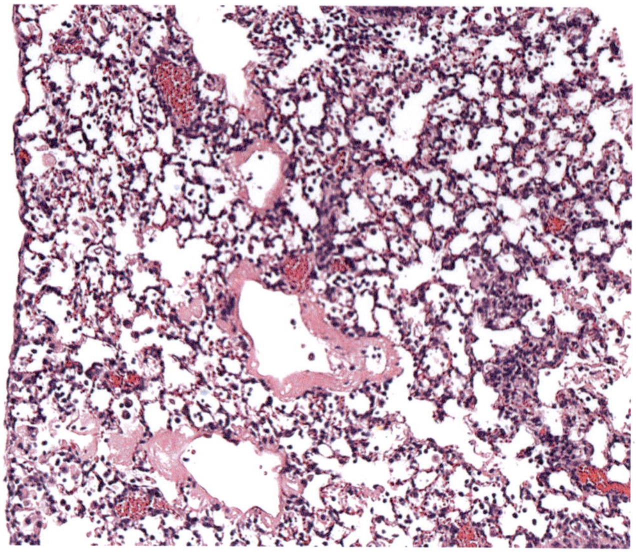

**Figure 2-36.** Hyaline membrane formation in the lung of a rat given a biologic. The alveolar ducts are lined by fibrinoid eosinophilic material, with a glassy appearance. Inflammatory cells are present in the alveoli, with focal interstitial inflammation. H&E.

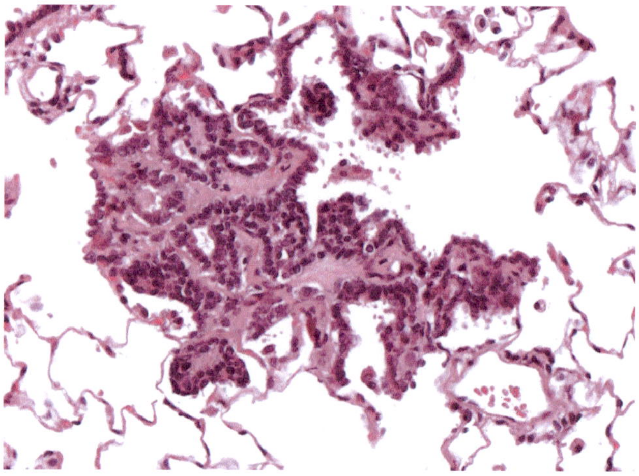

**Figure 2-37.** Ciliated cuboidal metaplasia in the lung of a rat. Focal alveoli at the bronchiolar–alveolar junction show septal thickening and are lined on both surfaces by cuboidal ciliated cells. This process also is known as bronchialisation. H&E.

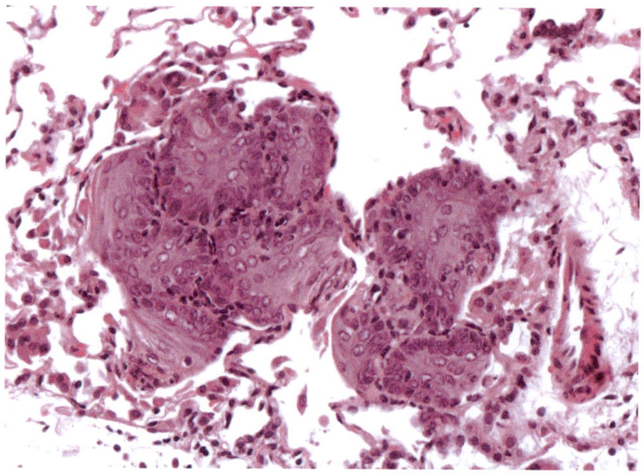

**Figure 2-38.** Squamous metaplasia of the bronchiolar–alveolar junction in a rat given a particulate compound. Marked squamous epithelial proliferation has partially occluded the airway, largely replacing the normal respiratory epithelium. This is well-differentiated squamous metaplasia, a protective response. H&E.

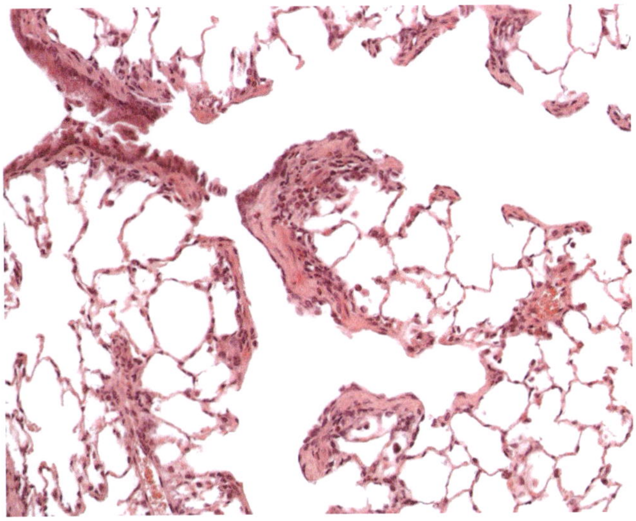

**Figure 2-39.** Collagenisation/fibrosis at the bronchiolar–alveolar junctions in a rat treated with a PDE inhibitor. Localised subepithelial collagen deposition with minimal fibrosis is present in the bronchiolar and alveolar duct walls. H&E.

## 2.8 Lungs

Pathologic changes in the lung generally result from an overload of clearance mechanisms, direct toxicity, and indirect toxicity due to metabolic activation or immune-mediated effects. They include:

- Increased alveolar macrophages, lipidoses, phospholipidoses, lipoproteinosis
- Epithelialisation—type II pneumocyte proliferation
- Alveolar mineralisation
- Alveolitis
- Alveolar injury—oedema, haemorrhage, necrosis, fibrosis
- Inflammation/thickening/pneumonitis/pneumonia
- Bronchiolar-associated lymphoid tissue hyperplasia/depletion
- Vascular/pleural changes
- Bronchioloalveolar hyperplasia
- Bronchioloalveolar adenoma/carcinomas
- Squamous metaplasia/epithelial cysts/keratinising epithelioma/squamous cell carcinoma
- Mesothelioma

Increases in the number or nature of alveolar macrophages are a common induced change in inhalation studies and indicate increased clearance of exogenous or endogenous substances. Macrophages may be localised to the alveoli near the alveolar ducts or diffusely distributed. They may contain a variety of substances, including test material, surfactant lipid, phospholipid, blood degradation products, pigments, and others (Fig. 2.40).

Foamy macrophage accumulation frequently is accompanied by alveolar inflammatory cells and thickening of the alveolar wall with inflammatory cells, type II pneumocyte proliferation, and slight increases in reticulin and collagen fibres (Fig. 2.41). Macrophages often form aggregates or granulomas composed of tightly packed and/or coalescing macrophages (Fig. 2.42). Cholesterol clefts often are seen within these granulomas, which may be induced by a variety of inhaled xenobiotics, including dusts, and also occur in systemic lipidosis (Fig. 2.43). Intravenously administered compounds, such as insoluble polysaccharides, induce localised angiocentric granulomas with epithelioid and foreign-body type giant cells. Procedure-related foreign-body granulomas containing exogenous and endogenous materials, such as fibres, fragments of epithelium, and adipocytes, are seen in intravenous injection and infusion studies (Fig. 2.44). Subcutaneous injection of vegetable oil as a vehicle can also result in lipid-containing macrophage accumulations and lipid granulomas in the lungs (Fig. 2.45).

Several conditions, discussed in the following text, result in a similar histopathological picture with aggregates or diffuse foamy macrophage infiltration. Overloading of macrophages results in rupture, with release of their contents into the alveoli and an associated inflammatory cell reaction.

Phospholipidosis manifests as diffuse or multifocal accumulations of foamy macrophages with secondary features, including eosinophilic alveolar material, type II pneumocyte proliferation, and infiltration with polymorphonuclear cells (Fig. 2.46). On transmission electron microscopy, macrophages contain electron-dense multilamellar bodies, which also are present in type II pneumocytes and Clara cells, as well as in circulating lymphocytes (Fig. 2.47). This condition typically is associated with cationic amphophilic compounds (CADs), such as amiodarone and chlorphentermine. Species and tissue specificities vary with these drugs. Very few drugs that produce phospholipidosis in rodents are capable of inducing significant phospholipidosis in humans, although amiodarone does induce the condition in rats and humans.

Lipoproteinosis is associated with exposure to dust, such as quartz, and refers to the accumulation of fine, eosinophilic PAS-positive material in the alveoli with increased numbers of large rounded foamy macrophages, which may rupture releasing lipoprotein. Secondary changes include type II pneumocyte proliferation and infiltration with polymorphonuclear cells. Electron microscopy shows that the material is composed predominantly of lamellar bodies consisting of surfactant from type II cells (Fig. 2.48).

Interstitial pneumonitis with lipid-laden macrophages occurs in rats fed a diet supplemented with cholesterol and cottonseed oil. Initially, macrophages accumulate in the alveoli, but later they may be seen in the subpleural, peribronchiolar, and perivascular regions. This is basically a hyperlipidaemia and also is seen with hypophysectomy and anorectic drugs, both of which reduce food intake and presumably cause hyperlipidaemia.

Mineralisation of the alveolar septae is induced by vitamin D analogues (Fig. 2.49). Dark bluish purple concretions are seen within the alveolar septae. Inflammatory cell infiltration, septal thickening with collagen, and alveolar macrophages sometimes are associated with these depositions.

Toxicity in the lungs may involve one or more areas, depending on the affected cell type(s). Type 1 pneumocytes and endothelial cells are targets for oxygen toxicity, which has implications for its therapeutic use in premature infants and adults with respiratory distress. Many agents produce respiratory injury by direct interaction of the reactive molecule with the target cells, causing cytolytic changes. Pulmonary toxicity also may be partially mediated through the release of certain proteins; for example, necrosis of the airway epithelium in ozone toxicity is associated with increased levels of

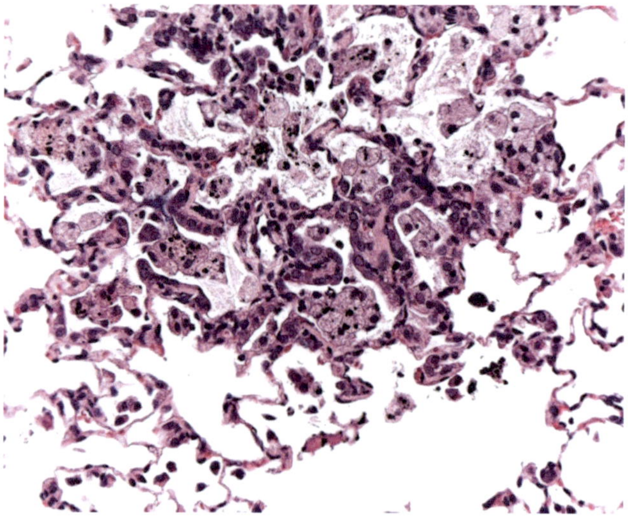

**FIGURE 2-40.** Focal pigmented macrophages containing variably sized black pigment granules in the lung of a rat given a black particulate material. The macrophages, some of which are ruptured, form aggregates. The alveolar septum displays type II pneumocyte proliferation. H&E.

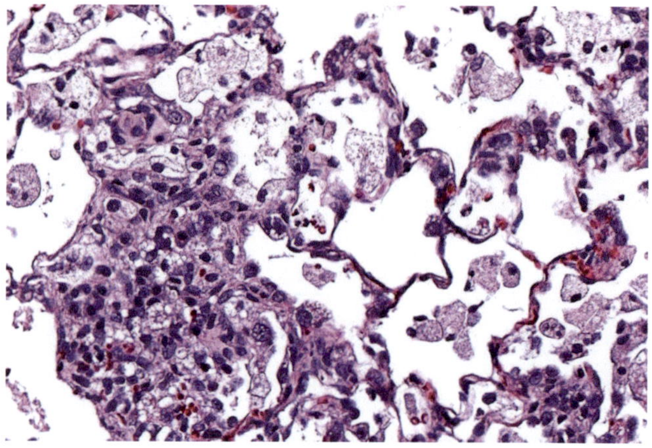

**FIGURE 2-41.** Foamy macrophages with type II pneumocyte proliferation in a rat lung. Large foamy macrophages are present in the alveoli; some of them have ruptured, releasing their contents. Some have coalesced to form an aggregate, and the alveolar septae show focal type II pneumocyte proliferation. H&E.

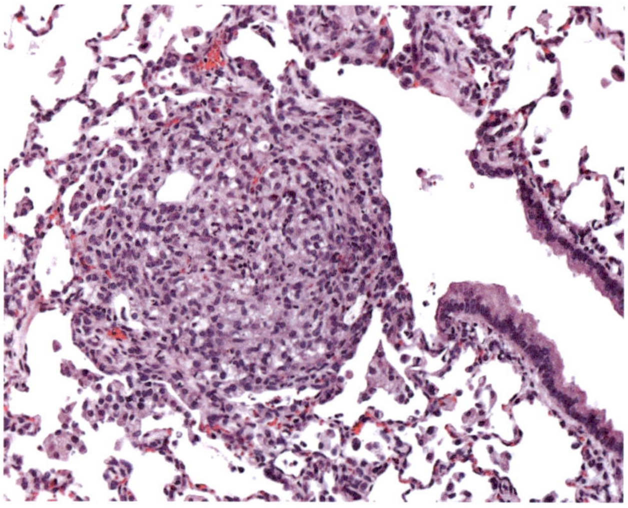

**FIGURE 2-42.** A large granuloma at the bronchiolar–alveolar junction in a rat lung. The granuloma comprises tightly packed large foamy macrophages with a few scattered neutrophils and lymphocytes. H&E.

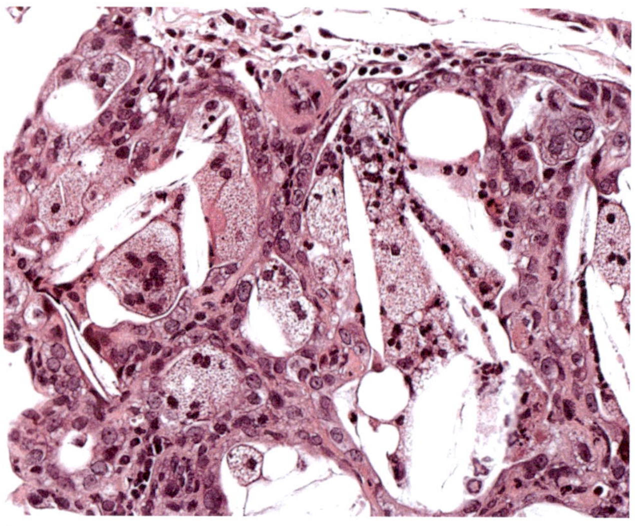

**FIGURE 2-43.** Cholesterol clefts in the lung of a rat with hyperlipidosis. A lesion consisting of coalescing large foamy macrophages is seen. Multinucleate cells, numerous cholesterol clefts, and small numbers of lymphocytes are present. H&E.

CGRP and activation of CGRP receptors and with neurokinin-1 receptor activation [33, 34].

Metabolic activation may occur either in the lung or elsewhere in the body with haematogenous transport of metabolites to the lung. If in the lung, it may occur subsequent to inhalation or blood-borne exposure to the test article. Many pulmonary toxicants are activated as a result of metabolism in the lung [35], where they generally are metabolised in the Clara cells; examples are 4-ipomeanol, carbon tetrachloride, and 3-methylindole.

Pulmonary oedema may be secondary to changes in other organ systems or may be the result of primary lung toxicity. In pulmonary oedema, the alveoli contain proteinaceous eosinophilic fluid with varying numbers of red and white blood cells, depending on the mechanism of induction and the inflammatory component (Fig. 2.50). Damage to endothelial cells by different mechanisms, such as their metabolism of α-naphthylthiourea and phenylthiourea, results in damage to capillaries and venules with marked pulmonary oedema. Administration of interleukin 2 causes 'vascular leak syndrome', characterised clinically by pulmonary oedema, pleural effusions, ascites, and other adverse effects, including pulmonary inflammation.

These effects are the result of cytotoxic vascular damage mediated directly by activated killer cells and cytotoxic T lymphocytes, with secondary release of inflammatory cytokines [36]. Many drugs produce pulmonary oedema in humans, either directly or through poorly understood immunogenic mechanisms.

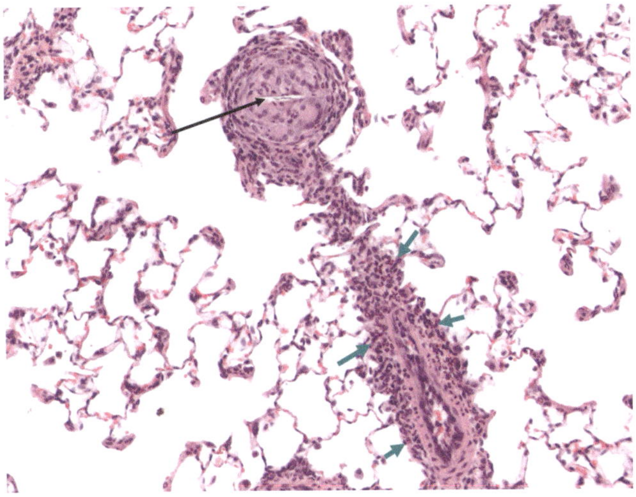

**Figure 2-44.** Foreign-body granuloma in the lung of a rat from a continuous intravenous infusion study. The granuloma contains a fibre (*black arrow*), and the blood vessel shows perivascular inflammatory cell infiltration (*green arrows*). Both are typical procedure-related lesions in rodent intravenous infusion studies. H&E.

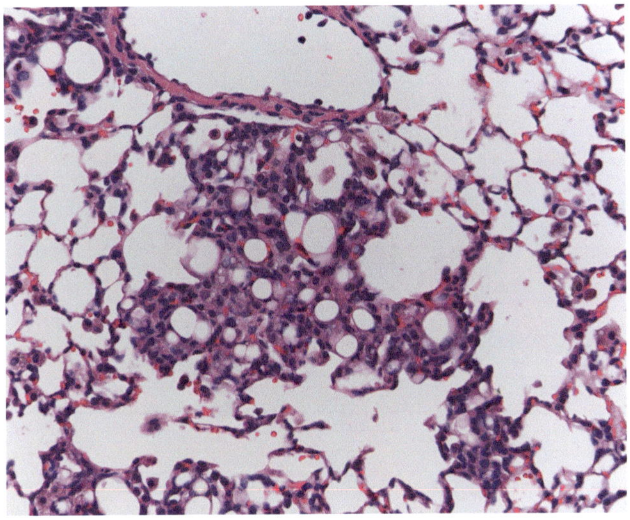

**Figure 2-45.** Perivascular/alveolar focus of macrophages containing lipid and pinkish-brown pigment. Large vacuoles resembling lipid are present in some cells. The rat was injected subcutaneously with an oil vehicle. H&E.

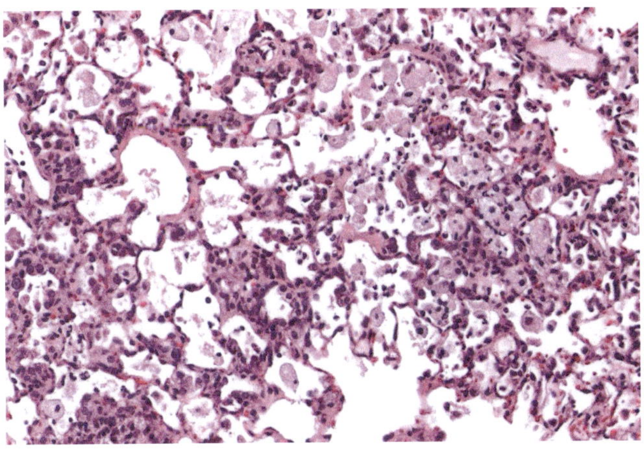

**Figure 2-46.** Phospholipidosis in the lung of a rat given a CAD. Diffuse infiltration of alveolar spaces with large foamy degenerating macrophages, as seen in this rat, is characteristic of phospholipidosis. The alveolar septae are markedly thickened with inflammatory cells and collagen, exhibiting type II pneumocyte proliferation. H&E.

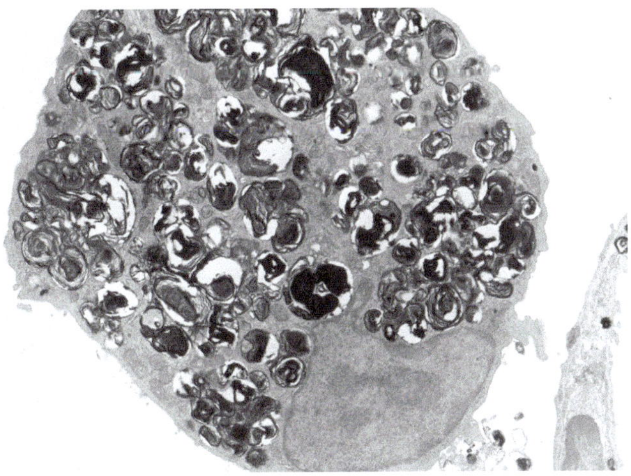

**Figure 2-47.** Numerous multilamellar bodies of various sizes and shapes in a pulmonary macrophage from a rat. These bodies are characteristic of phospholipidosis and may be seen in a wide variety of organs (Transmission electron microscopy).

Eosinophilic crystals in the alveoli, often accompanied by macrophages containing red blood cells or pigment, as well as neutrophils, are sequelae of focal haemorrhage (Fig. 2.51). Alveolitis of this type often is seen as a background finding.

Hyaline membranes lining the alveolar ducts are an uncommon response seen with some xenobiotics and strongly positive with PAS staining (Fig. 2.36). Some compounds, including Toll-like receptor agonists, produce a marked inflammatory response, with macrophage

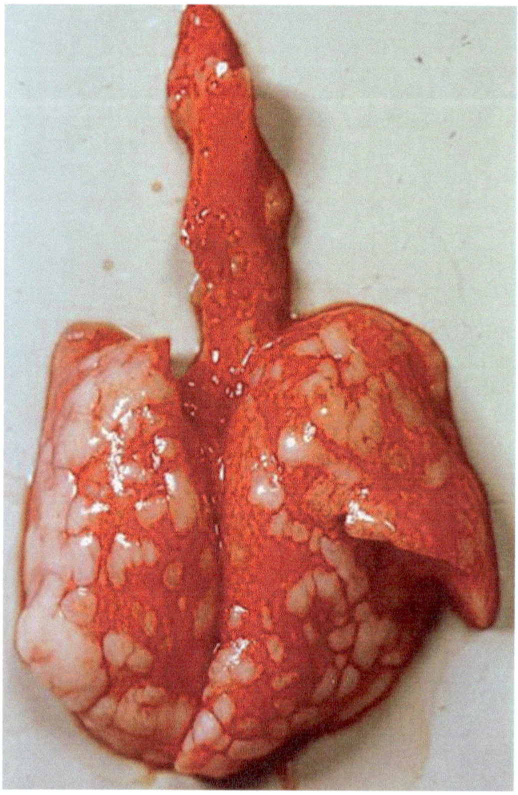

**FIGURE 2-48.** Lipoproteinosis has caused numerous large raised pale coalescing areas on the lungs of this mouse. These correlated histologically with aggregates of foamy macrophages. H&E.

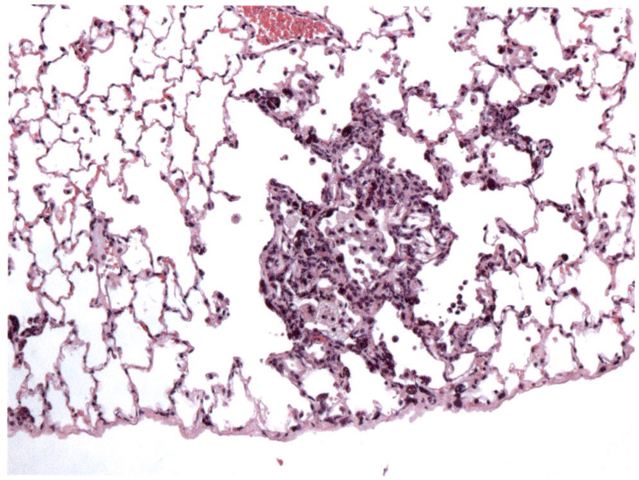

**FIGURE 2-49.** Mineralisation in the lung of this rat was induced by a vitamin D analogue. The change appears as multifocal dark bluish purple concretions in the alveolar septum, which is thickened by inflammatory cells and eosinophilic material. Foamy pigmented macrophage aggregates are present in the alveoli. H&E.

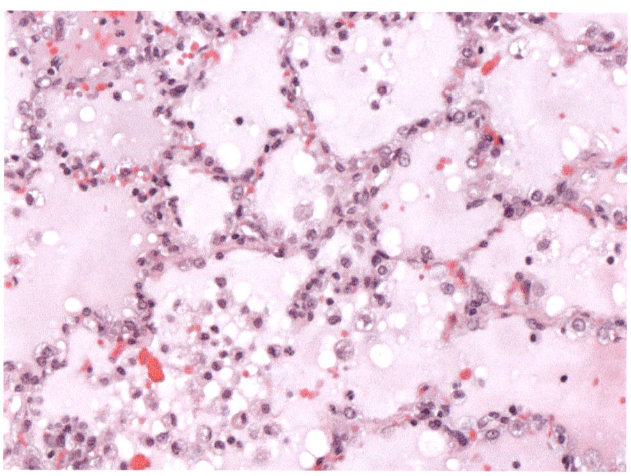

**FIGURE 2-50.** Pulmonary oedema in the lung of a rat. The alveoli are flooded with eosinophilic proteinaceous fluid. Scattered within the fluid are red blood cells and macrophages. The alveolar septum is thickened with intracapillary inflammatory cells in a few areas. H&E.

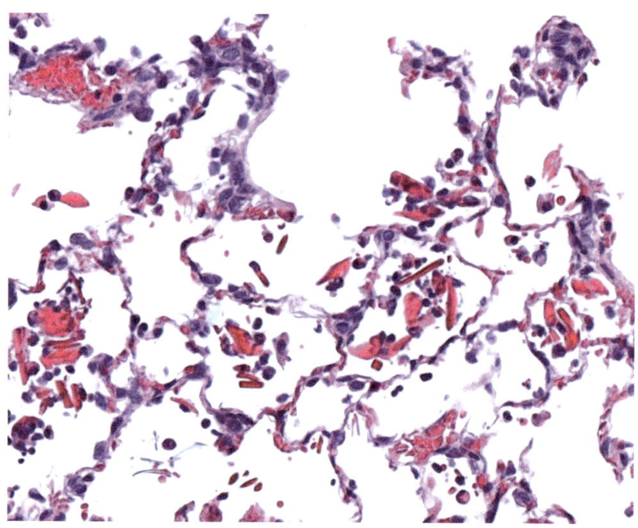

**FIGURE 2-51.** Alveolitis in the lung of a rat. Within the alveoli are several eosinophilic crystals composed of haematoidin. Scattered macrophages containing either pigment or red blood cells also are present. H&E.

aggregates in the alveoli and varying numbers of lymphocytes, plasma cells, and neutrophils within the alveoli and alveolar walls, causing interstitial thickening (Fig. 2.52).

Marked haemorrhage and necrosis of the alveolar walls are induced by paraquat, which selectively targets type I and II alveolar cells because of their possession of a polyamine uptake system. Females are less susceptible to free radical toxicity because of the stimulatory effect of estradiol on antioxidant mechanisms.

Damage to the alveolar walls results in fibrinous exudate and interstitial and alveolar inflammation (Fig. 2.53). If the damage is extensive, alveolar fibrosis develops as a sequel. Antisense oligonucleotides cause pneumonitis and subsequently alveolar fibrosis. Bleomycin produces interstitial pneumonitis, with extensive fibrosis as a sequel. Because of this effect on the lung parenchyma, it is used to create experimental models of alveolar fibrosis (Figs. 2.54 and 2.55).

Immunosuppression, resulting in impaired defence mechanisms, may result in secondary bacterial and fungal infections. Inhaled corticosteroids cause depletion of the lymphoid tissues associated with the airways (e.g. nasal-associated lymphoid tissue, bronchus-associated lymphoid tissue) (Fig. 2.56), and secondary alveolitis or bronchopneumonia may develop, often localised or confined to one lung lobe.

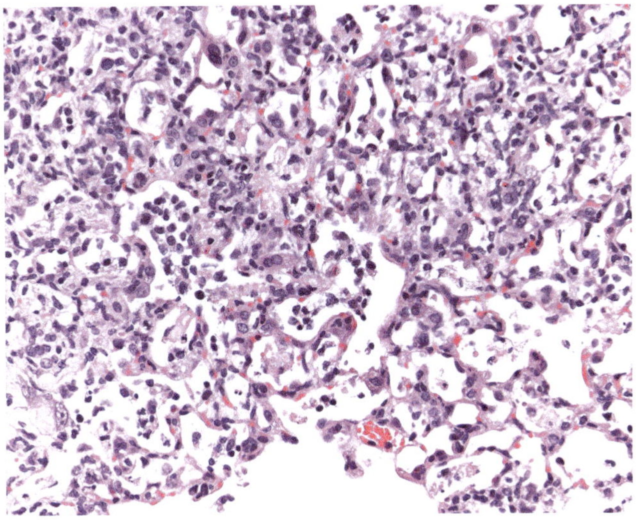

**Figure 2-52.** Interstitial inflammation in the lung of a mouse treated with a biologic. Marked interstitial thickening with chronic inflammatory cells and eosinophilic material, probably collagen, is present. Peribronchiolar and perivascular lymphocytic infiltration can be seen. H&E.

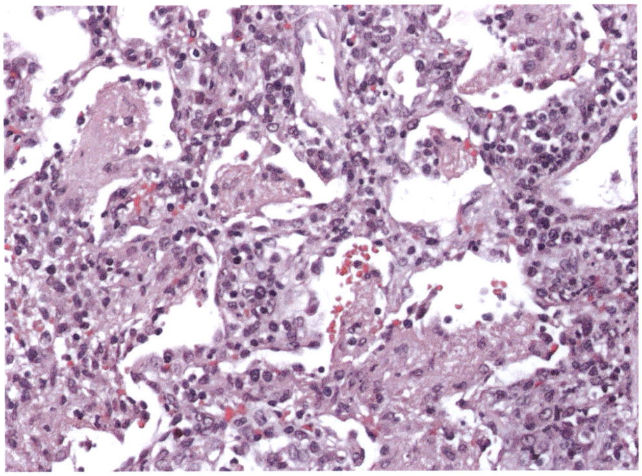

**Figure 2-53.** Fibrinous pneumonia in a rat lung. There is marked thickening of the alveolar septae with chronic inflammatory cells. The alveoli contain large amounts of fibrinoid inflammatory exudate, which often adheres to the septae and is starting to undergo fibrosis. H&E.

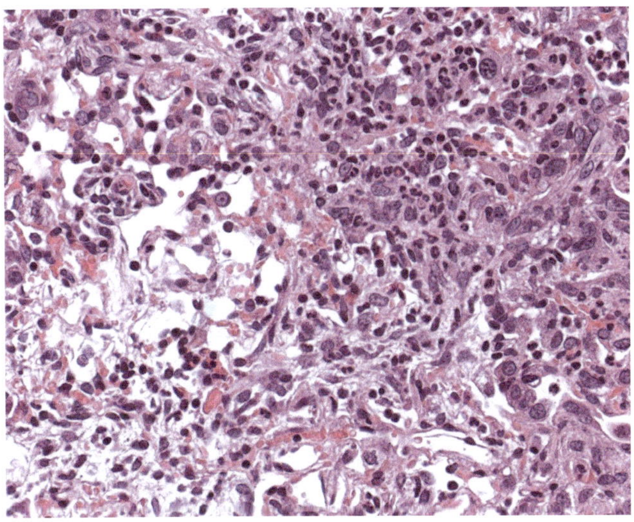

**Figure 2-54.** Interstitial pneumonitis and fibrosis in the lung of a rat treated with bleomycin. Mixed inflammatory cell infiltration, type II pneumocyte proliferation, and fibrosis have obscured the normal alveolar architecture. This is typical of bleomycin-induced lung pathology. H&E.

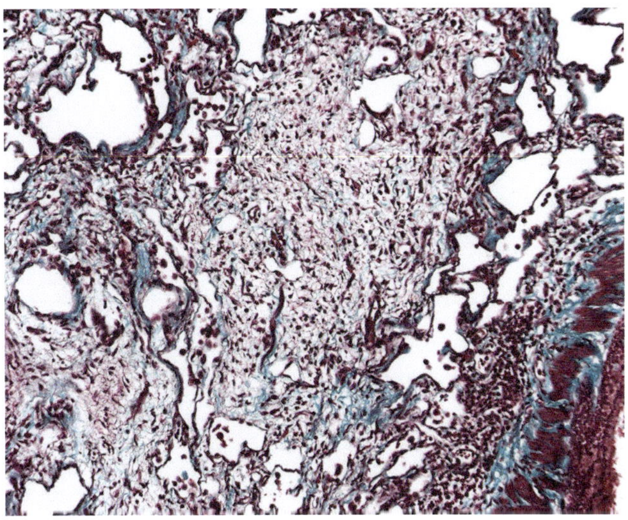

**Figure 2-55.** Alveolar fibrosis from the lung of a rat treated with bleomycin. Fibroblasts and collagen appear as a green fibrous matrix that has replaced the normal alveolar septae, with scattered inflammatory cells seen as dark red nuclei. Muscle and epithelia also are stained dark red (Masson's trichrome).

Stimulation of respiratory-associated lymphoid tissue, independent of inflammatory changes in the lungs, has been described in various species with Toll-like receptor agonists, with accompanying stimulation of associated lymph nodes (Fig. 2.57). PDE-4 inhibitors also cause immunostimulation of lymph nodes, partially as a result of inflammatory changes in the lungs.

Overstimulation of immune mechanisms occasionally may result in an adverse effect. The most common hypersensitive responses in the lung are types I and III. In type I, initial exposure results in production of IgE, which binds to mast cells and basophils, resulting in an eosinophil-mediated inflammation. In type III hypersensitivity, repeated exposure results in the development of antibodies and subsequent deposition of antigen–antibody complexes in the lung that fix complement and lead to inflammation. Beryllium has induced a type IV response in dogs, but in rats beryllium merely induces a foreign-body response, as there is no involvement of sensitised T cells in the lesion.

Non-immunologically mediated pulmonary disease may mimic immunologically mediated disease. Certain chemicals stimulate epithelial irritant receptors and cause secretion of inflammatory mediators without antibody involvement, resulting in a pseudoallergic reaction resembling type I hypersensitivity; examples include formaldehyde and ozone.

Misdosing may result in a variety of findings. In rats, oesophageal perforation during gavage can cause deposition of the test article in the thoracic cavity. Pleuritis, pericarditis, perithymic inflammation, and abscess are the common sequelae of intrathoracic dosing. If the article is an irritant, necrosis of the thoracic organs develops, initially involving the surface of the organ.

PDE-4 inhibitors induce pleural inflammation with fibrosis and development of adhesions between lung lobes in rats (Fig. 2.58). Macroscopically, adhesions between lung lobes are seen, with the pleura showing thickening with fibrosis and collagen deposition.

Vasculitis of the pulmonary vessels occurs with a variety of vasodilators, including PDE-4 inhibitors. Histologically, varying degrees of perivascular and vascular inflammation and mural necrosis with different proportions of cell types are seen (Fig. 2.59).

Compounds that cause degenerative changes in the myocardium, such as industrial chemicals, may induce similar degenerative findings in intrapulmonary blood vessels that are composed of cardiac muscle. Myofiber vacuolation, degeneration, and inflammatory cell infiltrate have been seen with an inhaled industrial chemical that caused similar lesions in the myocardium (Fig. 2.60).

Hyperplastic and neoplastic lesions in the lungs are induced in rodents by a wide variety of genotoxic and nongenotoxic compound classes administered by inhalation or orally. In mice, surveys have shown that most of these tumours are positive for surfactant apoprotein, indicative of a type II pneumocyte origin [37]. Bronchioloalveolar hyperplasia arises from the alveolar type II cells and/or bronchiolar ciliated respiratory or secretory cells (Fig. 2.61) [8]. This may be classified as alveolar, bronchiolar, or mixed based on cell morphology. When induced, these hyperplasias form a morphological and biological continuum of changes with bronchioloalveolar adenomas and carcinomas. To assess their relationship to the test article and possible carcinogenic potential, all bronchioloalveolar proliferative lesions should be evaluated together. Although different morphological tumour types, such as solid, papillary, and alveolar, have been described, it may be difficult, and is of limited use, to subclassify the tumours based on histologic pattern, as two or more patterns can be present within the same tumour (Figs. 2.62 and 2.63).

Lung tumours have been induced in mice by a wide range of genotoxic and nongenotoxic compounds, including nitrosamines, metals, industrial chemicals, and pharmaceuticals. Many of these nongenotoxic

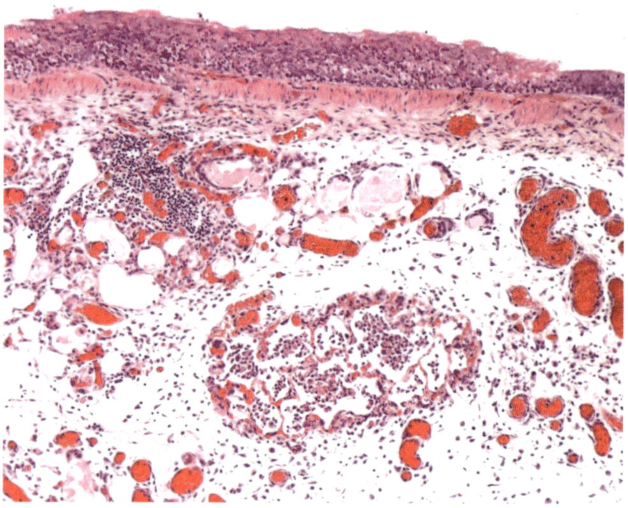

**Figure 2-56.** Lymphoid depletion in the lung of a rat given a corticosteroid. The bronchiolar-associated lymphoid tissue shows marked depletion, with a single focus of lymphocytes and a few scattered inflammatory cells remaining. H&E.

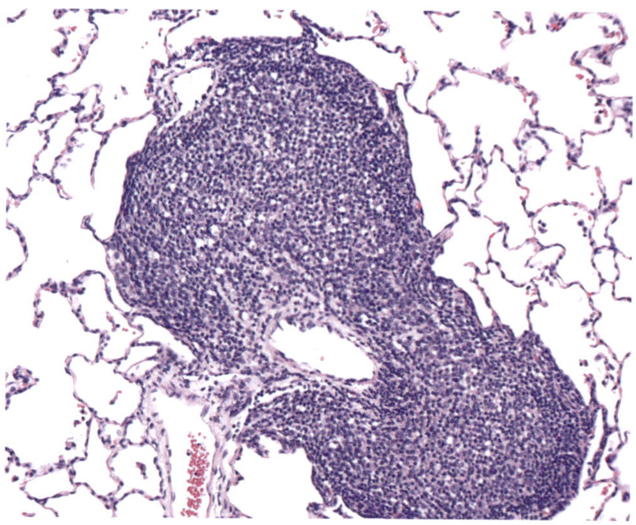

**Figure 2-57.** Marked perivascular lymphocytic infiltration is present in lung of this dog. The animal received an immunostimulant.

compounds, such as metronidazole, have been shown to be of no significance to humans at therapeutic doses. This is possibly because mice have larger numbers of Clara cells which contain a mouse-specific P450 isoform 2f2, resulting in higher levels of metabolism of many compounds and generation of metabolites that increase Clara cell turnover [38].

Squamous metaplasia in the lower conducting airways and alveoli occurs when proliferation of the existing cell type provides insufficient protection (Fig. 2.64). This occurs typically in response to inhalation of particulate matter, such as silica.

Along with squamous metaplasia, pulmonary keratinising cysts, cystic keratinising epitheliomas, and squamous cell carcinomas in rats form a continuum of lesions that are induced classically by prolonged exposure to inhaled particles or aerosols, such as talc, quartz, nickel oxide, and diesel exhaust. These changes result from initial squamous metaplasia of alveolar or bronchiolar cells, with subsequent neoplastic transformation and proliferation to form tumours. Morphologically, keratinising cysts are circumscribed cystic lesions lined by a layer of squamous epithelium without excessive proliferative changes (Fig. 2.65). Cystic keratinising epitheliomas demonstrate peripheral growth into alveolar spaces, numerous mitoses, and proliferating walls. Squamous cell carcinomas are highly invasive, with varying degrees of differentiation and keratin formation (Fig. 2.66).

Mesotheliomas are caused by a range of agents in a number of species including man. Asbestos, fibrous silicates, and thorium dioxide are associated with these tumours in man. In addition to asbestos, many compounds including bromine-containing chemicals, nitrosourea, and acrylamide induce peritoneal mesotheliomas in F344 rats (Fig. 2.67).

In dog safety studies, focal pulmonary subpleural lesions which include alveolar fibrosis, macrophage aggregates, alveolar type II hyperplasia, and squamous metaplasia are a common background finding. The lesions are possibly related to old infections with Filaroides or Toxocara species [39] and are of no biological significance. However, a high incidence of these lesions in treated animals may be misinterpreted by pathologists unfamiliar with background pathology in laboratory beagles (Fig. 2.68).

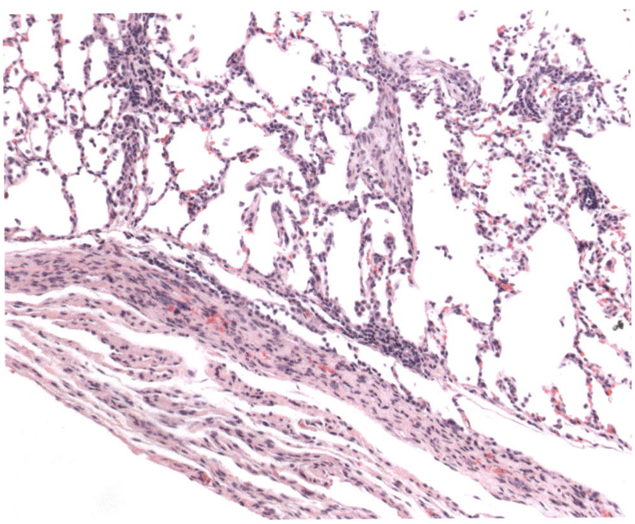

**Figure 2-58.** Pleural fibrosis of the lung in a rat treated with a PDE-4 inhibitor. Pleural collagen deposition, fibrosis, and adhesions are present. Mild alveolar inflammation and alveolar duct fibrosis are seen in the subpleural parenchyma. H&E.

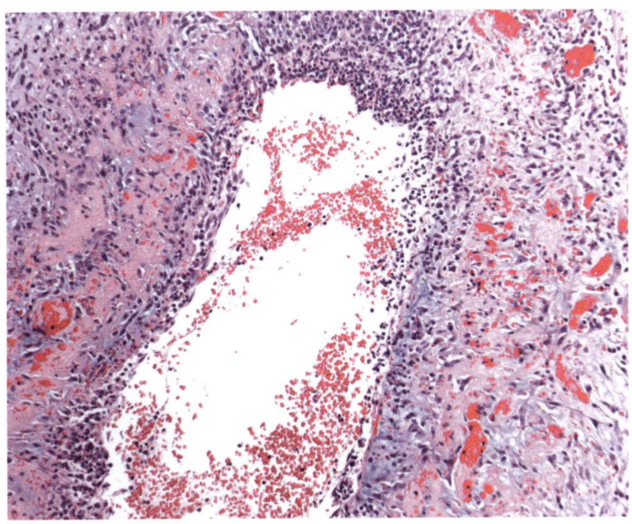

**Figure 2-59.** Necrotic vasculitis of a pulmonary vessel in a rat given a PDE-4 inhibitor. Severe fibrinoid mural necrosis and thickening of the vessel are seen, with marked inflammation and haemorrhage. These vasculitides are characteristic of PDE-4 inhibitors in rats. H&E.

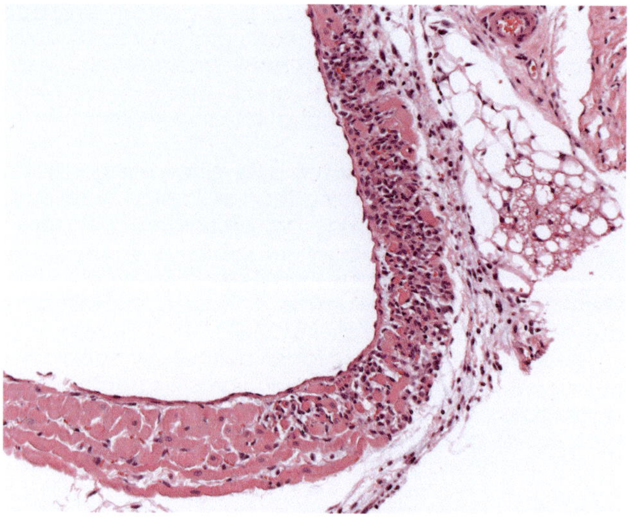

**Figure 2-60.** Pulmonary artery from a rat given an industrial chemical, showing focal degeneration of the myofibers. The affected fibres appear more eosinophilic and contracted, with loss of normal architecture. Associated lymphocytic and macrophage infiltration is present. H&E.

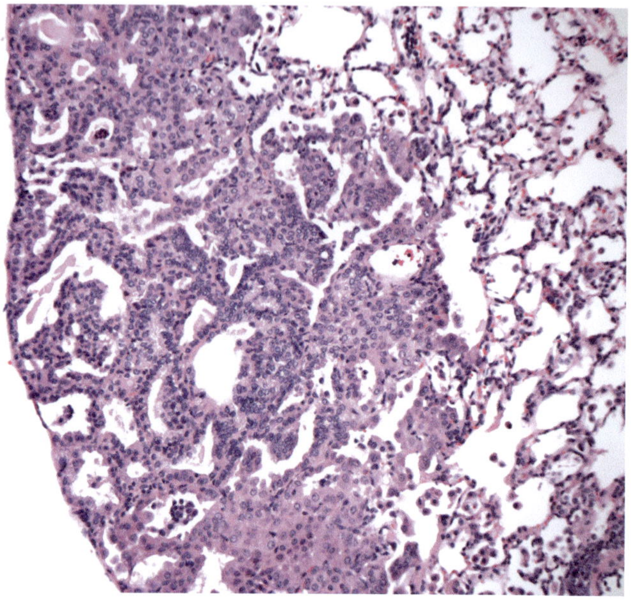

**Figure 2-61.** Bronchiolar alveolar hyperplasia in a mouse lung. Note the localised proliferation of large round cells thickening the alveolar septae. The lesion is too diffuse to qualify as an adenoma. H&E.

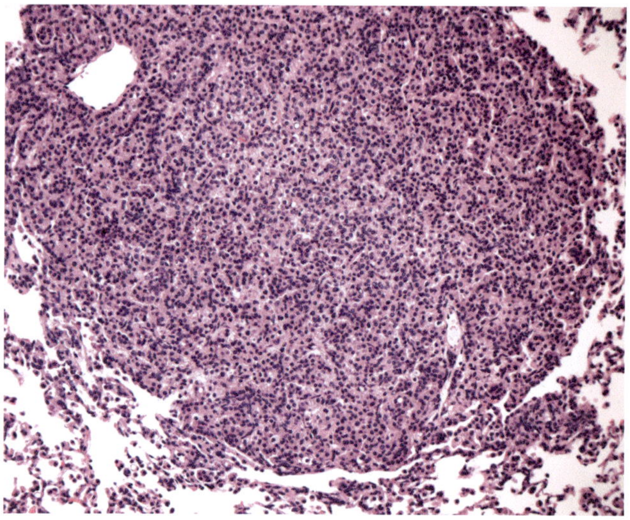

**Figure 2-62.** This bronchiolar–alveolar adenoma from a mouse lung is well circumscribed and solid. It is composed of well-differentiated round and cuboidal cells forming nests and acinar structures. H&E.

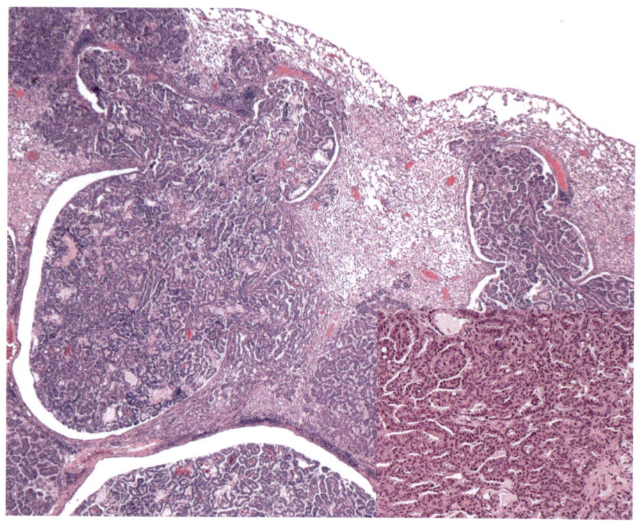

**Figure 2-63.** Bronchiolar–alveolar carcinoma in a mouse lung. This large, highly invasive tumour has invaded the airways. The tumour cells are basophilic and form papillary and acinar structures. H&E.

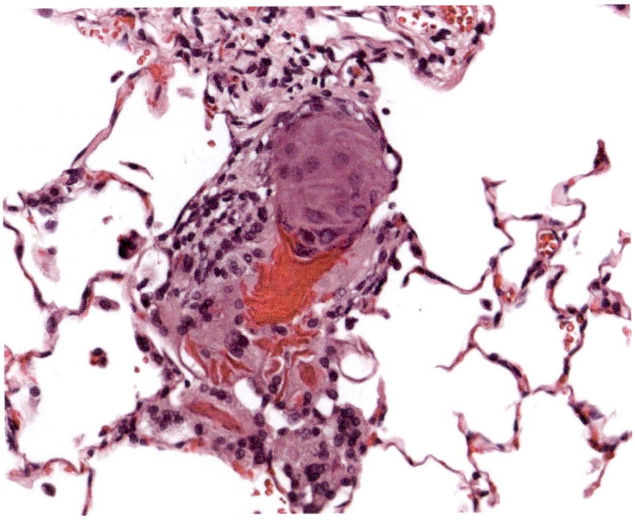

**Figure 2-64.** Focal squamous metaplasia of the alveolar wall, with keratin production. Coalescing aggregates of foamy macrophages are present around the lesion. H&E.

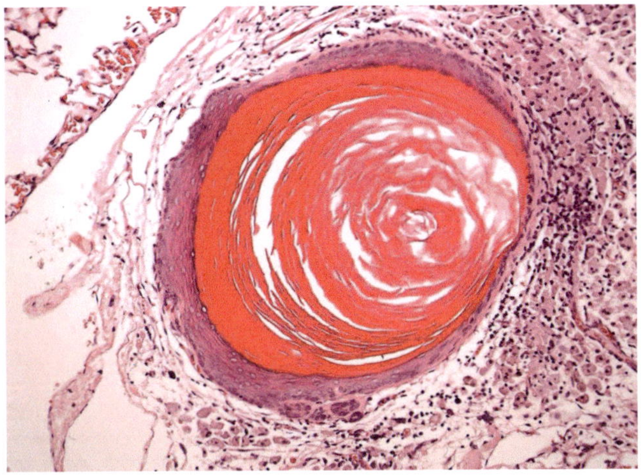

**Figure 2-65.** Keratin cyst in a rat lung, with foamy macrophage infiltration in the surrounding parenchyma. The cyst is lined by squamous epithelium of varying thickness and contains concentric lamellae of keratin. These are induced by particulate matter. H&E.

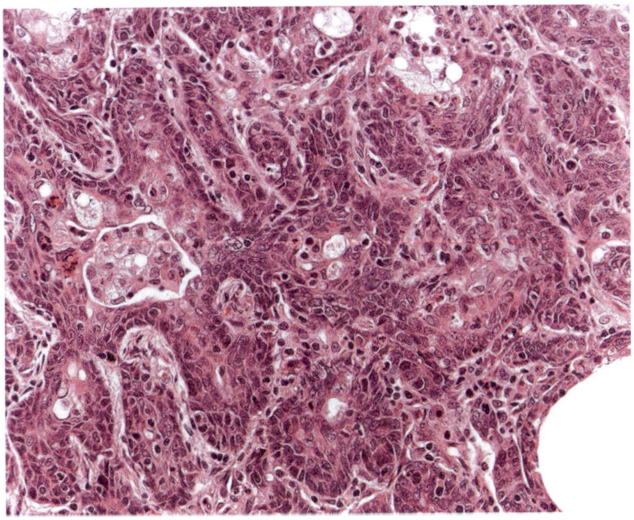

**Figure 2-66.** Squamous cell carcinoma from a rat lung. Large moderately differentiated epithelioid cells are forming nests, with spaces containing foamy macrophages. The tumour cells have large open nuclei, and several mitoses are evident. H&E.

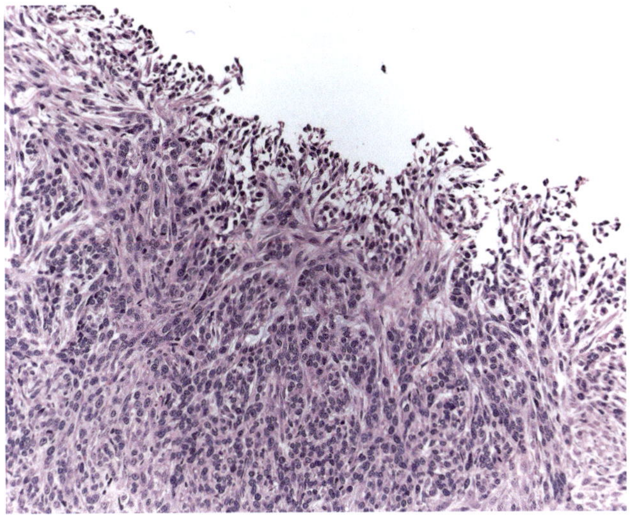

**Figure 2-67.** Malignant mesothelioma, from a mouse, which has invaded the thoracic wall. The tumour is composed of fronds and sheets of round and oval cells with large nuclei and scanty cytoplasm. Fibres are associated with development of these tumours. H&E.

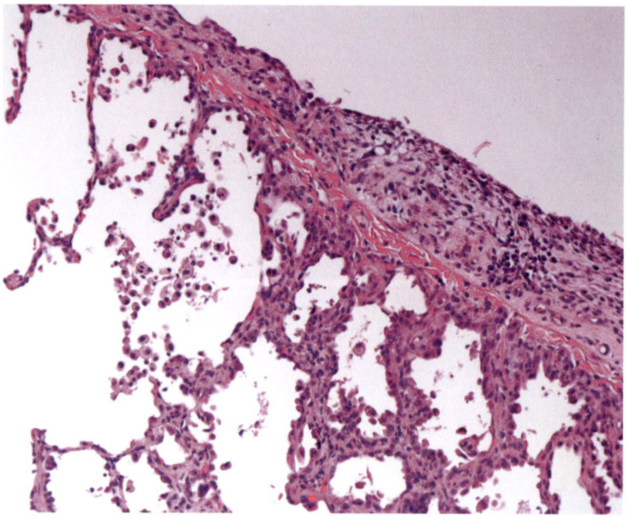

**FIGURE 2-68.** Fibrosing alveolitis in a dog. Pleural inflammation and thickening with subpleural alveolar fibrosis, as seen here, are typical of this lesion. Scattered foamy alveolar macrophages are present in the alveoli.

## References


1. Kimbell JS, Gross EA, Richardson RB, Conolly RB, Morgan KT. Correlation of regional formaldehyde flux predictions with the distribution of formaldehyde-induced squamous metaplasia in F344 rat nasal passages. Mutat Res. 1997;380:143–54.
2. Kimbell JS. Nasal dosimetry of inhaled gases and particles: where do inhaled agents go in the nose? Toxicol Pathol. 2006;34:270–3.
3. Kimbell JS, Gross EA, Joyner DR, Godo MN, Morgan KT. Application of computational fluid dynamics to regional dosimetry of inhaled chemicals in the upper respiratory tract of the rat. Toxicol Appl Pharmacol. 1993;121:253–63.
4. Kimbell JS, Godo MN, Gross EA, Joyner DR, Richardson RB, Morgan KT. Computer simulation of inspiratory airflow in all regions of the F344 rat nasal passages. Toxicol Appl Pharmacol. 1997;145:388–98.
5. Kimbell JS, Subramaniam RP, Gross EA, Schlosser PM, Morgan KT. Dosimetry modeling of inhaled formaldehyde: comparisons of local flux predictions in the rat, monkey, and human nasal passages. Toxicol Sci. 2001;64:100–10.
6. Kaewamatawong T, Kawamura N, Okajima M, Sawada M, Morita T, Shimada A. Acute pulmonary toxicity caused by exposure to colloidal silica: particle size dependent pathological changes in mice. Toxicol Pathol. 2005;33:743–9.
7. Harkema JR, Carey SA, Wagner JG. The nose revisited: a brief review of the comparative structure, function, and toxicologic pathology of the nasal epithelium. Toxicol Pathol. 2006;34:252–69.
8. Renne R, Brix A, Harkema J, Herbert R, Kittel B, Lewis D, et al. Proliferative and nonproliferative lesions of the rat and mouse respiratory tract. Toxicol Pathol. 2009;37:5S–73.
9. Young JT. Histopathologic examination of the rat nasal cavity. Fundam Appl Toxicol. 1981;1:309–12.
10. Morgan KT. Approaches to the identification and recording of nasal lesions in toxicology studies. Toxicol Pathol. 1991;19:337–51.
11. Kai K, Sahto H, Yoshida M, Suzuki T, Shikanai Y, Kajimura T, Furuhama K. Species and sex differences in susceptibility to olfactory lesions among the mouse, rat and monkey following an intravenous injection of vincristine sulphate. Toxicol Pathol. 2006;34:223–31.
12. Harkema JR. Comparative aspects of nasal airway anatomy: relevance to inhalation toxicology. Toxicol Pathol. 1991;19:321–36.
13. Harkema JR. Comparative pathology of the nasal mucosa in laboratory animals exposed to inhaled irritants. Environ Health Perspect. 1990;85:231–8.
14. Buckley LA, Jiang XZ, James RA, Morgan KT, Barrow CS. Respiratory tract lesions induced by sensory irritants at the RD50 concentration. Toxicol Appl Pharmacol. 1984;74:417–29.
15. Monticello TM, Morgan KT, Uraih L. Nonneoplastic nasal lesions in rats and mice. Environ Health Perspect. 1990;85:249–74.
16. Lewis JL, Nikula KJ, Sachetti LA. Induced xenobiotic-metabolizing enzymes localized to eosinophilic globules in olfactory epithelium of toxicant-exposed F344 rats. Inhal Toxicol. 1994;6:422–5.
17. Renne RA, Gideon KM, Harbo SJ, Staska LM, Grumbein SL. Upper respiratory tract lesions in inhalation toxicology. Toxicol Pathol. 2007;35:163–9.
18. Genter MB, Owens DM, Deamer NJ. Distribution of microsomal epoxide hydrolase and glutathione S-transferase in the rat olfactory mucosa: relevance to distribution of lesions caused by systemically-administered olfactory toxicants. Chem Senses. 1995;20:385–92.
19. Genter MB, Deamer NJ, Blake BL, Wesley DS, Levi PE. Olfactory toxicity of methimazole: dose-response and structure-activity studies and characterization of flavin-containing monooxygenase activity in the Long-Evans rat olfactory mucosa. Toxicol Pathol. 1995;23:477–86.
20. Dejonghe S, Lammens L, Raoof A, Steemans K, Broeckaert F, Verbeeck J, et al. Lethal rhinitis/sinusitis in rodents by aspiration of formulation in gavage studies: importance of evaluation of the nose. Exp Toxicol Pathol. 2008;61:410.
21. Maronpot RR, Miller RA, Clarke WJ, Westerberg RB, Decker JR, Moss OR. Toxicity of formaldehyde vapor in B6C3F1 mice exposed for 13 weeks. Toxicology. 1986;41:253–6.
22. Takagi M, Shiraiwa K, Kusuoka O, Tamura K. A case of olfactory neuroblastoma induced in a rat by N-nitrosobis(2-hydroxypropyl)amine. J Toxicol Pathol. 2010;23:111–4.
23. Renne RA, Gideon KM. Types and patterns of response in the larynx following inhalation. Toxicol Pathol. 2006;34:281–5.
24. Lewis DJ. Morphological assessment of pathological changes within the rat larynx. Toxicol Pathol. 1991;19:352–7.
25. Lewis DJ, Prentice DE. The ultrastructure of rat laryngeal epithelia. J Anat. 1980;130:617–32.

26. Kaufmann W, Bader R, Ernst H, Harada T, Hardisty J, Kittel B, et al. 1st international ESTP expert workshop: "Larynx squamous metaplasia." A re-consideration of morphology and diagnostic approaches in rodent studies and its relevance for human risk assessment. Exp Toxicol Pathol. 2009;61:591–603.

27. Osimitz TG, Droege W, Finch JM. Toxicologic significance of histologic change in the larynx of the rat following inhalation exposure: a critical review. Toxicol Appl Pharmacol. 2007;225:229–37.

28. Kambara T, McKevitt TP, Francis I, Woodfine JA, McCawley SJ, Jones SA, et al. Eosinophilic inclusions in rat Clara cells and the effect of an inhaled corticosteroid. Toxicol Pathol. 2009; 37:315–23.

29. Sturgess J, Reid L. The effect of isoprenaline and pilocarpine on (a) bronchial mucus-secreting tissue and (b) pancreas, salivary glands, heart, thymus, liver and spleen. Br J Exp Pathol. 1973;54:388–403.

30. Haworth R, Woodfine J, McCawley S, Pilling AM, Lewis DJ, Williams TC. Pulmonary neuroendocrine cell hyperplasia: identification, diagnostic criteria and incidence in untreated ageing rats of different strains. Toxicol Pathol. 2007;35:735–40.

31. Sunday ME, Willett CG. Induction and spontaneous regression of pulmonary neuroendocrine cell hyperplasia in a hamster model. Chest. 1992;101:21S.

32. Gopinath C, Prentice DE, Lewis DJ. Atlas of experimental toxicological pathology. Lancaster: MTP Press Limited; 1987. p. 11–22.

33. Oslund KL, Hyde DM, Putney LF, Alfaro MF, Walby WF, Tyler NK, et al. Activation of calcitonin gene-related peptide receptor during ozone inhalation contributes to airway epithelial injury and repair. Toxicol Pathol. 2009;37:805–13.

34. Oslund KL, Hyde DM, Putney LF, Alfaro MF, Walby WF, Tyler NK, et al. Activation of neurokinin-1 receptors during ozone inhalation contributes to epithelial injury and repair. Am J Respir Cell Mol Biol. 2008;39:279–88.

35. Smith BR, Brian WR. The role of metabolism in chemical-induced pulmonary toxicity. Toxicol Pathol. 1991;19:470–81.

36. Zhang J, Wenthold Jr RJ, Yu ZX, Herman EH, Ferrans VJ. Characterization of the pulmonary lesions induced in rats by human recombinant interleukin-2. Toxicol Pathol. 1995;23:653–66.

37. Pilling AM, Mifsud NA, Jones SA, Endersby-Wood HJ, Turton JA. Expression of surfactant protein mRNA in normal and neoplastic lung of B6C3F1 mice as demonstrated by in situ hybridization. Vet Pathol. 1999;36:57–63.

38. Strupp C, Banas DA, Cohen SM, Gordon EB, Jaeger M, Weber K, Relationship of metabolism and cell proliferation to the mode of action of fluensulfone-induced mouse lung tumors: analysis of their human relevance using the IPCS framework 1, Toxicol Sci. 2012;128:284-294.

39. Scudamore C. Beagle dog. In: McInnes EF, editor. Background lesions in laboratory animals: a colour atlas. Edinburgh: Saunders Elsevier; 2012. p. 37–44.

# 3 The Liver

Importance of hepatotoxicity in toxicity studies is briefly discussed. Various induced lesions occurring in the liver of experimental animals, such as degeneration, necrosis, inclusions, pigmentation, hypertrophy, hyperplasia, and tumours, are illustrated, and their relative importance is discussed. Significance of adaptive responses is also discussed.

## 3.1 Introduction

The liver is frequently identified as a target organ in toxicity studies; this is partly attributable to its anatomical location and functional complexity. Its close association with the digestive system makes it vulnerable to exposure from many toxicants from the digestive tract, which is the first port of entry [1]. Several endogenous and exogenous toxicants arrive in the liver through the circulation. Many toxins, pharmaceuticals, agrochemicals, chemicals, nutritive additives, contaminants from food and drinks, endogenous breakdown products, and hormones all pass through the liver, evoking adaptive or injurious responses.

Because the liver is frequently a target for toxicity and carcinogenesis in rodents, assessment of potential hepatotoxic risk to humans is of considerable importance [2–7]. Numerous toxicants react with the liver and result in hepatotoxicity. Hepatotoxicity is classified in different ways; a simple classification is provided here:

- Intrinsic
- Idiosyncratic
- Direct
- Indirect
- Hypersensitivity
- Aberrant metabolism

Intrinsic hepatotoxicity is often predictable, affects a large proportion of exposed individuals, is dose-related, and in most cases produces similar effects in experimental animals and humans [8]. There are two types, direct and indirect hepatotoxicity. Direct hepatotoxicity occurs when cell injury is produced by the agent or its metabolite directly, resulting in metabolic and functional disturbances [9]. Some directly bind with macromolecules and cause cell injury, as with metals like phosphorus and iron salts. Others require metabolic biotransformation to toxic metabolites that cause cell injury. Halocarbons like carbon tetrachloride and chloroform come under this category. The reactions are mediated by the Cyp family of enzymes.

Indirect hepatotoxicity occurs when agents interfere with certain metabolic pathways that in turn cause overload and subsequent subcellular injury. Steatosis caused by ethionine falls under this. Here the hepatocyte is overloaded with lipid and develops cytotoxicity. Cholestasis due to interference with the excretory mechanism is also an example of indirect toxicity.

Idiosyncratic hepatotoxicity affects only a small proportion of exposed individuals; the majority remain unaffected. These toxicities do not show a clear dose response and are

C. Gopinath, V. Mowat, *Atlas of Toxicological Pathology*,
DOI 10.1007/978-1-62703-998-7_3, 

often not predicted by experimental animal studies. Allergic reactions or hypersensitivity can be involved, as in halothane toxicity in humans. In another type, the toxicity is manifested in only a small proportion of the exposed individuals, in which toxicity occurs owing to formation of a toxic metabolite because of presence of an aberrant metabolic pathway [8–10]. Toxicity does not occur in the majority of exposed individuals. Experimental animal studies cannot predict this type of toxicity.

Several external factors can influence hepatotoxicity. Nutritional status, age, sex, level of drug-metabolising enzymes (DME) in the liver, glutathione, and other essential metabolites all can influence or modify hepatotoxicity [11]. There is marked interspecies differences in susceptibility, so information from as wide a range of species as is practical should be obtained [12].

Most liver injuries are dose and time related. Cell membrane injury, organelle damage, changes in intracellular lipid, glycogen, fluid, and essential metabolites along with mesenchymal and sinusoidal cell alterations occur during hepatotoxicity. Minor structural alterations are reflected by changes in cell functions such as protein synthesis, lipid and carbohydrate metabolism, and secretory and excretory status. The changes can be monitored by invasive and noninvasive tests that help to assess severity and progress. Structural changes assessed histologically and function test results do not always correlate with each other in toxicity studies.

Exposure of the liver to a number of xenobiotics can result in noninjurious changes that are not adverse. Changes in subcellular organelles occurring as a response to cellular overload are usually of a hypertrophic nature, in order to cope with continuous overload of the external agent. These changes are not deleterious and occur because of persistence of the xenobiotic agent. The result is liver enlargement, increase in liver weight often associated with hepatocyte hypertrophy, and induction of drug-metabolising enzymes. Stoppage of exposure usually resolves the changes in liver weight and morphology, and organelles return to normality.

Hepatic metabolism of xenobiotics can be enhanced by induction of the enzyme systems. DME systems can be modified by inducers or inhibitors in experimental conditions. Such modifications can have profound effects on hepatotoxicities produced by agents like carbon tetrachloride, chloroform, or halothane (increase or decrease in necrogenic potentialities) [13].

This chapter mainly describes various morphological changes seen in laboratory animals used in toxicity studies. Toxic injuries of the liver often tend to appear with a zonal distribution. The classic terminology of centrilobular, midzonal, and periportal locations is still in vogue, although acceptance of the hepatic acinus has displaced the concept of a liver lobule arranged around a central vein. The pathogenesis of liver changes is better understood in light of the concept of the anatomical and physiological basis of a liver acinus.

The zonal distribution of hepatic injuries is not always understood. Factors such as circulatory predisposition due to relative anoxia or hypercarbia in areas away from arterial blood supply are relevant in some cases. Specific affinities due to binding by the parent compound or its metabolites are considerations. The relative concentrations/availability of drug-handling enzymes and other aspects of cellular function that mediate toxicity are important factors in determining the location of the injury [14, 15].

The induced lesions affecting liver are summarised:

- Hydropic degeneration
- Fatty change (steatosis)
- Necrosis
- Apoptosis
- Glycogen alterations
- Nuclear changes
- Cytoplasmic inclusions
- Pigmentation
- Hypertrophy
- Atrophy
- Hyperplasia
- Foci of cellular alterations
- Cystic degeneration
- Sinusoidal dilation/peliosis
- Leucocytosis
- Cholangitis
- Bile duct hyperplasia
- Oval cell proliferation
- Cholangiofibrosis
- Cirrhosis
- Liver tumours

## 3.2 Hydropic Degeneration

Affected liver cells appear swollen/distended with vacuoles or clear spaces in the cytoplasm, sometimes replacing the entire cytoplasm, and cells appear ballooned. The nucleus remains central. Frequently the affected cells are adjacent to areas of necrosis. The loss of cell membrane integrity leads to fluid accumulation within the cell. Carbon tetrachloride injury results in hydropic degeneration of the centrilobular cells, along with other changes, in rodents (Figs. 3.1 and 3.2). Carbon disulphide given to rats pretreated with phenobarbitone sodium will result in marked hydropic degeneration of centrilobular hepatocytes [16]. The change is reversible, but it can progress to necrosis.

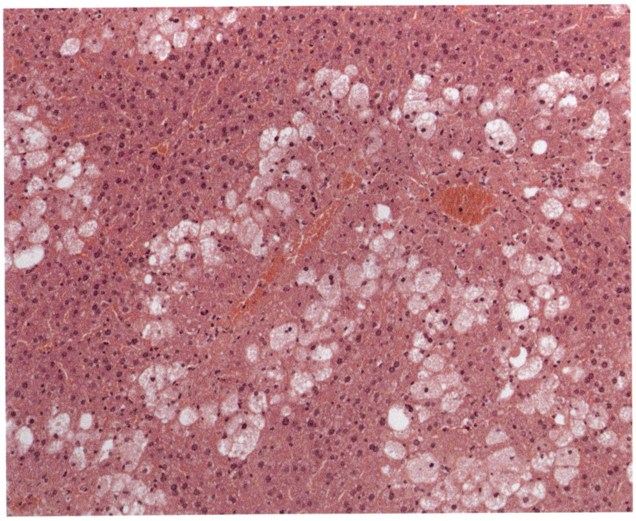

**Figure 3-1.** Hydropic degeneration, liver, in a rat treated with carbon tetrachloride. Note ballooned hepatocytes surrounding necrotic centrilobular hepatocytes. The cells are swollen with clear cytoplasm and central nuclei. Haemotoxylin and eosin (H&E).

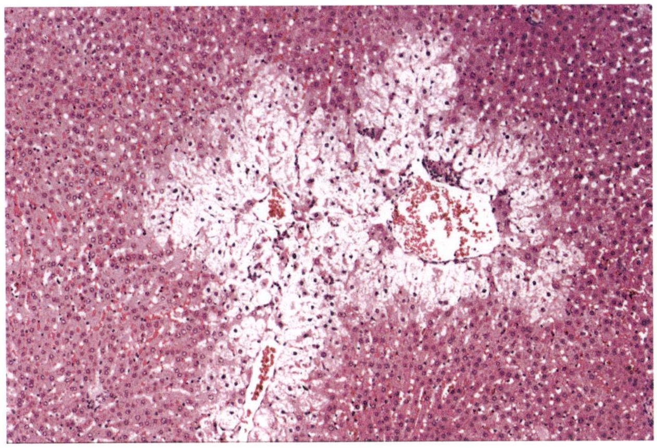

**Figure 3-2.** Hydropic degeneration, centrilobular, liver, in a rat. H&E.

## 3.3 Fatty Change (Steatosis)

Cytoplasmic vacuolation due to the presence of lipid in the liver cells is fatty change. This is a common finding in rodent livers. Vacuoles in the cytoplasm can be large and are referred to as macrovesicular, or they can be multiple small/fine vacuoles within the hepatocyte cytoplasm, when they are termed microvesicular vacuolation (Fig. 3.3). Tetracycline and aflatoxin produce the microvesicular type, and methotrexate produces macrovesicular vacuolation [8]. The vacuolation is frequently zonal, appearing as centrilobular or periportal and rarely as midzonal or diffuse (Figs. 3.4–3.6). Fatty change can be diffuse when it affects large areas without a zonal distribution or focal/multifocal distribution (Fig. 3.7). Fatty change, when extensive, tends to displace the nuclei of the affected cells to the periphery. The presence of lipid can be confirmed by fat stains in frozen sections. Phosphorus causes periportal fat, carbon tetrachloride causes centrilobular lipid, and choline deficiency results in midzonal fatty change in the rodent liver. Ethionine induces diffuse fatty change. Organelle injury, metabolic disorder, or deficiency of lipotropic factors all cause fatty change in the liver. The change is reversible. Presence of periportal lipid is normal in female rats. If the change is severe and persistent, it can lead to necrosis, fibrosis, inflammation, and nodular hyperplasia as with choline deficiency.

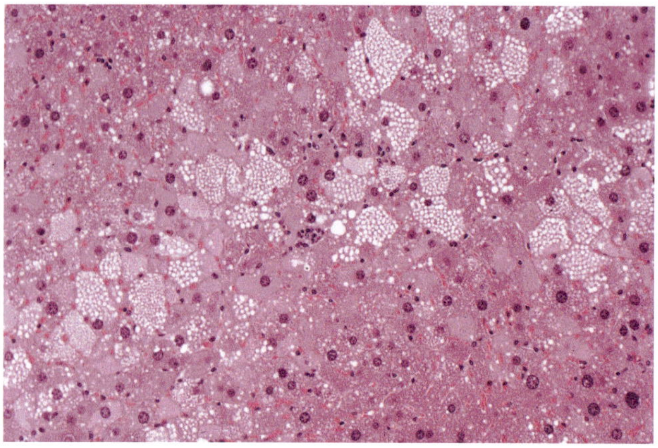

**Figure 3-3.** Hepatocellular vacuolation, microvesicular, in a mouse. Hepatocytes with intracytoplasmic fine vacuolation and nuclei peripherally displaced. H&E.

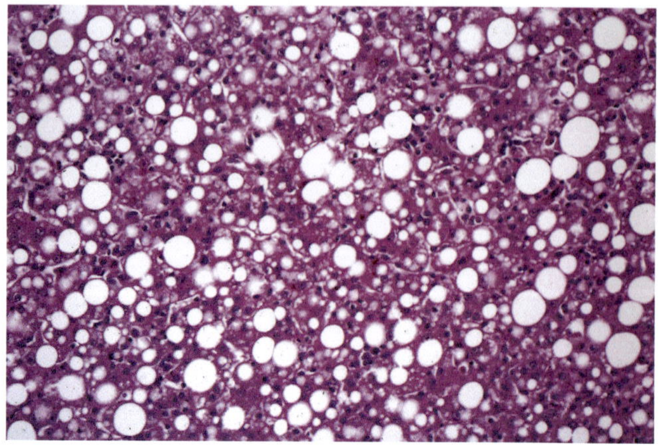

**Figure 3-4.** Hepatocellular macrovesicular vacuolation, diffuse, in a rat treated with an agrochemical agent. H&E.

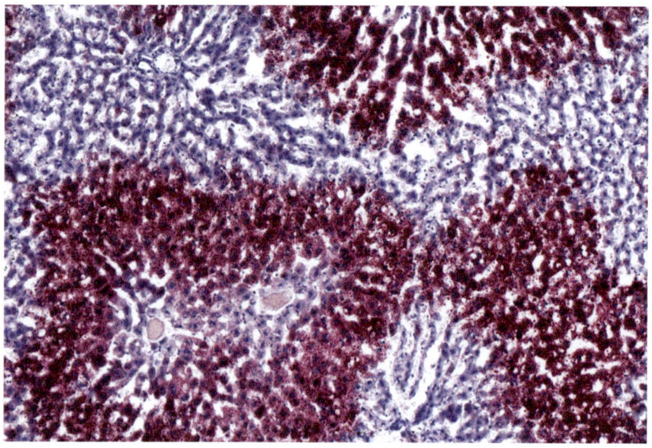

**Figure 3-5.** Lipid deposition, midzonal hepatocytes, in a mouse treated with a novel pharmaceutical. Frozen section, Oil red O (ORO).

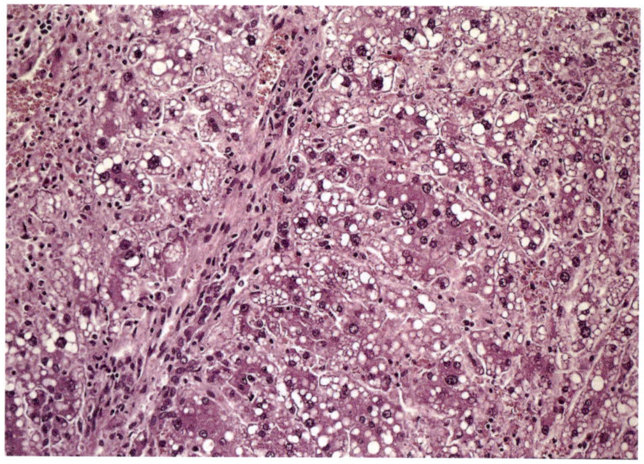

**Figure 3-6.** Hepatocellular vacuolation, macrovascular, diffuse, in a dog. Some evidence of interstitial fibrosis. H&E.

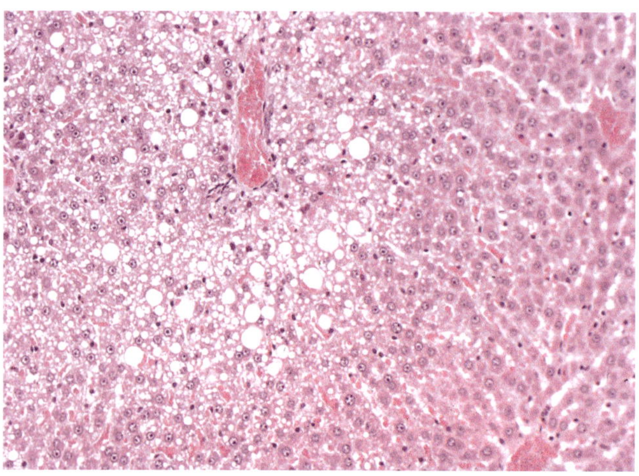

**Figure 3-7.** Hepatocellular vacuolation, periportal, in a rat. H&E.

## 3.4 Necrosis

Hepatocellular death, while still attached to the remaining normal parenchyma, is necrosis. Generally hepatic necrosis is coagulative in type, and induced necrosis is usually of a zonal distribution (i.e. centrilobular, periportal, or midzonal) (Figs. 3.8–3.10). Occasionally necrosis can be focal or diffuse, involving large areas of the liver. Carbon tetrachloride, chloroform, copper salts, tannic acid, and dimethylnitrosamine (DMN) all cause centrilobular necrosis [17]. One of the early steps in necrosis is loss of cell membrane integrity and accumulation of intracellular calcium. In classic zonal necrosis induced by agents like carbon tetrachloride or chloroform, hepatocytes around the central vein reveal coagulative necrosis surrounded by hepatocellular degeneration and more peripherally by a zone of inflammatory cells. Other agents evoke little inflammatory response. The necrotic zone reveals loss of glycogen, and plasma liver-specific enzymes are increased (Fig. 3.11). The reticular framework remains intact. Recovery from zonal necrosis is rapid and complete. If injury is mild, repair by regeneration takes place quickly, resulting in no scar formation. However, in more serious injuries, as produced by DMN, the necrosis is associated with haemorrhage, endothelial damage, and collapse of the reticular framework (Fig. 3.12) [18]. This is followed by repair with inflammation/fibrosis and often lobular distortion (Fig. 3.13). In severe cases the necrotic zones merge with adjacent lobules, resulting in bridging necrosis. Periportal necrosis is produced by agents like phosphorus, ferrous sulphate, or allyl formate and in some species aflatoxin [8]. Midzonal necrosis is rare and can be produced by ngaione, beryllium, and furosemide. Diffuse necrosis is noted with galactosamine (Fig. 3.14). Focal necrosis is often spontaneous and rare as an induced result. Manganese chloride and biliary obstruction can result in focal necrosis (Fig. 3.15) [19].

On rare occasions, in dogs centrilobular injury progresses to fibrosis and inflammation along with the presence of proliferating bile ducts in the centrilobular zone (personal observation). Single cell necrosis (piecemeal necrosis) is noticed in rats given paracetamol. Repeated administration of hepatotoxins like chloroform does not potentiate necrogenic effects. In experimental conditions, subsequent doses produce a diminishing response as the regenerating hepatocytes are more resistant to continued dosing of the hepatotoxin [20].

In the mouse another type of necrosis occasionally occurs as distinct from coagulative necrosis. Initially the affected cells appear swollen with intracytoplasmic multiple small vacuoles, followed by appearance of erythrocytes within the cytoplasm (Fig. 3.16). Cell nuclei appear normal, but soon the affected cell disappears leaving an empty space, which becomes filled with blood (Fig. 3.17). Sinusoids appear distended giving a punched-out appearance in the parenchyma (Fig. 3.18).

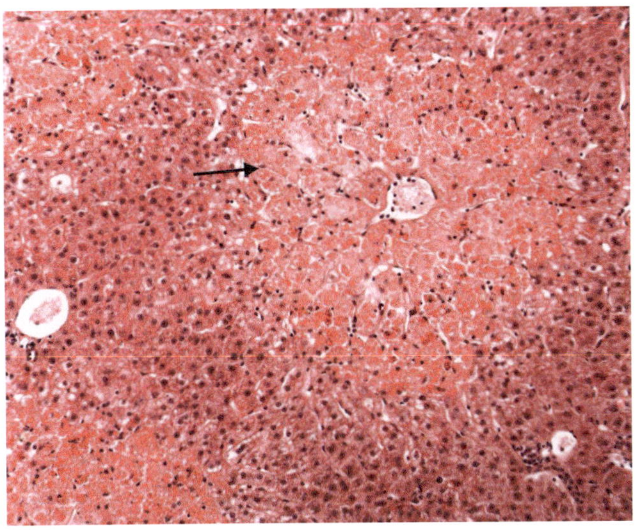

**Figure 3-8.** Hepatocellular necrosis, centrilobular, in a monkey treated with an industrial chemical. Note absence of any inflammatory response (*arrow*). H&E.

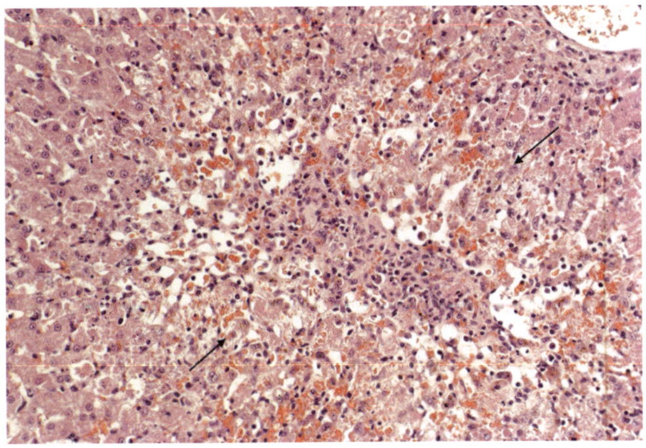

**Figure 3-9.** Hepatocellular necrosis, centrilobular, in a rat. Note loss of hepatocytes, inflammatory cell infiltration, and haemorrhage (*arrows*) in the centrilobular zone. H&E.

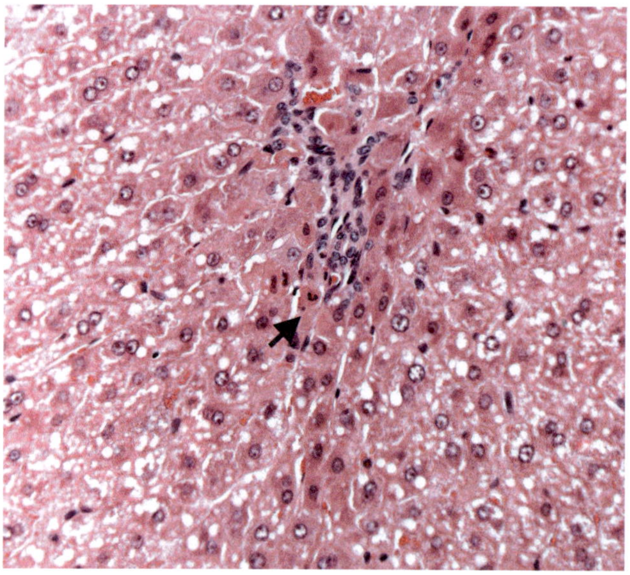

**FIGURE 3-10.** Hepatocellular degeneration/necrosis, periportal (*arrow*), in a rat treated with an agrochemical agent. Hepatocellular vacuolation of cells from other zones is present. H&E.

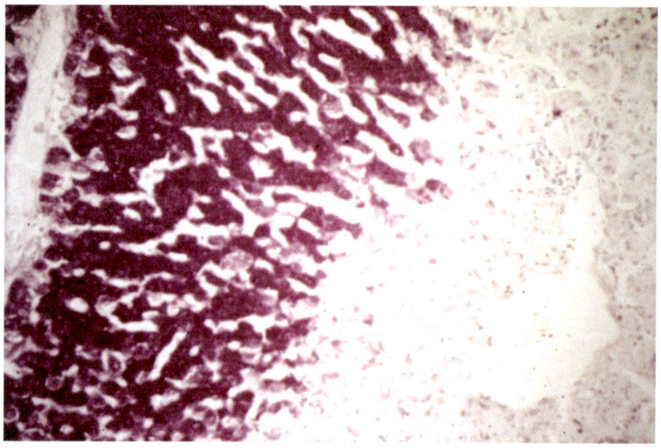

**FIGURE 3-11.** Hepatocellular necrosis and loss of glycogen staining, centrilobular. Periodic acid–Schiff (PAS).

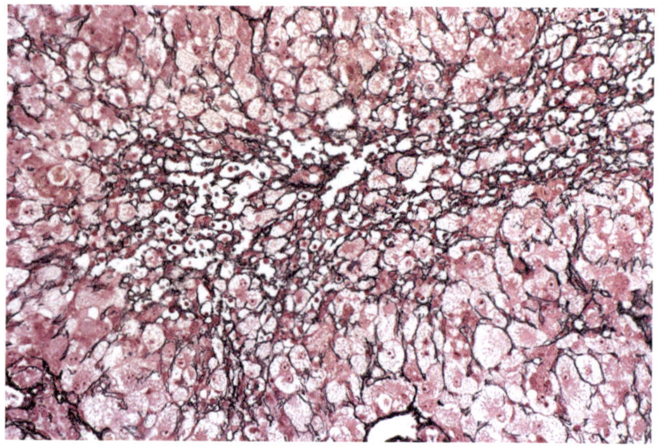

**FIGURE 3-12.** Hepatocellular necrosis and loss, centrilobular hepatocytes. Note reticulin collapse and duplication in a rat treated with an inhalation anaesthetic. Gordon's silver staining.

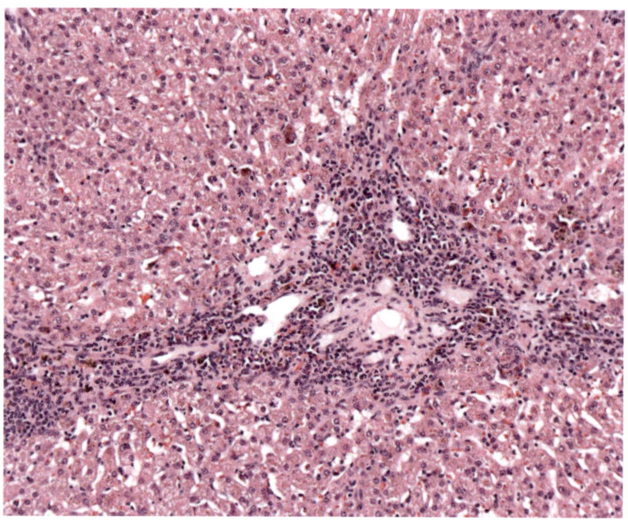

**FIGURE 3-13.** Fibrosis/inflammation, centrilobular, liver, in a dog treated with an industrial chemical. Note loss of hepatocytes and presence of pigmented macrophages, centrilobular. H&E.

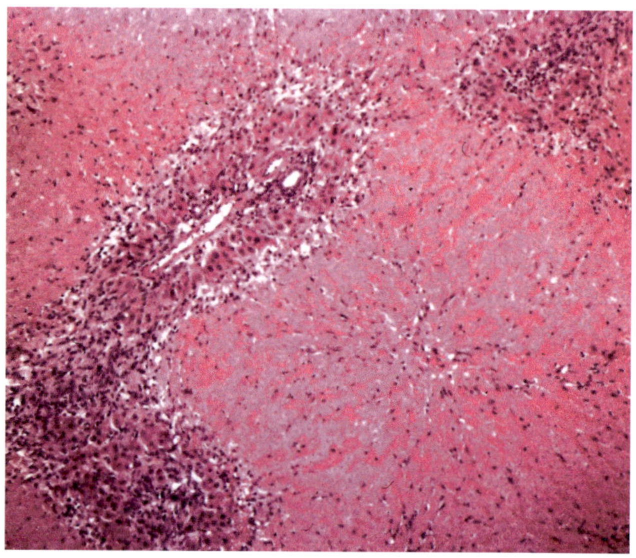

**FIGURE 3-14.** Necrosis, panlobular (diffuse), liver, in a rat. Only a few periportal hepatocytes have survived. H&E.

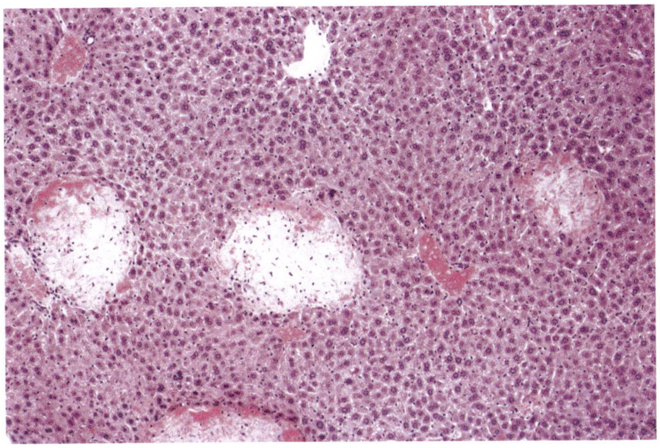

**FIGURE 3-15.** Necrosis, multifocal, liver, in a rat. Foci of necrotic hepatocytes irregularly distributed within the parenchyma. H&E.

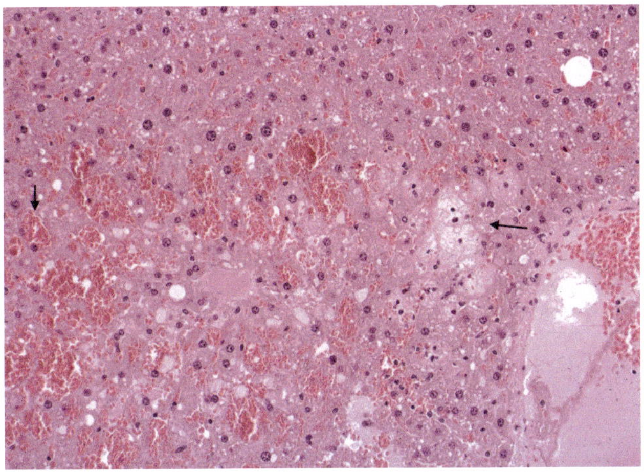

**FIGURE 3-16.** Hepatocellular necrosis, atypical, in a mouse. Degenerating and necrotic hepatocytes appear swollen (*arrows*), pale eosinophilic with loss of structural details, some hepatocytes with intracytoplasmic erythrocytes. H&E.

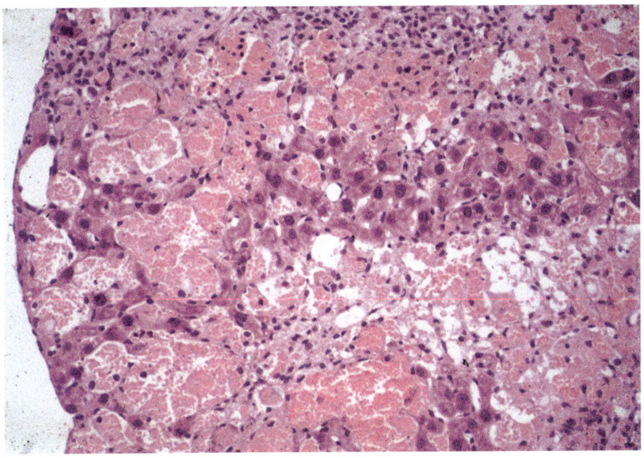

**FIGURE 3-17.** Hepatocellular necrosis, atypical, in a mouse. Distended sinusoidal spaces with blood with hepatocyte loss are present. H&E.

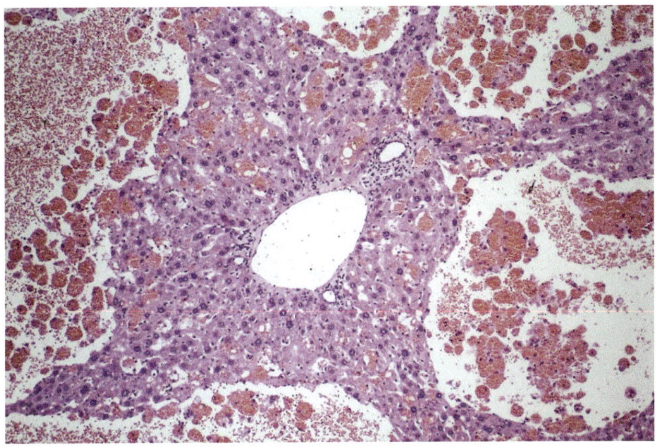

**FIGURE 3-18.** Hepatocellular necrosis, atypical, in a mouse. Large vascular spaces replace lost hepatocytes containing blood, giving a punched-out appearance. H&E.

## 3.5 Apoptosis

Apoptosis occurs in the liver as in other organs and is a process of cell deletion following growth/regression and regulatory response balancing the cell population. This can be seen in the liver where retardation of growth by some cytotoxic agents or radiation is induced. Apoptosis is also seen during regression of hyperplasia induced by promoting agents in rodents on withdrawal of the dosing. Administration of cyproterone acetate to rats causes hepatic enlargement. Withdrawal of dosing results in loss of liver weight accompanied by abundant apoptosis [21]. Ischaemic hepatic injury caused by portal venous ligation also results in apoptosis [22]. The apoptotic cell assumes a spherical/ovoid shape and stains eosinophilically, revealing specks of pyknotic nuclear fragments (Fig. 3.19). Bodies often appear intracytoplasmic. The apoptotic cells reveal membrane-bound cell fragments and intact organelles, and the nucleus shows fragmentation. Apoptosis can be confirmed by special staining such as the TUNEL (terminal deoxynucleotidyl transferase dUTP [deoxyuridine triphosphate] nick end labelling) method.

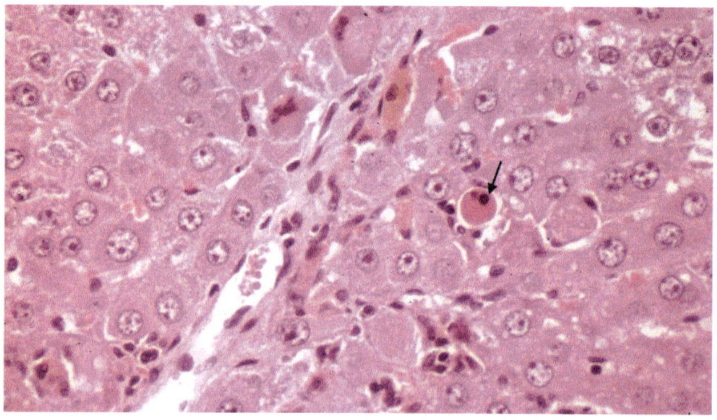

**Figure 3-19.** Apoptosis, liver, in a rat. Note shrunken, spheroidal eosinophilic cells with nuclear fragments *(arrow)*. H&E.

## 3.6 Nuclear Changes

With loss of hepatocytes, as in the case of DMN toxicity, the remaining parenchyma shows increased mitotic figures, probably representing a regenerative response. Pyridine derivatives cause increased mitotic activity without necrosis. Sudden anoxia produces a transient increase in mitotic activity in the rodent liver (personal observation). Isolated mitotic figures are normal in the liver. When they occur more frequently than normal in microscopic fields (two or more), they should be recorded (Fig. 3.20).

Aflatoxin and pyrrolizidine alkaloids cause karyomegaly and cytomegaly of the hepatocytes (Fig. 3.21). Hepatocytes with multiple nuclei are induced by dioxin and some other chemicals [18, 23]. Multinucleated cells occur by fusion rather than by cell division (Fig. 3.22) [24]. Intranuclear crystalline deposits (eosinophilic) are seen in lead toxicity.

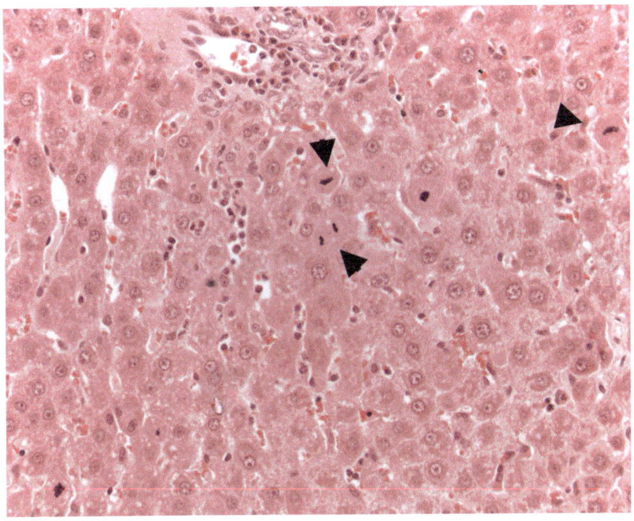

**Figure 3-20.** Increased mitotic figures (*arrowheads*), hepatocytes, in a rat. H&E.

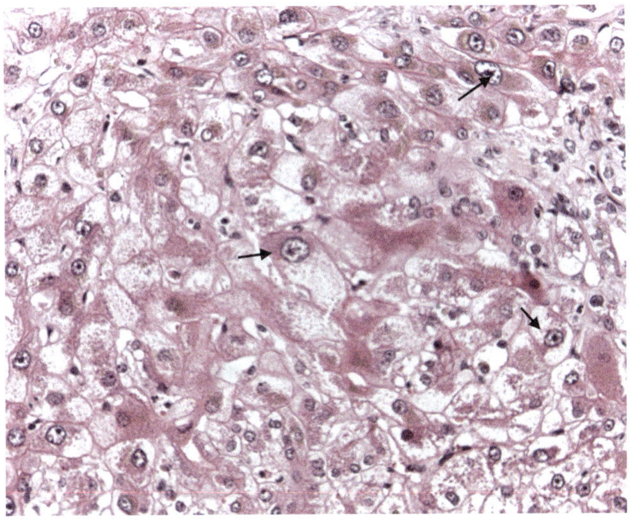

**Figure 3-21.** Cytomegaly and karyomegaly (*arrows*), liver, in a horse suffering from ragwort poisoning. H&E.

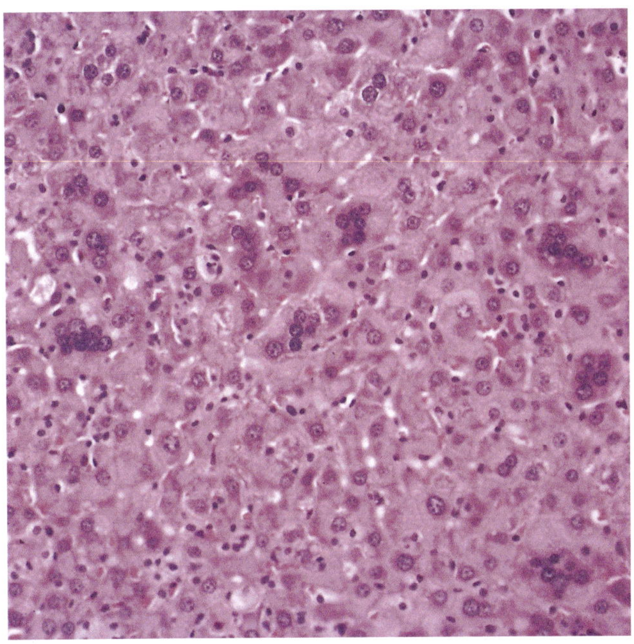

**Figure 3-22.** Multinucleated hepatocytes, in a rat treated with a novel pharmaceutical agent. H&E (With kind permission from Springer Science + Business Media B.V [49]).

## 3.7 Intracytoplasmic Inclusions

Intracytoplasmic inclusions are frequently seen in subacute or chronic studies. They appear as eosinophilic inclusions, sometimes membrane bound (secondary lysosomes), and occur in dogs and rodents (Fig. 3.23). On occasions the inclusions stain positive with periodic acid–Schiff (PAS) and are diastase resistant. They occur in different locations and may be periportal, centrilobular, or scattered irregularly within the lobules. On rare occasions they are more basophilic. Treatment with certain agrochemicals that induce proliferation of endoplasmic reticulum sometimes results in inclusion bodies with a concentric whorling pattern (Fig. 3.24). On electron microscopy these were found to be whorls of proliferating endoplasmic reticulum. Intracytoplasmic inclusions can occur in neoplastic hepatocytes within hepatocellular adenomas, in some rodent studies. In mice eosinophilic inclusions noted within the hepatocellular nuclei were found to be cytoplasmic invaginations. Accumulation of cytokeratin is reported in hepatocyte cytoplasm in rats treated with certain antifungal agents [25].

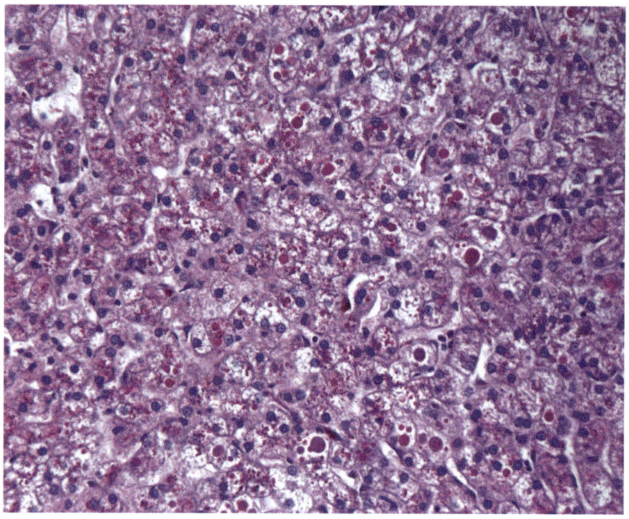

**Figure 3-23.** Intracytoplasmic eosinophilic inclusions, hepatocytes, and Kupffer cells, in a rat. H&E.

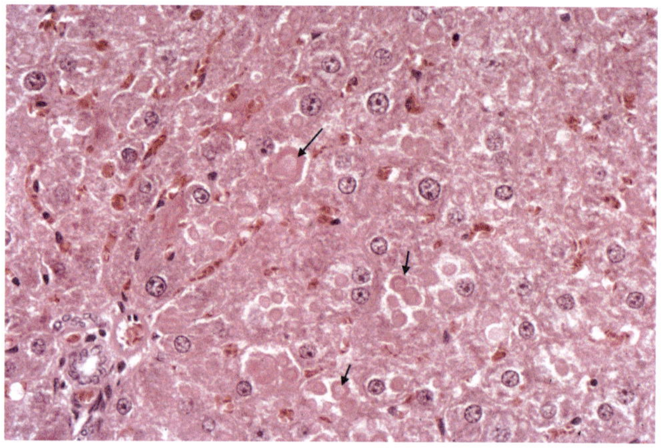

**Figure 3-24.** Intracytoplasmic inclusions, whorl pattern (*arrows*), hepatocytes, in a rat treated with an agrochemical agent. H&E.

## 3.8 Pigments

Endogenous and exogenous pigments occur in the liver. In cholestatic or obstructive jaundice, bile pigment occurs in the canaliculi as plugs, both in dogs and in rodents. Porphyria (compound induced) in dogs shows biliary plugs and porphyrin deposits in hepatocytes and Kupffer cells (Fig. 3.25). Haemosiderin pigmentation appears in liver cells and in Kupffer cells in haemolytic episodes. Lipofuscin pigments usually occur centrilobularly in hepatocytes in pericanalicular locations (Fig. 3.26). Administration of iron-containing compounds also reveals iron-positive pigments. Certain agrochemicals have induced iron pigmentation in hepatocytes and Kupffer cells in rat livers (Fig. 3.27).

Exogenous pigments of varying colours are seen in the livers of animals treated with various agents that are either pigmented themselves or have metabolites that are pigmented. Vincamine alkaloids and certain antimalarial drugs cause pigmentation in the liver (Fig. 3.28).

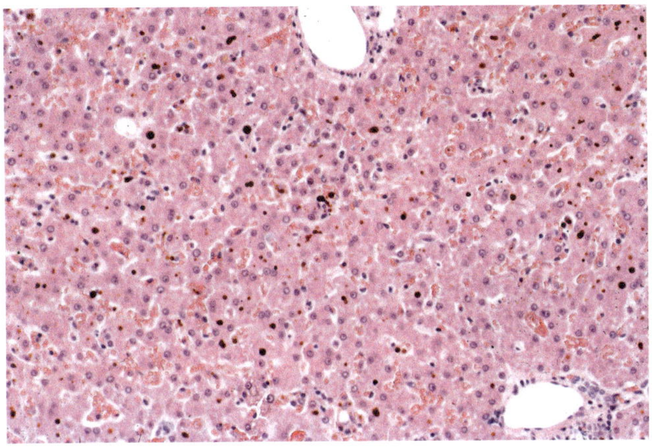

**FIGURE 3-25.** Porphyrin pigment in hepatocytes, canaliculi, and Kupffer cells, in a dog treated with an antifungal agent. H&E.

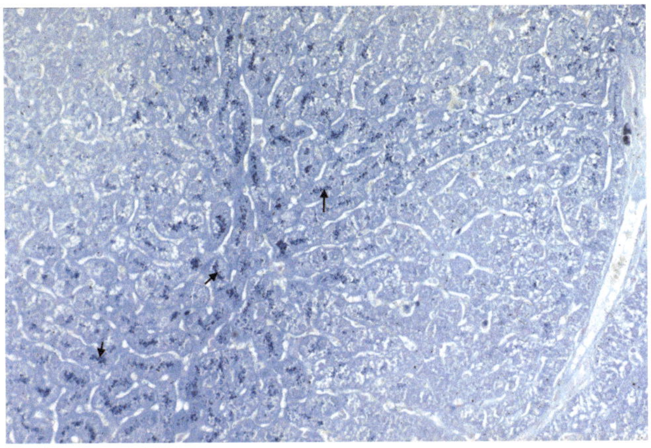

**FIGURE 3-26.** Lipofuscin deposition, hepatocytes, in a rat. Note intracytoplasmic and pericanalicular (*arrows*) deposits. Schmorl's stain.

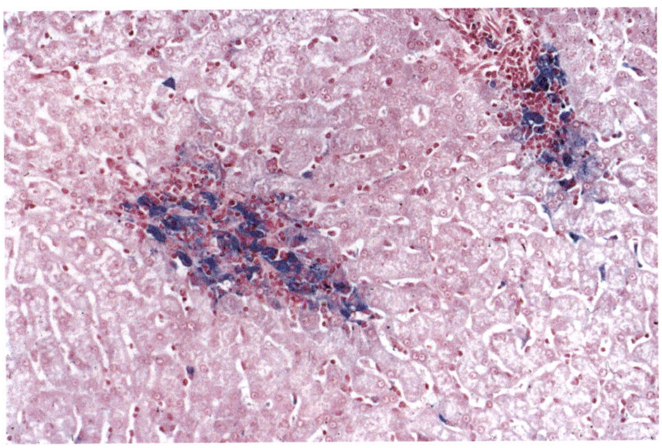

**FIGURE 3-27.** Iron pigment in macrophages and hepatocytes, centrilobular, in a rat treated with an industrial chemical. Perl's stain.

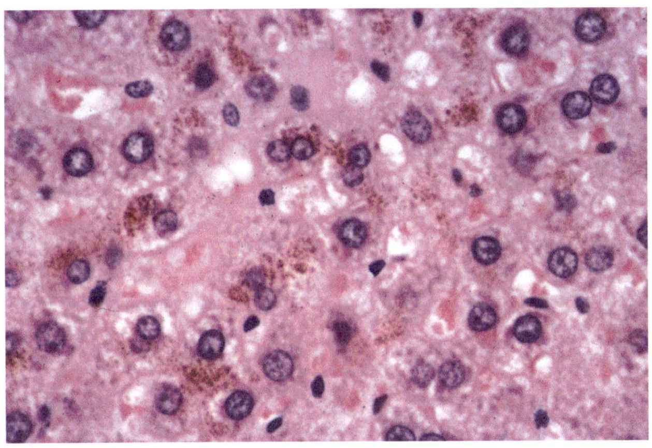

**FIGURE 3-28.** Brown granular pigment, hepatocytes, in a rat treated with a vincamine alkaloid. H&E.

A rare bluish pigment in Kupffer cells was noted in rats treated with an antimalarial agent (Fig. 3.29). Administration of substances containing carotenoid pigments causes deep orange discoloration of the livers. On haematoxylin and eosin (H&E) staining, the pigments are not observed because they are lipid soluble and dissolve out during processing, but they can be seen in frozen sections as brownish pigment (Fig. 3.30). In overspill situations exogenous pigments occur in perivascular macrophages in portal areas and around the central vein (Fig. 3.31). Copper toxicity results in Cu-containing pigments in liver cells and Kupffer cells, along with pigments derived from the blood [26, 27]. Dark brown pigment was seen in bile ducts and in Kupffer cells in rats treated with an industrial chemical (Fig. 3.32)

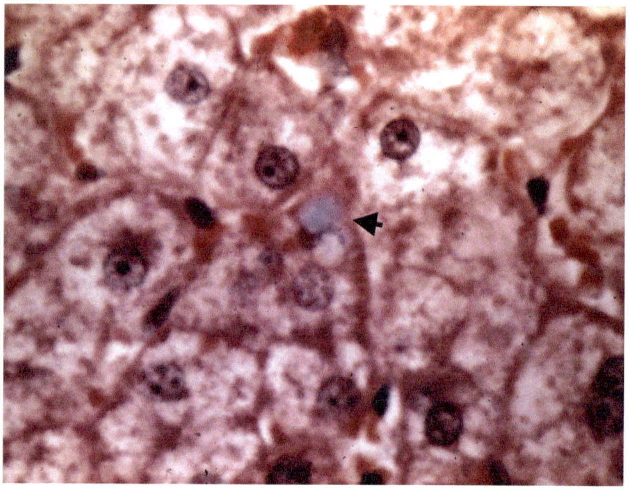

**Figure 3-29.** Blue pigment, Kupffer cells (*arrowhead*), in a rat treated with an antimalarial agent. H&E.

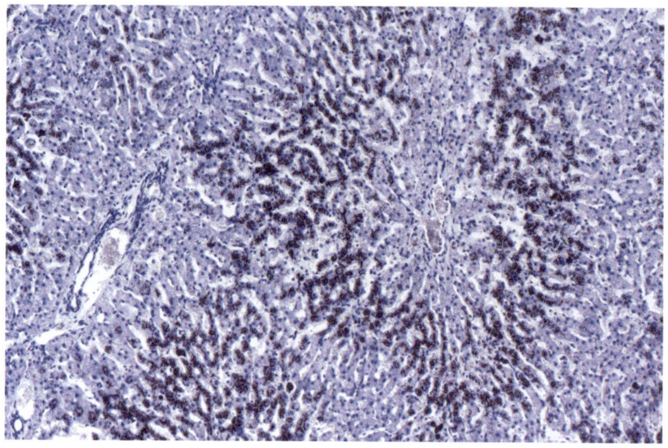

**Figure 3-30.** Brown pigment in hepatocytes, in a rat treated with a carotenoid pigment. Frozen section. Haematoxylin.

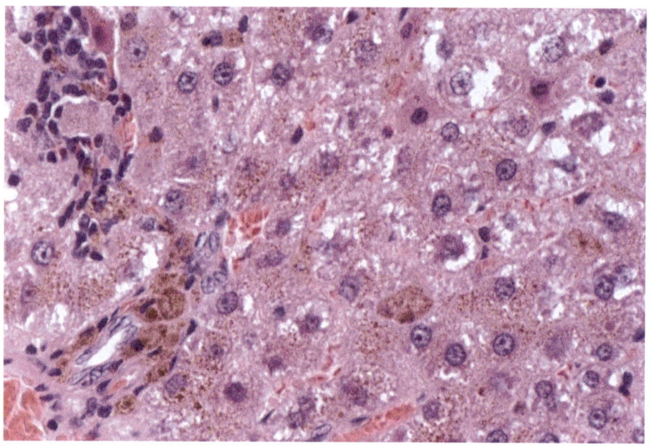

**Figure 3-31.** Brown pigment, hepatocytes, Kupffer cells, and macrophages, in a dog treated with a herbicide. H&E.

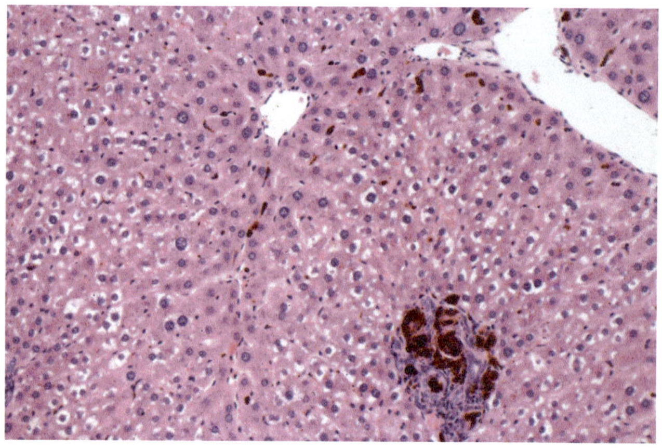

**Figure 3-32.** Dark brown pigment in Kupffer cells and in bile ducts, in a rat. H&E.

## 3.9 Mineralisation

Mineralisation is an infrequent lesion in the liver. Rarely, postnecrotic dystrophic mineralisation can be seen with a focal distribution.

## 3.10 Hepatocellular Hypertrophy

Centrilobular hepatocyte hypertrophy is a common adaptive response of the liver to a number of xenobiotics including many pharmaceuticals, agrochemicals, and others (Fig. 3.33). This is a cellular response to overload of test substance. The cell responds by proliferation of smooth endoplasmic reticulum and drug-metabolising enzyme induction (family of cytochrome P450 enzymes). Centrilobular cells are hypertrophied with a pale granular appearance. The change is accompanied by an increase in liver weight. Phenobarbitone sodium is one of the agents that produces centrilobular hypertrophy in rodent livers [28]. The change is reversible on withdrawal of the treatment [29].

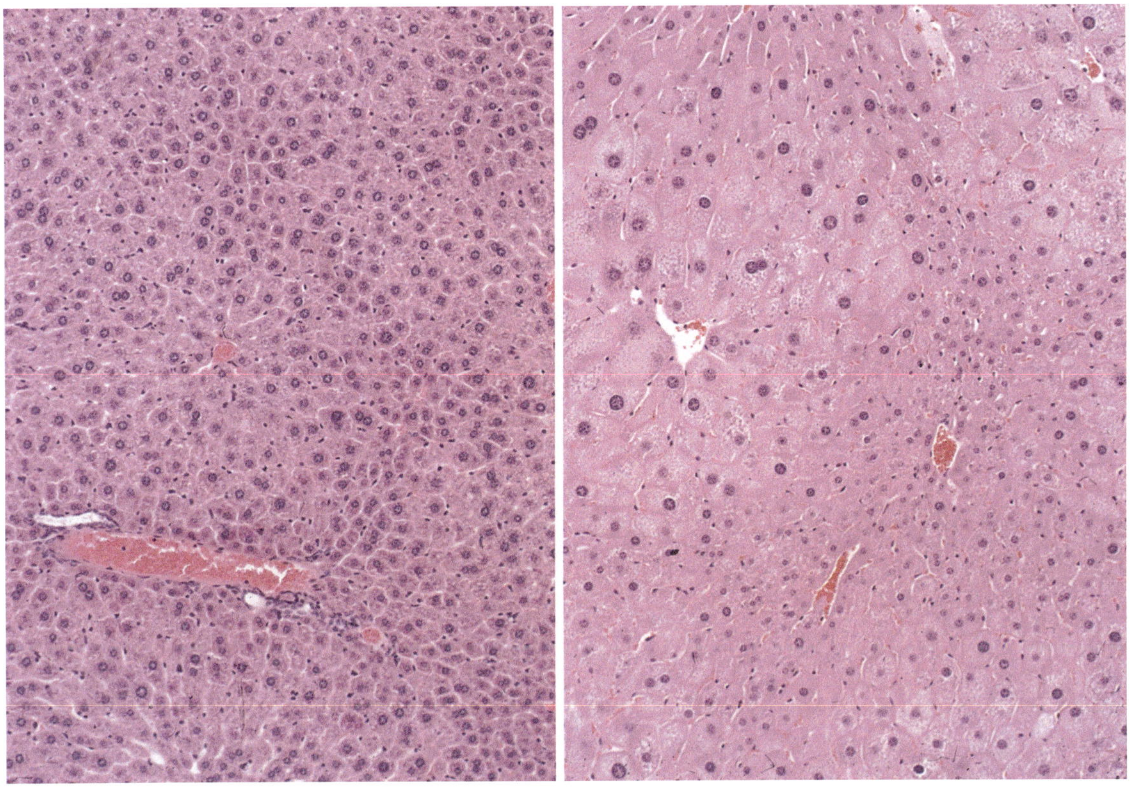

**Figure 3-33.** Hepatocellular hypertrophy, centrilobular, in mouse treated with a xenobiotic. The picture on the left is normal for comparison. H&E.

Hypolipidaemic agents like clofibrate induce hepatocellular hypertrophy owing to peroxisome proliferation. Affected cells appear more eosinophilic with granular cytoplasm (Fig. 3.34). The hypertrophy can be centrilobular, but it can involve other zones and sometime occurs diffusely. Panzonal diffuse hypertrophy is more difficult to recognise (Figs. 3.35 and 3.36). Peroxisome proliferation can be confirmed by electron microscopy or by immunohistochemical methods such as catalase staining (Fig. 3.37) [30]. The associated liver weight increase is much more pronounced than that associated with agents producing smooth

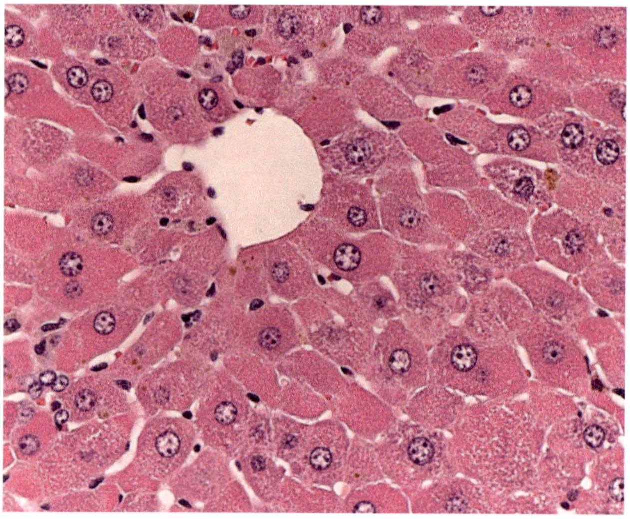

**Figure 3-34.** Hepatocellular hypertrophy and increased eosinophilia (granular), centrilobular, in a rat treated with a peroxisome proliferator-activated receptor (PPAR) agonist. H&E.

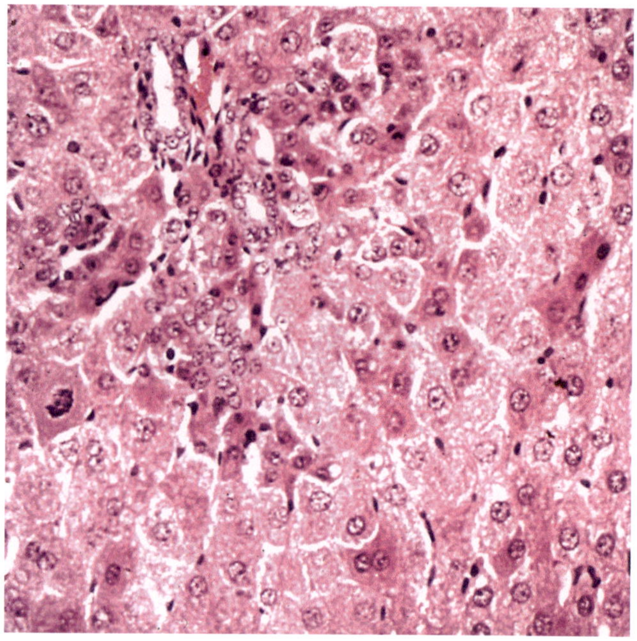

**Figure 3-35.** Hepatocellular hypertrophy, panlobular (diffuse), in a rat treated with an agrochemical agent. Note minimal increase in bile ducts in portal areas. H&E (With kind permission from Springer Science + Business Media B.V [49]).

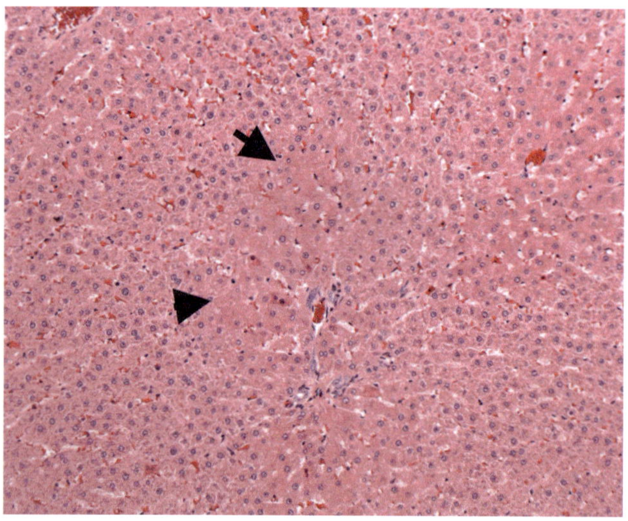

**Figure 3-36.** Hepatocellular hypertrophy, periportal (*arrowheads*), in a rat treated with an industrial chemical. H&E.

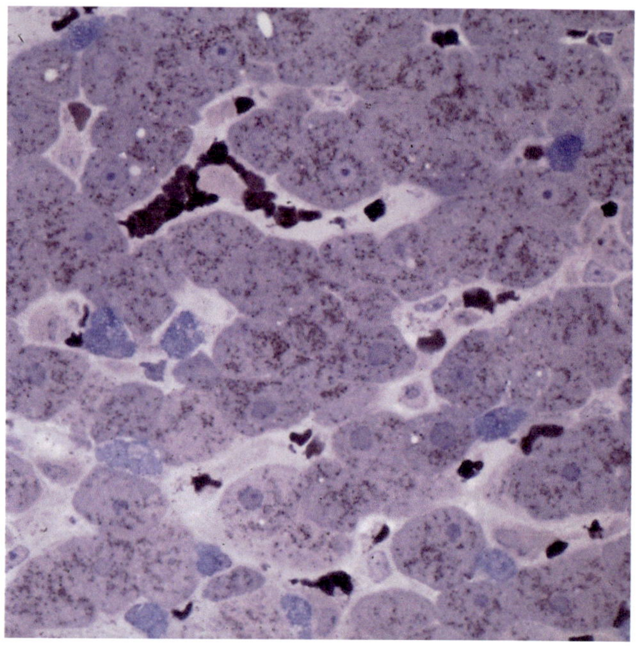

**Figure 3-37.** Catalase-positive granules in hepatocytes, in a rat treated with a hypolipidaemic agent. Enzyme histochemistry.

endoplasmic reticulum (SER) proliferation (Fig. 3.38). In hepatic enlargement induced by agents causing peroxisome proliferation, if treatment is prolonged, brownish pigment in Kupffer cells is an accompanying change.

With hypertrophy caused by SER or peroxisome proliferation, if treated for long periods, the liver undergoes proliferation and develops hepatocellular tumours in rodents. Agents inducing mitochondrial proliferation can also give rise to hypertrophy and increased liver weight. Increases in liver weight in short-term toxicity studies are a useful indicator of hypertrophy, which may progress to hyperplasia and even neoplasia in long-term rodent studies [2, 31].

Hepatic enlargement can be due to hepatocellular hypertrophy, hyperplasia, tumours, fatty change, and storage of substances like glycogen. Excessive glycogen in the liver cell causes fine vacuolation with irregular borders, giving a rarefied appearance to the cytoplasm (Fig. 3.39). The presence can be confirmed by staining for glycogen. Extensive glycogen accumulation as seen with steroid treatment causes affected hepatocytes to become distended with clear cytoplasm. Treatment with certain antibiotics results in formation of glycogen lakes within the cell cytoplasm, pushing the rest of the organelles to one side (Fig. 3.40).

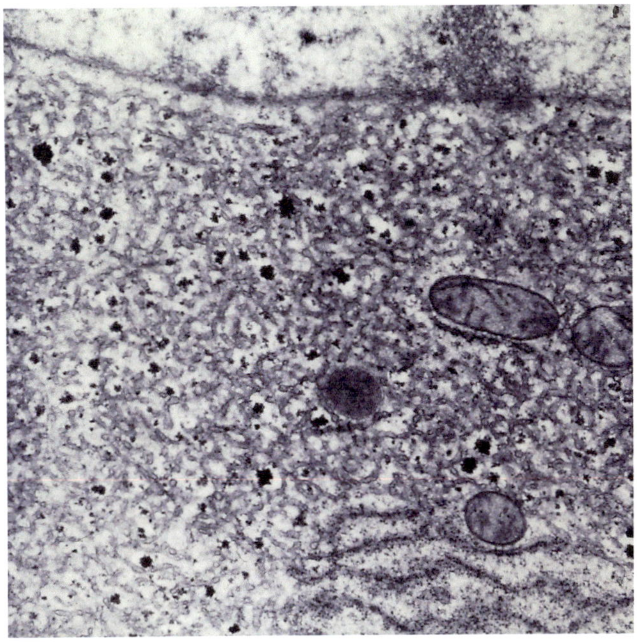

**Figure 3-38.** SER proliferation, hepatocyte, in a rat treated with phenobarbitone sodium. Electron micrograph.

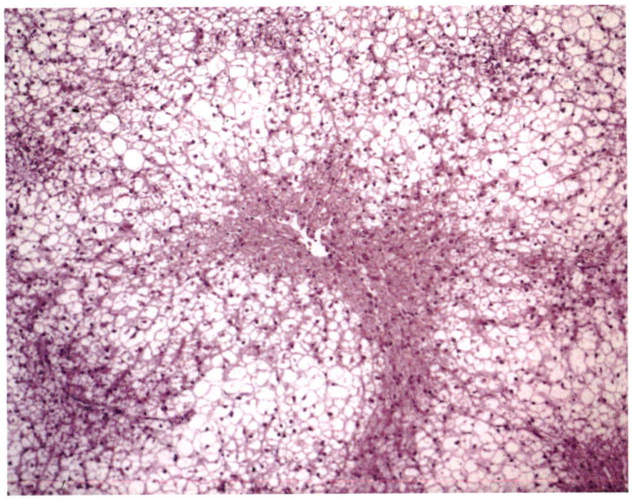

**Figure 3-39.** Cytoplasmic rarefaction, hepatocytes mainly periportal, in a dog treated with a glucocorticoid. H&E.

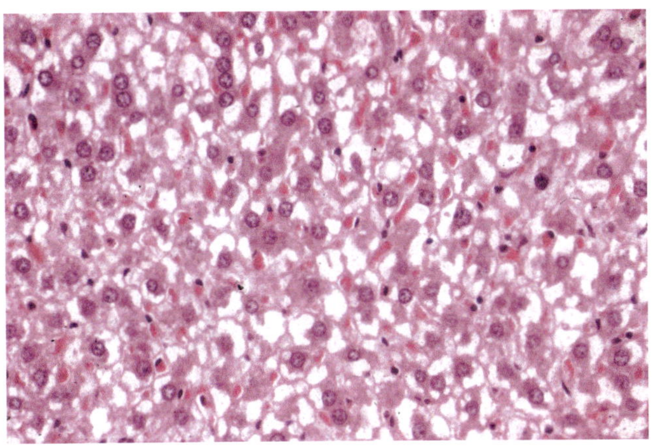

**Figure 3-40.** Hepatocyte with cytoplasmic clumping and glycogen lakes, in a rat treated with an antibiotic. H&E.

## 3.11 Hyperplasia

Hyperplasia can affect hepatocytes, bile ducts, and endothelial cells. Hepatocellular hyperplasia is well described [32]. Hepatocellular hyperplasia can be simple, zonal, regenerative, or diffuse nodular.

Simple hyperplasia often goes unnoticed by the pathologists because it is difficult to recognise morphologically. This often follows hepatocyte hypertrophy induced by promoting agents like phenobarbitone or clofibrate. On DNA analysis or by employing techniques to reveal cells in phases of cell division, such as bromodeoxyuridine (BrdU) or proliferating cell nuclear antigen (PCNA) staining, the presence of silent hyperplasia may be demonstrated. Continued exposures by promoting agents for long periods result in neoplasia in rodent livers.

Zonal hyperplasia is a rare phenomenon in which cells of specific zones of the hepatic lobule undergo hyperplasia. Certain synthetic sex steroids can induce zonal hyperplasia in rat liver. Affected cells appear more basophilic, with vesicular nuclei and the presence of increased mitotic figures (Fig. 3.41).

### 3.11.1 Regenerative Hyperplasia

Repeated and persistent hepatic injury with loss of hepatocytes results in compensatory hyperplasia in the adjacent parenchyma. Hyperplasia coexists with necrosis, fibrosis, or inflammation. Hyperplastic hepatocytes are more basophilic with vesicular/open nuclei, and they appear as islands or nodules often surrounded by fibrosis (Fig. 3.42).

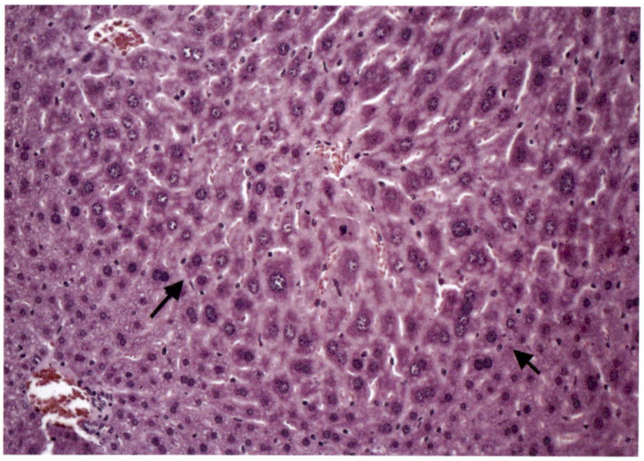

**Figure 3-41.** Hepatocyte hyperplasia, centrilobular, in a rat treated with a steroid. Note hypertrophy, increased basophilia (*arrows*), and increase in mitotic figures. H&E.

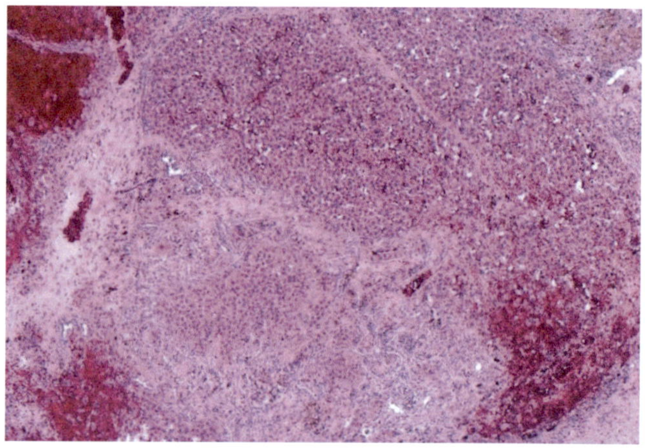

**Figure 3-42.** Hepatocellular hyperplasia, regenerative, in a rat treated with a novel pharmaceutical agent. Note areas of necrosis, fibrosis, inflammation, and haemorrhage adjacent to islands/nodules of small basophilic hepatocytes. H&E.

### 3.11.2 Diffuse Nodular Hyperplasia

The change appears in chronic studies and the affected liver has an irregular/nodular surface. The change occurs as a result of persistent hepatocellular injury and represents compensatory hyperplasia on overdrive. Choline-deficient diets in rodents cause extensive lipidosis with ongoing loss of hepatocytes, and in later stages there is multifocal regenerative hyperplasia involving large areas of the liver. Hyperplastic areas appear as islands or nodules of smaller-sized hepatocytes replacing the lobular pattern of normal liver. There is also internodular fibrosis and inflammatory cell infiltration (Fig. 3.43). The nodules vary in size but are mostly smaller than a lobule. Bile salts and other agents given for a long period result in diffuse nodular hyperplasia in rats [18].

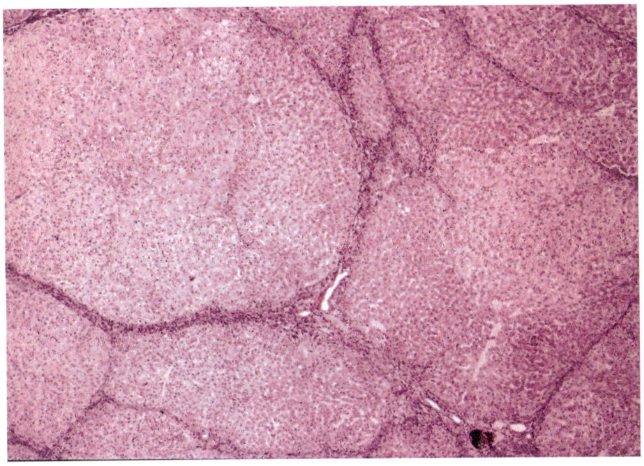

**FIGURE 3-43.** Nodular hyperplasia, diffuse, liver, in a rat treated with bile salt. Different-sized islands of hepatocytes, each surrounded by fibrosis/inflammation. H&E.

## 3.12 Foci of Cellular Alteration

Groups of hepatocytes revealing different cytoplasmic staining affinities when compared with the surrounding normal parenchyma are referred to as foci of cellular alteration. These changes are mainly described in rodent livers either in older animals as spontaneous change or in rodents from chronic studies [7, 33]. Foci of cellular alterations are induced by potent genotoxic carcinogens like aflatoxin, diethylnitrosamine (DEN), or nitrosomorpholine [34–36].

A large number of nongenotoxic agents, such as promoting agents like phenobarbitone sodium or peroxisome proliferators like clofibrate on long-term exposure, produce increased incidences of altered foci. The foci appear with different phenotypic expressions, such as eosinophilic, basophilic, clear cell, amphophilic, or mixed cell foci (Figs. 3.44–3.47). A number of histochemical markers are used to characterise these foci, and they reveal a variety of different affinities among them.

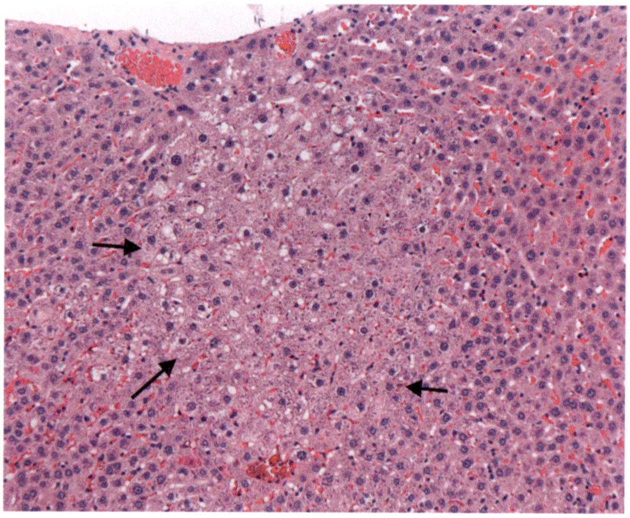

**Figure 3-44.** Altered hepatocytes, eosinophilic, focus (*arrows*), in a rat. H&E.

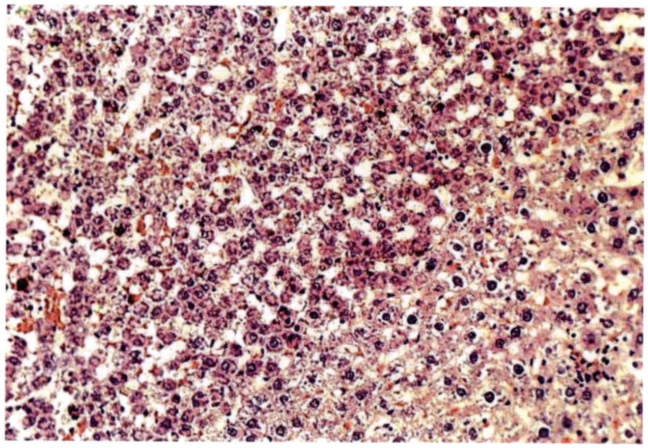

**Figure 3-45.** Altered hepatocytes, basophilic, focus, in a rat. H&E.

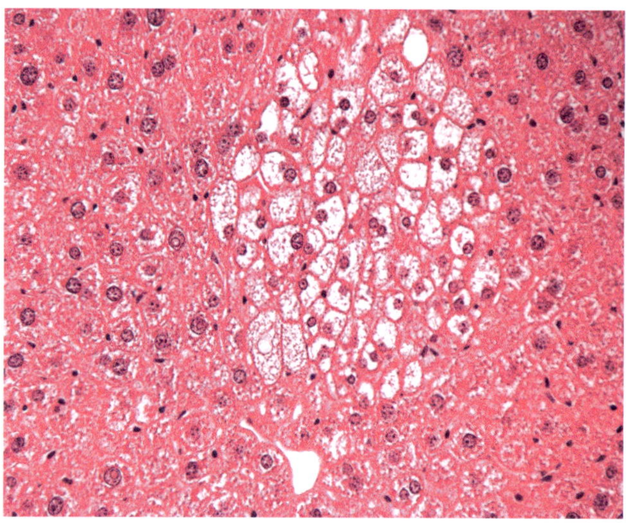

**Figure 3-46.** Altered hepatocytes, clear cells, focus, in a rat. H&E.

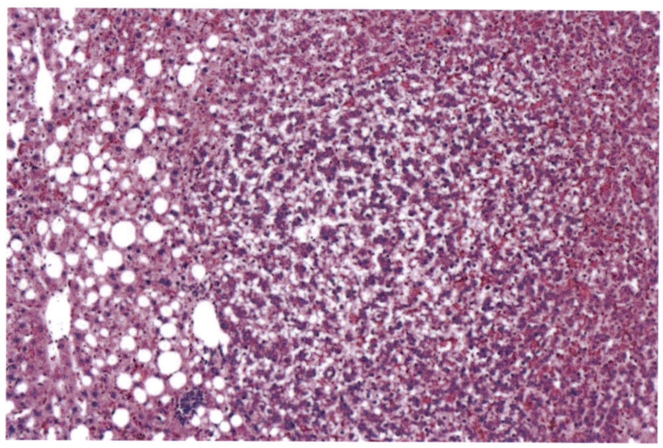

**Figure 3-47.** Altered hepatocytes, mixed cells, focus, in a rat. Mixture of basophilic, eosinophilic, and clear cells. H&E.

γ-Glutamyl-transferase (GGT), glucose-6-phosphate dehydrogenase, glutamate-S-transferase, PAS, and iron storage are among the methods used (Figs. 3.48 and 3.49). The foci reveal a higher proliferative index. In experimental carcinogenesis schemes, the foci are considered as putative preneoplastic lesions [36]. Aflatoxin exposure produces basophilic foci, and nitrosomorpholine produces eosinophilic or clear cell foci as early indicators.

Altered foci appear as spontaneous lesions in old rodents, albeit at a low incidence rate. In female F344 rats incidence of basophilic (tigroid) foci are relatively high with no increase in hepatocellular tumours, suggesting that they are not preneoplastic. Several nongenotoxic xenobiotics are capable of inducing altered foci in the liver. In this context they cannot be termed as putative preneoplastic, as only negligible numbers (<2 %) end up as tumours. In many instances, 2-year bioassays only show increases in altered foci with no progression to neoplasia (personal observation). During the recording of altered foci, they need to be graded on severity depending on the number and size of the foci. During analysis different types of foci are analysed separately [37].

Another condition seen in rat livers in long-term studies is the presence of foci of cystic degeneration (spongiosis hepatis). A group of ballooned cells appear with pale pink cytoplasm and flattened peripheral nuclei. These foci are of Ito cell origin and some xenobiotics cause increased incidences of this age-related lesion [38, 39].

Perivascular and hepatic sinusoidal leucocytosis was seen in monkeys and dogs treated with certain biotechnical products (Fig. 3.50). Multifocal granulomas were induced in mice livers treated with a biological agent (Fig. 3.51).

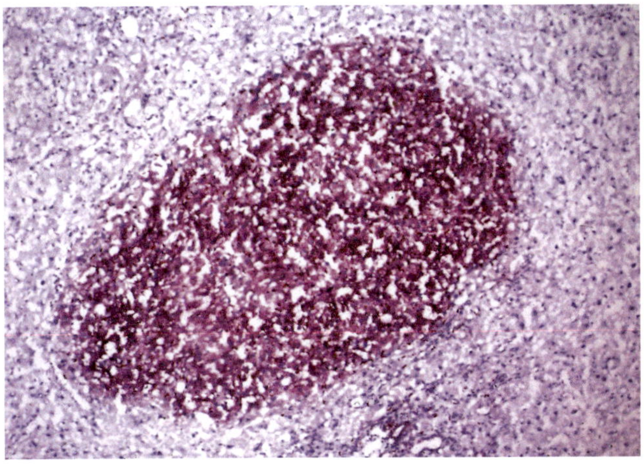

**Figure 3-48.** Altered hepatocytes, γ-glutamyl-transferase, focus, in a rat. Enzyme histochemistry.

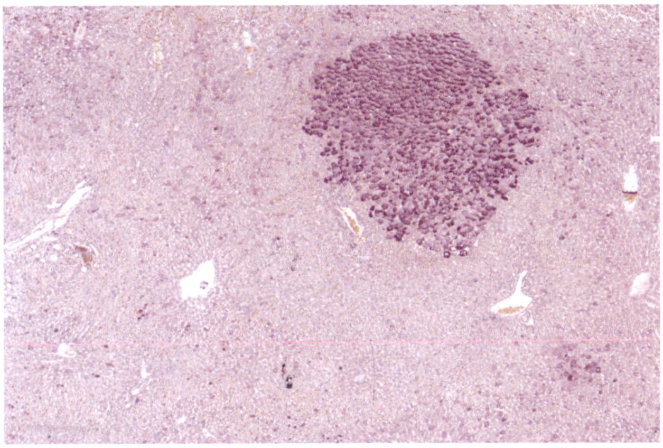

**Figure 3-49.** Altered hepatocytes, focus, in a rat, PAS-positive, diastase-resistant focus of hepatocytes embedded within a glycogen-depleted parenchyma. PAS.

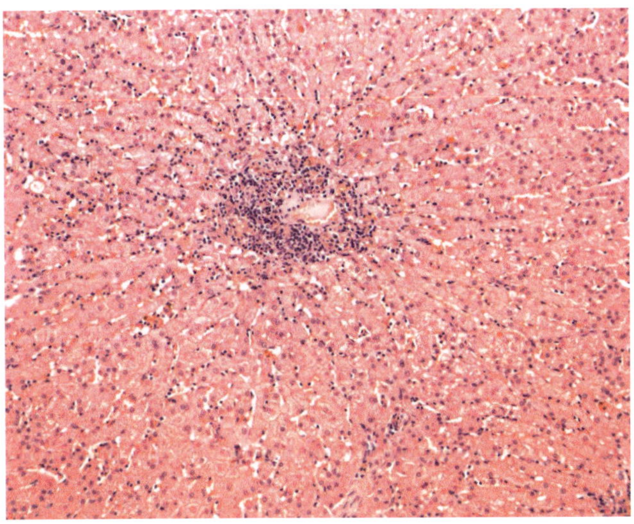

**Figure 3-50.** Leucocytosis, sinusoidal and centrilobular, liver, in a dog treated with a novel biotechnical product. H&E.

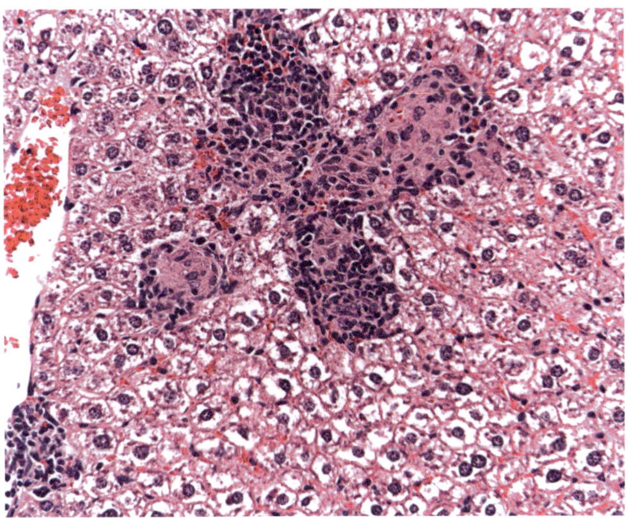

**Figure 3-51.** Granulomas, liver, in a mouse treated with a biological agent. Multiple granulomas are mainly composed of histiocytes within liver parenchyma. H&E.

## 3.13 Bile Duct Hyperplasia

In rodents this is a common response to biliary irritation/injury induced by toxicants or their metabolites excreted through the bile (Figs. 3.52 and 3.53). The initial response is damage to biliary epithelium and inflammation (cholangitis), soon followed by proliferation of bile ducts (Fig. 3.54). In some instances portal areas reveal extensive inflammation, fibroblastic proliferation, and bile duct hyperplasia (Figs. 3.55 and 3.56). The bile ductular proliferation sometimes extends into the parenchyma and is occasionally accompanied by oval cell proliferation. Cholangitis can progress into peribiliary fibrosis. In rodents bile duct hyperplasia sometimes develops into cystic hyperplasia in which the ducts are dilated/cystic and lined by flattened epithelium. In F344 rats, bile duct hyperplasia is a spontaneous change in older rats.

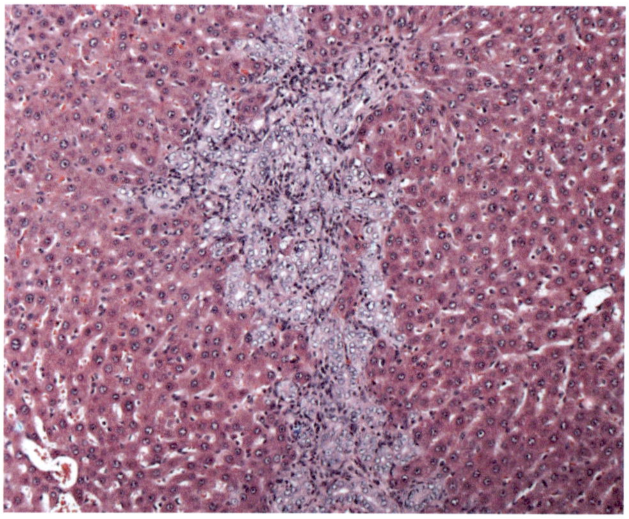

**Figure 3-52.** Bile duct hyperplasia, in a rat. Note increase in numbers of bile ductules and inflammatory cells, portal area. H&E.

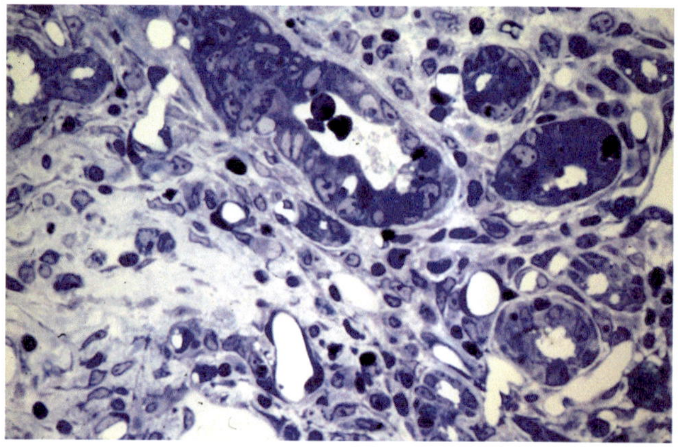

**Figure 3-53.** Bile duct hyperplasia, in a rat. Increased numbers of bile ductules are lined by hypertrophic epithelium, with vesicular nuclei and reduced lumens. Resin section, toluene blue.

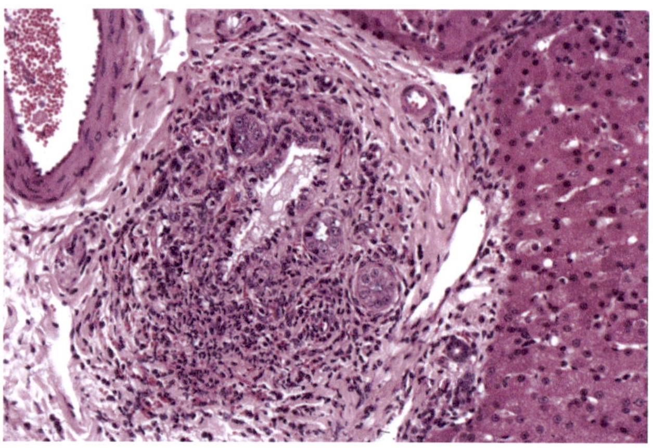

**Figure 3-54.** Cholangitis, liver, in a dog treated with an antihypertensive agent. Note necrosis of epithelium, inflammation of the wall, and periductular connective tissue. H&E.

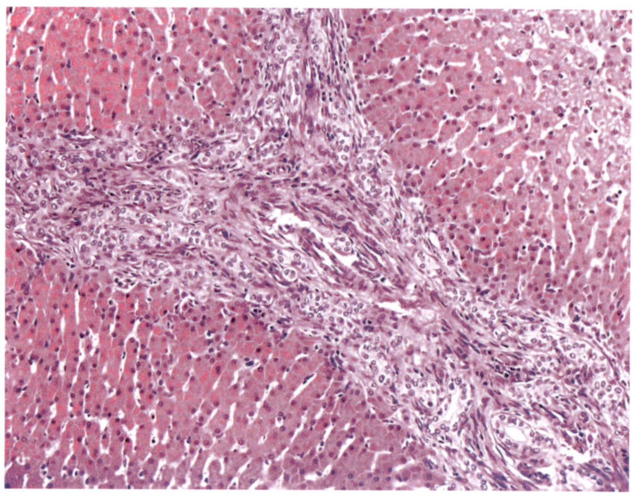

**Figure 3-55.** Bile duct hyperplasia, inflammation, and fibrosis, liver, in a dog treated with a xenobiotic. Increased number of bile ductules, interlobular fibrosis with inflammation. H&E.

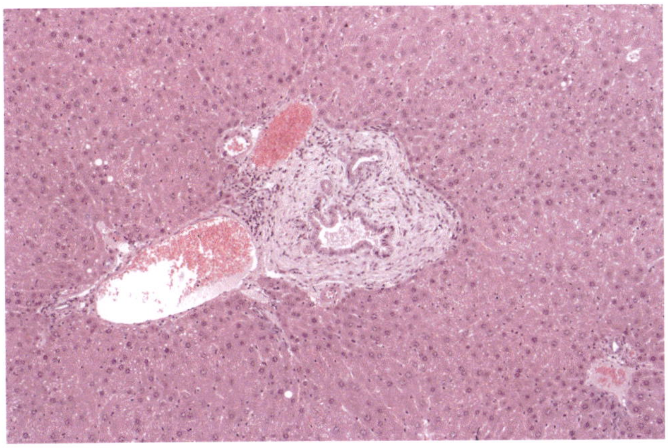

**FIGURE 3-56.** Periductular fibrosis, liver, in a rat. H&E.

## 3.14 Oval Cell Proliferation

Oval cell proliferation is a distinct lesion in which undifferentiated basophilic cells with scanty cytoplasm and elongated/ovoid nuclei appear in and around portal areas and within lobules (Fig. 3.57). They tend to form into ducts, suggesting that they are precursors of bile ducts. The cells are primitive and pluripotential, capable of differentiating into bile ducts and hepatocytes. They are easily induced by genotoxic agents like 2-acetylaminofluorene (2-AAF), DEN, and aflatoxin [40]. Oval cell proliferation can extend into the parenchyma.

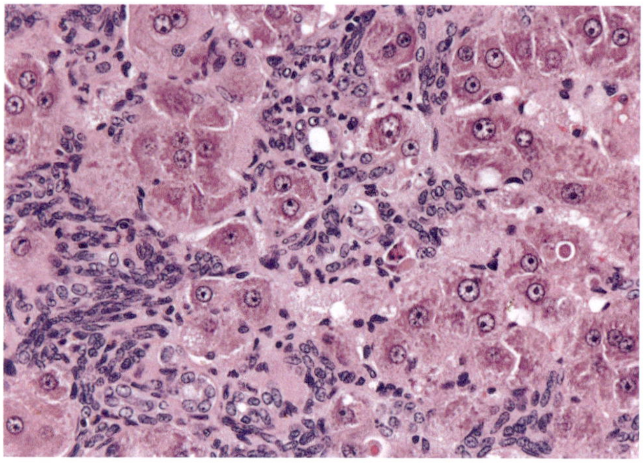

**Figure 3-57.** Oval cell proliferation, liver, in a rat. Note intralobular and portal proliferation of undifferentiated basophilic cells with scanty cytoplasm and ovoid elongated nuclei. Occasional bile ductular differentiation and single cell necrosis are seen. H&E.

## 3.15 Cholangiofibrosis

Cholangiofibrosis is an interesting lesion seen in rats treated with certain genotoxic and nongenotoxic agents like 2-AAF, dimethylaminoazobenzene (DAB), and coumarin [18]. The change is characterised by proliferation of atypical bile ducts showing intestinal metaplasia of epithelium, excessive mucus production, and distension of the ducts. There is interstitial fibrosis and inflammation and considerable extension of portal areas. In severe cases large areas of the parenchyma are displaced by cholangiofibrosis (Figs. 3.58 and 3.59). The lesion can progress into cholangiocarcinoma with features of cholangiofibrosis. The changes are only described in rats.

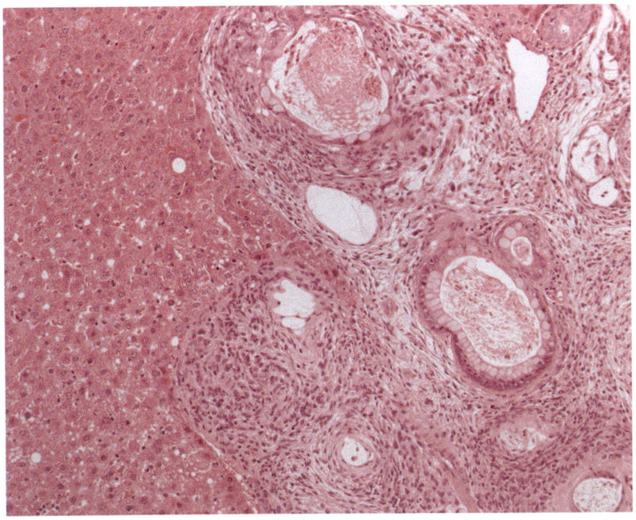

**FIGURE 3-58.** Cholangiofibrosis, liver, in a rat. Distended bile ducts are lined by columnar epithelium and goblet cells and contain mucus. Periductular fibrosis and inflammation causing expansion into the parenchyma. H&E.

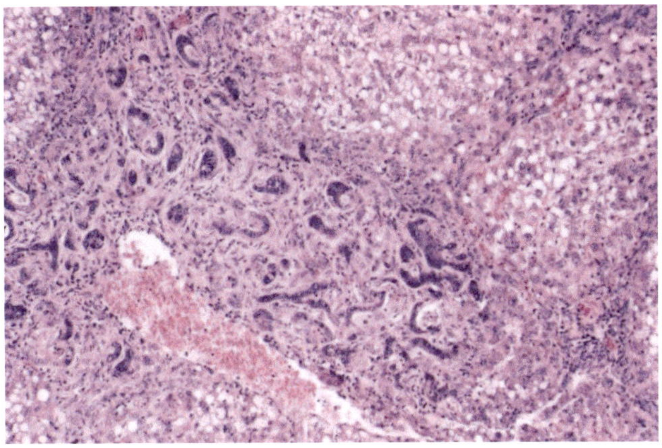

**FIGURE 3-59.** Cholangiofibrosis, liver, in a rat treated with 2-acetylaminofluorene (2-AAF). Note proliferation of atypical bile ductules lined by columnar epithelium and goblet cells (intestinal metaplasia), interstitial fibrosis, and inflammation. The lesion extends interlobularly. H&E.

## 3.16 ItoCell Prominence or Hyperplasia

Increased numbers of Ito cells occur scattered in the parenchyma in dogs treated with carotenoid pigments. Prominent Ito cells appear in the sinusoidal lining with vacuolated/clear cytoplasm (Fig. 3.60).

Increased incidence of serous glandular metaplasia of bile ducts is seen in mice treated with certain xenobiotics (Fig. 3.61).

Treatment with an industrial chemical in mice has produced increased numbers of prominent sinusoidal lining cells with hyperchromatic nuclei (Fig. 3.62). Focal sinusoidal dilation, usually located subcapsularly, is seen in rats treated with steroids (Fig. 3.63). Marked dilation along with atrophy of hepatic cords results in peliosis hepatis (Fig. 3.64). Intravenous administration of a nutrient supplement to rats produced lipoid granulomas in the liver (Fig. 3.65).

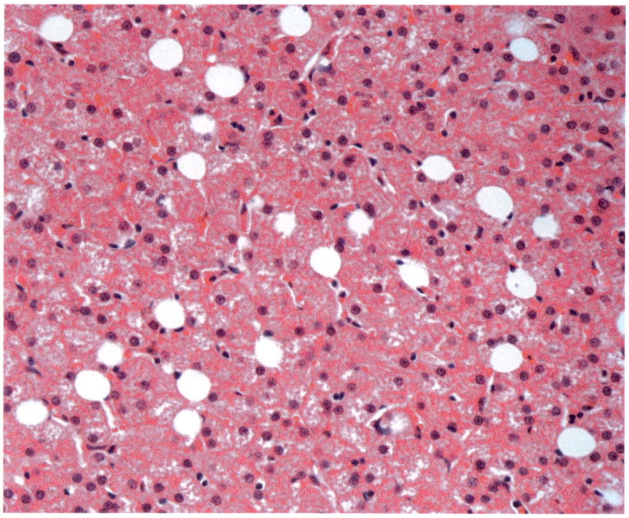

**Figure 3-60.** Increase in Ito cells, liver, in a dog treated with a carotenoid pigment. Perisinusoidal cells are distended with vacuolated cytoplasm and peripheral crescentic nuclei. H&E.

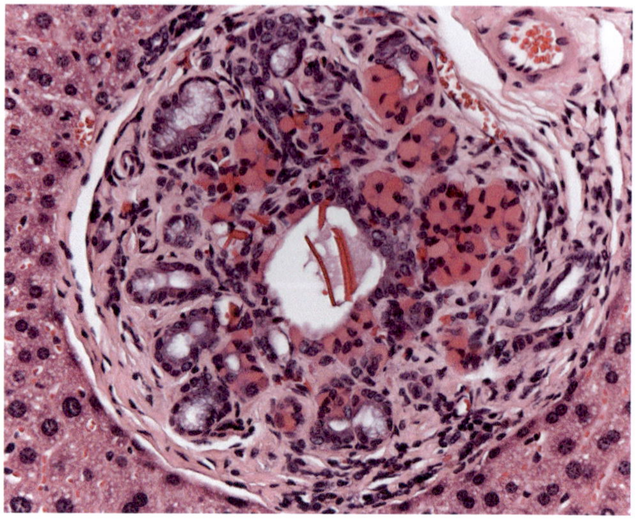

**Figure 3-61.** Serous glandular metaplasia, bile duct, in a mouse. Note increased number of bile ducts, some with serous glands (eosinophilic). Eosinophilic crystalline deposits are seen in the lumen. H&E.

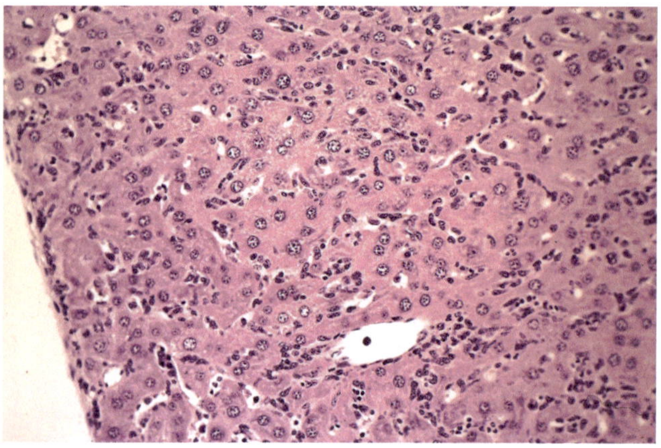

**Figure 3-62.** Hyperplasia, sinusoidal (endothelial) cells, liver, in a mouse treated with an industrial chemical. Minimal leucocytosis is also present. H&E.

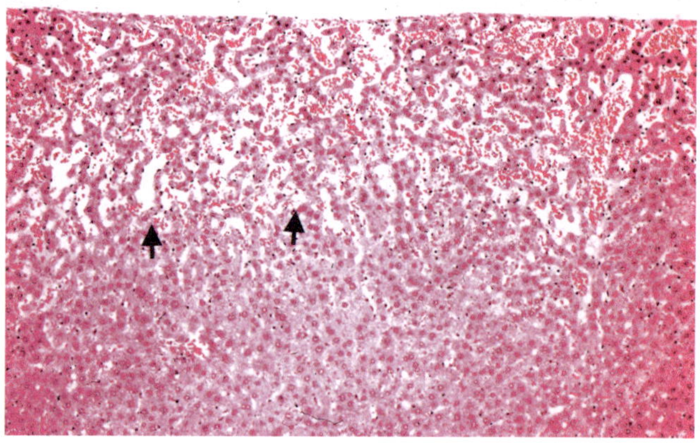

**Figure 3-63.** Focal sinusoidal dilation (*arrows*), subcapsular, liver, in a rat treated with a steroid. H&E.

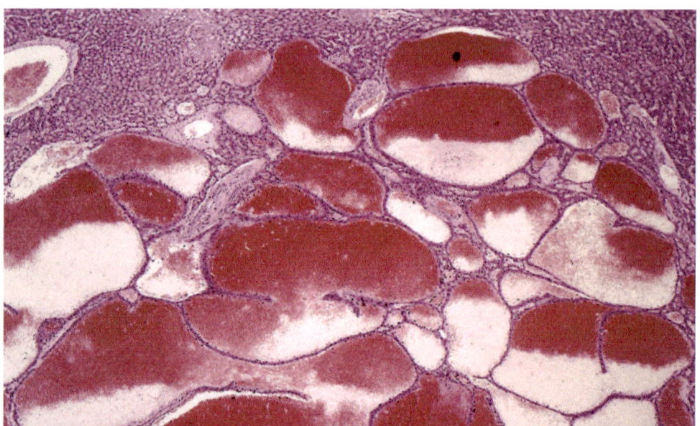

**Figure 3-64.** Peliosis hepatis, liver, in a rat. Note cystic dilation of vascular spaces lined by atrophic hepatocytes in a cordlike pattern. H&E.

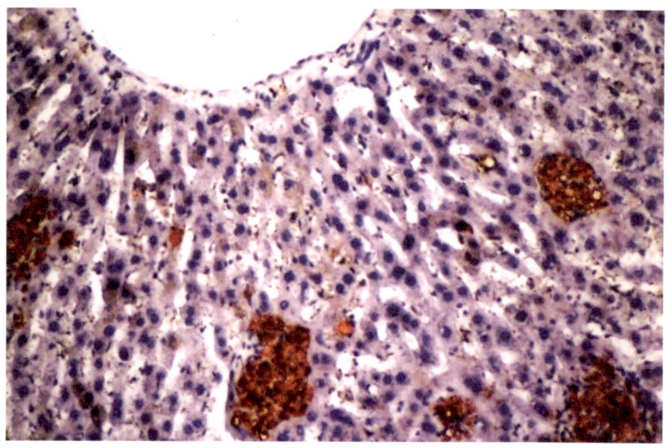

**Figure 3-65.** Lipid granuloma, liver, in a rat given intravenous administration of a nutrient supplement. Multifocal granulomas with lipid containing macrophages are seen. Frozen section, ORO.

## 3.17 Cirrhosis

In routine toxicity studies cirrhosis is seldom encountered. Cirrhosis is a progressive lesion that develops following repeated and persistent injury to the liver, resulting in nodular hyperplasia and interstitial fibrosis (Fig. 3.66). The concurrent cell injury, nodular hyperplasia, and fibrosis cause structural disorientation and circulatory disturbance. This evokes further cell loss due to ischaemia thus perpetuating hyperplasia and continuing cell destruction. Cirrhosis is progressive after circulation becomes disorientated. 2-AAF can cause cirrhosis in rat liver. There are experimental models using repeated administration of carbon tetrachloride and other chemicals [41–43].

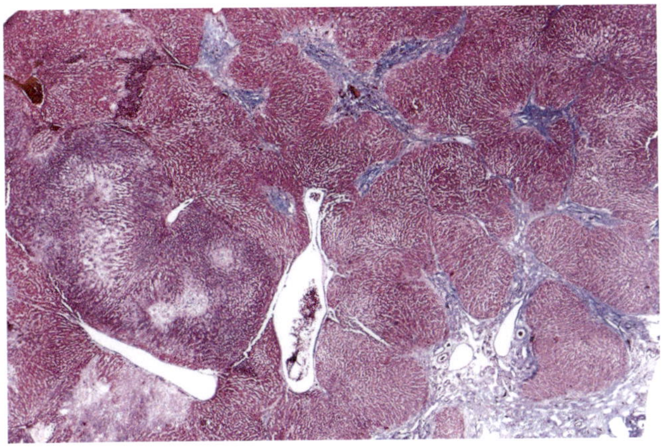

**Figure 3-66.** Cirrhosis, liver, in a rat treated with an industrial chemical for long periods. Note nodular hyperplasia, internodular fibrosis, lobular pattern, neovascularisation in the fibrous strands. Masson's trichrome.

## 3.18 Neoplasia

Hepatocellular adenomas and carcinomas are easily induced by a number of genotoxic and nongenotoxic agents in rodents. The interest is with those induced by nongenotoxic agents. Most hepatocellular tumours produced by nongenotoxic agents in rodents are found to be of little importance from a safety point of view, owing to their species-specific features, safety margins available, and lack of similar pathways in humans. Thus a large number of xenobiotics result in increased incidences of hepatocellular adenomas in rodents, evoking these owing to their capacity for cytochrome P450 induction and promoting effects. The doses by which these induce rodent tumours are too high to be significant to human safety. Similarly many hypolipidaemic agents that induce peroxisomes also produce liver tumours in rodents. Again such agents pose no human safety issues.

Rodent hepatocellular adenomas vary in size from just above a lobule to several centimetres. Morphologically, they are compressive nodules, but their autonomic growth in the absence of an initial evoking stimulus is not established because regulatory carcinogenicity studies are dosed until the end of study. They do not have a dose-free recovery period to establish their reversibility (Fig. 3.67). Thus for these hepatocellular adenomas reported in rodent carcinogenicity studies, doubt exists about their biological nature as true neoplasms.

Hepatocellular carcinomas are induced by genotoxic carcinogens like DEN, 2-AAF, and aflatoxin (Figs. 3.68–3.70). Tamoxifen, a potent antiestrogen, induces very high incidences of hepatocellular carcinomas in rats [44]. Some nongenotoxic agents (peroxisome proliferators) also are known to induce both benign and malignant hepatocellular tumours in rodents [45].

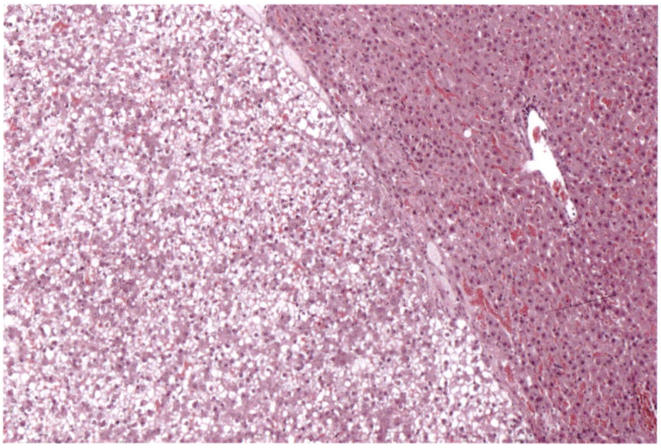

**FIGURE 3-67.** Hepatocellular adenoma, in a rat. A well-circumscribed hepatocellular lesion is causing compression. Neoplastic cells are uniform with clear cytoplasm. H&E.

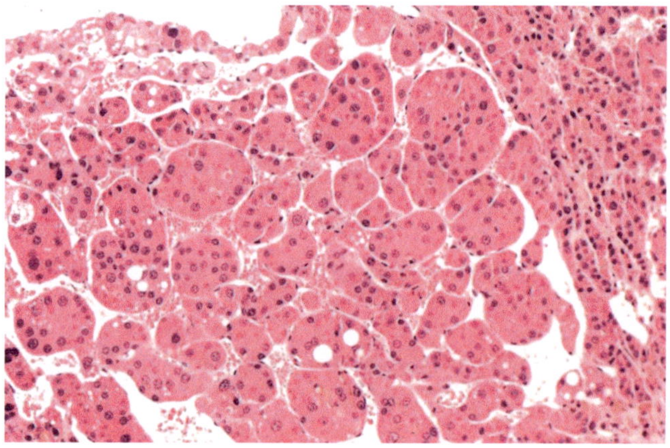

**FIGURE 3-68.** Hepatocellular carcinoma, in a mouse. Note neoplastic hepatocytes arranged in irregular multicellular chords and trabeculae. H&E.

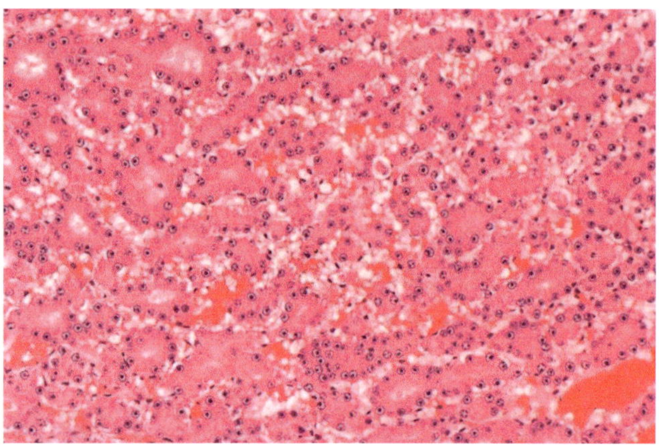

**FIGURE 3-69.** Hepatocellular carcinoma, in a rat. Note neoplastic hepatocytes arranged in irregular multicellular chords and pseudoglandular patterns. H&E.

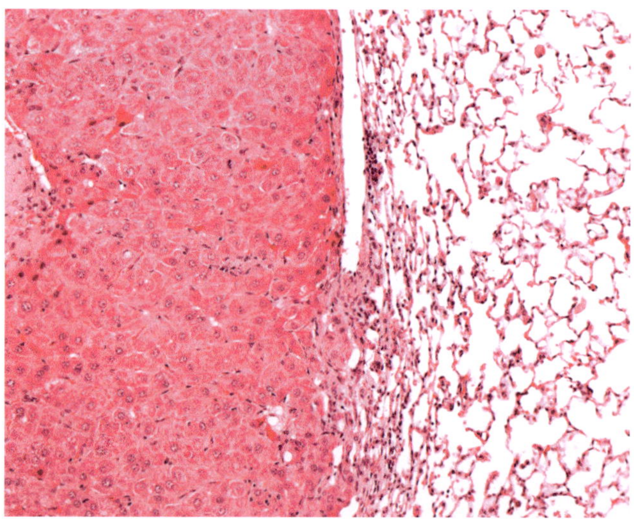

**FIGURE 3-70.** Hepatocellular carcinoma, metastasis, into the lung, in a mouse. H&E.

### 3.18.1 Cholangiocarcinomas

Cholangiocarcinoma is a malignant tumour of bile duct origin, revealing a ductular pattern with moderate to marked amounts of stroma. These often show local invasion and distant metastases. A cholangiofibromatous type of cholangiocarcinoma also occurs in rats. Sometimes they are difficult to differentiate from severe cases of cholangiofibrosis (Fig. 3.71). Most often, these are induced by genotoxic agents like 2-AAF, but they can also be induced by nongenotoxic agents on rare occasions (personal observation). These tumours can display distant metastases in the lungs and lymph nodes (Fig. 3.72).

Another inducible neoplasm arising in the liver is haemangiosarcoma. Proliferating endothelial cells arising from the sinusoidal lining replace liver parenchyma. The neoplastic endothelial cells form irregular vascular channels separated by collagenous interstitium. The tumour cells appear plump with vesicular nuclei and abundant mitoses. Tumours reveal areas of necrosis and haemorrhage. Vinyl chloride induces such tumours in the liver in experimental animals.

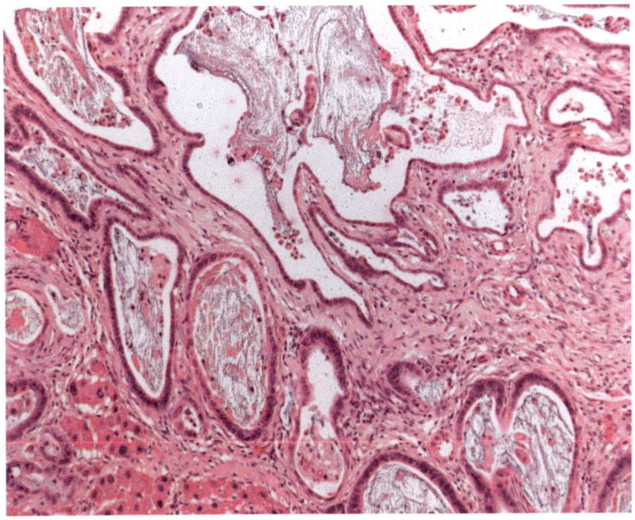

**Figure 3-71.** Cholangiocarcinoma, cholangiofibrotic type, in a rat. Note distended bile ducts with atypical epithelium, mucous secretion, interstitial fibrous stroma. H&E.

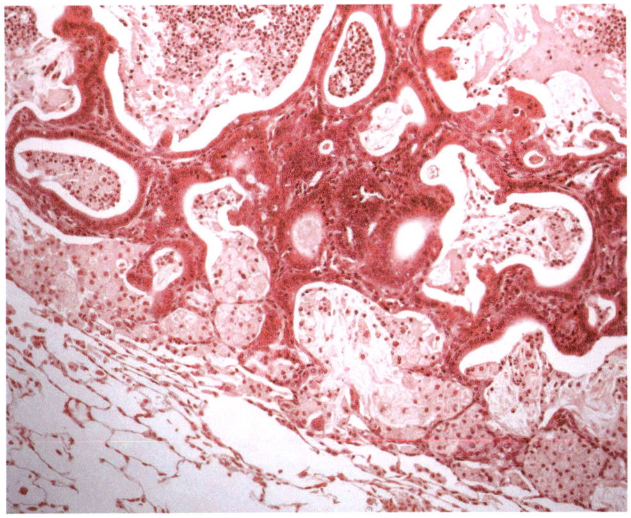

**Figure 3-72.** Cholangiocarcinoma, metastasis into the lung, in a rat. Cholangiofibrotic type. H&E.

## 3.19 Gall Bladder

The gall bladder can show toxic lesions on rare occasions. Cystic mucinous hyperplasia is reported in dogs treated long term with synthetic progestogens (Fig. 3.73) [46]. The mucosa was thick and the lumen was distended with mucus. Mucosal ulceration was noted in a dog study with a hormonal receptor antagonist (Fig. 3.74). A similar finding along with extensive fibrosis of the gall bladder wall was seen in mice from a chronic study using a growth factor inhibitor (Fig. 3.75). Cholecystitis is reported in dogs treated with 3-hydroxy-3-methylglutaryl coenzyme A (HMG CoA) reductase inhibitors [47]. Gall bladder adenomas are reported in mice treated long term with PPAR agonists [48].

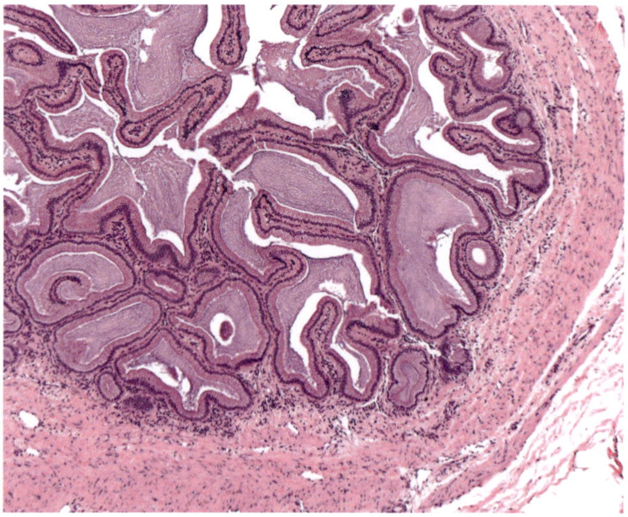

**FIGURE 3-73.** Cystic mucinous hyperplasia, gall bladder, in a dog treated long-term with a synthetic progestogen. H&E.

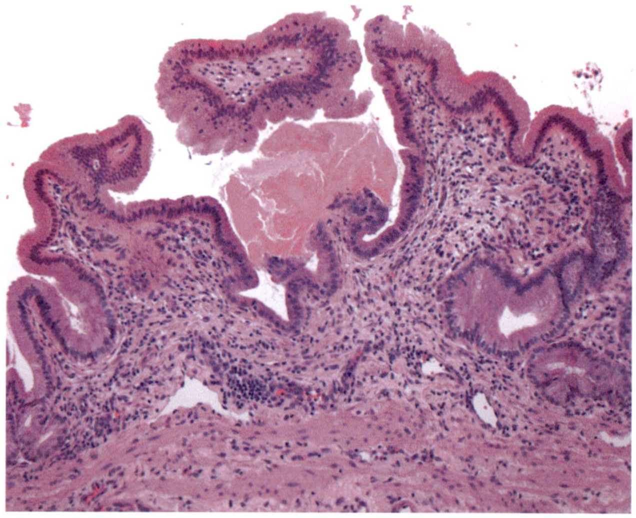

**FIGURE 3-74.** Ulceration mucosal, gall bladder, in a dog treated with a hormonal receptor antagonist. H&E.

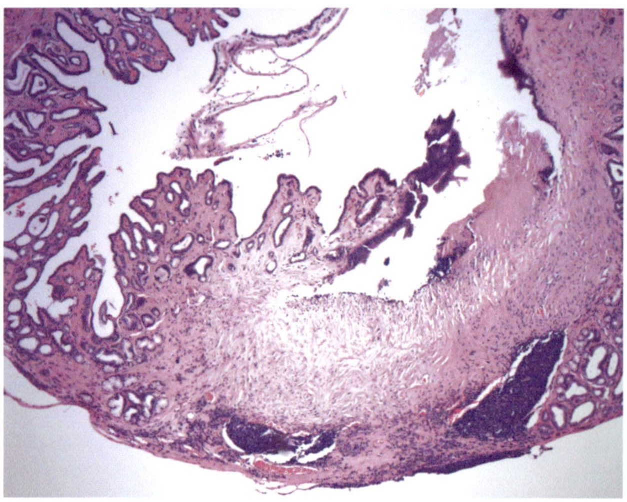

**FIGURE 3-75.** Ulceration, fibrosis, gall bladder, in a mouse from a chronic study using a growth factor inhibitor. H&E.

## References


1. Cullen JM. Mechanistic classification of liver injury. Toxicol Pathol. 2005;33:6–8.
2. Boobis AR, Cohen SM, Doerrer NG, Galloway SM, Haley PJ, Hard GC, et al. A data-based assessment of alternative strategies for identification of potential human cancer hazards 2. Toxicol Pathol. 2009;37:714–32.
3. Carmichael N, Bausen M, Boobis AR, Cohen SM, Embry M, Fruijtier-Polloth C, et al. Using mode of action information to improve regulatory decision-making: an ECETOC/ILSI RF/HESI workshop overview 1. Crit Rev Toxicol. 2011;41:175–86.
4. Hall AP, Elcombe CR, Foster JR, Harada T, Kaufmann W, Knippel A, et al. Liver hypertrophy: a review of adaptive (adverse and non-adverse) changes—conclusions from the 3rd International ESTP Expert Workshop. Toxicol Pathol. 2012; 40:971–94.
5. Holsapple MP, Pitot HC, Cohen SM, Boobis AR, Klaunig JE, Pastoor T, et al. Mode of action in relevance of rodent liver tumors to human cancer risk 7. Toxicol Sci. 2006;89:51–6.
6. Dambach DM, Andrews BA, Moulin F. New technologies and screening strategies for hepatotoxicity: use of in vitro models. Toxicol Pathol. 2005;33:17–26.
7. Harada T, Maronpot RR, Morris RW, Stitzel KA, Boorman GA. Morphological and stereological characterization of hepatic foci of cellular alteration in control Fischer 344 rats. Toxicol Pathol. 1989;17:579–93.
8. Zimmerman HJ, Ishak KG. Hepatotoxic injury due to drugs and toxins. In: MacSween RN, Antony PP, Scheur PJ, editors. Pathology of the liver. London: Churchill Livingstone; 1979. p. 335.
9. Plaa GL. Toxic responses of the liver. In: Doull H, Klasse CD, Amdur MO, editors. Casarett and Doull's toxicology. London: Macmillan; 1980. p. 206.
10. Zimmerman HJ. Chemical injury and its detection. In: Plaa GL, Hewitt WRP, editors. Toxicology of the liver. New York: Raven; 1982.
11. Jollow DJ, Mitchell JR, Zampaglione N, Gillette JR. Bromobenzene-induced liver necrosis. Protective role of glutathione and evidence for 3,4-bromobenzene oxide as the hepatotoxic metabolite. Pharmacology. 1974;11:151–69.
12. Foster JR. Spontaneous and drug-induced hepatic pathology of the laboratory beagle dog, the cynomolgus macaque and the marmoset. Toxicol Pathol. 2005;33:63–74.
13. Gopinath C, Ford JH. The role of microsomal hydroxylases in the modification of chloroform hepatotoxicity in rats. Br J Exp Pathol. 1975;56:412–22.
14. Richard JD, Parker JS, Lobenhofer EK, Burka LT, Blackshear PE, Vallant MK, et al. Transcriptional profiling of the left and median liver lobes of male F344/N rats following exposure to acetaminophen. Toxicol Pathol. 2005;33:111–7.
15. Malarkey DE, Johnson K, Ryan L, Boorman G, Maronpot RR. New insights into functional aspects of liver morphology. Toxicol Pathol. 2005;33:27–34.
16. Margos L, Butler WH. Effect of phenobarbitone and starvation on hepatotoxicity in rats exposed to carbon disulfide. Br J Ind Med. 1972;29:95–8.
17. Rouiller C. Experimental toxic injury of the liver. In: Rouiller C, editor. The liver, vol. 2. New York: Academic; 1964. p. 335.
18. Butler WH. Experimental liver injury. In: MacSween RN, Antony PP, Scheur PJ, editors. Pathology of the liver. London: Churchill Livingstone; 1979. p. 55.
19. Gopinath C, Prentice DE, Street AE, Crook D. Serum bile acid concentration in some experimental liver lesions of rat. Toxicology. 1980;15:113–27.
20. Thorpe E, Gopinath C, Jones RS, Ford EJ. The effect of chloroform on the liver and the activity of serum enzymes in the horse. J Pathol. 1969;97:241–51.
21. Bursch W, Lauer B, Timmermann-Trosiener I, Barthel G, Schuppler J, Schulte-Hermann R. Controlled death (apoptosis) of normal and putative preneoplastic cells in rat liver following withdrawal of tumor promoters. Carcinogenesis. 1984;5:453–8.
22. Kerr JF. Shrinkage necrosis: a distinct mode of cellular death. J Pathol. 1971;105:13–20.
23. Scampini G, Nava A, Newman AJ, Della TP, Mazue G. Multinucleated hepatocytes induced by rifabutin in rats. Toxicol Pathol. 1993;21:369–76.
24. Jones G, Butler WH. A morphological study of the liver lesion induced by 2,3,7,8-tetrachlorodibenzo-p-dioxin in rats. J Pathol. 1974;112:93–7.
25. Denk H, Franke WW, Eckerstorfer R, Schmid E, Kerjaschki D. Formation and involution of Mallory bodies ("alcoholic hyalin") in murine and human liver revealed by immunofluorescence microscopy with antibodies to prekeratin. Proc Natl Acad Sci U S A. 1979;76:4112–6.
26. Ishmael J, Gopinath C, Howell JM. Experimental chronic copper toxicity in sheep. Histological and histochemical changes during the development of the lesions in the liver. Res Vet Sci. 1971;12:358–66.
27. Haywood S. The effect of excess dietary copper on the liver and kidney of the male rat. J Comp Pathol. 1980;90:217–32.
28. Elrick MM, Kramer JA, Alden CL, Blomme EAG, Bunch RT, Cabonce MA, et al. Differential display in rat livers treated for 13 weeks with phenobarbital implicates a role for metabolic and oxidative stress in nongenotoxic carcinogenicity. Toxicol Pathol. 2005;33:118–26.
29. Williams GM, Iatropoulos MJ. Alteration of liver cell function and proliferation: differentiation between adaptation and toxicity. Toxicol Pathol. 2002;30:41–53.
30. Pruimboom-Brees IM, Brees DJJE, Shen AC, Keener M, Francone O, Amacher DE, et al. Using laser scanning cytometry to measure PPAR-mediated peroxisome proliferation and beta oxidation. Toxicol Pathol. 2005;33:86–91.
31. Maronpot RR, Yoshizawa K, Nyska A, Harada T, Flake G, Mueller G, et al. Hepatic enzyme induction: histopathology. Toxicol Pathol. 2010;38:776–95.
32. Thoolen B, Maronpot RR, Harada T, Nyska A, Rousseaux C, Nolte T, et al. Proliferative and nonproliferative lesions of the rat and mouse hepatobiliary system. Toxicol Pathol. 2010;38: 5S–81.
33. Harada T, Maronpot RR, Morris RW, Boorman GA. Observations on altered hepatocellular foci in National Toxicology Program two-year carcinogenicity studies in rats. Toxicol Pathol. 1989;17: 690–706.
34. Bannasch P, Moore MA, Klimek F, Zerban H. Biological markers of preneoplastic foci and neoplastic nodules in rodent liver. Toxicol Pathol. 1982;10:19–34.
35. Williams GM, Watanabe K. Quantitative kinetics of development of N-2-fluorenylacetamide-induced, altered (hyperplastic) hepatocellular foci resistant to iron accumulation and of their reversion or persistence following removal of carcinogen. J Natl Cancer Inst. 1978;61:113–21.

36. Kushida M, Kamendulis LM, Peat TJ, Klaunig JE. Dose-related induction of hepatic preneoplastic lesions by diethylnitrosamine in C57BL/6 mice. Toxicol Pathol. 2011;39:776–86.
37. Maronpot RR, Harada T, Murthy AS, Boorman GA. Documenting foci of hepatocellular alteration in two-year carcinogenicity studies: current practices of the National Toxicology Program. Toxicol Pathol. 1989;17:675–83.
38. Bannasch P, Bloch M, Zerban H. Spongiosis hepatis. Specific changes of the perisinusoidal liver cells induced in rats by N-nitrosomorpholine. Lab Invest. 1981;44:252–64.
39. Karbe E, Kerlin RL. Cystic degeneration/spongiosis hepatis in rats. Toxicol Pathol. 2002;30:216–27.
40. Tatematsu M, Ho RH, Kaku T, Ekem JK, Farber E. Studies on the proliferation and fate of oval cells in the liver of rats treated with 2-acetylaminofluorene and partial hepatectomy. Am J Pathol. 1984;114:418–30.
41. Kang JS, Morimura K, Salim EI, Wanibuchi H, Yamaguchi S, Fukushima S. Persistence of liver cirrhosis in association with proliferation of nonparenchymal cells and altered location of alpha-smooth muscle actin-positive cells. Toxicol Pathol. 2005;33:329–35.
42. Low TY, Leow CK, Salto-Tellez M, Chung MC. A proteomic analysis of thioacetamide-induced hepatotoxicity and cirrhosis in rat livers. Proteomics. 2004;4:3960–74.
43. Nuber R, Teutsch HF, Sasse D. Metabolic zonation in thioacetamide-induced liver cirrhosis. Histochemistry. 1980;69: 277–88.
44. Greaves P, Goonetilleke R, Nunn G, Topham J, Orton T. Two-year carcinogenicity study of tamoxifen in Alderley Park Wistar-derived rats. Cancer Res. 1993;53:3919–24.
45. Klaunig JE, Babich MA, Baetcke KP, Cook JC, Corton JC, David RM, et al. PPARalpha agonist-induced rodent tumors: modes of action and human relevance. Crit Rev Toxicol. 2003;33:655–780.
46. Nelson LW, Kelly WA. Progestogen-related gross and microscopic changes in female beagles. Vet Pathol. 1976;13: 143–56.
47. Walsh KM, Rothwell CE. Hepatic effects in beagle dogs administered atorvastatin, a 3-hydroxy-3-methylglutaryl coenzyme A reductase inhibitor, for 2 years. Toxicol Pathol. 1999;27: 395–401.
48. Waites CR, Dominick MA, Sanderson TP, Schilling BE. Nonclinical safety evaluation of muraglitazar, a novel PPARalpha/gamma agonist. Toxicol Sci. 2007;100:248–58.
49. Gopinath C, Prentice DE, Lewis DJ. The liver. In: Atlas of experimental toxicological pathology. Boston: MTP Press Limited; 1987. p. 43–60.

# 4 The Alimentary System and Pancreas

The alimentary system is continuously exposed to a wide range of xenobiotics in daily life, and oral administration, either by gavage or dietary admixture, is the commonest route of treatment in safety assessment studies. For this reason, and because of the length and diversity of the gastrointestinal tract, it is one of the most commonly targeted body systems. Owing to the varied functions and structure of different components of the tract, a wide range of test materials can affect one or more regions of the tract through a variety of mechanisms. Toxicity can result from the effects of the test material on contact surfaces, such as changes due to irritation in the stomach and intestines. In addition, absorption may lead to more complex toxicologic effects, with localised or systemic results including cell destruction or impairment of normal cell division, function, or defence mechanisms. The high turnover of intestinal epithelial cells makes them susceptible to radiomimetic effects. Secondary mechanisms such as hormonal perturbations, alteration of bacterial flora, and effects via the autonomic nervous system can also result in indirect or secondary toxicity in various sections of the tract. Compounds excreted through bile have a higher exposure and potentially higher toxicity in the intestines. Induced changes can also be secondary to vascular effects.

## 4.1 The Oral Cavity

Oral mucosa irritation studies are used for the safety assessment of dental products and sometimes for therapeutics intended for administration by the sublingual or oral route. Models include most common laboratory species. Irritation is scored using a system similar to that used in dermal irritation studies. The hamster cheek pouch model is used for oral carcinogenesis testing.

The oral cavity is not a common site for induced toxicity in laboratory species. Changes due to direct contact, such as those caused by irritation, are infrequent in the oral cavity, presumably because exposure is limited during oral gavage and modulated during dietary administration. The oral cavity also displays well-developed defence mechanisms, which include the protective effects of saliva and squamous epithelium. Toxicologic changes seen in the oral cavity usually follow systemic absorption and involve a wide range of mechanisms, including electrolyte level alterations, hormonal actions, targeting of receptors, and antimitotic activity. Some agents also induce changes in the teeth by direct and indirect mechanisms. Various types of toxicologic changes are seen in the oral cavity:

- Pigment changes
- Stomatitis, erosion, or ulceration
- Mucosal atrophy
- Oral epithelial hyperplasia
- Gingival hyperplasia
- Papillomas or squamous cell carcinomas

Compounds that alter skin pigmentation can produce similar changes in the oral mucosa in both humans and laboratory animals. Pigmentation changes may be due to

C. Gopinath, V. Mowat, *Atlas of Toxicological Pathology*,
DOI 10.1007/978-1-62703-998-7_4, 

stimulation of melanogenesis resulting in increased numbers of melanocytes, as is seen with pyrimethamine and chloroquine [1], or may be due to local development of drug–pigment complexes, as seen with chlorpromazine. Accumulation of a xenobiotic may also cause pigmentation, as is seen with silver in rats and humans [2, 3]. Loss of pigmentation in the oral mucosa has been induced in dogs by a platelet aggregation inhibitor [4].

Stomatitis is induced by a wide range of classes of compound. Cytotoxic and cytostatic anticancer agents cause erosions owing to their antimitotic activity on the epithelium. Drugs targeting epithelial antigens, such as tyrosine kinase inhibitors and anti-epidermal growth factor receptor monoclonal antibodies (anti-EGFR mAbs), are also associated with the development of gingival erosions and necrosis (Fig. 4.1) [5]. Tyrosine kinase inhibitors like sunitinib can also induce atrophy of the lingual epithelium [5]. Gingival erosions and ulceration, with collagen necrosis and epithelial hyperplasia, have been reported in monkeys with a polychlorinated biphenyl [6]. Compounds causing alteration of salivary gland secretion can lead indirectly to inflammatory changes in the oral cavity. Similarly, immunosuppressive agents such as azathioprine predispose to secondary infections both by altering immune defence mechanisms and by inducing epithelial atrophy and ulceration.

Growth factors, such as epidermal growth factor (EGF) and insulin-like growth factor (IGF), and other biologics induce epithelial hyperplasia of the oral mucosa and tongue in rats and monkeys [7, 8]. Immunosuppressants also can increase the incidence of papilloma virus-induced focal oral epithelial hyperplasia in dogs.

Sublingual blood sampling in rodents, a common procedure in many laboratories, results in a low level of procedural changes in the tongue, predominantly haemorrhage and myofibre degeneration with regeneration. The incidence and severity of these findings can be exacerbated by myotoxic compounds. Myofibre vacuolation and degeneration in the tongue can occur with phospholipidotics, as part of a generalised myopathy.

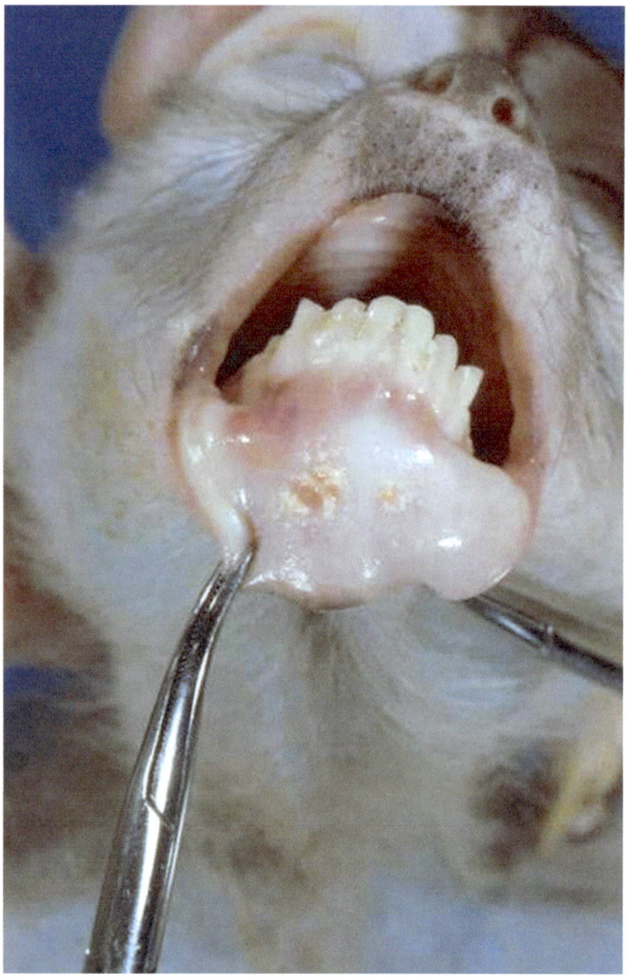

**Figure 4-1.** Buccal mucosal erosions in a monkey from a short-term toxicity study. Shallow erosions, bordered by yellow-white fibrinous material, are present on the buccal mucosa. Such lesions can be induced by EGF inhibitors and viral diseases.

Gingival hyperplasia, one of the few treatment-related changes seen in the oral cavity in safety assessment studies, is most prominent in life. It is induced by a variety of compound classes, including calcium channel blockers (*e.g.* lacidipine), anticonvulsants (*e.g.* diphenylhydantoin), and immunosuppressants (*e.g.* cyclosporine). Humans and several other species are often affected. Decreased salivary IgA secretion in some patients and impairment of T-cell function with immunosuppressants, leading to bacterial overgrowth, are proposed contributory factors with some pharmaceuticals. At necropsy, the change appears as firm, nodular gingival masses partially occluding the teeth in dogs (Fig. 4.2). Histologically, the epithelium is markedly hyperplastic, with hyperparakeratosis and formation of rete pegs. Submucosal oedema, fibroblast proliferation, myxomatous degeneration, and junctional infiltration with lymphocytes and plasma cells are common histologic features of this lesion. Proposed pathogenetic mechanisms include altered fibroblastic and proliferative activity, with possible selection of a subpopulation of fibroblasts.

Although viral papillomas occur spontaneously in young beagles, administration of immunosuppressants such as inhaled corticosteroids often increases the numbers of oral papillomas and focal oral epithelial hyperplastic lesions in treated animals. Histologically, these appear as sessile or polypoid proliferations of stroma covered by hyperplastic epithelium, with varying degrees of inflammatory cell infiltration (Fig. 4.3).

Several industrial chemicals, including benzene, tetrachloroazobenzene, and certain polychlorinated biphenyls (dioxin-like compounds), induce gingival squamous hyperplasia and squamous cell carcinomas in rats, some targeting particularly the junctional epithelium of the molars [9–11]. Smoking is associated with oral squamous cell carcinomas in humans, as is chewing of tobacco or betel nut in certain parts of the world.

### 4.1.1 Teeth

Induced changes seen in the teeth are:

- Pigmentation changes
- Ameloblastic degeneration
- Odontoblastic degeneration
- Pulp necrosis
- Ameloblastic epithelial hyperplasia

In safety assessment studies, degenerative changes in the teeth are most often detected either in young animals, in which the teeth are immature, or in rodents, in which the incisors continue to grow throughout life. Induced changes in the teeth are usually detected in life; the rodents' incisors may be pale, thin, discoloured, striated, or break easily (Figs. 4.4 and 4.5).

Effects on the teeth can be due to direct effects on multiplying cell populations, as is seen with anticancer agents such as vincristine and cyclophosphamide, or can be due to indirect mechanisms such as calcium chelation. For example, tetracyclines form complexes with calcium in the teeth, with subsequent hypoplasia. Pigmentation changes of the teeth in humans and laboratory animals are seen with fluorine and with a number of pharmaceuticals, such as tetracycline and minocycline.

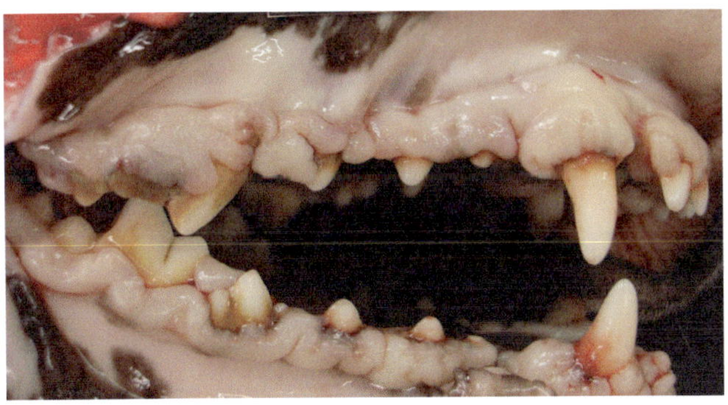

**Figure 4-2.** Dog from a short-term toxicity study given a calcium channel blocker. The gingiva is markedly swollen, partially occluding the teeth. Haemorrhage is evident around the canines.

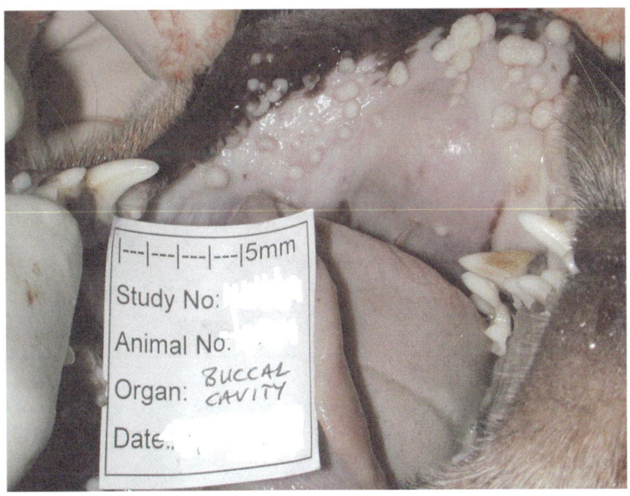


**Figure 4-3.** Multiple papillomas of varying sizes are present at the junction of skin and buccal mucosa in a dog given an immunosuppressant in a short-term study.

Xenobiotics may target ameloblasts, odontoblasts, or both. Ameloblastic degeneration has been recorded with industrial chemicals, antimitotics, antivirals, and many other classes of compounds. Anticancer agents such as cyclophosphamide and N-nitroso-N-methylurea, a genotoxic carcinogen, induce odontogenic lesions. Histologically, this change can feature degeneration, necrosis, and/or apoptosis of ameloblasts, with disorganisation and thinning of the ameloblastic layer (Fig. 4.6). If exposure is chronic, the ameloblastic layer may be completely atrophic. The resulting defects in enamel production appear grossly as discolouration or pallor, with increased chipping or fractures of the teeth.

Tyrosine kinase inhibitors, which target vascular endothelial growth factor (vEGF), and fibroblast growth factor receptors affect both ameloblasts and odontoblasts, also causing haemorrhage and necrosis of the dental pulp [5, 12]. Industrial chemicals can induce similar changes (Figs. 4.7 and 4.8). Parathormone-related peptide (PTHrP) of malignancy has been associated with increased fractures of incisors, appearing histologically as hypercalcification of dentin and reduced odontoblast height [13, 14]. Anticonvulsants such as diphenylhydantoin affect normal tooth growth in the rat in addition to causing gingival hyperplasia. They can also cause effects in the teeth secondary to inflammatory and degenerative changes of the gingival epithelium. Diabetic humans and animal models have a higher incidence of dental caries, which predisposes to periodontal disease [15].

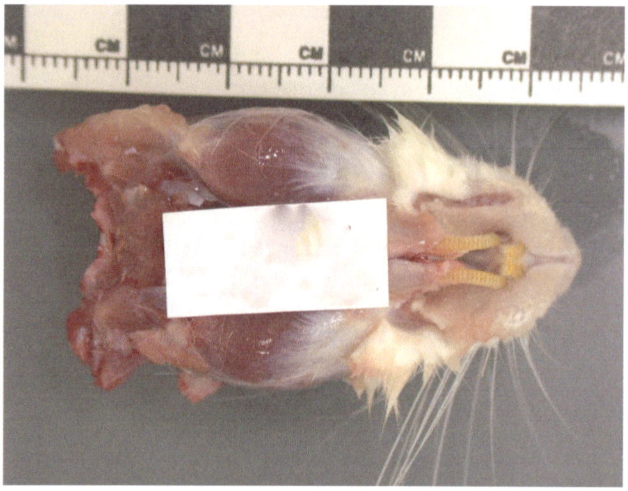

**Figure 4-4.** Striation of the upper and lower incisors is present in the teeth of a rat from a short-term study, with the teeth being yellower than usual. Tetracycline produces similar lesions.

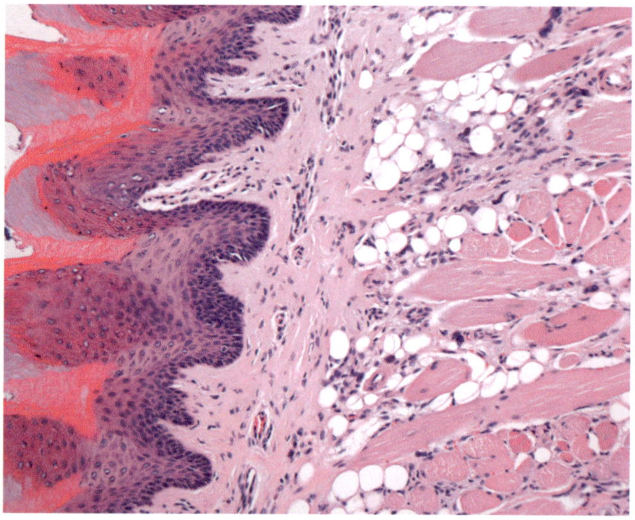

**Figure 4-5.** Vacuolar myopathy in the tongue from a rat given a phospholipidotic. Multifocal lipidotic vacuolation, inflammatory cell infiltration, and shrunken degenerating eosinophilic myofibres are evident. H&E.

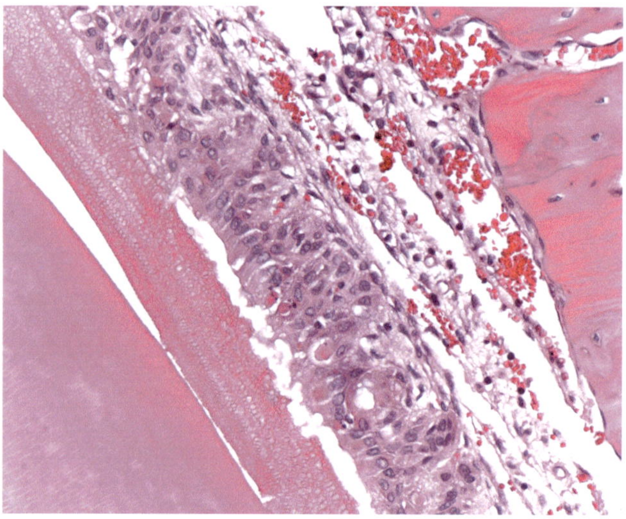

**Figure 4-6.** Ameloblast degeneration in the incisors of a rat. The ameloblast layer is disorganised and shows cell loss, with some apoptotic figures present. A range of chemicals, pharmaceuticals, and biologics can induce these changes. H&E.

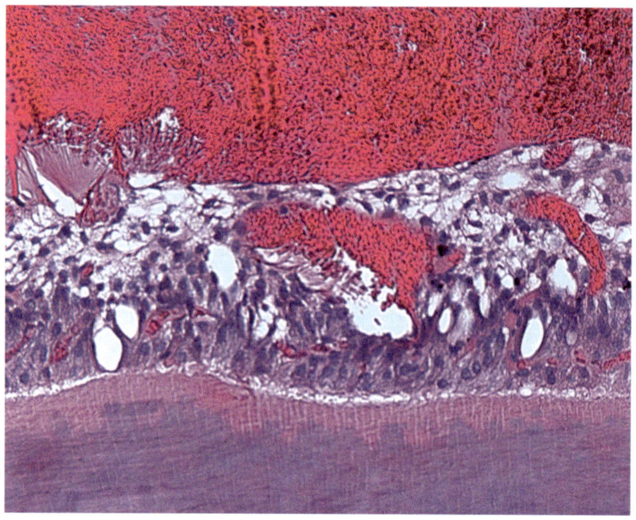

**Figure 4-7.** Odontoblast degeneration in the incisors of a rat. The odontoblast layer is disorganised, with vacuolation and some cell loss. This change was associated with administration of a chemical. H&E.

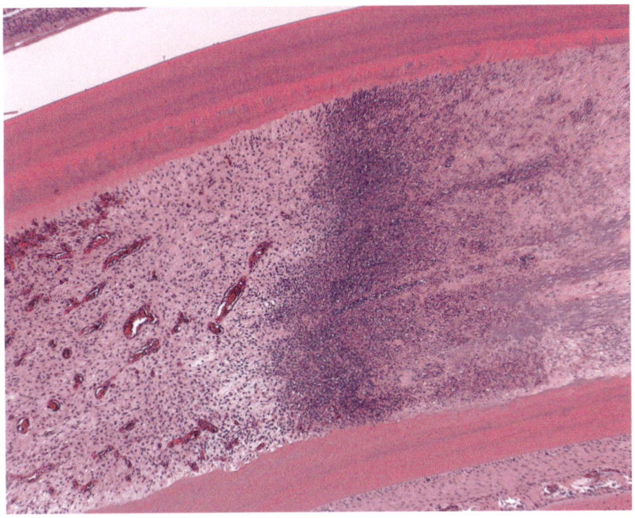

**Figure 4-8.** Pulp cavity necrosis in the incisor of a rat given an industrial chemical. The pulp cavity of the incisor is normal on the left and completely necrotic on the right, with loss of cellular detail. A darker zone of degenerating inflammatory cells is present between the healthy and necrotic pulp tissue. H&E.

## 4.2 Salivary Glands

Most mammals have three major pairs of salivary glands. The parotids, located most ventrally, produce a serous, watery secretion. The submandibular (maxillary, mandibular) glands have mixed serous and mucous acini with, accordingly, mixed secretion. Sexual dimorphism of this salivary gland is present in rodents, with the granular ducts being far more prominent in males. The sublingual gland, which is closely associated with the submandibular gland anatomically, produces predominantly mucoid secretions.

These glands have a variety of important functions, including lubricating food, initiating starch digestion, modulating oral microbial flora, and regulating function and maturing of other tissues. Saliva comprises a variety of substances including mucin, amylase, electrolytes, lysozymes, and growth factors (epidermal growth factor, EGF; nerve growth factor, NGF). Toxicologic effects vary between the salivary glands because of differences in physiological secretory control, with sublingual glands lacking sympathetic innervation. Changes seen in the submandibular gland are often mediated by effects on the nervous system or hormonal alterations.

Several types of changes are seen in the salivary glands:

- Acinar basophilia
- Acinar vacuolation, degeneration, or atrophy
- Acinar hypertrophy
- Granular duct changes
- Ductal changes: vacuolation, squamous metaplasia

Acinar basophilic foci are seen as a spontaneous change in the parotid salivary glands of rats, with an age-related increase in incidence. Phosphodiesterase inhibitors induce acinar hypertrophy and basophilia of the parotid glands, with mucous acinar hypertrophy of the submandibular and sublingual glands [16]. Theophylline causes enlargement of acinar nuclei and of the basophilic basal portion of the acinar cells; this enlargement is presumably due to increased cyclic AMP, which results in increased secretion [17]. Acinar vacuolation and degeneration can be induced by antineoplastic agents, which cause degeneration of acinar cells, accompanied by varying degrees of inflammatory cell infiltration (Figs. 4.9 and 4.10). DL-ethionine toxicity in rats causes shrinking of the parotid glands with nuclear pyknosis, karyorrhexis, cytoplasmic vacuolation, and duct dilation [18]. Recovery can occur after cessation of treatment. The rat parotid gland has been found to be the most sensitive to irradiation of all three glands, with low regenerative capacity [19].

Acinar atrophy is induced by reduced food consumption, powdered or liquid diets, β-adrenergic antagonists, and denervation (Fig. 4.11) [20]. The diuretic furosemide is associated with atrophic changes. Histologically, decreased numbers of secretion granules are seen in the acinar cells, with decreased cell height and vacuolation. Duct ligation induces acinar atrophy secondary to blockage. Sunitinib, a tyrosine kinase inhibitor, induced acinar atrophy and degranulation in primates and rats [5].

Administration of β-adrenergic agonists, opioid receptor agonists, or antihistamines such as doxylamine results in acinar hypertrophy (Fig. 4.12). Salivary secretion involves both α-and β-catecholamine receptors, so β-agonists and pilocarpine induce hypertrophy of the submandibular and parotid glands in the rat, whereas the sublingual gland does not demonstrate this response. These effects are generally reversible and can be inhibited by β-blockers such as propranolol.

Granular duct changes in the mandibular salivary gland can reflect reduced or increased serous secretion. Because granular duct morphology is androgen-dependent, castration results in feminisation of the gland in males, with testosterone causing masculinisation in females. Thyroxine and adrenocortical hormones also stimulate the male granular ducts, and deficiency of these hormones results in atrophy.

Hyperplasia of the intercalated ducts has been induced in rats given a steroid with oestrogenic and progestagenic properties, appearing histologically as increased numbers of microcystic ducts surrounded by myoepithelial cells [21]. EGF results in salivary ductal epithelial hyperplasia in rats [7].

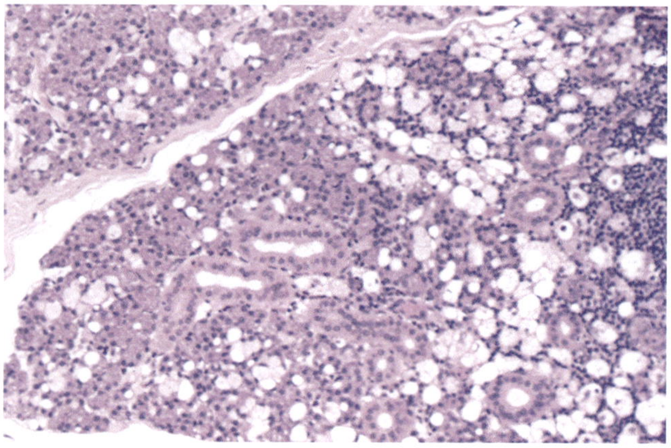

**FIGURE 4-9.** Submandibular salivary gland from a monkey following administration of a novel antineoplastic agent. The coarse acinar vacuolation is associated with mononuclear cell infiltrates. H&E. (With kind permission from Springer Science + Business Media B.V [20]).

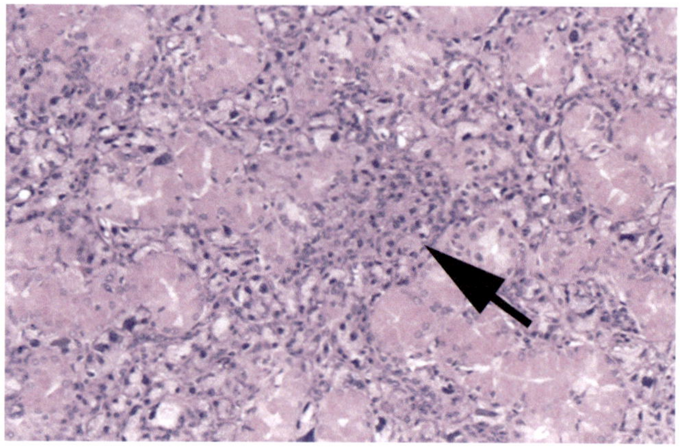

**FIGURE 4-10.** Submandibular salivary gland from a rat treated with an industrial chemical, showing focal atrophy of acinar cells (*arrow*). H&E. (With kind permission from Springer Science + Business Media B.V [20]).

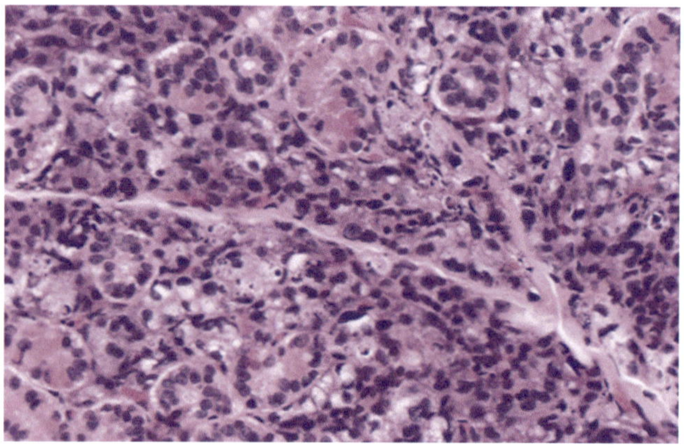

**FIGURE 4-11.** Single-cell degeneration and atrophy of serous acini from the submandibular salivary gland of a rat treated with a novel antibiotic neoplastic agent. H&E. (With kind permission from Springer Science + Business Media B.V [20]).

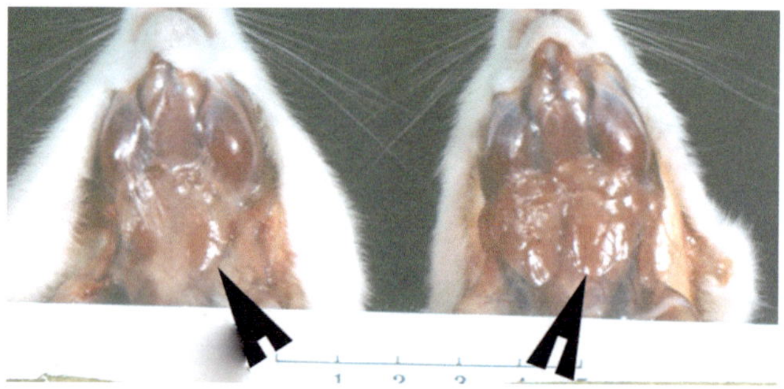

**FIGURE 4-12.** Hypertrophy of rat submandibular salivary glands (*arrow heads*) following administration of a β-sympathomimetic agonist. Compared with the glands of an untreated animal on the left, the glands on the right are grossly enlarged. (With kind permission from Springer Science + Business Media B.V [20]).

## 4.3 Oesophagus

Induced lesions of the oesophagus are rare in preclinical safety studies. Local oesophageal irritant potential of drugs is routinely assessed in a number of models, including the dog, cat, and pig. The test drugs are placed in the oesophagus by endoscopy and allowed to dissolve. Histopathologic examination is performed after 3–6 days, and ulcerogenic activity is assessed on the basis of the degree of inflammation and ulceration.

In toxicity studies, the following lesions may be seen in the oesophagus:

- Epithelial atrophy
- Hyperkeratosis
- Hyperplasia
- Inflammation
- Myofibre degeneration
- Megaoesophagus
- Mucosal gland hypertrophy
- Impaction
- Erosion, ulceration, necrosis
- Papillomas or squamous cell carcinomas

Epithelial atrophy is an uncommon induced finding, but it has been seen in primates given sunitinib; it was characterised by thinning, hypereosinophilia, and nuclear pyknosis resulting in parakeratosis [5]. Drugs with antimitotic activity also can cause thinning and atrophy [22].

Hyperkeratosis is seen in rodents with anorexia and is also induced by deficiency of zinc or vitamin A. Epithelial hyperplasia in rats can be induced by chronic alcohol administration and mesuprine hydrochloride, a β-adrenergic receptor stimulator (Fig. 4.13). Raf inhibitors are associated with hyperplasia of the oesophageal epithelium, probably through alteration of the mitogen-activated protein kinase (MAPK) pathway, which results in cell proliferation [23].

In rodents, a low level of myofibre degeneration sometimes presents as a background finding in oral gavage studies, without oesophageal perforation. Compounds affecting musculature at other sites, including phospholipidotics, sometimes cause myofibre degeneration in the smooth muscle of the oesophagus in rodents. Histologically, lesions are typical of myopathy, comprising eosinophilic degenerating fibres and regenerative basophilic fibres with centrally positioned chains of nuclei. Inflammatory cell infiltrate may be present in the musculature but is not usually a significant feature. If myopathy is severe, muscle weakening can result in megaoesophagus and dilation (Fig. 4.14). Induced megaoesophagus is often secondary to neurotoxicants such as acrylamide, which causes dilation of the oesophagus in dogs due to nerve damage.

Steroids induce mild hypertrophy of the oesophageal mucous glands in dogs. Glands appear larger and slightly more eosinophilic than in controls. Mucous cells are mildly hypertrophic, partially occluding the acinar lumen (Fig. 4.15).

In rodents, impaction of the oesophagus may be caused by food (powdered diet), bedding, or administration of capsules, resulting in inflammation and erosion or ulceration. Effects due to irritation are rare because of the short transit time in the oesophagus, but if passage is delayed or capsules containing irritant compounds are retained and ruptured, erosion and ulceration of the oesophagus can result and may lead to perforation.

During gavage studies, dosing can result in perforation and the sudden death of the animal. Perforation alone is sometimes detected at necropsy, without a histologic correlation in the oesophagus. If (as often happens) the animal does not die immediately, varying degrees of inflammation and/or abscessation are seen in the cervical region or thoracic cavity, with pleuritis or pericarditis, depending on the area of oesophageal rupture and deposition of test material.

Spontaneous tumours of the oesophagus are rare but can be induced in rodents by genotoxic chemicals such as methyl nitrosourea and nitrosomethylbenzylamine, which cause hyperplasia, papillomas, and squamous cell carcinomas of the oesophagus [24].

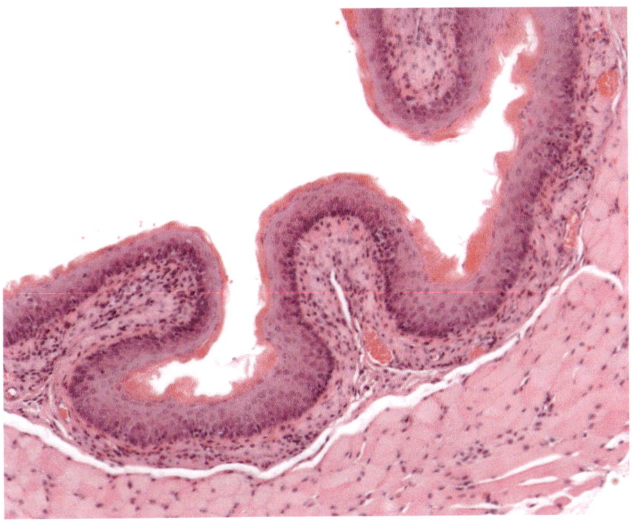

**Figure 4-13.** In a transgenic mouse given methyl nitrosourea, the oesophageal epithelium is hyperplastic and hyperkeratotic, with mild inflammatory cell infiltration in the lamina propria. H&E.

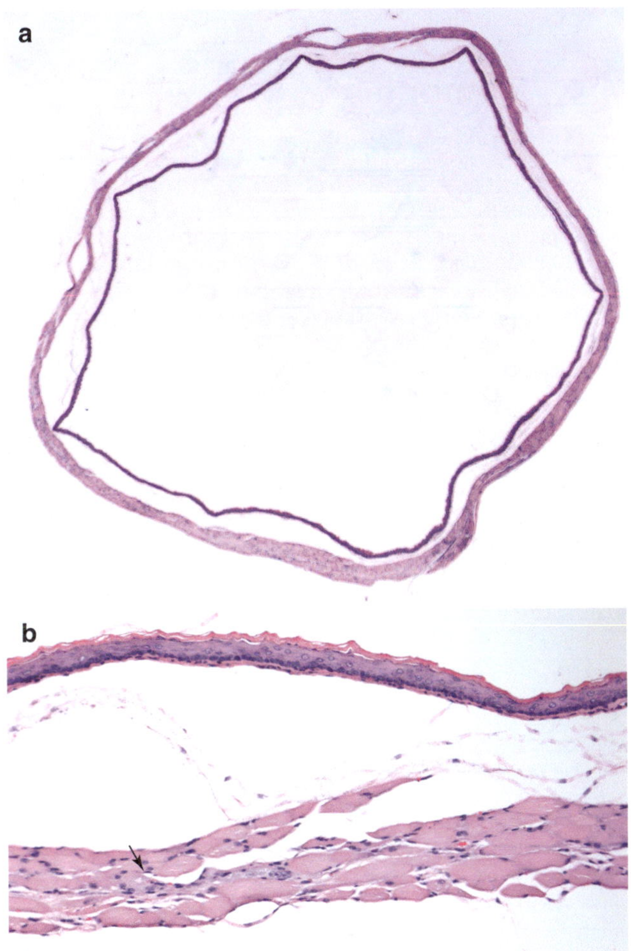


**Figure 4-14.** (**a**) Megaoesophagus in a rat from a long-term study with a phospholipidotic. The oesophagus is markedly dilated, with varying thickness of the muscle wall. H&E. (**b**) At a higher power, the muscle wall is thin, with degenerating, pale, vacuolated myofibres (*arrow*), and basophilic, regenerating myofibres with central nuclei. H&E.

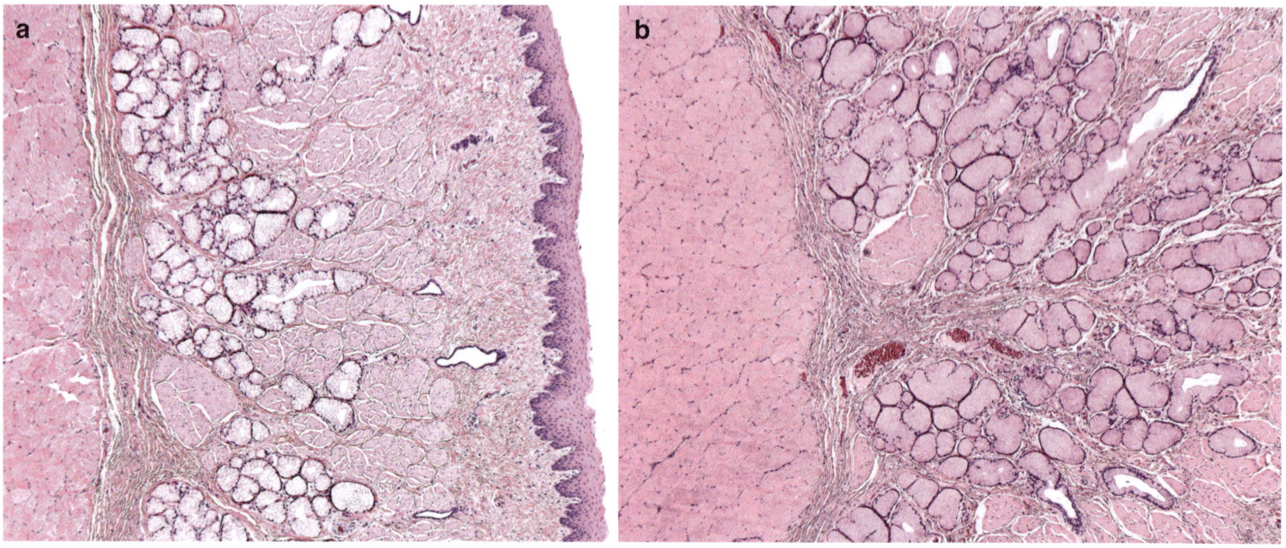

**Figure 4-15.** (**a**) Normal oesophagus from a control dog; note the size of the submucosal mucous glands. H&E. (**b**) Dog given a steroid on a short-term study. Submucosal oesophageal glands appear larger than in the control. Mucous cells are hypertrophic and slightly eosinophilic and occlude the acinar lumen. H&E.

## 4.4 Stomach

The stomach is one of the commonest sites in the alimentary tract for induced changes, as a result of its prolonged exposure to the unaltered test material. In rodents, changes are often seen in the nonglandular forestomach because of its storage function. Some of the factors that influence gastric toxicity are pH, rate of gastric emptying, fasting or feeding state, and the physical properties of the test article. The level of enterohepatic circulation also affects the extent of gastric damage, as exemplified by indomethacin in dogs. Sensitivity to different compound classes varies with species, dogs generally being more sensitive than primates or minipigs.

### 4.4.1 The Rodent Forestomach

Listed are induced changes in the rodent forestomach:

- Hyperkeratosis
- Hyperplasia
- Inflammation
- Erosion, ulceration
- Papillomas, squamous cell carcinoma

Dietary deficiency of vitamin A and zinc are associated with hyperkeratosis and hyperplasia of the rodent nonglandular stomach, with zinc deficiency characteristically causing parakeratosis with retention of nuclei in the keratin layer.

Hyperkeratosis and hyperplasia of the rodent forestomach are frequently seen in gavage and dietary studies (Fig. 4.16). These can be an adaptive response to mild irritation, secondary to cytotoxicity, or due to a direct proliferative effect. If these changes are due to irritation, degrees of inflammatory cell infiltration, epithelial vacuolation, intraepithelial and subepithelial vesiculation, and rete peg formation may also be present. Changes are sometimes localised to the limiting ridge or are more prominent there. More severe irritation results in erosion or ulceration with necrosis (Fig. 4.17). Induced erosion and ulceration of the stomach are often focal, so thorough examination at necropsy and accurate sampling of abnormalities are essential for the detection of small lesions. Many classes of drugs, food additives, and chemicals are associated with changes of this type; agents include sodium metabisulphite, butylated hydroxyanisole (BHA), and a range of phenols and acids. Prolonged administration of some of these nongenotoxic agents, such as BHA, results in development of squamous cell carcinomas. The mechanism of tumour development with these agents is epigenetic, resulting from increased cell proliferation secondary to chronic cytotoxicity. With HMG-CoA reductase inhibitors and Raf inhibitors, a direct proliferative effect results in epithelial hyperplasia [23]. Systemic administration of pharmaceuticals can also result in forestomach hyperplasia, as is seen with intravenous acetaminophen [25]. Hyperkeratosis and epithelial hyperplasia in rats and mice can be caused by prostaglandin E1 analogues such as misoprostol [26, 27]. It has been suggested that different areas of the rodent forestomach possibly react differently to chemicals because of varying levels of activating enzymes.

Forestomach hyperplasia and squamous cell carcinomas have been recorded in alloxan-induced diabetic rats. These lesions are considered to be due to *Candida albicans* infection, and they can be potentiated by tetracycline therapy [28]. Control of blood glucose reduces their incidence [29]. Many genotoxic carcinogens, including nitrosamines such as methyl nitrosourea, induce papillomas and squamous cell carcinomas of the nonglandular stomach (Figs. 4.18 and 4.19).

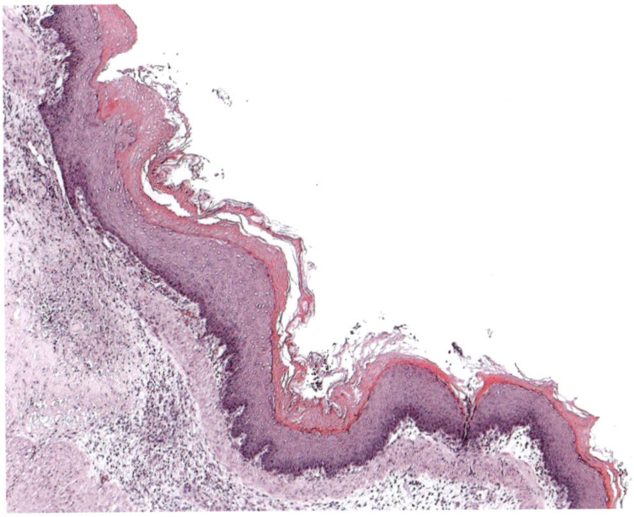

**FIGURE 4-16.** Hyperplasia and hyperkeratosis of the nonglandular stomach in a rat. Minor irritation is associated with these adaptive changes. H&E.

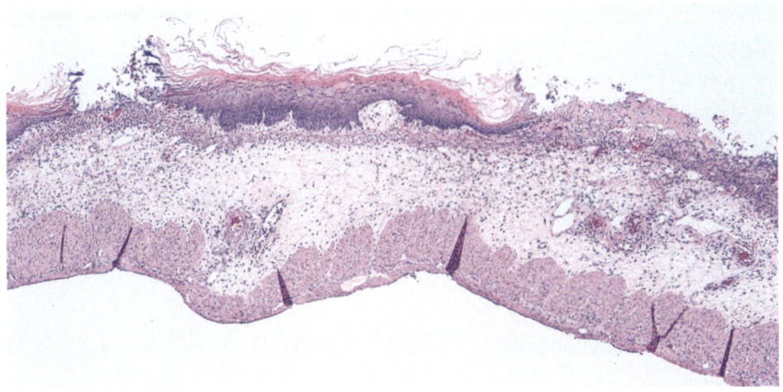

**FIGURE 4-17.** Ulceration of the nonglandular stomach in a rat. The squamous epithelium is extensively ulcerated and necrotic, with oedema and inflammation of the submucosa. The focal area of remaining epithelium is hyperkeratotic and hyperplastic, with rete pegs growing into the submucosa. H&E.

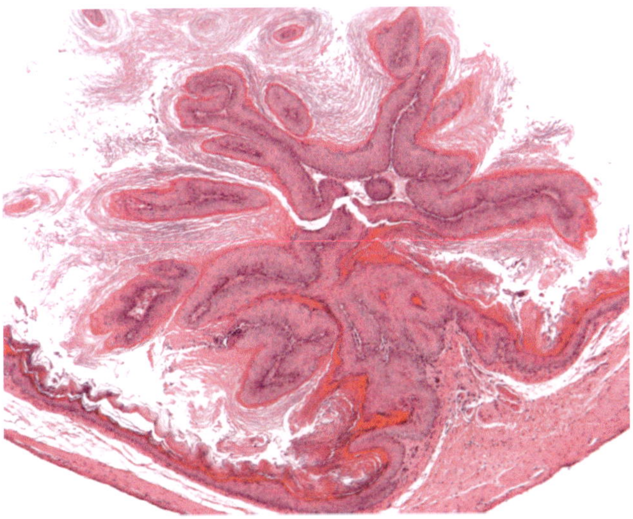

**FIGURE 4-18.** Papilloma of the nonglandular stomach in a transgenic mouse given methyl nitrosourea. The tumour consists of branching stromal proliferations covered by hyperplastic and hyperkeratotic squamous epithelium. H&E.

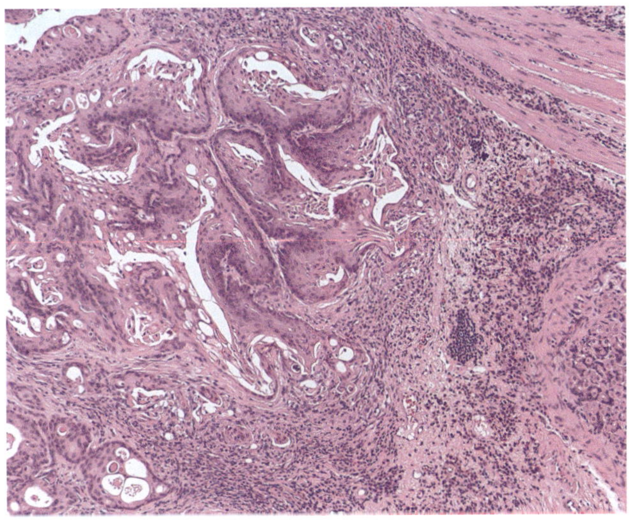

**FIGURE 4-19.** Gastric squamous cell carcinoma in a rat from a long-term study. Nests of neoplastic, moderately differentiated squamous cells have invaded the submucosa. Marked lymphoplasmacytic infiltration is seen in the submucosa and between muscle bands. H&E.

## 4.4.2 The Glandular Stomach

The glandular mucosa is composed of a variety of cell types, Histologically, the surface columnar epithelium forms pits or foveolae. These pits communicate with the gastric glands , which are divided into isthmus, neck and base. Some of the commonest cell types are mucous cells, parietal cells which produce hydrochloric acid and chief cells which produce pepsinogen. Gastric acid section is stimulated by histamine produced by enterochromaffin cells, which are stimulated by gastrin produced by the antral G cells. Somatostatin from antral D cells inhibits gastrin production in response to a variety of stimuli including low gastric pH, calcitonin gene-releasing peptide, norepinephrine and other neurohumoral factors. Cell proliferation in the gastric mucosa takes place principally in the isthmus or superficial gastric glands, with cells migrating both superficially and to the lower regions of the mucosa. The mucosa has a number of protective mechanisms including the mucus-bicarbonate layer and the epithelial barrier. Toxicity is exerted through a variety of mechanisms including disruption of protective barriers, antimitotic activity, direct irritation. Indirect effects are exerted via a variety of effects including disruption of hormonal , humoral and nervous control mechanisms.

These induced changes are seen in the glandular stomach:

- Mineralisation
- Pigment deposition
- Hyalinisation
- Increased globule leucocytes
- Chief cell degeneration
- Parietal cell degeneration
- Parietal cell hyperplasia
- Intestinal metaplasia
- Erosion, ulceration
- Foveolar/adenomatous/mucosal hyperplasia
- Enterochromaffin-like (ECL) cell hyperplasia, tumours
- Adenomas, adenocarcinomas

Mineralisation of the glandular stomach is associated with increased plasma calcium levels and can be induced by vitamin D analogues, gadolinium III, and tyrosine kinase inhibitors [30–32]. Histologically, mineralisation is seen in the fundic mucosa, muscularis, and blood vessel walls (Fig. 4.20). This finding also occurs in uremic gastropathy due to chronic renal disease in rodents and dogs.

Accumulation of pigment and pigmented macrophages in the glandular crypts occurs with iron-containing compounds administered orally (Fig. 4.21). Hyalinisation of the pyloric stomach has recently been recorded in mice given corticosteroids. This change appears as collagen deposits in the lamina propria, and is considered to represent an expansion of collagen-rich extracellular matrix [33].

An unusual change sometimes seen in the glandular mucosa is an increase in globule leucocytes, often in the region of the fundus adjacent to the limiting ridge. This change is induced by a range of agents, including kinin inhibitors [personal observation], polyethylene glycol, iron lactate, and industrial compounds containing heavy metals [34, 35]. These cells are considered to be of mast cell lineage, and their granules have been shown with Giemsa stain and toluidine blue stain; they stain positively for rat mast cell protease II [35]. Increases in globule leucocytes often occur in combination with increased eosinophils in the lamina propria (Fig. 4.22).

Less commonly occurring induced lesions include atrophy of chief and parietal cells. Degeneration of parietal cells in the dog has been observed with novel $H_2$ antagonists [20]. Some proton pump inhibitors also induce parietal cell vacuolation and single-cell necrosis [36]. Decreased parietal cells have been observed in cynomolgus monkeys treated with polychlorinated biphenyls, associated with a diffuse hypertrophy and hyperplasia of the mucinous gastric mucosa [6]. Parietal cell degeneration has been observed in our laboratory with an industrial chemical (Fig. 4.23). Anticancer agents with cytotoxic or cytostatic effects can cause cell loss of gastric glandular epithelium.

Parietal cell hyperplasia occurs in rats given pentagastrin [37]. $H_2$ antagonists, antacids, and proton pump blockers have a similar trophic effect through increased gastrin levels.

Proliferation of cells lining the basal areas of gastric glands, possibly atypical Paneth cells or hyperplastic eosinophilic chief cells, is recorded with $H_2$ blockers such as loxtidine and industrial chemicals [personal observation] (Fig. 4.24). Cells are large, with eosinophilic granules and a basal nucleus. This change is believed to be a metaplasia [17].

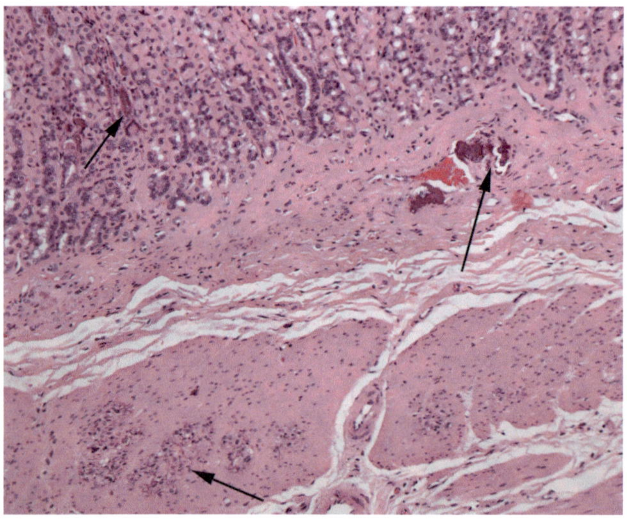

**Figure 4-20.** Mineralisation in the stomach of a rat from a long-term study. Pinkish-purple mineral deposits are present in the mucosa, muscularis, and blood vessel walls (*arrows*). Mineralisation is associated with increased blood calcium levels and can be induced by vitamin D analogues. H&E.

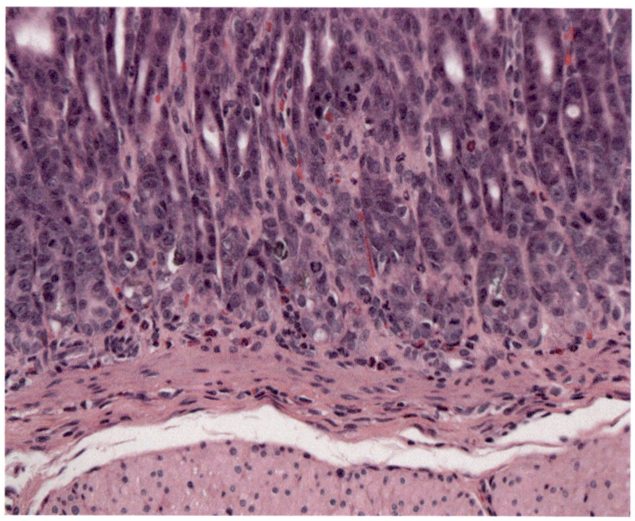

**Figure 4-21.** Rat given an iron-containing compound in a short-term study. Dark-brown granules are present in some of the glandular epithelial cells, with minimal eosinophilic infiltration in the lamina propria. H&E.

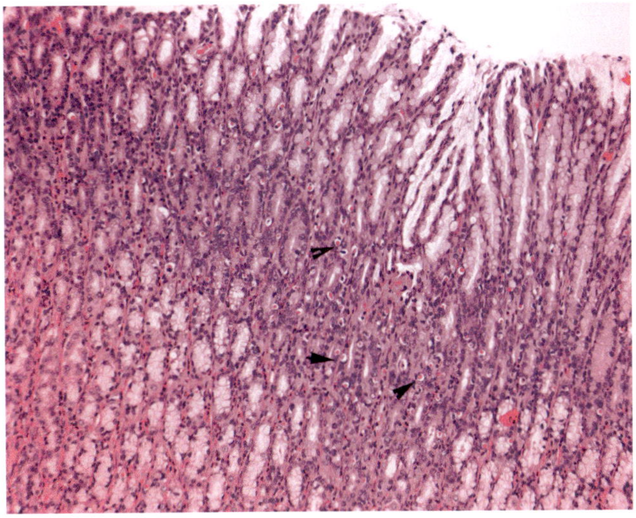

**Figure 4-22.** Increased globule leucocytes in the glandular stomach of a rat. Increased numbers of eosinophilic globule leucocytes (*arrowheads*) are present, predominantly in the foveolar region near the limiting ridge. A range of chemicals and biologically active compounds can cause this change. H&E.

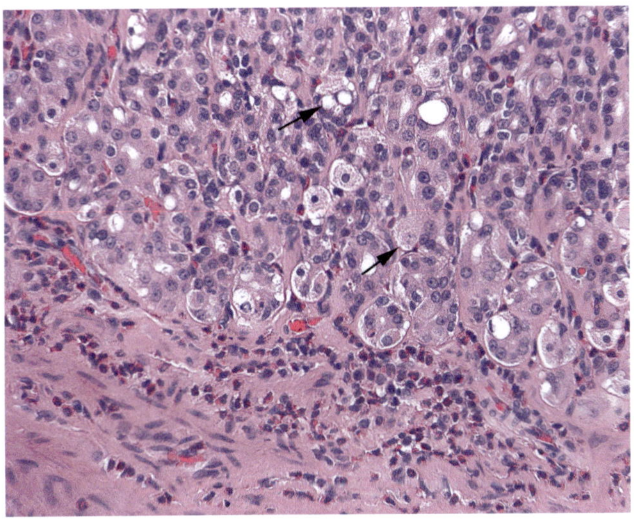

**Figure 4-23.** Parietal cell degeneration in the glandular stomach of a rat. The glands display vacuolation and degeneration of isolated parietal cells (*arrows*), sometimes leaving eosinophilic debris. H&E.

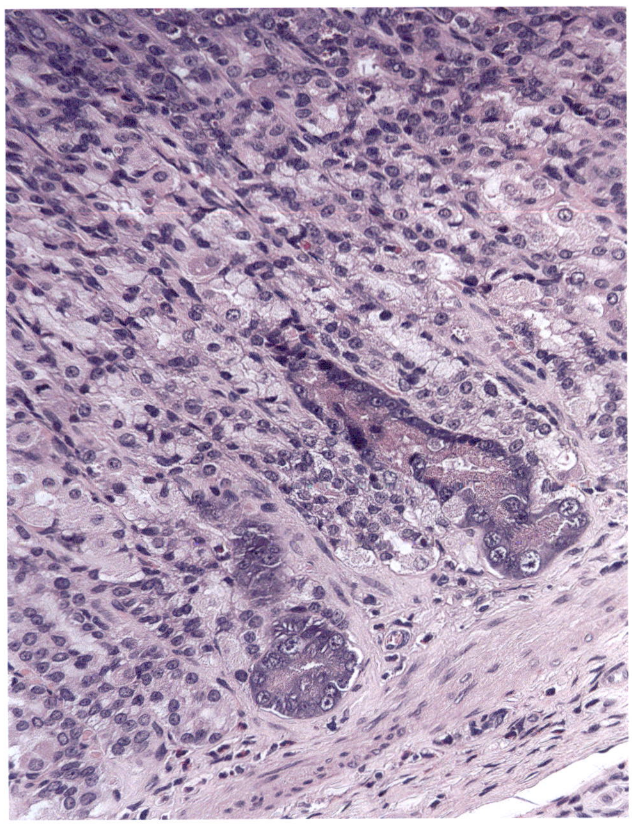

**Figure 4-24.** Intestinal metaplasia in a rat glandular stomach. The normal glandular cells have been replaced by larger, basophilic, Paneth-like cells with apical zymogen granules and basal basophilic nuclei. H&E.

Many chemical and pharmaceutical groups cause erosion and ulceration of the glandular mucosa (Fig. 4.25). NSAIDs are probably the class of compounds most closely associated with gastric ulceration. It has been suggested that these drugs can be classified into three groups based on the extent and severity of the gastric lesions they induce:

I. Drugs that induce mucosal haemorrhage (*e.g.* cyclophosphamide, methotrexate)
II. Drugs that induce mucosal haemorrhage and ulcers (*e.g.* aspirin)
III. Drugs that induce mucosal haemorrhage, erosion, ulcers, and damage to the small intestine (*e.g.* phenylbutazone and indomethacin)

Histologically varying degrees of erosion and ulceration are seen, accompanied by inflammation and haemorrhage. Perforation is a common sequel with high doses or chronic administration, followed by peritonitis and intestinal adhesions in rodents.

Lesions may be produced by two different mechanisms: direct contact with the mucosa or systemic toxicity after absorption. The ulcerogenic effect of NSAIDs is widely accepted as being due to reduction of prostaglandin synthesis by cyclooxygenase inhibition, with both COX-1 and COX-2 inhibition required [38–41]. The reduction in protective prostaglandin levels and gastric acid levels potentially leaves the mucosa susceptible to vasoconstrictors such as lipoxygenases. Expression of COX-1 and COX-2 prostaglandins varies between different cell populations and areas of the stomach [42]. Direct contact with NSAIDs also decreases mucus and bicarbonate release in the mucosa, contributing to their ulcerogenic effects. Aspirin inhibits cyclooxygenase activity, and after deacetylation it produces salicylate, which affects mucosal barrier function. Dogs are more sensitive than rats to NSAID toxicity, with monkeys being the least sensitive of the three species. Steroids also induce gastric ulceration if given over long periods or at a high dose, at least partially through inhibition of prostaglandin synthesis, and they can delay healing of gastric ulcers even at nonulcerogenic doses [43, 44].

Other drugs such as diuretics, angiotensin-converting enzyme (ACE) inhibitors, and angiotensin II antagonists induce gastric lesions by means of severe electrolyte imbalances. Bile salts in the stomach break down gastric mucosal permeability and solubilise the outer lipid bilayer of surface epithelium, predisposing to erosions and ulcer development.

Foveolar hyperplasia, an unusual change that occurs with various compounds, manifests as increased thickness of the foveolar region. This occurs in rats given neurokinin antagonists and in dogs and monkeys given a prostaglandin $E_1$ analogue [45]. Hypertrophy and hyperplasia of mucous neck cells occur with irritants, prostaglandins, and $\gamma$-interferon [46]. Administration of epidermal growth factor to (Fig. 4.26) monkeys causes epithelial hyperplasia, with replacement of differentiated cells by less-differentiated cell types [8]. Adenomatous hyperplasia in older mice is a well-documented spontaneous change, which may demonstrate penetration of the lamina propria by hyperplastic glands but does not progress to neoplasia. Antisecretory agents can increase the incidence of this spontaneous change.

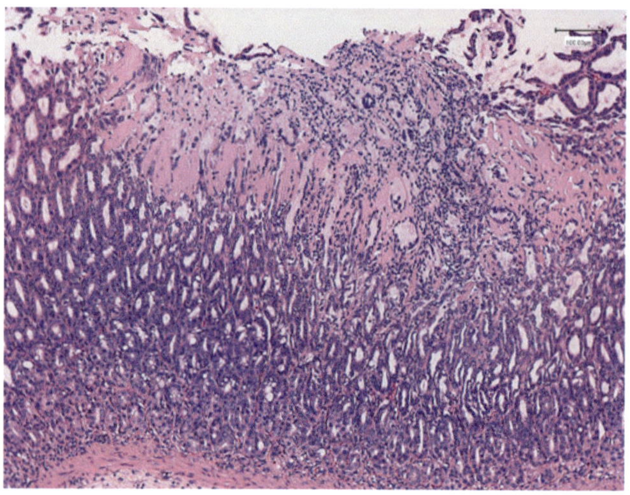

**Figure 4-25.** Erosions in the glandular stomach of a rat. The foveolar mucosa is necrotic, with eosinophilic material and inflammatory cell debris. Such lesions are caused by many compound classes including NSAIDS, chemicals, and phosphodiesterase (PDE) inhibitors. H&E.

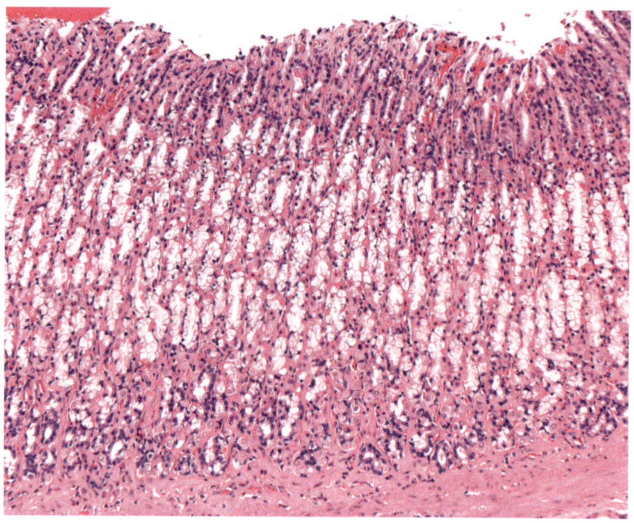

**Figure 4-26.** Increased mucous cells in the glandular stomach of a rat. Mucous cells are increased in number and size, forming a broad band below the foveolar region. These changes can be a response to minimal irritation. H&E.

Arteritis of the gastric blood vessels can occur as part of a generalised vascular syndrome in dogs with idiopathic polyarteritis and rodents with polyarteritis. In rodents, it is often associated with severe nephropathy. Phosphodiesterase 4 (PDE4) inhibitors cause vasculitis in several laboratory species (Fig. 4.27). Antibiotics, cytotoxics, and cardioactive agents, among others, can induce gastric vascular injury in rodents.

Enterochromaffin-like (ECL) cell proliferation in rodents is caused by certain compound classes that reduce acid secretion from parietal cells, such as histamine ($H_2$) blockers (*e.g.* ranitidine) and proton pump inhibitors (*e.g.* omeprazole). The resulting compensatory hypergastrinaemia stimulates ECL cell proliferation and, if treatment is prolonged, carcinoid tumour development. ECL cells are not easily distinguished on H&E sections but can be identified by silver stains such as Grimelius' method, or by immunohistochemical staining for neuron-specific enolase or chromogranin A (Fig. 4.28). Electron microscopy reveals characteristic electron-dense granules containing peptides in the cell cytoplasm ECL proliferation and tumours with.

Adenomas occasionally occur as spontaneous tumours in rodents. They are usually polypoid or sessile and moderately differentiated, consisting of proliferating glands (Fig. 4.29). Induction of gastric adenocarcinomas in laboratory animals, notably rodents, with diethylnitrosamine (DEN) and N-nitrosamine compounds is well documented. Irradiation and opioids are also known to induce these tumours. Epidemiologic surveys have also linked nitrosamines with these tumours in humans. *Helicobacter pylori* infection is strongly associated with gastric carcinomas in humans but not with spontaneous tumours in animals. Animal models of gastric carcinoma use *Helicobacter* species as well as carcinogens to induce tumours, with the Mongolian gerbil considered the closest model [47].

Morphologically, gastric adenocarcinomas may vary from well-differentiated types with tubular or papillary features to those with signet ring or trabecular patterns. Penetration through the submucosa is generally accepted as proof of malignancy for these tumours, without penetration of the serosa.

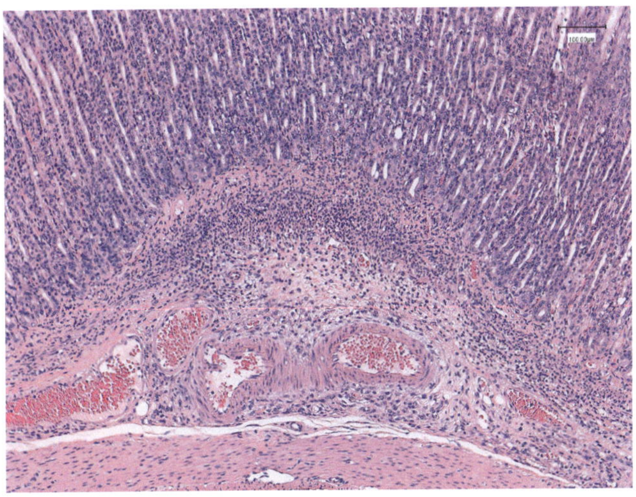

**Figure 4-27.** Arteritis of the submucosal blood vessels in a rat stomach. Mild adventitial thickening and lymphocytic infiltration are seen around a submucosal artery. The lamina propria is markedly infiltrated by granulocytes. Arteritis can be secondary to renal disease or may be induced by agents including PDE inhibitors. H&E.

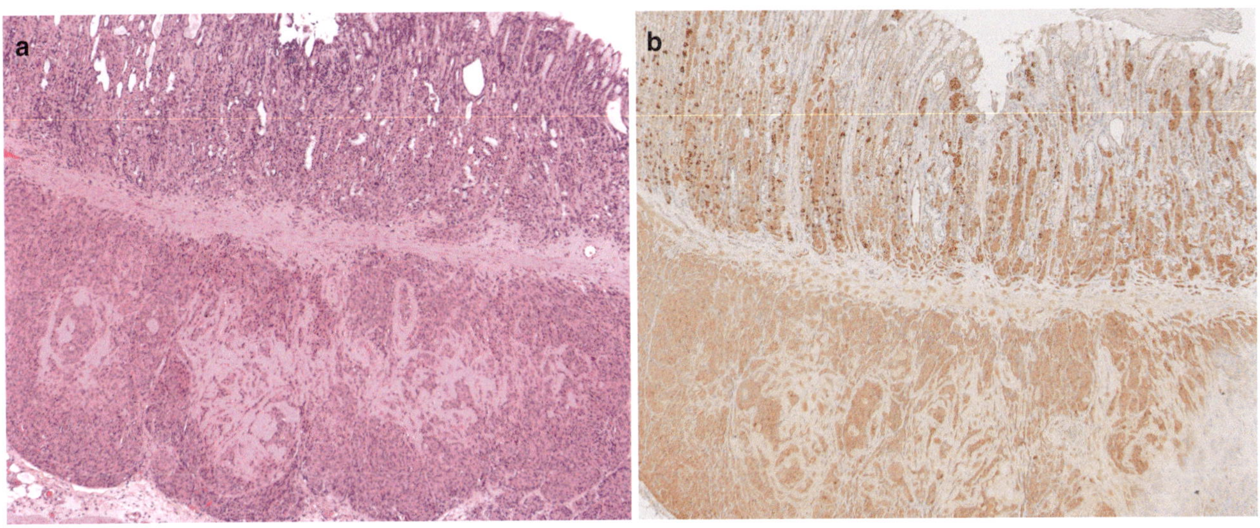



**Figure 4-28.** (**a**) Carcinoid in the stomach of a rat. An infiltrative tumour is present in the mucosa and submucosa. Cells are oval to spindle-shaped with oval nuclei and eosinophilic cytoplasm. H&E. (**b**) Most cells in the carcinoid are positive for chromogranin A. Enterochromaffin-like (ECL) cells are best visualised with chromogranin A staining. These tumours can occur spontaneously but are often associated with histamine and proton pump blockers. Immunohistochemical staining for chromogranin A.

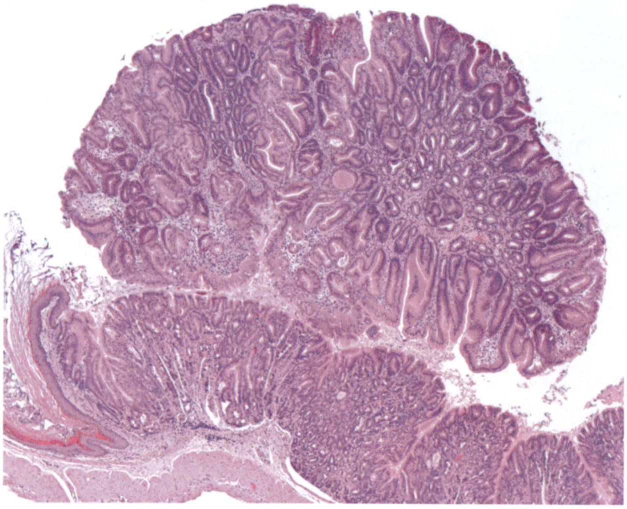

**Figure 4-29.** Adenoma in the glandular stomach of a rat. The tumour appears polypoid and consists of moderately differentiated glands. The stroma is infiltrated by lymphocytes. H&E.

## 4.5 Small Intestines

Many changes are seen in the small intestines:

- Villous atrophy or stunting
- Villous hypertrophy
- Hypertrophy of muscularis
- Villous or mucosal hyperplasia
- Brunner's gland hypertrophy
- Brunner's gland degeneration
- Erosion, ulceration, inflammation
- Storage enteropathies
- Lymphangiectasis
- Adenoma/adenocarcinoma

Villous atrophy or stunting appears histologically as a reduction of size or height of the villi (Fig. 4.30). Fasting in rats causes villous atrophy as a physiological response. Hypophysectomy also induces villous atrophy in rats, with reduced numbers of enterocytes and goblet cells. Villous atrophy as an induced change occurs through increased loss of enterocytes and/or impaired enterocyte replacement. Several classes of compounds cause atrophy or stunting of the villi. Anticancer agents (*e.g.* cis-platinum in mice) and antiviral agents (*e.g.* acyclovir in dogs) induce villous stunting by mitotic inhibition.

Routine loss of enterocytes can be increased through damage by various mechanisms, resulting in degeneration or increased apoptosis. Villous stunting may also accompany chronic inflammation. As an adaptive response in chronic exposure, villous stunting is often accompanied by increased glandular proliferation in the crypt area which results in glandular hyperplasia, as is seen with exposure to the fungicide folpet (Fig. 4.31).

Alternatively, inhibition of mitosis in the crypt cells causes delayed replacement of enterocytes, resulting in reduced height and size of the villi. Increased loss and delayed replacement may be present together with the use of cytostatics and cytotoxics like methotrexate. In mice, cis-platinum and cytosine arabinoside reduce crypt cell production and increase apoptosis. Triparanol in rats produces villous atrophy.

Mucosal hypertrophy and hyperplasia are induced by a number of physiological stimuli and a variety of xenobiotics. The villi, the mucosal glands, or both may be involved. Partial enterectomy, increased feeding, and increased dietary fibre all induce mucosal hyperplasia. The administration of hormones such as thyroxine and growth hormone, EGFs, steroids, and many other agents is associated with mucosal thickening in one or more regions of the intestines. Villous hypertrophy is often noticed as thickening of the affected region at necropsy. Histologically, the villi appear longer and protrude further into the lumen (Fig. 4.32). Epithelial hyperplasia in monkeys can be induced by administration of EGF [8]. Some PDE inhibitors can cause mucosal hyperplasia [16]. Alpha-adrenergic agonists have been associated with intussusception in rats, presumably due to increased peristalsis, without histological changes [20].

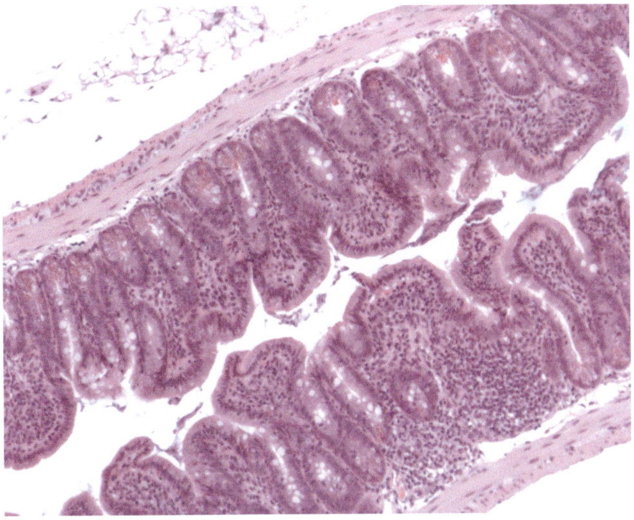

**Figure 4-30.** Villous stunting in the duodenum of a rat. The villi are shorter and thicker than normal. Anticancer agents, antivirals, agrochemicals, and growth factor inhibitors can cause this change. H&E.

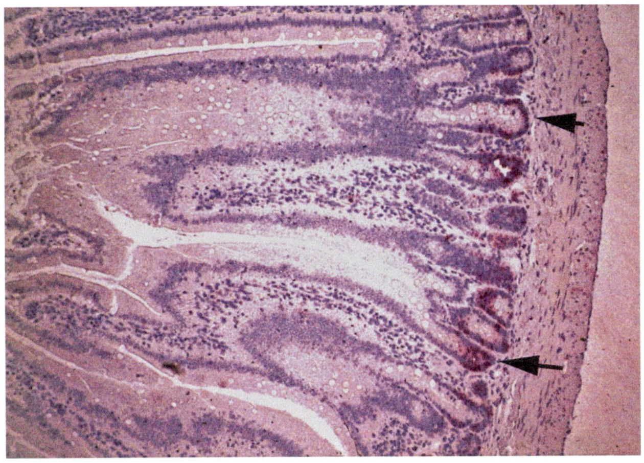

**Figure 4-31.** Glandular epithelial proliferation in a rat. Increased numbers of cells positive for bromo-2'-deoxyuridine (BrdU, a marker for cell proliferation) are seen in the glandular crypts (arrows). H&E. (With kind permission from Springer Science + Business Media B.V [20]).

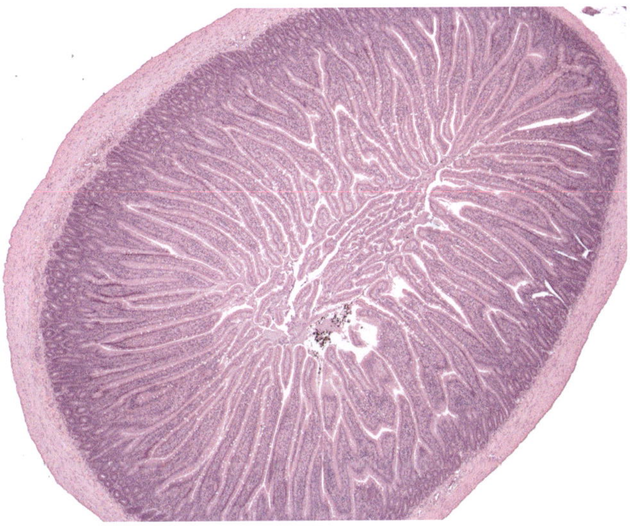

**Figure 4-32.** Villous hypertrophy in the duodenum of a rat. The villi are longer than normal, almost obliterating the lumen and causing the duodenum to appear thickened macroscopically. This change can be physiological or can be induced by several drugs and hormones. H&E.

Smooth muscle hypertrophy resulting in thickening of the muscularis is an unusual intestinal finding (Fig. 4.33). This change can be surgically induced by partial luminal occlusion [48].

Vacuolation of Brunner's glands in the dog has been described with a β-adrenergic receptor blocker, atenolol [17]. Hypertrophy of Brunner's glands in the rat can be induced by novel peptides that act via receptors on these glands. The change manifests as diffuse mild hypertrophy of the Brunner's glands, often detectable only by direct comparison with controls (Fig. 4.34). Necrosis and inflammation of Brunner's glands can be induced by classes of compounds such as growth factor inhibitors (*e.g.* vascular endothelial growth factor [VEGF] inhibitors) because of their antiangiogenic action (Fig. 4.35). However, adenosis of Brunner's glands has also been described in rats given VEGF inhibitors, with extension of hyperplastic Brunner's glands into the muscularis and serosa [49].

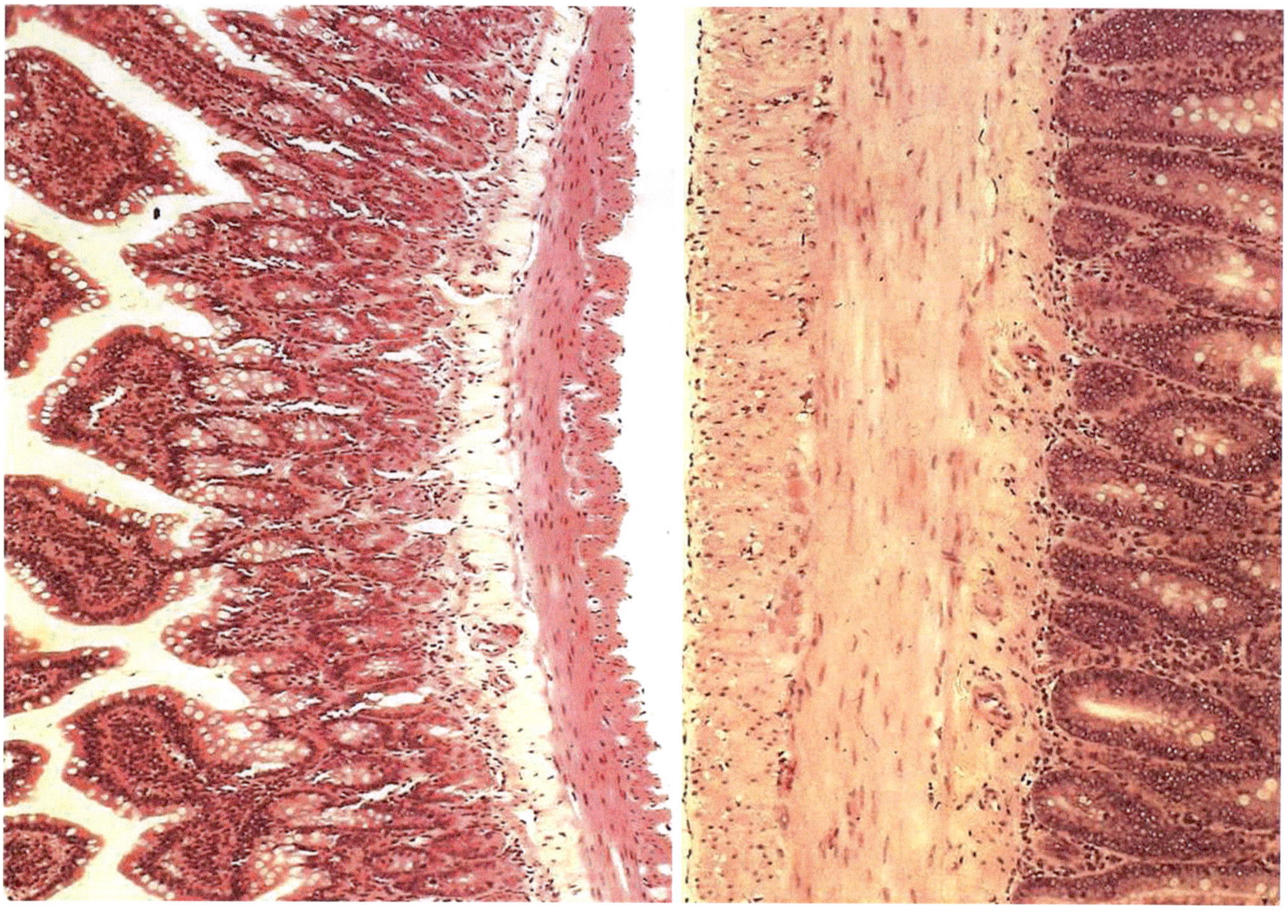

**Figure 4-33.** Hypertrophy of the muscularis in a rat (*right*). A normal jejunum from a control animal is shown on the *left*. Both the concentric and longitudinal muscle layers are markedly thickened in the hypertrophic jejunum. H&E.

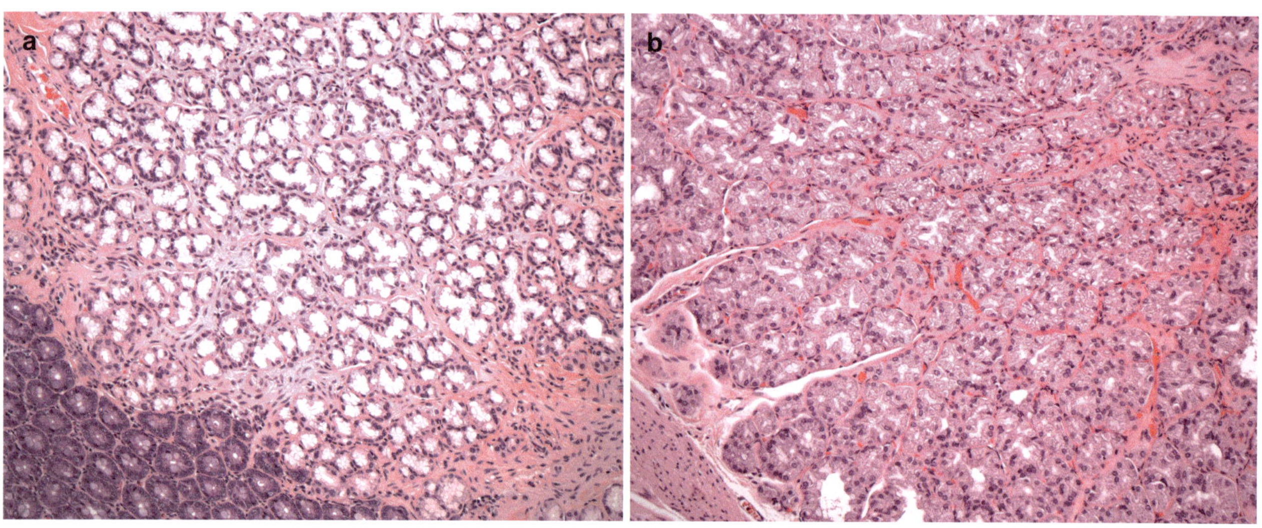


**Figure 4-34.** (**a**) Normal Brunner's glands in a rat. H&E. (**b**) Brunner's gland hypertrophy in a rat. The Brunner's gland cells appear larger and more eosinophilic than those of the control. H&E.

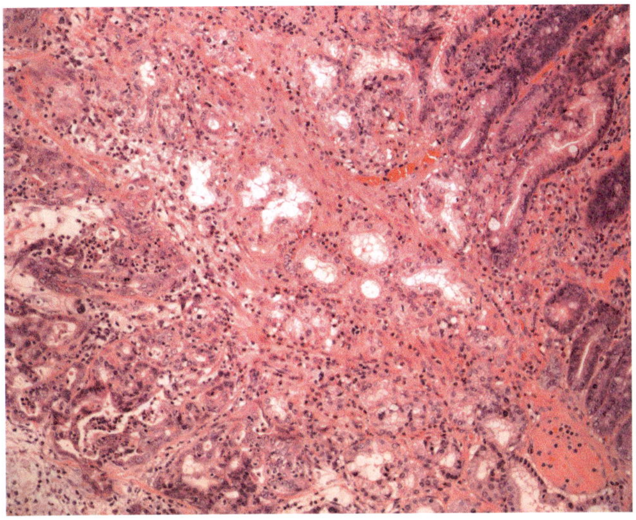

**Figure 4-35.** Degeneration of Brunner's glands in the rat. Degeneration, inflammation, and atrophy of the glands are apparent. Basophilic cells with large nuclei in some glands indicate ongoing regeneration. Growth factor inhibitors can induce this change. H&E.

Erosions and ulceration, accompanied by inflammation, are induced in the small intestines by direct irritation or via absorption and systemic effects. Specific areas of the small intestine are preferentially affected based on physiological variations and the agent's mode of action. For example, EGF receptor inhibitors cause erosions and ulcers of the antroduodenal junction (Fig. 4.36). EGF is produced by the Brunner's glands and plays a role in the repair and healing of duodenal ulcers [50]. This region is susceptible to erosions owing to the overspill of gastric acids. NSAIDs also typically cause lesions in the duodenum. Cysteamine is used in rats to create duodenal ulcer models because of its cytotoxic effects. Cysteamine acts by generating reactive oxygen species and possibly decreasing the defence activity of antioxidative enzymes; its ulcerogenic effect is potentiated by iron overload [51, 52]. Differential expression of cyclooxygenase (COX)-1 and COX-2 receptors in different areas of the ileum explains the localisation of lesions in the distal ileum with COX-2 inhibitors [53].

Storage and accumulation of a variety of orally administered compounds or their products can occur in the villi (Fig. 4.37). Vacuolation due to lipid accumulation is seen with puromycin, antiobesity drugs, and tetracyclines. Lipid droplets are seen within macrophages at the villous tip, sometimes with droplets lying free in the lamina propria after macrophage rupture. Cationic amphiphilic drugs (CADs) such as amiodarone can cause a similar change because of their phospholipidotic effect. This effect is due to their structure, which gives them hydrophobic and hydrophilic properties, coupled with the presence of a cationic amine group. High-fat diets are associated with vacuolation in the absorptive cells of the small intestine. Pigmented test articles of many types can also accumulate in the macrophages within the lamina propria (Fig. 4.38).

Lymphangiectasis in all species results from obstruction of the lymph flow, appearing morphologically as dilated villous lacteals and dilated subcapsular lymphatics in the mesenteric lymph nodes. This condition is considered to result from impaired lipid transport [54]. Dilated lacteals with no histologic changes in the mesenteric lymph nodes have been observed in rats given a novel antihypertensive agent [20]. Dilated lacteals have also been recorded in monkeys given an immunomodulator (Fig. 4.39) [20].

Mesenteric and serosal lipid granulomas due to lymphatic rupture are seen in spontaneous lymphangiectasia, which in dogs is associated with protein-losing enteropathy. Blocked lymphatics in the mesentery sometimes rupture, resulting in lipid granuloma formation.

Focal atypical hyperplasia occasionally occurs as a background finding in mice and can resemble adenomatous polyps. The prevalence of these lesions can be increased by dietary manipulation and by drugs and chemicals. Adenomas and adenocarcinomas of the small intestines are infrequent background findings in rodents.

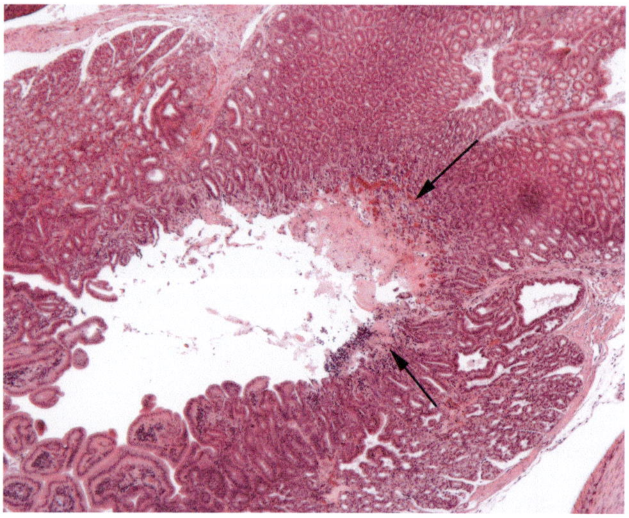

**Figure 4-36.** Mucosal erosion in the duodenum of a rat. The gastroduodenal junction shows focal, superficial necrosis of the duodenal villi and antral mucosa, with eosinophilic material and cell debris (*arrows*). This area is particularly susceptible to ulceration because of acid overspill.

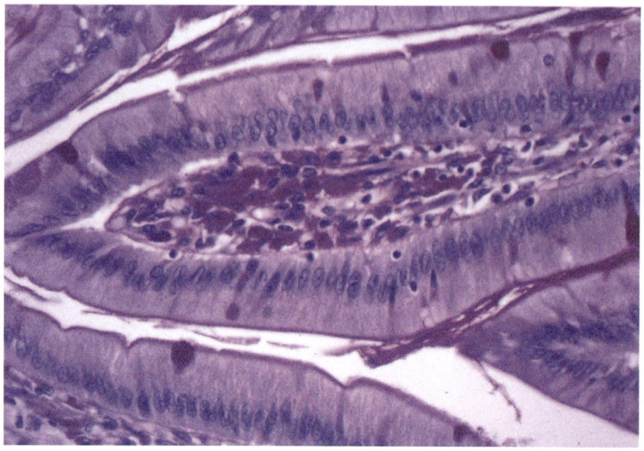

**Figure 4-37.** Histiocytes in the lamina propria of the duodenum from a rat given a plant extract orally. The material has accumulated in histiocytes and stains positively with mucopolysaccharides. No evidence of degenerative change is visible. Periodic acid–Schiff (PAS) stain. (With kind permission from Springer Science + Business Media B.V [20]).

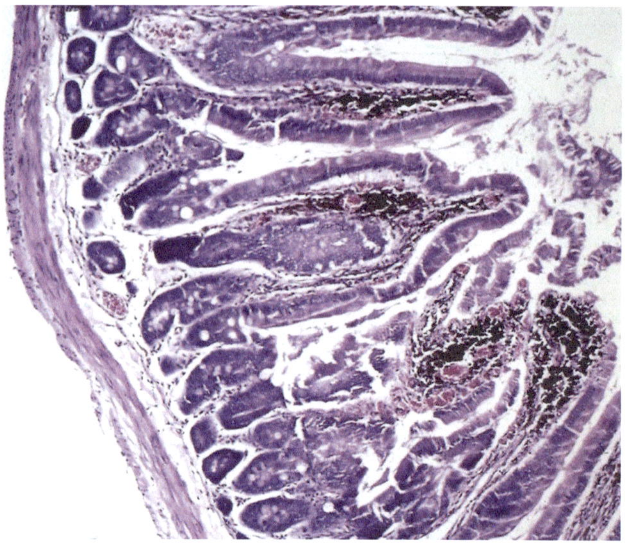

**Figure 4-38.** Pigment accumulation in histiocytes in the lamina propria at the tips of the villi in a rat following oral administration of a hair dye. H&E. (With kind permission from Springer Science + Business Media B.V [20]).

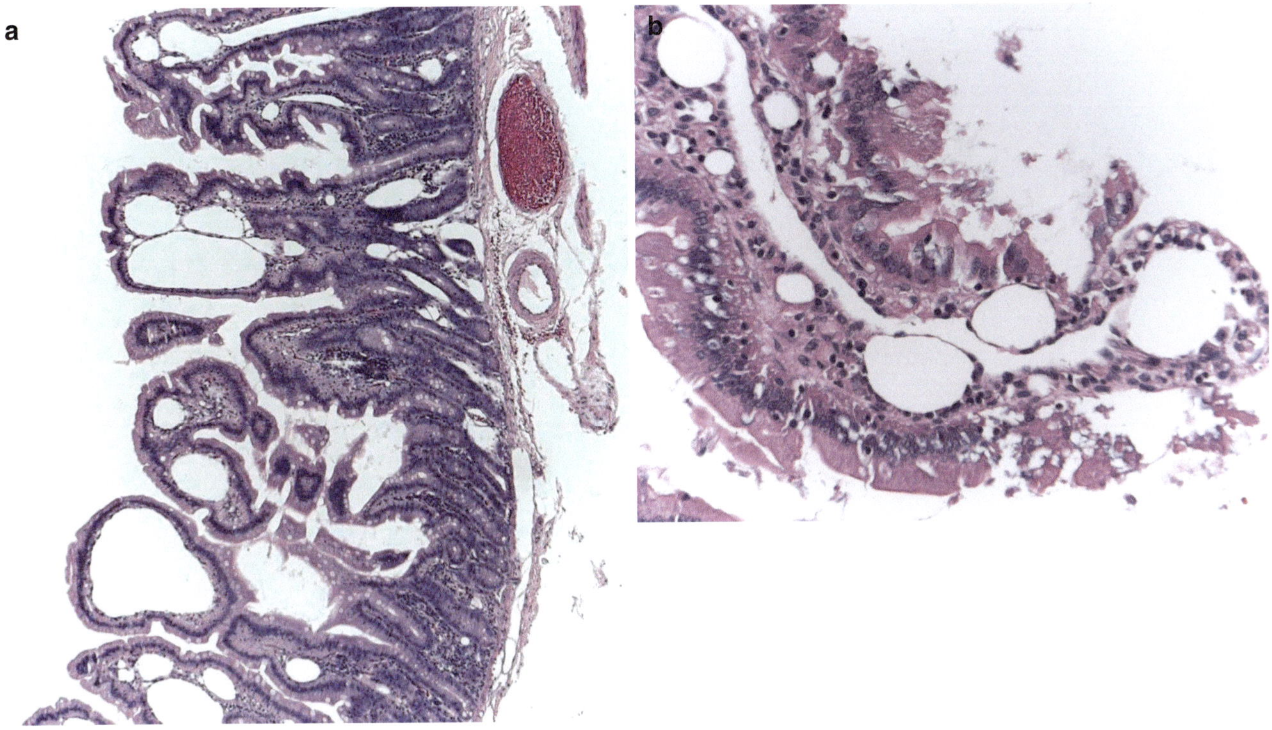

**Figure 4-39.** (**a**) Lymphangiectasia in the duodenum of a monkey given minocycline. Lacteals are markedly dilated at the villous tips. H&E. (**b**) At a higher magnification, it can be seen that the lacteals are markedly dilated, distending the villi, but an inflammatory reaction is not obvious. H&E.

## 4.6 Large Intestines

The range of changes seen in the large intestine is small, as the mucosa has limited responses to xenobiotics. However, the concentration of xenobiotics is higher here than in the small intestine, and transit time is longer, so the exposure potential in the large intestine is high. Species variation is also a factor, with susceptibilities varying between rodents and nonrodents, and between rodent species. Induced changes in the large intestines are listed below:

- Erosion, ulceration, inflammation, necrosis
- Pigment or test material in epithelium and lamina propria
- Mucosal hypertrophy, goblet cell hypertrophy
- Mucosal hyperplasia
- Adenoma or adenocarcinoma

Erosions and ulceration are induced by many classes of drugs and some chemicals, being classically associated with NSAIDs (Figs. 4.40 and 4.41). If changes are ulcerative, perforation followed by peritonitis may occur. Among the antibiotics causing haemorrhagic colitis in hamsters and rabbits are lincomycin and clindamycin. Histologically, haemorrhagic, necrotic typhlitis is seen. Diffuse, severe haemorrhagic necrosis of the caecal mucosa sometimes occurs in control rats on intravenous infusion studies, with no evidence of bacterial infection (Fig. 4.42). This change possibly may be related to stress, although alterations in blood flow also are a possibility.

Administration of carageenans or dextrans results in ulceration, predominantly in the caecum. In the rat, these ulcers can involve the circumference of the intestine, resulting in stricture. Dextran sodium sulphate induces colitis in mice and is widely used as a model of inflammatory bowel disease [55]. Selective p-38 MAPK inhibitors cause mucosal epithelial necrosis and linear haemorrhage of the caecum and colon in the dog, but not in other laboratory species. Histologically, lymphocyte apoptosis and necrosis in the gut-associated lymphoid tissue (GALT) is the earliest and most prominent histopathologic change observed, followed by neutrophilic infiltration and acute inflammation of the lymph nodes and spleen, and multifocal mucosal epithelial necrosis and linear haemorrhages in the colon and caecum [56].

Test materials and pigments can be taken up by the mucosal epithelial cells and by macrophages in the lamina propria, where the macrophages accumulate (Fig. 4.43). Industrial chemicals can accumulate in the lamina propria, eliciting a macrophagic response with foreign-body giant cells (Fig. 4.44).

Hypertrophy and hyperplasia can be seen as adaptive changes in the presence of compounds that change intestinal microflora (*e.g.* antibiotics, sugar alcohols) and with increased fibre and other dietary manipulations. The caecum is particularly sensitive to such alterations and undergoes adaptive enlargement. Prominent caecal enlargement is often detected at necropsy, but it may be associated with no histologic changes or only mild mucosal hypertrophy (Fig. 4.45). Early changes induced by this mechanism will generally reverse once the stimulus is removed.

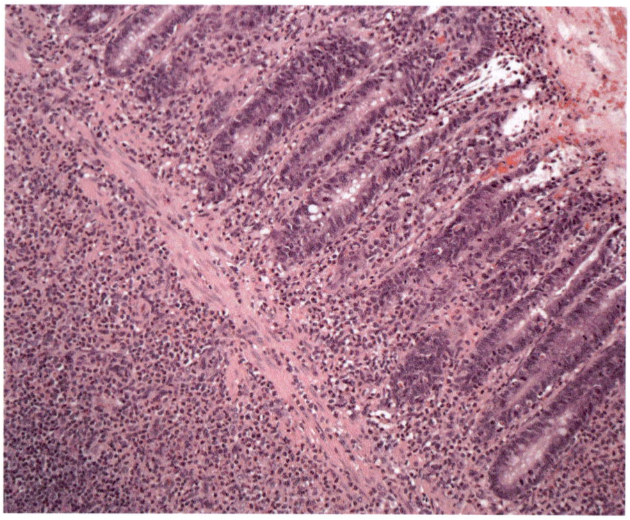

**Figure 4-40.** Inflammation and erosion of the caecum in a mouse. Marked granulocytic infiltration of the mucosa and muscularis is present. The superficial mucosa is eroded, with haemorrhage and inflammatory debris in the lumen. H&E.

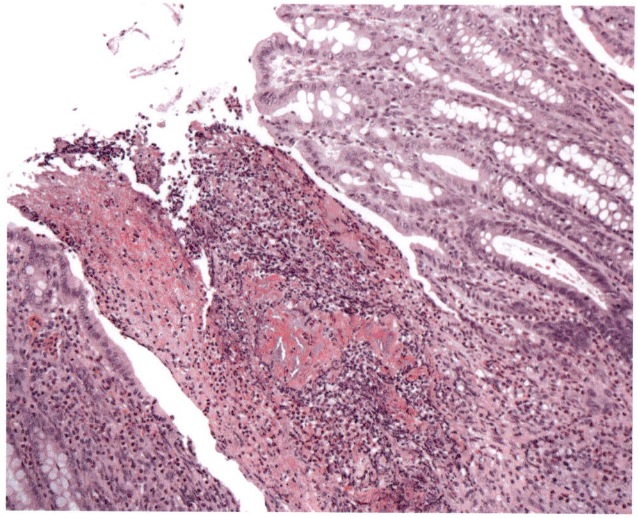

**Figure 4-41.** Focal ulceration of the colonic mucosa in a rat. Localised necrosis of the mucosa is present, with cellular debris and fibrin. H&E.

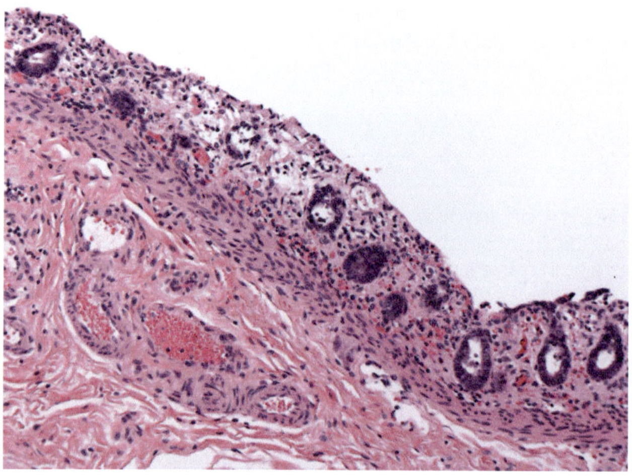

**Figure 4-42.** Necrosis and atrophy of the caecal mucosa. The mucosa is atrophic, with loss of the superficial mucosa. The remainder shows glandular loss, with some glands containing cell debris, with mucosal oedema and inflammation of the stroma. H&E.

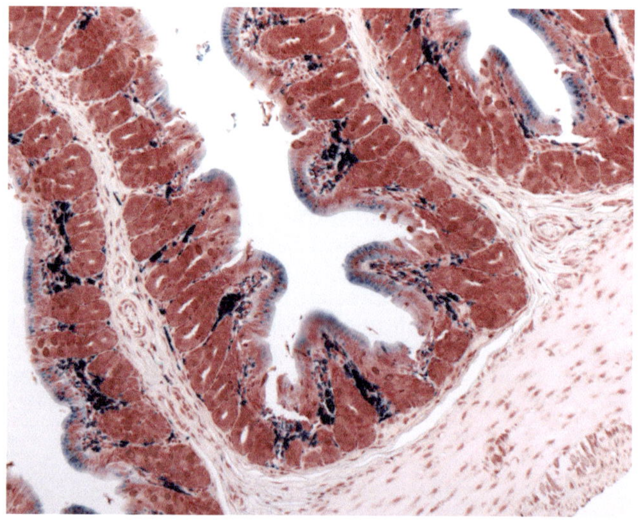

**Figure 4-43.** Iron-containing material in the caecal mucosa of a rat. Iron-containing pigment, staining dark blue with the use of Perls' technique, is present within the enterocytes and within macrophages in the lamina propria. Perls' stain.

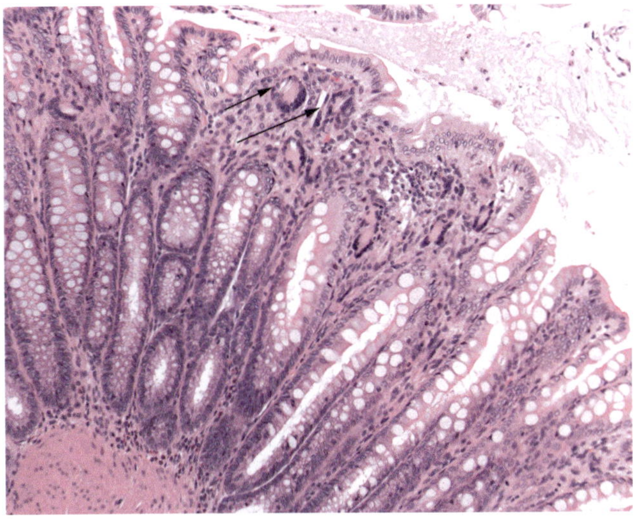

**FIGURE 4-44.** Accumulation enteropathy with foreign-body reaction in the rectum of a rat. Several foreign-body giant cells are present in the lamina propria, some containing crystals (*arrows*). A few crystalline clefts, representing accumulation of the test material, are present in the connective tissue. H&E.

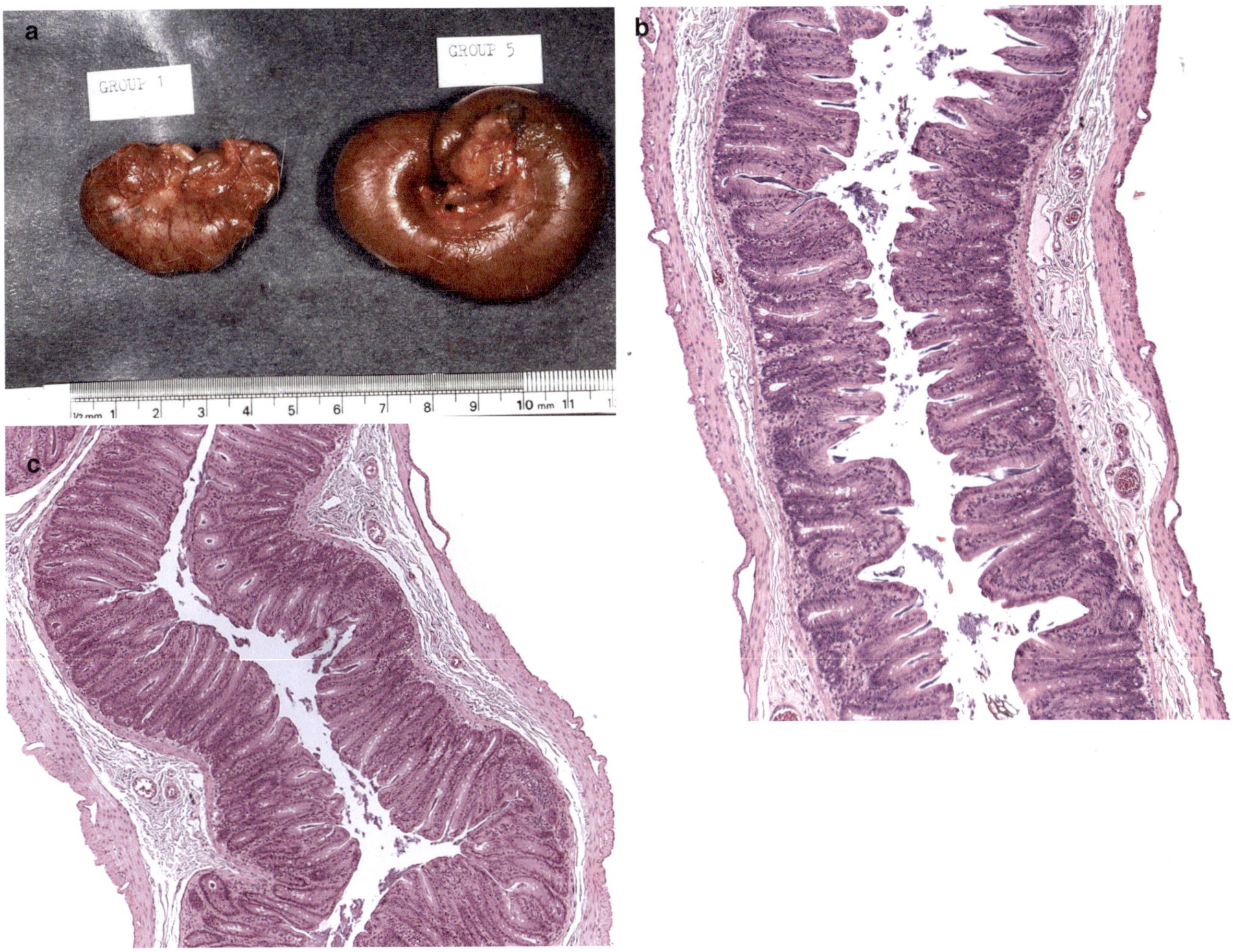


**FIGURE 4-45.** (**a**) Normal and enlarged caeca from a short-term rat study. The treated caecum on the right is markedly larger than the control. This finding does not always have a histologic correlation. (**b**) Normal caecum from a rat. Note the height of the mucosa. H&E. (**c**) Caecal hypertrophy in a rat. The caecal mucosa appears much thicker than the control mucosa, with diffuse hypertrophy of the epithelial cells. Alteration of caecal flora can result in this adaptive response. H&E.

Mucosal hyperplasia of the colon and caecum has been recorded with a phosphodiesterase inhibitor [16]. Bile salts and acids damage colonic epithelium, possibly through alterations in sphingomyelinase activity, causing inflammation, oedema, and necrosis. The result is increased mitotic activity and epithelial hyperplasia, with the bile salts thus promoting the development of colon carcinoma [20, 57].

Numerous experimental models of inflammatory bowel disease are used, although none are ideal. In cotton-top tamarins, the condition is spontaneous. Dextran sodium sulphate is widely used to induce this syndrome in rodents and results in crypt loss, ulceration, inflammation, epithelial hyperplasia, and dysplasia (Fig. 4.46). A number of transgenic or knockout mice with specific genes that target inflammatory mediators are also used as models.

Administration of high doses of carageenans or dextrans is associated with the formation of polypoid adenomas and adenocarcinomas in the distal colon and rectum. With carageenans, the mechanism of tumorigenesis is unclear. Changes in bacterial flora, tumour initiation, tumour promotion, and increased cell proliferation secondary to inflammation and degenerative changes have all been suggested. Known carcinogens like 1,2-dimethylhydrazine and azoxymethane induce atypical hyperplasias and intestinal tumours. Non-oral routes of administration can also result in intestinal tumours; for example, chronic inhalation studies with 1-bromopropane have demonstrated an increase in adenomas in rats [58].

Adenomas may be sessile, polypoid, or localised and consist of proliferating tubular glands without invasion of the basement membrane. Varying degrees of dysplasia, atypia, and pseudostratification may be present (Fig. 4.47).

Adenomas and adenocarcinomas of the large intestines in laboratory species are of particular interest because of their significance in humans. In mice, metal-containing compounds administered orally over long periods have been associated with marked inflammation, mild focal mucosal hyperplasia, and the formation of diverticula in the caecum and colon. The diverticula appear to become blocked and develop into large, cystlike structures that are often multiloculated, contain mucus, and are lined by flattened or atrophic epithelium. Glandular hyperplasia and dysplasia are not characteristic features but may be seen occasionally. In many cases, these cystic lesions expand and penetrate between the muscularis fibres into the peritoneal cavity, although invasion of the cavity and metastasis to other abdominal organs generally does not follow (Fig. 4.48). This continuum of lesions does not include polypoid hyperplasia and adenomas, and the difference between cystic hyperplasia and carcinomas is often not clear-cut, being based on penetration of the muscularis rather than on the morphology of the lesions. Induction of these lesions is often specific to the mouse; other laboratory species do not develop similar lesions with these compounds. Based on the lack of metastases, and the mouse specific-nature of the lesions, they are now considered to be diverticula rather than adenocarcinomas.

The role of inflammatory factors, bacteria, and other agents in the development of colon tumours in various species (including humans) has been extensively studied. In humans and many other species, inflammatory factors play a major role in tumour development. Administration of antitumor necrosis factor (TNF) $\alpha$, interleukin (IL)-10, or $T_{reg}$ factors has been found to cause remission of colon cancer in mice, highlighting the importance of these cytokines in the development of large intestinal tumours [59].

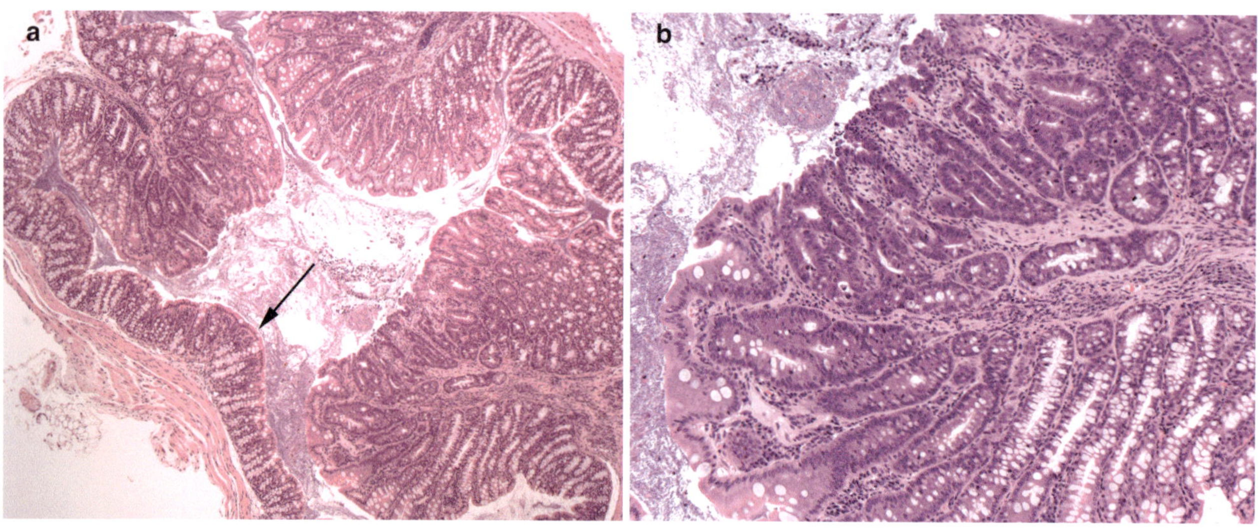


**Figure 4-46.** (**a**) Mucosal hyperplasia in a mouse colon. The mucosa on the left is normal (*arrow*). The colonic mucosa on the right is thickened, with loss of normal mucosal architecture, and hypertrophy and hyperplasia of the mucosal cells. H&E. (**b**) The colon of the same animal seen at a higher magnification shows focal regenerative hyperplasia, comprising several basophilic glands with lymphoplasmacytic infiltration of the stroma. The mucosal surface is focally irregular, probably indicating a healed erosion. H&E.

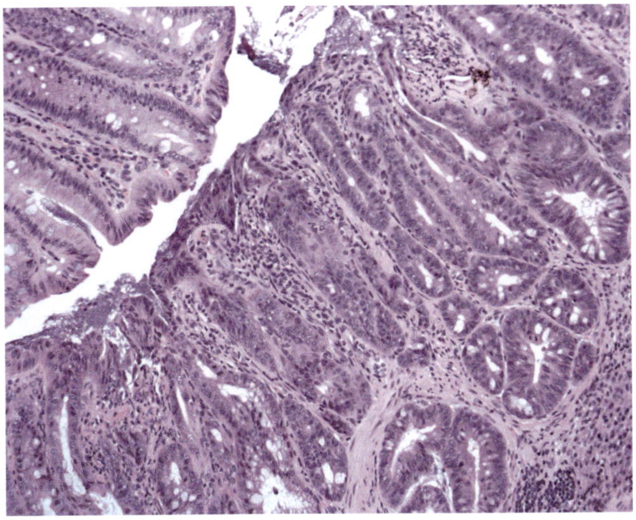

**FIGURE 4-47.** Caecal adenoma in a mouse. Glandular proliferation, disorganisation, and loss of architecture are evident, with lymphoplasmacytic infiltration of the stroma. Mild dysplasia, layering of epithelium, and several mitoses are characteristics of this lesion. H&E.

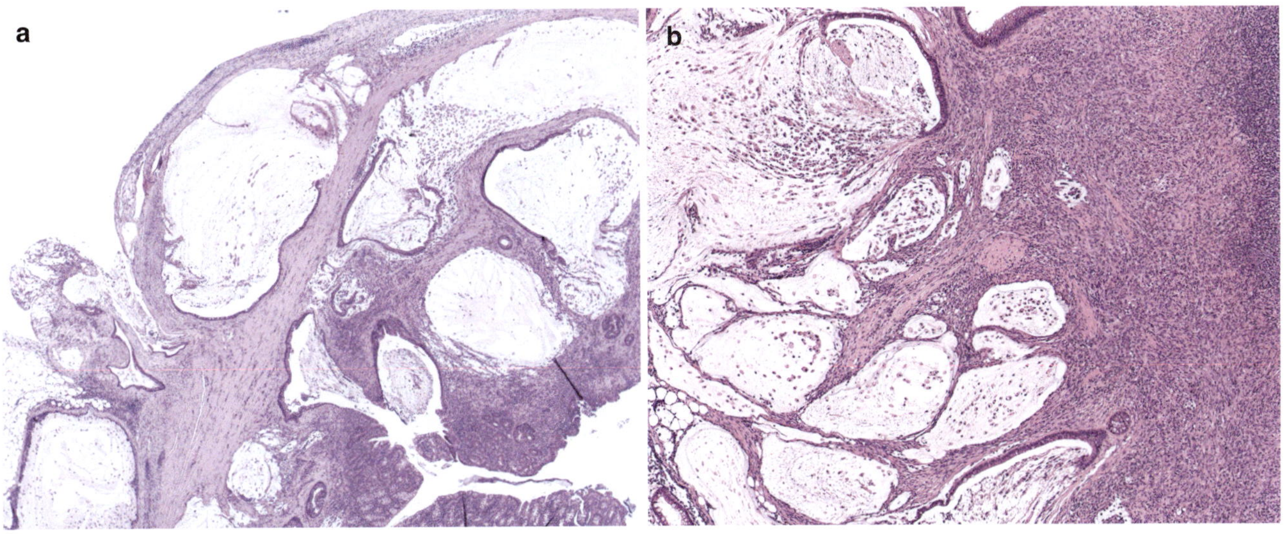

**FIGURE 4-48.** (**a**) Colonic lesion in a mouse. The tumour consists predominantly of large, mucus-containing cystic structures that have penetrated the muscularis and are invading the abdominal cavity. The tumour is poorly cellular, and the glands are generally well differentiated. H&E. (**b**) Higher magnification shows that the epithelium lining these cysts is cuboidal in some areas, but is often completely absent. The cysts contain mucus and cell debris. Marked chronic inflammation of the muscularis is present. H&E.

## 4.7 The Exocrine Pancreas

The pancreas is a compact gland in humans, nonhuman primates, hamsters, and dogs; it is mesenteric (multifocal) in rats, mice, and rabbits. Toxicologic changes in different species are to some extent influenced by anatomical and physiological variations. The pancreatic duct opens into the common bile duct in rats and mice, while it opens directly into the duodenum in humans, dogs, and rabbits. In dogs and primates, efferent blood vessels from the islets of Langerhans supply most of the exocrine pancreas, regulating its function. In rats, more of the blood supply to the acini is direct.

The pancreatic acinar unit is a tubuloalveolar structure consisting of a single layer of pyramidal cells with luminal microvilli. A flat epithelial cell, the centriacinar cell, lines the lumen of the acinus and forms a continuum with the intercalating duct.

Cholecystokinin (CCK), gastrin, prolactin, somatotropin, corticosteroids, and thyroxine are trophic to acinar cells. Vascular endothelium regulates pancreatic growth, so disturbances in blood supply cause aberrant growth.

Lesions of the exocrine pancreas are rare but can be induced by direct and indirect mechanisms, as drug-metabolising enzymes are present in the exocrine pancreas. There are various types of induced pancreatic acinar lesions:

- Degranulation
- Degeneration
- Atrophy

- Apoptosis
- Necrosis
- Pancreatitis
- Basophilic and hypertrophic foci
- Hyperplasia
- Hepatic metaplasia
- Adenoma or adenocarcinoma
- Nesidioblastosis

Degranulation of acinar cells occurs in a variety of pathologic conditions and also can be induced as a primary or secondary change. The loss of cytoplasmic apical zymogen granules makes the affected cells smaller and more basophilic (Figs. 4.49 and 4.50). Acinar cells can lose their granularity because of stress, fasting, poor general condition, or treatment with agents such as furosemide [60]. Protein deprivation and copper deficiency also induce loss of granularity. A variety of hormonal alterations, including hypophysectomy and administration of glucagon, induce the loss of zymogen granules. If exposure is prolonged, normal levels of apoptosis can increase or acinar atrophy can develop. Degranulation and apoptosis are associated with sunitinib, a tyrosine kinase inhibitor [5].

Acinar atrophy occurs spontaneously in rodents, especially older animals, or it can be induced by treatment. Affected cells and acini are smaller, appear basophilic, and are reduced in numbers. Fibrosis, inflammation, and duct proliferation can accompany acinar loss in rats. The change can affect isolated lobules or can appear more diffuse (Fig. 4.51). In advanced cases in mice and dogs, lobules can disappear and be replaced by diffuse adipose tissue (Fig. 4.52). In extreme cases, only islets, vasculature, and a few ductules may remain. In dogs, pancreatic atrophy is accompanied by clinical insufficiency. Atrophy can be induced by hypophysectomy, starvation, protein depletion, ethionine, and induced copper deficiency [61, 62]. Gatifloxacin, a fluoroquinolone antibiotic, induces atrophy in dogs and cynomolgus monkeys.

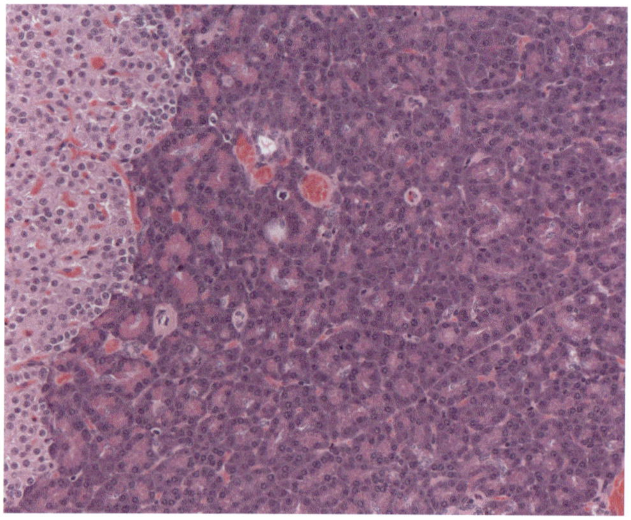

**Figure 4-49.** Degranulation of pancreatic acini in a rat treated with a novel pharmaceutical agent. The affected acinar cells appear basophilic owing to the loss of zymogen granules. H&E.

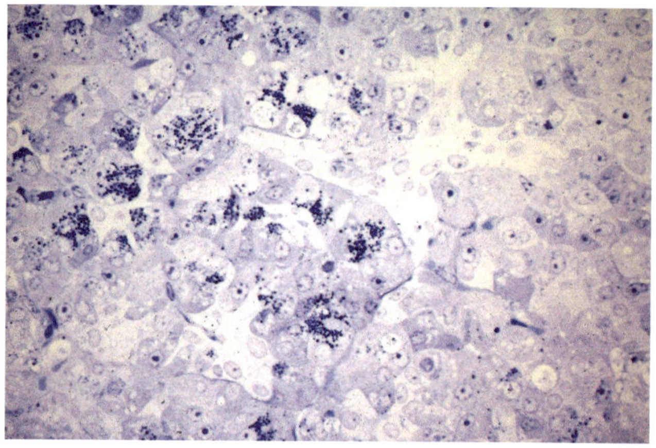

**Figure 4-50.** Pancreas from a rat showing acinar degranulation and occasional apoptotic cells. Blue-stained zymogen granules are present in only a few acinar cells. 1 μ section. Toluidine blue (With kind permission from Springer Science+Business Media B.V [20]).

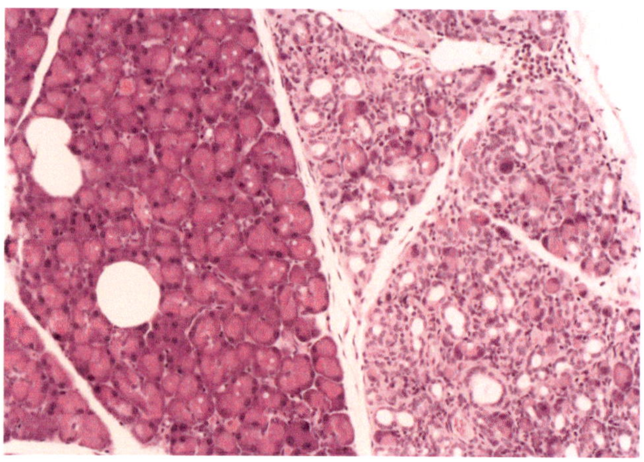

**Figure 4-51.** Focal acinar atrophy in a rat. The lobule on the right shows loss of acinar cells, with an apparent increase in ducts and interstitial cell infiltration. The lobule on the left appears normal. H&E.

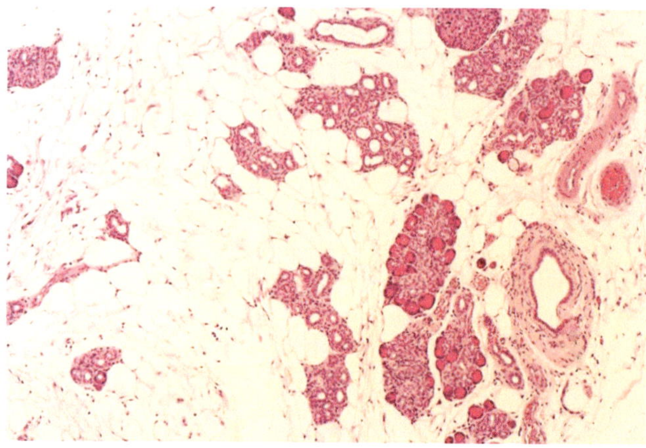

**Figure 4-52.** Diffuse acinar atrophy in the pancreas of a mouse. Acinar cells are lost, replaced by interstitial adipose tissue, with preservation of ducts and islets. H&E.

Apoptosis occurs spontaneously at a low rate in dogs and rodents. Apoptotic cells appear as shrunken, ovoid, eosinophilic bodies with dark nuclear fragments situated intracytoplasmically (Fig. 4.53). With electron microscopy, they appear as membrane-bound aggregates of organelles and fragmented nuclear remnants (Fig. 4.54). The rate of apoptosis can be enhanced by treatment with certain xenobiotics.

Acinar cell vacuolation has been reported in animals treated with cyclosporin A, caerulein, and puromycin [63]. Cytoplasmic vacuolation can occur due to lipid accumulation, as in treatment with ethionine or ethyl alcohol (Figs. 4.55 and 4.56). Zinc deficiency leads to degenerative vacuolation as a result of lipid accumulation and prominence of lysosomes. Certain fungicides have produced similar lesions [20]. Some acinar vacuolation is due to autophagy [64]. Puromycin treatment causes acinar vacuolation through autophagic changes, with lysosomes containing groups of degenerating organelles (Fig. 4.57). Vacuoles appear translucent.

Systemic phospholipidosis also causes vacuolation of acinar cells. In such instances, the presence of multilamellatar inclusions is confirmatory for phospholipidosis. A type of interstitial vacuolation has been observed in monkeys treated with a novel antibiotic in our laboratories, with vacuolated macrophages accumulating in the interstitium. The vacuolation appeared to be due to a storage phenomenon, as similar vacuoles also were present in phagocytic cells elsewhere [20].

Pancreatic necrosis occurs as single-cell, focal, or more diffuse to extensive haemorrhagic necrosis with inflammation and fat necrosis (Fig. 4.58). Lesions pass quickly though the stage of coagulative necrosis to liquefaction because of the high content of hydrolytic enzymes. Escaping enzymes digest the surrounding lipocytes, resulting in fat necrosis. Haemorrhagic necrosis is seldom seen in rats but does occur in dogs and mice. Intraperitoneal injection of 4-hydroxyaminoquinoline-1-oxide (4-HAQO) or puromycin results in necrosis. Mice fed on choline-deficient diets and D-ethionine develop haemorrhagic necrosis. Ethionine toxicity in rats is more severe in females and is potentiated in males by the administration of oestrogen. Azaserine, aflatoxin, actinomycin D, ethanol, and copper deficiency all induce pancreatic damage. Sodium taurocholate induces acute pancreatitis, indicating a possible role for bile in the pathogenesis of this syndrome [65].

When the oral administration of ethanol is accompanied by a high-fat diet, the result is a spectrum of lesions that include hypogranulation, fat necrosis, mononuclear cell infiltration, fibrosis, acinar atrophy, ductal dilatation, and intraductal mucus or proteinaceous plugs [66]. Azathioprine, furosemide, methyldopa and rifamycin damage pancreatic acini (Fig. 4.59). Pancreatic necrosis is generally followed by inflammation and fibrosis, sometimes with duct hyperplasia (Fig. 4.60). Manganese treatment in rats results in pancreatitis. Caerulein and glucagon also produce pancreatitis in rodents [67]. Serum amylase and lipase are useful for monitoring pancreatic damage.

Hypertrophy of acinar cells around the islets is a spontaneous finding in several laboratory species, possibly owing to a higher blood supply in peri-islet areas. Hypertrophic peri-islet cells are usually more eosinophilic than the rest of the parenchyma, with more zymogen granules and a different enzymatic content than the surrounding acini (Fig. 4.61).

Basophilic foci of the pancreas can be spontaneous or induced [68]. The incidence of spontaneous basophilic foci increases with age. Focal hypertrophy of the acini is induced by treatment with azaserine and 4-HAQO, with the affected groups of acinar cells appearing hypertrophic and more basophilic (Fig. 4.62). This change represents a focal reduction in zymogen granules, sometimes accompanied by an increase in rough endoplasmic reticulum or enlarged parabasal nuclei.

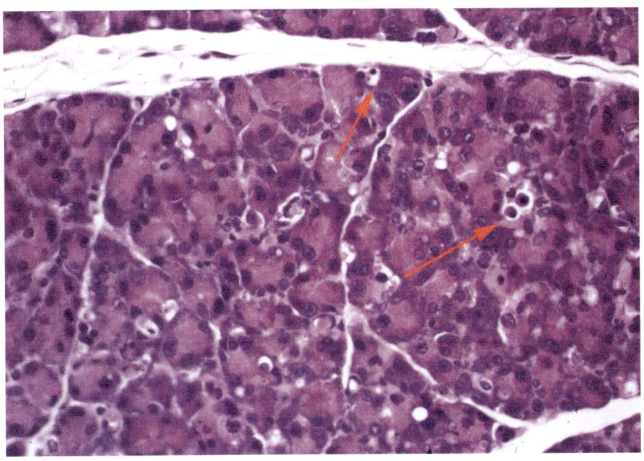

**Figure 4-53.** Pancreas showing apoptosis of acinar cells induced in a rat following inhalation of an industrial chemical. The apoptotic cells appear as rounded eosinophilic bodies with basophilic nuclear fragments (*arrows*). H&E.

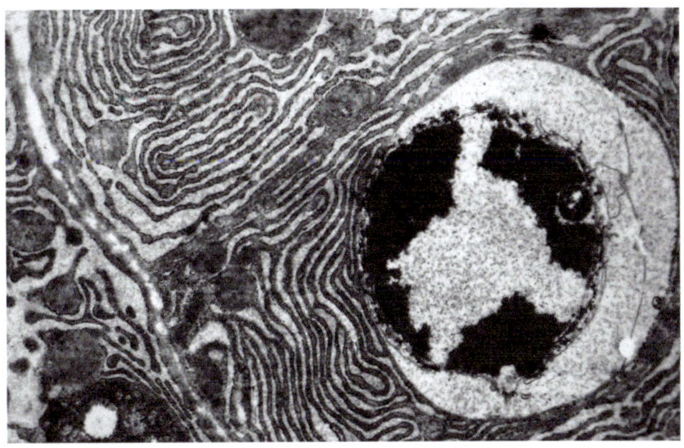

**Figure 4-54.** Apoptosis in the pancreas of a monkey. An apoptotic inclusion within the cytoplasm of an acinar cell. Transmission electron micrograph (With kind permission from Springer Science+Business Media B.V [20]).

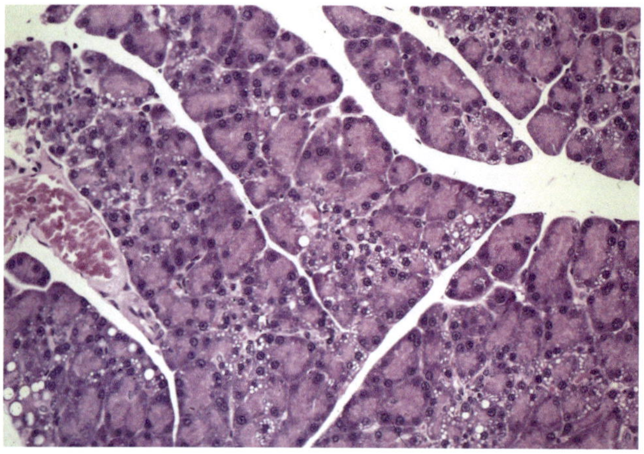

**Figure 4-55.** Fatty change characterised by fine vacuolation in acinar cells of a rat treated with a novel fungicide. The affected cells contain few zymogen granules. Other acinar cells appear unaffected. H&E. (With kind permission from Springer Science + Business Media B.V [20]).

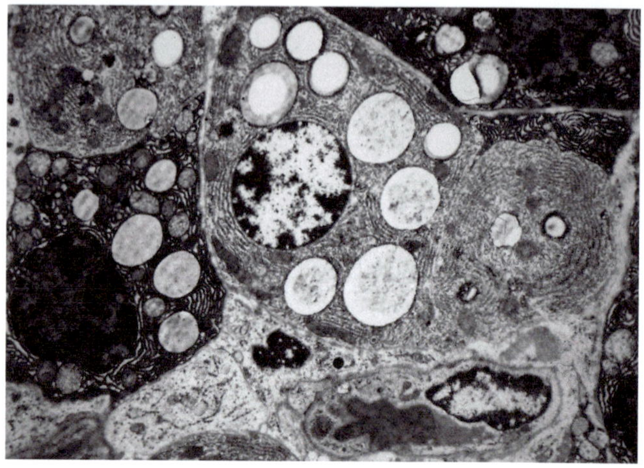

**Figure 4-56.** Fat droplets in rat pancreatic acinar cells, from the same study as Fig. 4.55. Note absence of zymogen granules. Transmission electron micrograph. (With kind permission from Springer Science + Business Media B.V [20]).

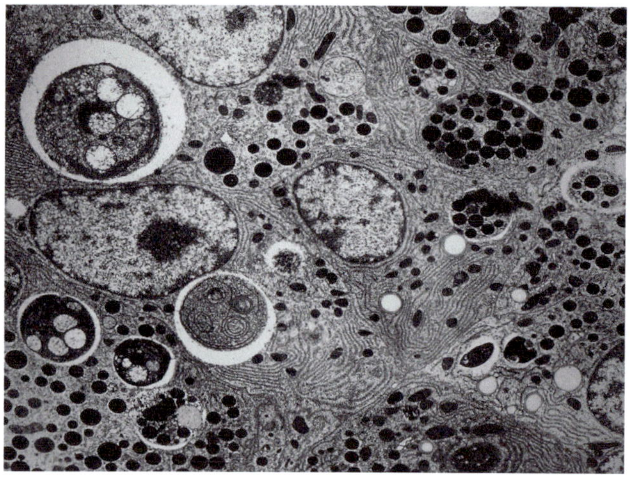

**Figure 4-57.** Intracytoplasmic lysosomal inclusions in acinar cells of the pancreas of a rat. Organelles are bound by lysosomal membranes. Electron micrograph.

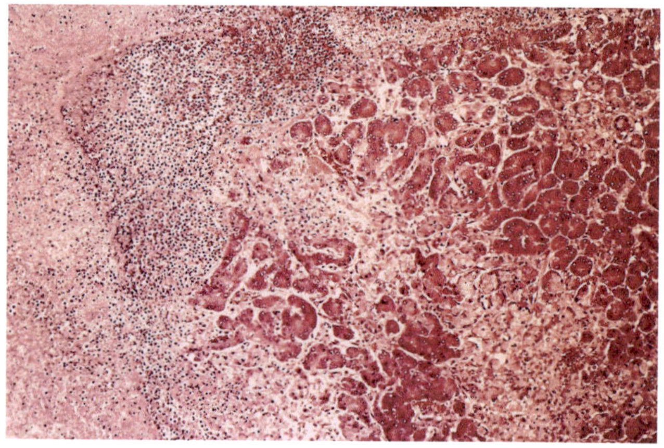

**Figure 4-58.** Necrotising pancreatitis in a dog. The marked liquefactive necrosis appears with inflammation and degenerating acini. H&E.

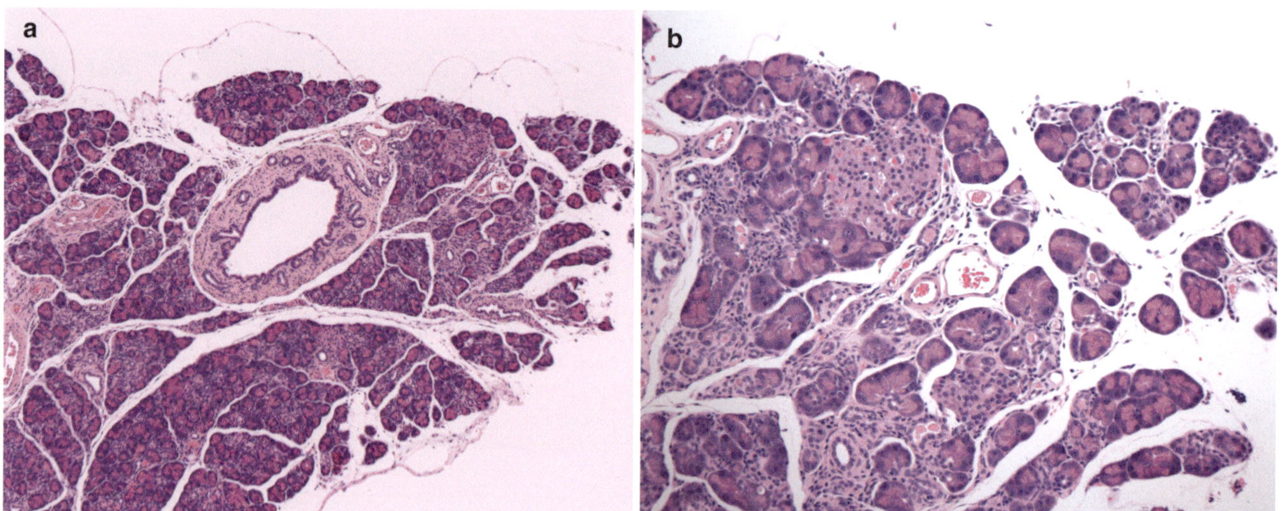


**Figure 4-59.** (**a**) Chronic pancreatitis in a rat given an industrial chemical; shown are a patchy loss of acini with interstitial inflammation and fibrosis. H&E. (**b**) At a higher magnification, degeneration and loss of acini, interstitial fibrosis, and inflammation can be seen. Islets are unaffected. H&E.

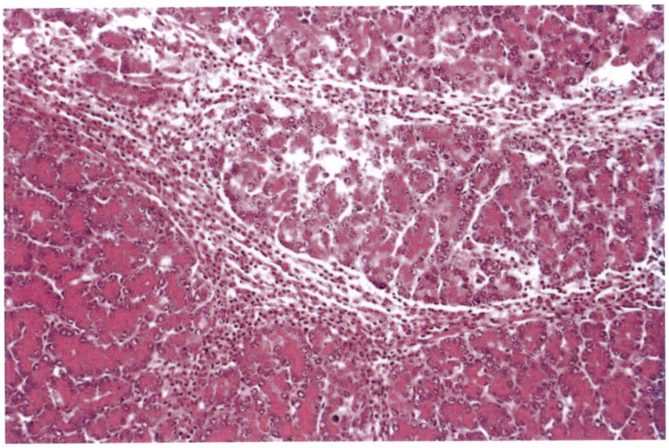

**Figure 4-60.** Pancreatitis in a monkey treated with a novel pharmaceutical agent, featuring a focal loss of acini with interstitial fibrosis and inflammation. H&E.

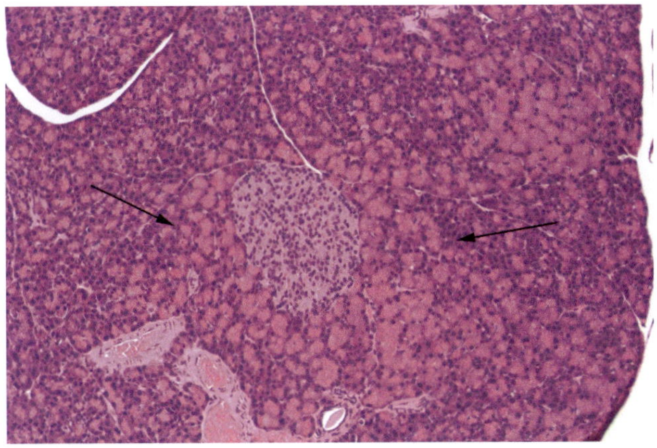

**Figure 4-61.** Eosinophilic, hypertrophic peri-islet acinar cells in a rat (*arrows*). These cells contain increased zymogen and altered enzyme profiles attributable to local factors including insulin and a higher blood supply. This finding is normal in several species. H&E.

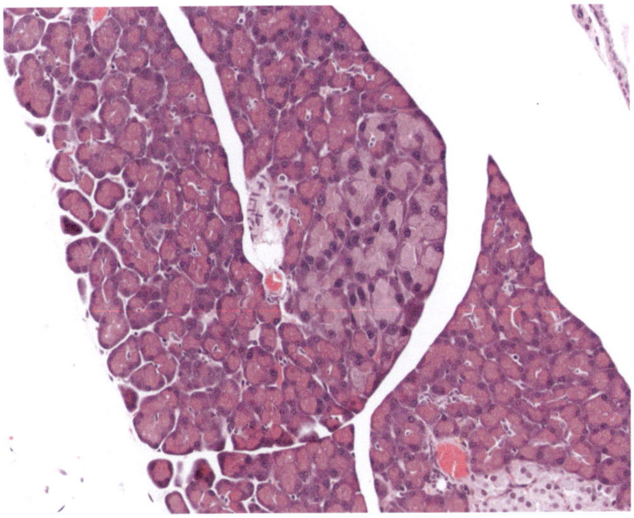

**Figure 4-62.** Basophilic acinar focus in a rat. Such a focus of enlarged basophilic cells is a common spontaneous finding in older rats but can also be induced by drugs and chemicals. H&E.

Pancreatic hepatocytes occur spontaneously, often around the margins of islets [69]. They are also induced by a protocol of copper depletion and repletion, or by orally or parenterally administered xenobiotics. Hepatocyte-like metaplasia or transdifferentiation of acinar cells to hepatocytes is seen in hamsters treated with N-nitroso*bis*(2-oxopropyl)amine and in rats treated with 2,6-dichloro-p-phenylenediamine [70, 71]. Hypolipidaemic agents such as ciprofibrate, a peroxisome proliferator-activated receptor (PPAR)α agonist, also induce this change in rats [72]. The altered acinar cells are usually located around the islets. They become large and eosinophilic, with the histologic features of hepatocytes, and are positive for liver-specific enzymes by immunohistochemical staining (Fig. 4.63). Cadmium chloride injected subcutaneously results in increased numbers of pancreatic hepatocytes in Fischer and Wistar rats, the altered cells being immunohistochemically positive for albumin and Connexin32, a gap-junction protein seen in hepatocytes [73]. Pancreatic hepatocytes may be associated with atrophic or inflammatory acinar changes.

Treatment of rats with raw soya flour, which contains a trypsin inhibitor, can induce focal hypertrophy and hyperplasia. The resulting overproduction of cholecystokinin (CCK) is trophic to pancreatic acini. Direct administration of CCK or similar synthetic peptides (*e.g.* pentagastrin) also results in acinar growth due to direct stimulation [62].

Eosinophilic foci are composed of hypertrophic cells containing increased numbers of zymogen granules, sometimes with enlarged parabasal nuclei. They are reported to have increased mitotic activity and are probably early focal hyperplastic lesions. Hyperplastic foci appear as distinct groups of acini with increased zymogen granules and a more eosinophilic appearance. The foci retain normal lobular architecture with ductules, but they can cause partial compression of the surrounding parenchyma (Fig. 4.64). Focal hyperplasia is induced by corn oil, CCK, raw soya flour, or carcinogens such as azaserine and 4-HAQO [74, 75].

Acinar-cell adenomas appear as well-demarcated and circumscribed areas of acinar cells causing compression. Loss of lobulation and ducts is seen within these lesions (Fig. 4.65). Adenomas are induced in mice by prolactinogenic agents and in rats by corn oil and soya flour, occurring as a continuum with hyperplasia. PPARα agonists induce acinar tumours, probably due to both PPARα activation in the liver and changes in bile composition and secretion, resulting in increased CCK secretion in the duodenum [76, 77]. Gabapentin, an anticonvulsant, is associated with acinar tumours in male rats [78].

Acinar-cell carcinomas can display different morphological patterns within the same tumour and may display evidence of local invasion. Acinar, ductular, and glandular patterns are noted, sometimes with scirrhous stroma (Fig. 4.66). Ductular patterns are seen in humans and hamsters, whereas rodents display mostly acinar carcinomas. Substances known to induce acinar carcinomas include 7,12-dimethylbenz(a)anthracene (DMBA), azaserine, clofibrate, nafenopin, and soya flour. Mice are resistant to tumours induced by corn oil and soya.

Lesions resembling nesidioblastosis are seen as a spontaneous change in dogs. The affected pancreas shows scattered foci of acinar atrophy and lymphocytic infiltration, along with ductular/endocrine complexes appearing as irregular linear tracts (Figs. 4.67 and 4.68) [79, 80]. A postinflammatory regenerative response is postulated. Considering the small group sizes used in regulatory studies, caution is required in interpreting higher incidences of this change in treated groups.

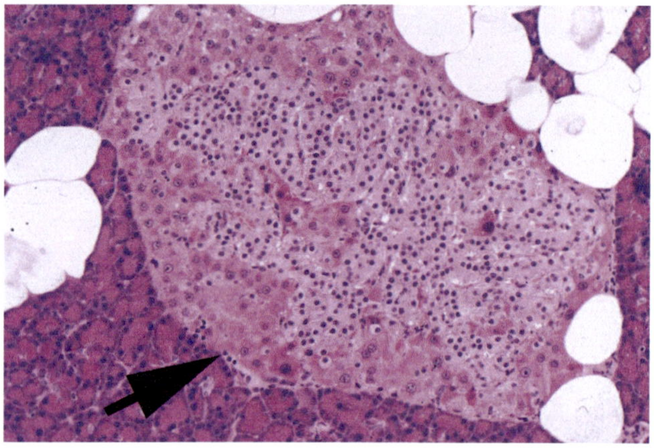

**Figure 4-63.** Hepatocyte-like cells in and around a rat pancreatic islet (*arrow*). The adjacent acinar and islet cells appear unaffected. These cells are believed to arise by transdifferentiation of acinar cells and have been induced in rats by the peroxisome proliferator ciprofibrate. H&E. (With kind permission from Springer Science + Business Media B.V [20]).

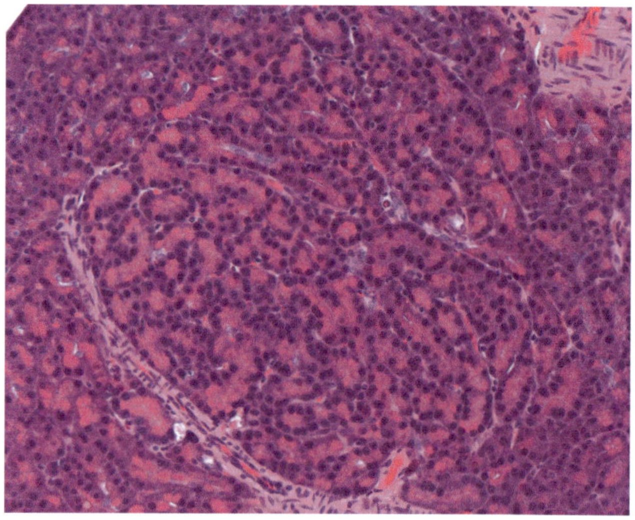

**Figure 4-64.** Acinar hyperplasia in a rat. Hyperplastic cells have a ductular arrangement, and the surrounding parenchyma is slightly compressed. H&E.

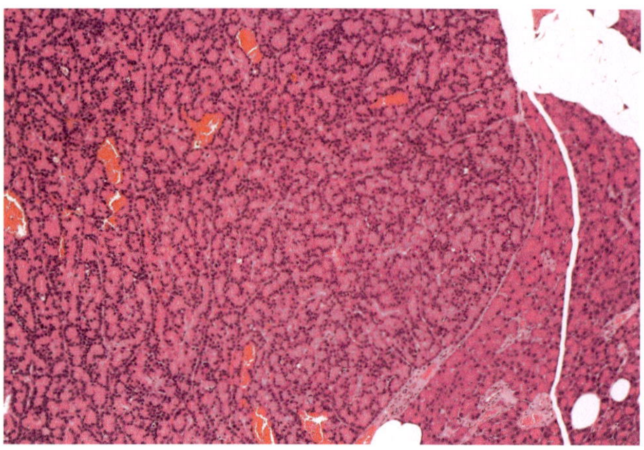

**Figure 4-65.** Adenoma in the exocrine pancreas of a rat. The tumour consists of tubular structures and appears more cellular than the surrounding parenchyma, which is slightly compressed. H&E.

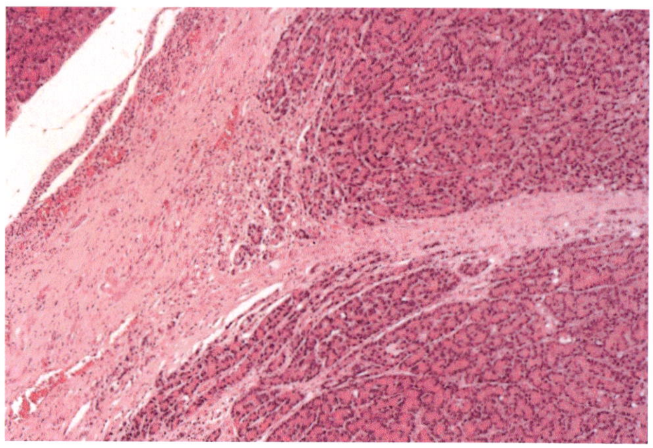

**Figure 4-66.** Carcinoma in the exocrine pancreas of a rat. Neoplastic acinar cells are invading the fibrous capsule. H&E.

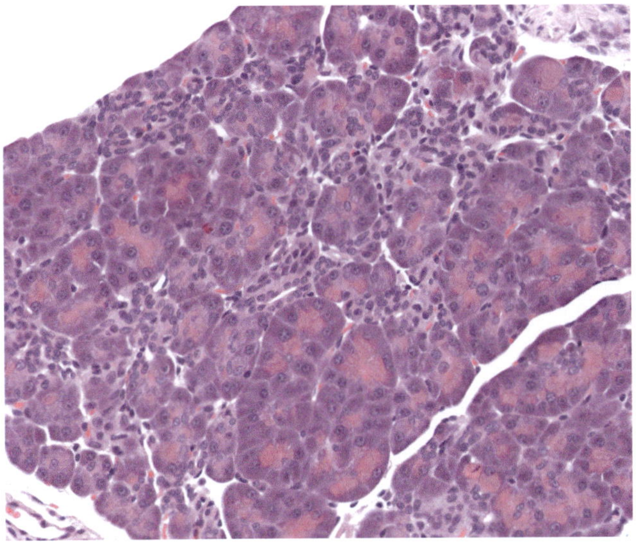

**Figure 4-67.** Nesidioblastosis-like lesion in the pancreas of a dog. Patchy acinar-cell degranulation and degeneration are accompanied by interstitial fibrosis, ductular proliferation, and mononuclear cell infiltration. Extra-islet cell proliferation is not identifiable without immunohistochemistry. H&E.

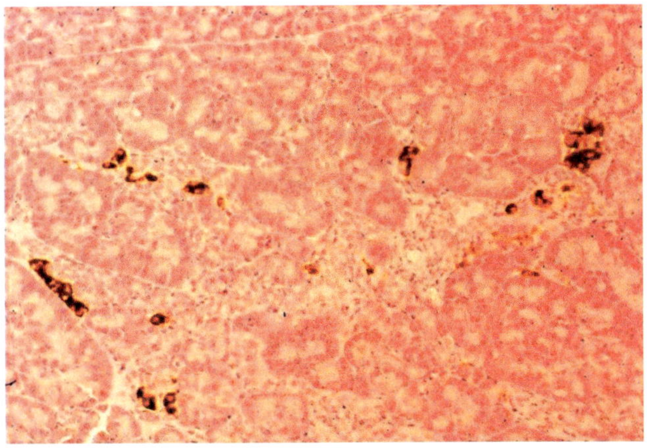

**Figure 4-68.** Immunohistochemical staining for insulin shows a nesidioblastosis-like lesion in the pancreas of a dog. Aggregates of insulin-positive cells of variable sizes are present within the fibrotic areas.

## References


1. Savage NW, Barber MT, Adkins KF. Pigmentary changes in rat oral mucosa following antimalarial therapy. J Oral Pathol. 1986;15:468–71.
2. Olcott CT. Experimental argyrosis; morphologic changes in the experimental animal. Am J Pathol. 1948;24:813–33.
3. Olcott CT. Experimental argyrosis: III. Pigmentation of the eyes of rats following ingestion of silver during long periods of time. Am J Pathol. 1947;23:783–91.
4. Walsh KM, Gough AW. Hypopigmentation in dogs treated with an inhibitor of platelet aggregation. Toxicol Pathol. 1989;17:549–53.
5. Patyna S, Arrigoni C, Terron A, Kim TW, Heward JK, Vonderfecht SL, et al. Nonclinical safety evaluation of sunitinib: a potent inhibitor of VEGF, PDGF, KIT, FLT3, and RET receptors. Toxicol Pathol. 2008;36:905–16.
6. Tryphonas L, Arnold DL, Zawidzka Z, Mes J, Charbonneau S, Wong J. A pilot study in adult rhesus monkeys (M. mulatta) treated with Aroclor 1254 for two years. Toxicol Pathol. 1986;14:1–10.
7. Breider MA, Bleavins MR, Reindel JF, Gough AW, de la Iglesia FA. Cellular hyperplasia in rats following continuous intravenous infusion of recombinant human epidermal growth factor. Vet Pathol. 1996;33:184–94.
8. Reindel JF, Pilcher GD, Gough AW, Haskins JR, de la Iglesia FA. Recombinant human epidermal growth factor1-48-induced structural changes in the digestive tract of cynomolgus monkeys (Macaca fascicularis). Toxicol Pathol. 1996;24:669–80.
9. Ramot Y, Vered M, Malarkey DE, Hooth MJ, Painter JT, Dayan D, et al. Immunohistochemical features of 3,3',4,4'-tetrachloroazobenzene-induced rat gingival lesions. Toxicol Pathol. 2012;40:577–92.
10. Yoshizawa K, Walker NJ, Jokinen MP, Brix AE, Sells DM, Marsh T, et al. Gingival carcinogenicity in female Harlan Sprague-Dawley rats following two-year oral treatment with 2,3,7,8-tetrachlorodibenzo-p-dioxin and dioxin-like compounds. Toxicol Sci. 2005;83:64–77.
11. National Toxicology Program. Toxicology and carcinogenesis studies of a mixture of 2,3,7,8-tetrachlorodibenzo-p-dioxin (TCDD) (CAS No. 1746-01-6), 2,3,4,7,8-pentac hlorodibenzofuran (PeCDF) (CAS No. 57117-31-4), and 3,3',4,4',5-pentachlorobiphenyl (PCB 126) (CAS No. 57465-28-8) in female Harlan Sprague–Dawley rats (gavage studies). Natl Toxicol Program Tech Rep Ser. 2006;(526):1–180.
12. Fletcher AM, Bregman CL, Woicke J, Salcedo TW, Zidell RH, Janke HE, et al. Incisor degeneration in rats induced by vascular endothelial growth factor/fibroblast growth factor receptor tyrosine kinase inhibition. Toxicol Pathol. 2010;38:267–79.
13. Kato A, Suzuki M, Karasawa Y, Sugimoto T, Doi K. PTHrP and PTH/PTHrP receptor 1 expression in odontogenic cells of normal and HHM model rat incisors. Toxicol Pathol. 2005;33:456–64.
14. Kato A, Suzuki M, Karasawa Y, Sugimoto T, Doi K. Histopathological study on the PTHrP-induced incisor lesions in rats. Toxicol Pathol. 2003;31:480–5.
15. Sano T, Matsuura T, Ozaki K, Narama I. Dental caries and caries-related periodontitis in type 2 diabetic mice. Vet Pathol. 2011;48:506–12.
16. Westwood FR, Iswaran TJ, Greaves P. Long-term effects of an inotropic phosphodiesterase inhibitor (ICI 153,110) on the rat salivary gland, harderian gland, and intestinal mucosa. Toxicol Pathol. 1991;19:214–23.
17. Markovits JE, Betton GR, McMartin DN, Turner OC. Gastrointestinal tract. In: Sahota PS, Popp JA, Hardisty JF, Gopinath C, editors. Toxicologic pathology: nonclinical safety assessment. Boca Raton: CRC Press; 2013. p. 251–312.
18. Ulmansky M, Rubinow A, Ungar H. Salivary gland regeneration after DL-ethionine poisoning. Lab Invest. 1969;20:230–3.

19. Denny PC, Ball WD, Redman RS. Salivary glands: a paradigm for diversity of gland development. Crit Rev Oral Biol Med. 1997;8:51–75.
20. Gopinath C, Prentice DE, Lewis DJ. The alimentary system and pancreas. In: Gopinath C, Prentice D, Lewis DJ, editors. Atlas of experimental toxicologic pathology. Lancaster: MTP Press; 1987. p. 61–76.
21. de Rijk EP, Ravesloot WT, Hafmans TG, van Esch E. Multifocal ductal cell hyperplasia in the submandibular salivary glands of Wistar rats chronically treated with a novel steroidal compound. Toxicol Pathol. 2003;31:1–9.
22. Tucker Jr WE, Macklin AW, Szot RJ, Johnston RE, Elion GB, de Miranda P, Szczech GM. Preclinical toxicology studies with acyclovir: acute and subchronic tests. Fundam Appl Toxicol. 1983;3:573–8.
23. Carnahan J, Beltran PJ, Babij C, Le Q, Rose MJ, Vonderfecht S, et al. Selective and potent Raf inhibitors paradoxically stimulate normal cell proliferation and tumor growth. Mol Cancer Ther. 2010;9:2399–410.
24. Fong LY, Lau KM, Huebner K, Magee PN. Induction of esophageal tumors in zinc-deficient rats by single low doses of N-nitrosomethylbenzylamine (NMBA): analysis of cell proliferation, and mutations in H-ras and p53 genes. Carcinogenesis. 1997;18:1477–84.
25. Reindel JF, Gough AW, Pilcher GD, Bobrowski WF, Sobocinski GP, de la Iglesia FA. Systemic proliferative changes and clinical signs in cynomolgus monkeys administered a recombinant derivative of human epidermal growth factor. Toxicol Pathol. 2001;29:159–73.
26. Dodd DC, Port CD, Deslex P, Regnier B, Sanders P, Indacochea-Redmond N. Two-year evaluation of misoprostol for carcinogenicity in CD Sprague–Dawley rats. Toxicol Pathol. 1987;15:125–33.
27. Port CD, Dodd DC, Deslex P, Regnier B, Sanders P, Indacochea-Redmond N. Twenty-one-month evaluation of misoprostol for carcinogenicity in CD-1 mice. Toxicol Pathol. 1987;15:134–42.
28. Sano T, Ozaki K, Kodama Y, Matsuura T, Narama I. Antimicrobial agent, tetracycline, enhanced upper alimentary tract Candida albicans infection and its related mucosal proliferation in alloxan-induced diabetic rats. Toxicol Pathol. 2012;40:1014–9.
29. Sano T, Ozaki K, Kodama Y, Matsuura T, Narama I. Prevention of proliferative changes of forestomach mucosa by blood glucose control with insulin in alloxan-induced diabetic rats. Cancer Sci. 2009;100:595–600.
30. Brown AP, Courtney CL, King LM, Groom SC, Graziano MJ. Cartilage dysplasia and tissue mineralization in the rat following administration of a FGF receptor tyrosine kinase inhibitor. Toxicol Pathol. 2005;33:449–55.
31. Rees J, Spencer A, Wilson S, Reid A, Harpur E. Time course of stomach mineralization, plasma, and urinary changes after a single intravenous administration of gadolinium(III) chloride in the male rat. Toxicol Pathol. 1997;25:582–9.
32. Spencer AJ, Wilson SA, Batchelor J, Reid A, Rees J, Harpur E. Gadolinium chloride toxicity in the rat. Toxicol Pathol. 1997;25:245–55.
33. McKevitt TP, Giffen P, Woodfine JA, McCawley SJ, Papworth SA, McGill P, et al. Hyalinization of the pyloric stomach in CD-1 mice following oral (dietary) administration of the corticosteroid agonists mometasone furoate, budesonide, and flunisolide. Toxicol Pathol. 2011;39:958–68.
34. Ueda Y, Tsuboi M, Ota Y, Makita M, Aoshima T, Nakajima M, Narama I. Gastric mucosal changes induced by polyethylene glycol 400 administered by gavage in rats. J Toxicol Sci. 2011;36:811–5.
35. Narama I, Ozaki K, Matsushima S, Matsuura T. Eosinophilic gastroenterocolitis in iron lactate-overloaded rats. Toxicol Pathol. 1999;27:318–24.
36. Nomura S, Yamaguchi H, Ogawa M, Wang TC, Lee JR, Goldenring JR. Alterations in gastric mucosal lineages induced by acute oxyntic atrophy in wild-type and gastrin-deficient mice. Am J Physiol Gastrointest Liver Physiol. 2005;288:G362–75.
37. Crean GP, Marshall MW, Rumsey RD. Parietal cell hyperplasia induced by the administration of pentagastrin (ICI 50,123) to rats. Gastroenterology. 1969;57:147–55.
38. Fiorucci S, Antonelli E, Morelli A. Mechanism of non-steroidal anti-inflammatory drug-gastropathy. Dig Liver Dis. 2001;33 Suppl 2:S35–43.
39. Wallace JL, McKnight W, Reuter BK, Vergnolle N. NSAID-induced gastric damage in rats: requirement for inhibition of both cyclooxygenase 1 and 2. Gastroenterology. 2000;119:706–14.
40. Takeuchi K, Tanaka A, Miyazawa T. [Pathogenesis of NSAID-induced gastric mucosal damage–search for primary events and role of COX inhibition]. Nihon Shokakibyo Gakkai Zasshi. 2002;99:751–9.
41. Zinkievich JM, George S, Jha S, Nandi J, Levine RA. Gastric acid is the key modulator in the pathogenesis of non-steroidal anti-inflammatory drug-induced ulceration in rats. Clin Exp Pharmacol Physiol. 2010;37:654–61.
42. Iseki S. Immunocytochemical localization of cyclooxygenase-1 and cyclooxygenase-2 in the rat stomach. Histochem J. 1995;27:323–8.
43. Luo JC, Shin VY, Liu ES, So WH, Ye YN, Chang FY, Cho CH. Non-ulcerogenic dose of dexamethasone delays gastric ulcer healing in rats. J Pharmacol Exp Ther. 2003;307:692–8.
44. Yokota A, Taniguchi M, Takahira Y, Tanaka A, Takeuchi K. Dexamethasone damages the rat stomach but not small intestine during inhibition of COX-1. Dig Dis Sci. 2007;52:1452–61.
45. Kramer Jr AW, Dougherty WJ, Belson AR, Iatropoulos MJ. Morphologic changes in the gastric mucosa of rats and dogs treated with an analog of prostaglandin E1. Toxicol Pathol. 1985;13:26–35.
46. Kang W, Rathinavelu S, Samuelson LC, Merchant JL. Interferon gamma induction of gastric mucous neck cell hypertrophy. Lab Invest. 2005;85:702–15.
47. Tsukamoto T, Mizoshita T, Tatematsu M. Animal models of stomach carcinogenesis. Toxicol Pathol. 2007;35:636–48.
48. Gabella G. Hypertrophy of visceral smooth muscle. Anat Embryol (Berl). 1990;182:409–24.
49. Ettlin RA, Kuroda J, Plassmann S, Hayashi M, Prentice DE. Successful drug development despite adverse preclinical findings. Part 2: examples. J. Toxicol Pathol. 2010;23:213–34.
50. Lugea A, Mourelle M, Domingo A, Salas A, Guarner F, Malagelada JR. Epidermal growth factor increases surface hydrophobicity and resistance to acid in the rat duodenum. Am J Physiol Gastrointest Liver Physiol. 2001;280:G774–9.
51. Khomenko T, Kolodney J, Pinto JT, McLaren GD, Deng X, Chen L, et al. New mechanistic explanation for the localization of ulcers in the rat duodenum: role of iron and selective uptake of cysteamine. Arch Biochem Biophys. 2012;525:60–70.
52. Khomenko T, Szabo S, Deng X, Ishikawa H, Anderson GJ, McLaren GD. Role of iron in the pathogenesis of cysteamine-induced duodenal ulceration in rats. Am J Physiol Gastrointest Liver Physiol. 2009;296:G1277–86.
53. Haworth R, Oakley K, McCormack N, Pilling A. Differential expression of COX-1 and COX-2 in the gastrointestinal tract of the rat. Toxicol Pathol. 2005;33:239–45.
54. Boyle MC, Crabbs TA, Wyde ME, Painter JT, Hill GD, Malarkey DE, et al. Intestinal lymphangiectasis and lipidosis in rats follow-

ing subchronic exposure to indole-3-carbinol via oral gavage. Toxicol Pathol. 2012;40:561–76.

55. Rose 2nd WA, Sakamoto K, Leifer CA. Multifunctional role of dextran sulfate sodium for in vivo modeling of intestinal diseases. BMC Immunol. 2012;13:41.

56. Morris DL, O'Neil SP, Devraj RV, Portanova JP, Gilles RW, Gross CJ, et al. Acute lymphoid and gastrointestinal toxicity induced by selective p38alpha map kinase and map kinase-activated protein kinase-2 (MK2) inhibitors in the dog. Toxicol Pathol. 2010;38:606–18.

57. Duan RD, Cheng Y, Tauschel HD, Nilsson A. Effects of ursodeoxycholate and other bile salts on levels of rat intestinal alkaline sphingomyelinase: a potential implication in tumorigenesis. Dig Dis Sci. 1998;43:26–32.

58. Morgan DL, Nyska A, Harbo SJ, Grumbein SL, Dill JA, Roycroft JH, et al. Multisite carcinogenicity and respiratory toxicity of inhaled 1-bromopropane in rats and mice. Toxicol Pathol. 2011;39:938–48.

59. Erdman SE, Poutahidis T. Roles for inflammation and regulatory T cells in colon cancer. Toxicol Pathol. 2010;38:76–87.

60. Kitagawa T, Ono K. Ultrastructure of pancreatic exocrine cells of the rat during starvation. Histol Histopathol. 1986;1:49–57.

61. Fell BF, King TP, Davies NT. Pancreatic atrophy in copper-deficient rats: histochemical and ultrastructural evidence of a selective effect on acinar cells. Histochem J. 1982;14: 665–80.

62. Maysten PD, Barrowman JA. Influence of chronic administration of pentagastrin on the pancreas in hypophysectomized rats. Gastroenterology. 1973;64:391–9.

63. Mareninova OA, Sung KF, Hong P, Lugea A, Pandol SJ, Gukovsky I, Gukovskaya AS. Cell death in pancreatitis: caspases protect from necrotizing pancreatitis. J Biol Chem. 2006;281:3370–81.

64. Grasso D, Ropolo A, Lo RA, Boggio V, Molejon MI, Iovanna JL, et al. Zymophagy, a novel selective autophagy pathway mediated by VMP1-USP9x-p62, prevents pancreatic cell death. J Biol Chem. 2011;286:8308–24.

65. Aho HJ, Koskensalo SM, Nevalainen TJ. Experimental pancreatitis in the rat. Sodium taurocholate-induced acute haemorrhagic pancreatitis. Scand J Gastroenterol. 1980;15: 411–6.

66. Tsukamoto H, Towner SJ, Yu GS, French SW. Potentiation of ethanol-induced pancreatic injury by dietary fat. Induction of chronic pancreatitis by alcohol in rats. Am J Pathol. 1988;131:246–57.

67. Greaves P. Liver and pancreas. Histopathology of preclinical toxicity studies. 4th ed. London: Academic; 2012. pp 489–500

68. Chiu T. Spontaneous hypertrophic foci of pancreatic acinar cells in CD rats. Toxicol Pathol. 1983;11:115–9.

69. Chiu T. Focal eosinophilic hypertrophic cells of the rat pancreas. Toxicol Pathol. 1987;15:1–6.

70. Rao MS, Subbarao V, Luetteke N, Scarpelli DG. Further characterization of carcinogen-induced hepatocytelike cells in hamster pancreas. Am J Pathol. 1983;110:89–94.

71. McDonald MM, Boorman GA. Pancreatic hepatocytes associated with chronic 2,6-dichloro-p-phenylenediamine administration in Fischer 344 rats. Toxicol Pathol. 1989;17:1–6.

72. Reddy JK, Rao MS, Qureshi SA, Reddy MK, Scarpelli DG, Lalwani ND. Induction and origin of hepatocytes in rat pancreas. J Cell Biol. 1984;98:2082–90.

73. Konishi N, Ward JM, Waalkes MP. Pancreatic hepatocytes in Fischer and Wistar rats induced by repeated injections of cadmium chloride. Toxicol Appl Pharmacol. 1990;104:149–56.

74. Eustis SL, Boorman GA. Proliferative lesions of the exocrine pancreas: relationship to corn oil gavage in the National Toxicology Program. J Natl Cancer Inst. 1985;75:1067–73.

75. Chiu T. Hypertrophic foci of pancreatic acinar cells in rats. Crit Rev Toxicol. 1985;14:133–57.

76. Klaunig JE, Babich MA, Baetcke KP, Cook JC, Corton JC, David RM, et al. PPARalpha agonist-induced rodent tumors: modes of action and human relevance. Crit Rev Toxicol. 2003;33:655–780.

77. Cattley RC, Popp JA, Vonderfecht SL. Liver, gallbladder, and exocrine pancreas. In: Sahota PS, Popp JA, Hardisty JF, Gopinath C, editors. Toxicologic pathology: nonclinical safety assessment. Boca Raton: CRC Press; 2013. p. 313–66.

78. Sigler RE, Gough AW, de la Iglesia FA. Pancreatic acinar cell neoplasia in male Wistar rats following 2 years of gabapentin exposure. Toxicology. 1995;98:73–82.

79. Katsuta O, Tsuchitani M, Narama I. Abnormal proliferation of pancreatic endocrine cells in beagle dogs. J Toxicol Pathol. 1992;5:67–76.

80. Son WC, Faki K, Mowat V, Gopinath C. Spontaneously occurring extra-islet endocrine cell proliferation in the pancreas of young Beagle dogs. Toxicol Lett. 2010;193:179–82.

# 5 The Urinary System

Induced lesions affecting kidney and urinary bladder are included. In kidneys, changes affecting glomeruli, tubules, interstitium, and papilla are illustrated. These include degenerative, inflammatory, reparative, and proliferative changes. A few examples of induced tumours of kidney and urinary bladder are described.

## 5.1 Kidney

### 5.1.1 Introduction

The kidney's role as the main organ for excretion makes it vulnerable to many agents excreted through urine. Its high blood flow makes it susceptible to exposure through circulation to many xenobiotics. Its role as a site for metabolic biotransformation (as with the liver) results in new toxic metabolites being produced, leading to nephrotoxicity. The kidney's role in reabsorption and its ability to concentrate fluid also pose problems for the relevant sections of nephrons, which become preferential sites for toxicity.

Nephrotoxins exert their effect on specific cell types along the course of the nephron depending on their particular affinities. In the early stages, these appear as distinct entities. However, in repeat-dose toxicity studies, or in more serious injury, the change extends to involve other parts of the nephron as secondary responses. End-stage toxicity takes a common path in spite of early lesions being specific to cell types of various sections of the nephron.

For descriptive purposes, the kidney is grouped into four zones, each containing different proportions of the nephrons. They are as follows:

1. The cortex consists mainly of proximal convoluted tubules (PCTs; S1 and S2 segments), distal convoluted tubules (DCT), and the outer end of collecting ducts (CDs) and projections of medullary rays with CDs and thick ascending limbs that extend into the cortex.
2. The outer strip of medulla mainly consists of the straight portion of the PCT (pars recta [PR] or S3). Thick ascending limbs and CDs appear in the medullary rays.
3. The inner strip of the medulla consists of thick ascending limbs, thin limbs of Henle, CDs, and loops of Henle.
4. The inner medulla/papilla consists of thin limbs and loops of Henle and CDs.

Renal changes are described with the previously discussed anatomical zones in mind wherever possible, but it must be stressed that in practice changes occur at more than one site. Many histochemical techniques, such as α-glutathione-S-transferase (α-GST), calbindin D28K, and aquaporin-2, are used to mark and identify specific segments of the nephron. Although serum creatinine and blood urea nitrogen are used as indicators of kidney dysfunction, they are not very sensitive indicators, and the changes noted can sometimes be of extrarenal origin. Examination of urine provides useful information regarding the stage of the kidney disease.

Although morphological changes are described as separate entities, in reality, many of the changes coexist in repeat-dose programmes of toxicity studies along with stromal and vascular changes. Because males and females have different susceptibilities to nephrotoxic agents, generally they must be assessed separately in routine

C. Gopinath, V. Mowat, *Atlas of Toxicological Pathology*,
DOI 10.1007/978-1-62703-998-7_5, © Springer Science+Business Media New York 2014

toxicity studies. The changes occurring in different parts of the nephron are:

- Glomerulonephritis/sclerosis
- Mesangial changes
- Chronic progressive nephrosis
- Tubular vacuolation
- Degeneration/necrosis
- Inclusions
- Pigments
- Dilation
- Mineralisation
- Crystalline nephropathy
- Interstitial nephritis
- Hypertrophy
- Hyperplasia
- Renal papillary necrosis
- Vascular changes
- Neoplasia

Proliferative lesions and nonproliferative lesions of the urinary system of rodents are well described [1].

### 5.1.2 Glomerular Changes

Glomerular injuries are somewhat rare in toxicity studies and can occur owing to direct or indirect effects. Haematoxylin and eosin (H&E)-stained paraffin sections are not always ideal to study glomerular changes because subtle changes can be missed. Perfusion fixation, examination by one μ-resin sections, electron microscopy, and special stains for defining changes in basement membranes and other structures are useful for critical analysis of glomerular injury. The use of periodic acid–Schiff (PAS) and silver stains is valuable in depicting the basement membrane and other outlines in the glomeruli. When referring to a single glomerulus, lesions can be termed 'segmental' or 'diffuse' depending on whether a segment or the entire glomerulus is affected. The terms 'focal' and 'global' are used to indicate distribution within the kidney. In glomerulonephritis, cellular proliferation and inflammatory cell components are involved (Fig. 5.1). Subdivisions, such as 'membranoproliferative' and 'crescentic', refer to morphological appearance rather than specific or separate entities because both can coexist within an affected kidney (Figs. 5.2 and 5.3). On most occasions, use of the term 'glomerulonephritis' alone is adequate in toxicologic pathology. Drug-induced glomerulonephritis frequently appears to be species- and strain-specific and its extrapolation to human safety is not often very meaningful.

Aminonucleoside of puromycin produces direct damage to foot processes that develop into progressive glomerulosclerosis [2]. Initially, basement membrane thickening, mesangial proliferation, and hyalinisation occur. Adriamycin causes glomerulosclerosis in rats [3]. Synthetic progestogens producing hyperglycaemia cause segmental glomerulosclerosis in the dog [4, 5]. Myserate acetate and Adriamycin cause glomerulonephritis by a direct effect. Snake venom, croton oil, and mitomycin C cause mesangiolysis and inflammation. Anthracyclines and human fibroblastic growth factors cause vacuolation of the glomerular epithelium [6]. Glomerular basement membrane changes can be clearly seen by silver techniques and also by the PAS method. Increases in collagen in late stages can be better visualised by trichrome staining (Fig. 5.4). Antisense oligonucleotides can cause mesangioproliferative glomerulonephritis, seen in mice and monkeys in our laboratories.

Indirect injury can result from agents causing immune-mediated injuries with resultant deposition of immune complexes in the basement membrane, detectable by electron microscopy (Fig. 5.5). D-Penicillamine, gold salts, and mercury are associated with indirect glomerular injury [7, 8]. Ampicillin in dogs has a similar effect [9]. Immune-based glomerular injuries in laboratory animals are difficult to interpret as predictors of human safety because they can be species specific. Glomerulonephritis must be differentiated from hyaline glomerulopathy, seen spontaneously in the mouse. There is loss of cellularity

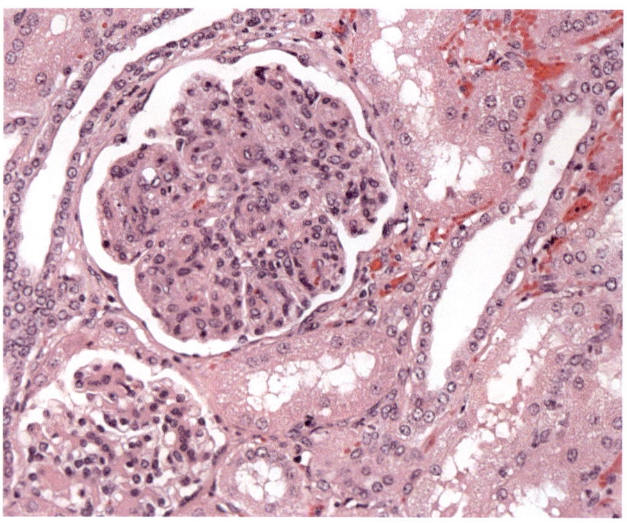

**Figure 5-1.** Glomerulonephritis, in a dog. Enlarged renal corpuscle, increased glomerular cellularity, focal thickening, and minimal inflammatory cells are seen. Haematoxylin and eosin (H&E).

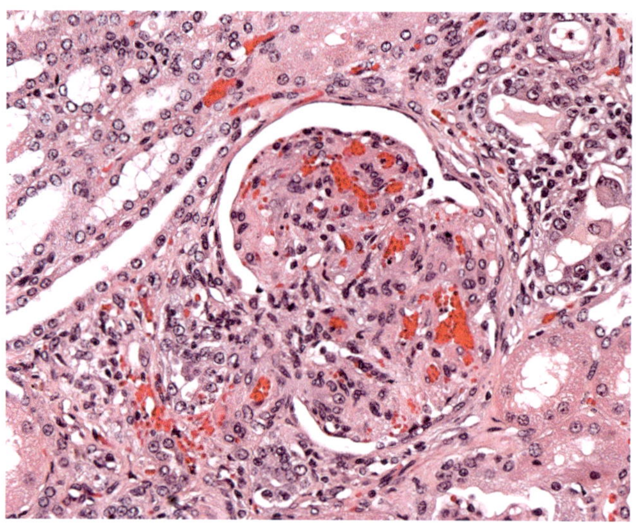

**Figure 5-2.** Glomerulonephritis, in a pig. Moderate mesangial thickening, increased cellularity, and inflammatory cells are seen. H&E.

and replacement of glomeruli with a pale pink homogenous matrix that stains positive with PAS and negative for amyloid.

Intravenous administration of substances like methylcellulose, gum acacia, lipoid materials, and polyvinyl alcohol results in particulate deposition in the mesangial cytoplasm (Fig. 5.6). Agents producing systemic phospholipidosis cause deposition of multilamellar bodies in the foot processes. In Schwartzman's reaction, extensive fibrin deposition occurs in the glomeruli (Fig. 5.7). Calcification following fibrin deposition was noticed in dogs treated with certain biologically active molecules (Fig. 5.8). Androgenic steroids induce metaplasia of epithelium of Bowman's capsule in rodents [10]. Hyperplasia of Bowman's capsule has been recorded in cynomolgus monkeys given human fibroblast growth factor [11].

Chronic progressive nephropathy (CPN; progressive glomerulonephritis) is an age-related spontaneous renal disease in rats, in which there is a markedly increased glomerular filtration rate with considerable damage to the nephrons. Marked proteinuria (mainly albuminuria) is associated with glomerulosclerosis, increased tubular basement membrane thickness, and periglomerular fibrosis. Associated tubular basophilia, atrophy, and loss of tubules occur. Focal tubular dilation with eosinophilic casts is frequently seen. Interstitial fibrosis, lymphocytic infiltration, cortical scarring, and tubular cysts are encountered. Advanced cases of CPN are associated with tubular hyperplasia. Factors like stress, dietary protein, high-caloric diets, sex steroids, several chemicals, and pharmaceutical agents all tend to exacerbate CPN [11]. Many nephrotoxic agents that produce specific lesions in parts of nephrons lose their specificity in chronic administration and result in kidneys morphologically similar to advanced cases of CPN. In many cases, one can only detect an increase in the severity and incidence of CPN. Thus, it is

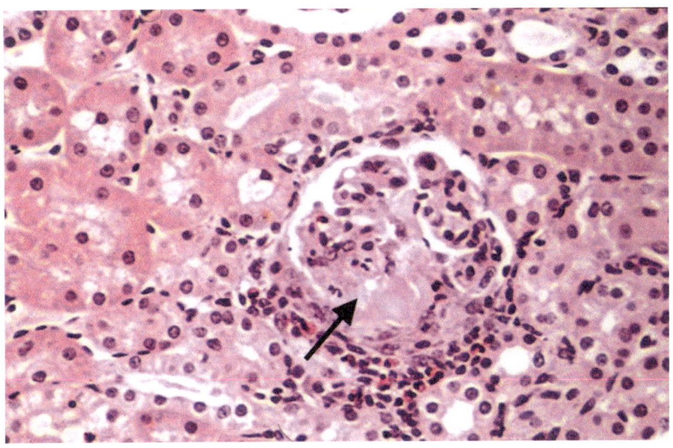

**Figure 5-3.** Glomerulonephritis, segmental, in a mouse. Area of hyalinisation (*arrow*) and areas with increased cellularity are seen. H&E.

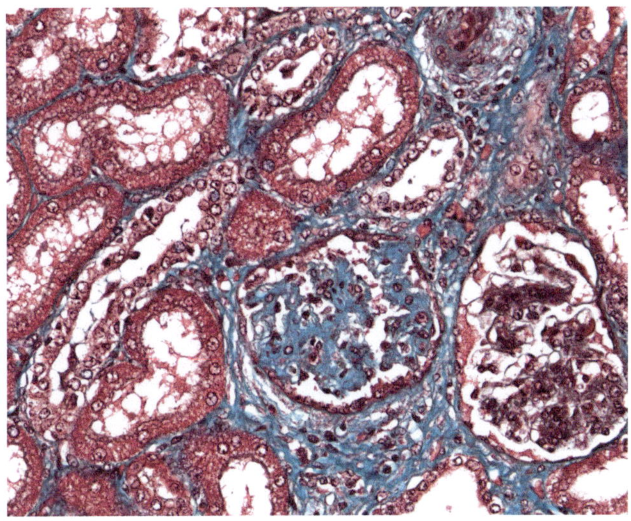

**Figure 5-4.** Glomerulosclerosis, in a pig. Note marked fibrosis of glomerular tufts and some interstitial fibrosis. Masson's trichrome.

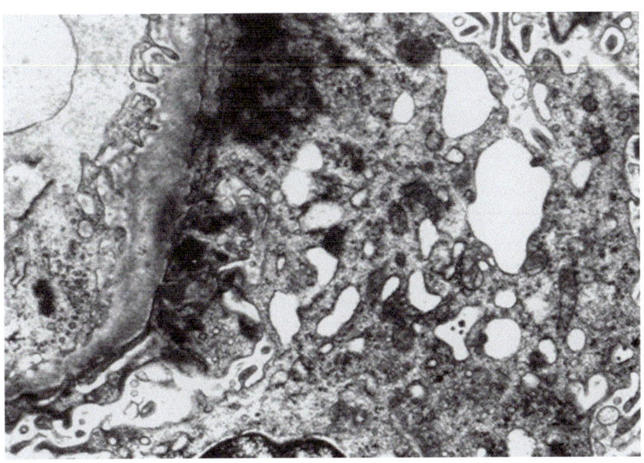

**Figure 5-5.** Glomerulonephritis, in a rat. Note electron-dense deposits in the basement membrane and foot processes. Electron micrograph.

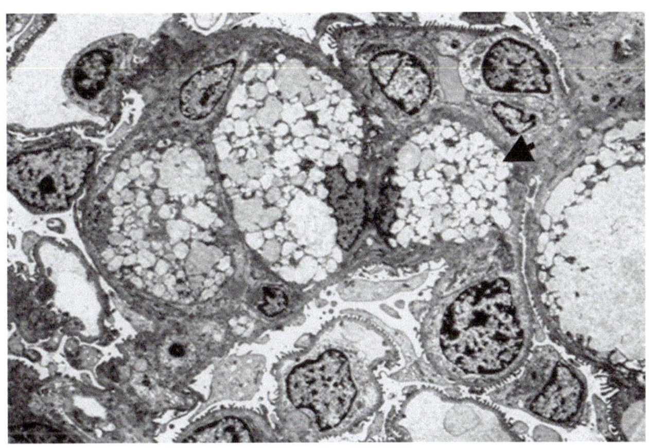

**Figure 5-6.** Mesangial storage, in a rat treated with intravenous administration of a high-molecular-weight compound. Note distended mesangial cells with granular/vesicular materials (*arrowhead*). Electron micrograph (With kind permission from Springer Science+Business Media B.V [5]).

important to carefully grade severity while reading chronic studies. Prolactin modifies CPN and many xenobiotics produce renal changes through changes in prolactin levels. Oestrogens seem to protect against development of CPN in rats.

Increases in the incidence and severity of nephropathy can be associated with an increase in renal tubular hyperplasia including atypical hyperplasia (preneoplastic lesions) and tumours in rats. The association between CPN and tubular hyperplasia and neoplasia has been extensively studied [12–17]. Evaluation of enhanced chronic nephropathy in rats must be based on case-by-case critical analyses of all available data, although in many instances, this is of little significance to human safety extrapolation [18].

Mice also suffer from spontaneous age-related chronic nephropathy. The lesions in mice appear more focal and show less interstitial changes. When compared with rats, chronic nephropathy in mice has been much less studied and reported.

### 5.1.3 Tubular Changes

The most frequently affected segment is the PCT; others are less affected. In rats, ischaemia and heavy metals tend to produce changes in the S3 segment, and gentamicin and other antibiotics target S2. Blood flow, transport of the agent, binding sites, and metabolic activity all contribute to the predilection sites of the induced changes. Toxic insults initially produce a series of reversible changes that progress to more irreversible changes and necrosis. The initial changes include loss of glycogen and microvilli, brush border, cell swelling, and vesiculation followed by nuclear changes and cell death. Vacuolation precedes necrosis in cyclosporine toxicity and is due to dilation of endoplasmic reticulum (Fig. 5.9) [19]. Zinc and ethylene glycol produce hydropic degeneration of the PCT. In cyclosporine toxicity, this is accompanied by the presence of eosinophilic granularity that represents secondary lysosomes (Fig. 5.10).

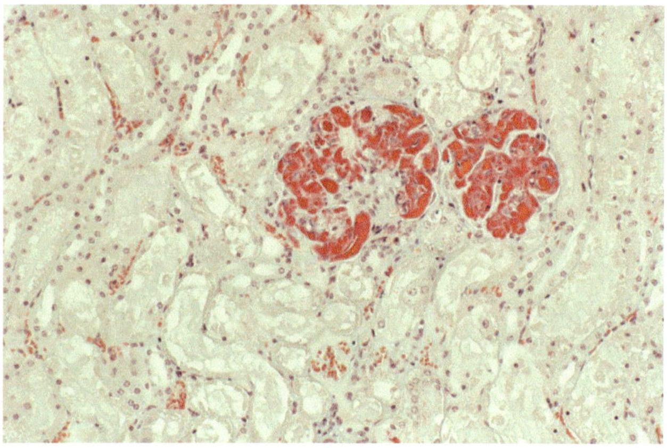

**Figure 5-7.** Fibrin thrombi in capillaries, in a rat. Martius scarlet blue (MSB).

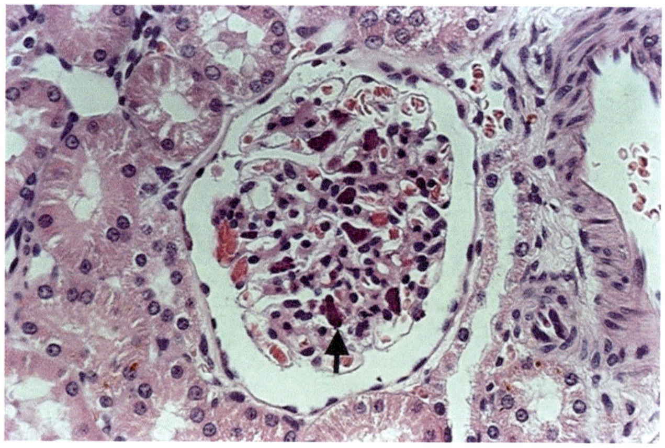

**Figure 5-8.** Glomerular mineralisation (*arrow*), in a dog, probably following fibrin deposition. H&E.

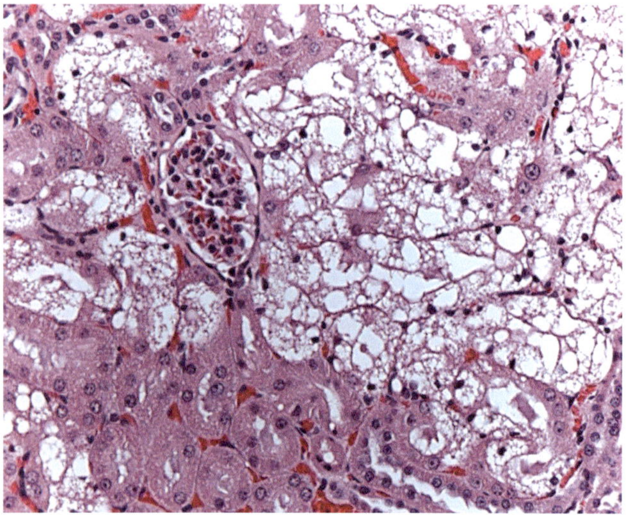

**Figure 5-9.** Tubular vacuolation, proximal convoluted tubules (PCTs), in a rat. Affected cells are swollen and finely vacuolated, and some have pyknotic nuclei. H&E.

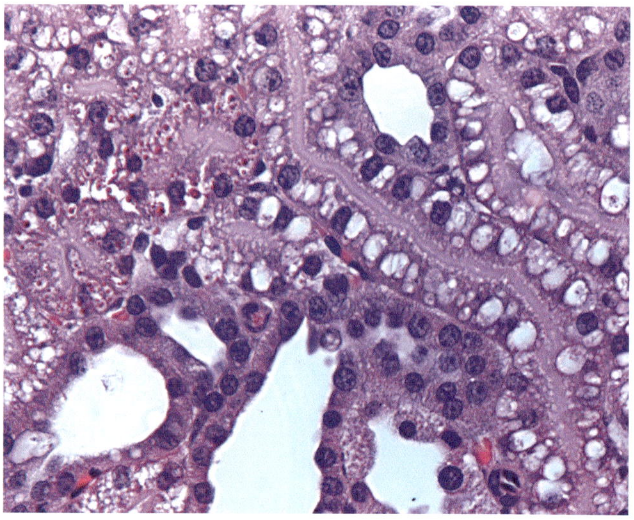

**Figure 5-10.** Tubular vacuolation with intracytoplasmic eosinophilic granules, proximal tubules, in a rat treated with an industrial chemical. H&E.

Vacuolation of the PCT due to lipid is a rare phenomenon and is an indication of toxic change (Fig. 5.11). Diffuse vacuolation of cortical tubules is seen in animals given high doses of hypertonic solutions of glucose or sugar and is referred to as 'osmotic nephrosis'. The change is reversible. A similar change is seen when radiocontrast agents are administered at high doses to different species of animals (Fig. 5.12). This is due to accumulation of the administered agent. The change is reversible but only slowly. Administration of cottonseed extracts produces vacuolation of PCT in monkeys. Clear cytoplasmic vacuolation is seen in the DCT and CDs of animals given agents producing hyperglycaemia. Vacuolation of the DCT is seen in rats given high doses of certain hydrocarbon derivatives (Fig. 5.13).

Tubular necrosis of various segments of PCT is produced by aminoglycoside antibiotics; cephalosporin; heavy metals like cadmium, mercury, lead, iron, and zinc; organohalides; and anticancer agents (Figs. 5.14 and 5.15) [19–21]. Aminoglycoside antibiotics and cisplatin target the PR, whereas organohalides, cadmium, and mercury affect the PCT. Gentamicin binds with the brush border and is taken up by endocytosis, causing lysosomal overload, myeloid body formation, vacuolation, increased apoptosis, and coagulative necrosis. This may be followed by exfoliation and cast formation. The location of the changes can be cortical when S1 and S2 are affected or it can be in the outer strip when S3 is affected. Necrosis is frequently accompanied by regenerative hyperplasia and regressive atrophy; both are represented by basophilic tubules. It is often difficult to differentiate between these. In regenerative changes, the basophilic tubules reveal vesicular nuclei and some evidence of proliferation. In some instances, necrotic areas also reveal interstitial fibrosis/inflammation (Fig. 5.16). Cortical tubular necrosis must be differentiated from a morphologically similar artefact in rat kidneys that is produced by postmortem change (Fig. 5.17). Tubular degeneration or necrosis is often accompanied by different types of casts that

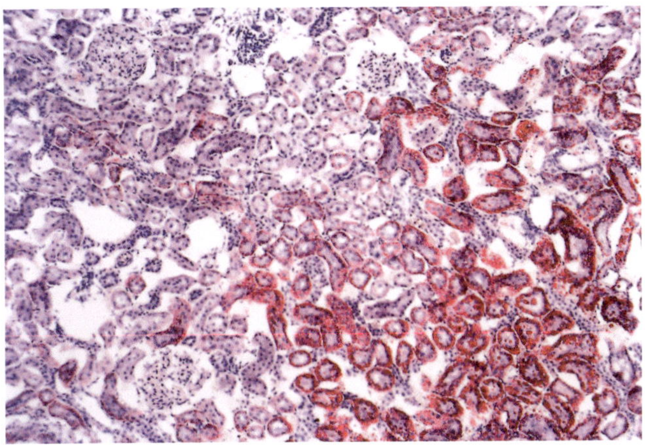

**Figure 5-11.** Lipid deposition, PCT, in a rat. Oil red O (ORO).

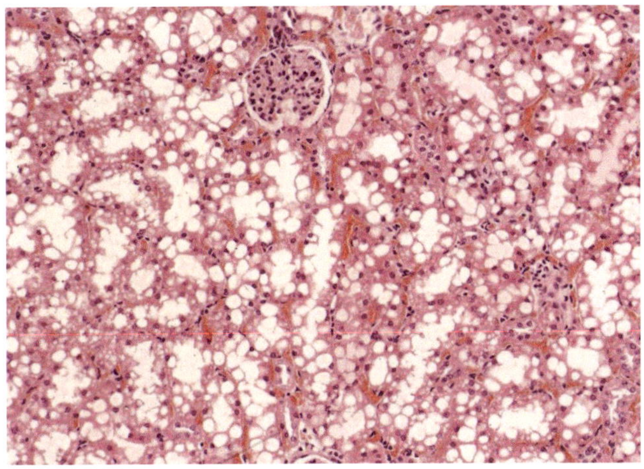

**Figure 5-12.** Vacuolation of cortical tubules, in a rat treated with a high dose of a radiocontrast agent. H&E.

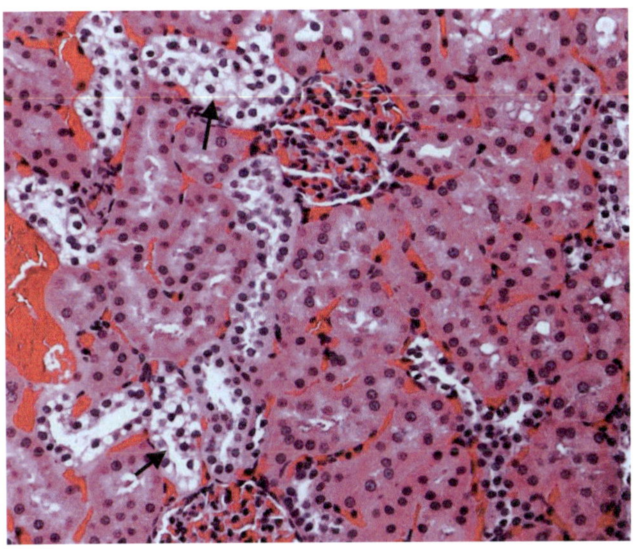

**Figure 5-13.** Vacuolation of distal convoluted tubules (*arrows*), in a rat treated with a hydrocarbon derivative. H&E.

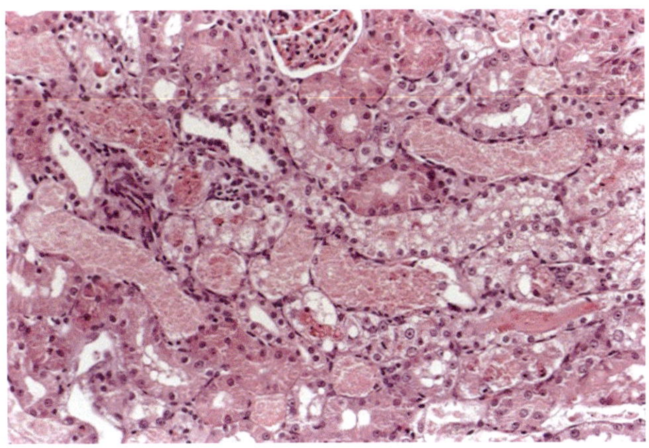

**Figure 5-14.** Necrosis and vacuolation, PCT, in a rat. Some tubules show casts and exfoliated cells. H&E.

vary from hyaline, granular, cellular, or mineralised casts.

Occasionally, intracytoplasmic inclusions are seen in toxicity studies. They are usually eosinophilic and granular as in cyclosporine toxicity [22]. Some of the inclusions are PAS positive (Fig. 5.18). Hyaline droplet infiltration of the PCT occurs in male rats exposed to a number of hydrocarbon derivatives including gasoline, jet fuels, limonene, lindane, and nitrotoluene (Fig. 5.19) [23, 24]. Female rats and other laboratory animal species are not affected by this change. Hyaline droplet accumulation is partly due to the male rat's inability to excrete $\alpha_2$-microglobulin. The xenobiotic in question binds with this protein and is stored in lysosomes. They resist catabolism, which results in overload and produces nephrosis in male rats. Under electron microscopy, the granules appear as irregular bodies associated with secondary lysosomes (Fig. 5.20). $\alpha_2$-microglobulin can be demonstrated by immunohistochemistry (Fig. 5.21) [24]. If the overload is persistent and prolonged, this will lead to degeneration and cast formation and can progress to regenerative hyperplasia and even renal tubular adenomas. This finding is of no human relevance because this is a male rat-specific lesion [25]. Hyaline droplets which are not linked to $\alpha_2$-microglobulin can be induced by other pharmaceutical agents. This can affect both sexes in rats and can also occur in other species of laboratory animals (Fig. 5.22).

Pigment deposition is seen in cortical tubules as a result of lipofuscin, hemosiderin, haemoglobin (in haemolytic crises), ferric iron, and in copper toxicity as copper bound with protein (Figs. 5.23–5.25). External pigments occur as result of the test compound or its metabolites accumulating, as with benzodiazepine and certain neuroleptics. Oestrogen treatment also results in pigmentation of the cortical tubules. Intranuclear inclusions are seen in lead and bismuth toxicity. Eosinophilic globular inclusions within the nuclei of cortical tubules are seen occasionally on treatment with certain pharmaceutical agents (Fig. 5.26) [5]. They do not progress to cellular degeneration but are slow to recover.

Certain xenobiotics that induce drug-metabolising enzymes and smooth endoplasmic reticular proliferation result in increased kidney weight and hypertrophy of the PR (Fig. 5.27). Similarly, some hypolipidaemic agents result in peroxisome proliferation in the PR.

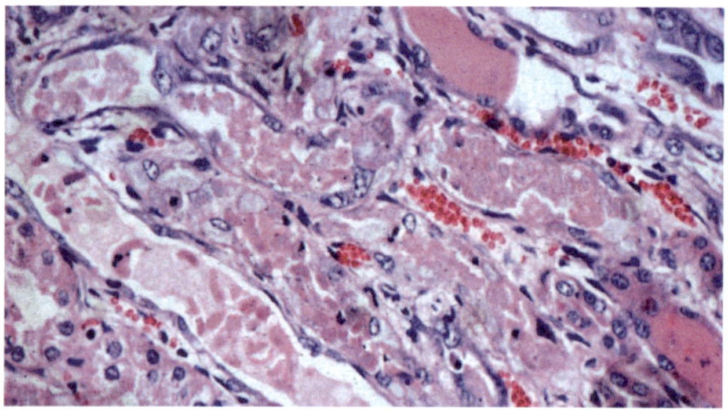

**Figure 5-15.** Tubular necrosis, pars recta, in a rat treated with an antibiotic agent. Tubular casts, exfoliated cells, and regenerating tubules are present. H&E.

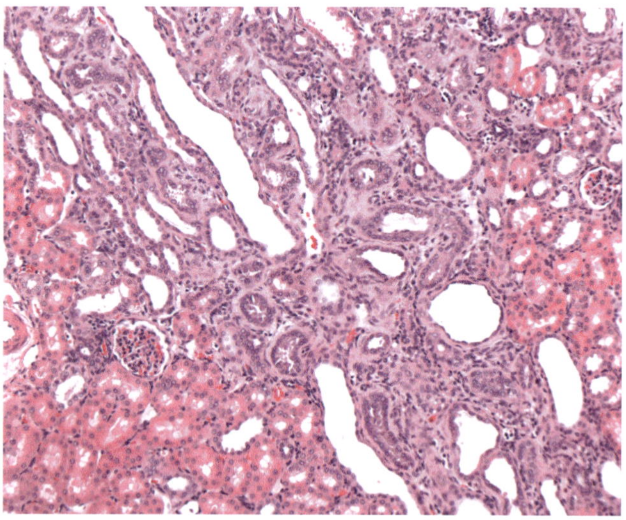

**Figure 5-16.** Basophilic tubules, dilated tubules, and interstitial fibrosis suggest repair in a rat treated with a nephrotoxic agent. H&E.

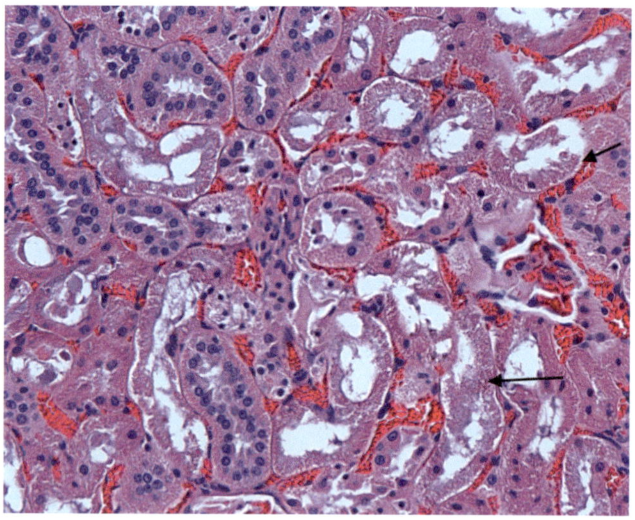

**Figure 5-17.** Tubular disruption (*arrows*), renal cortex (artefactual), in a rat; represents postmortem artefact-mimicking necrosis. H&E.

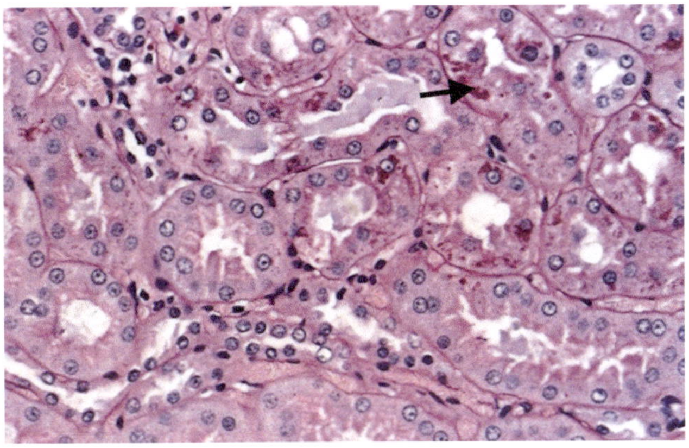

**Figure 5-18.** Intracytoplasmic inclusions (*arrow*), periodic acid–Schiff (PAS) positive, diastase resistant, cortical tubules, in a rat treated with an agrochemical agent. PAS.

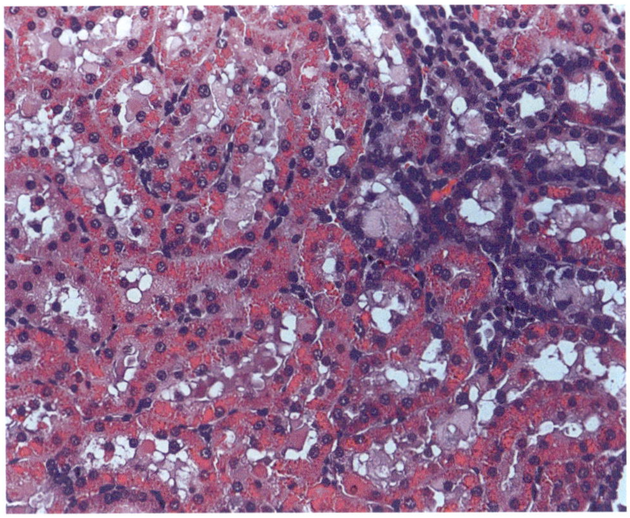

**Figure 5-19.** Hyaline droplet infiltration, proximal tubules, in a male rat treated with a hydrocarbon derivative. H&E.

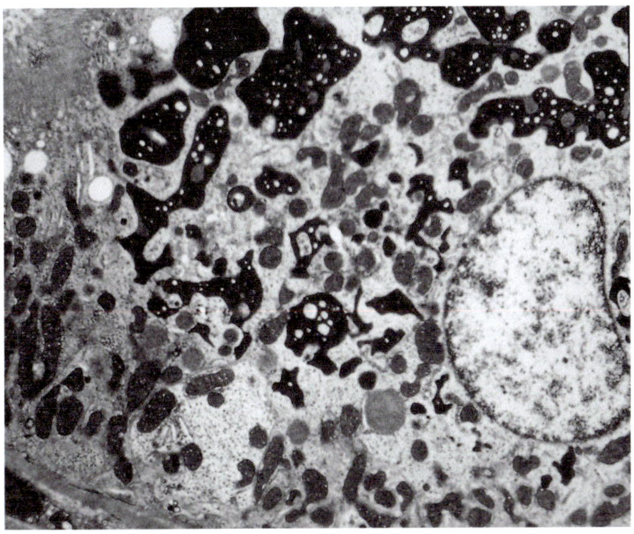

**Figure 5-20.** Intracytoplasmic heterogeneous granular inclusions, PCT. Electron micrograph (With kind permission from Springer Science + Business Media B.V [5]).

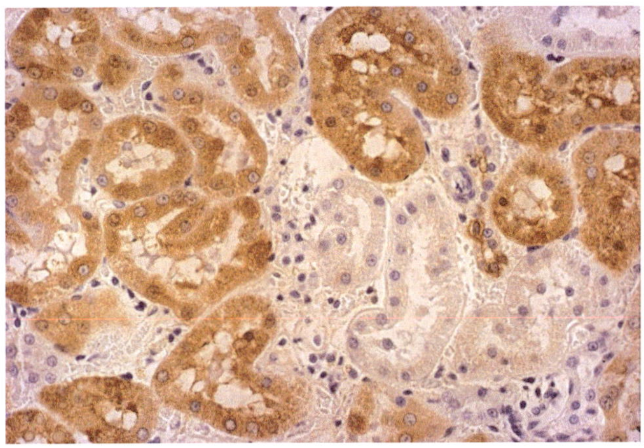

**Figure 5-21.** $\alpha_2$-microglobulin staining of PCT, in a rat treated with a hydrocarbon derivative. Immunohistochemistry.

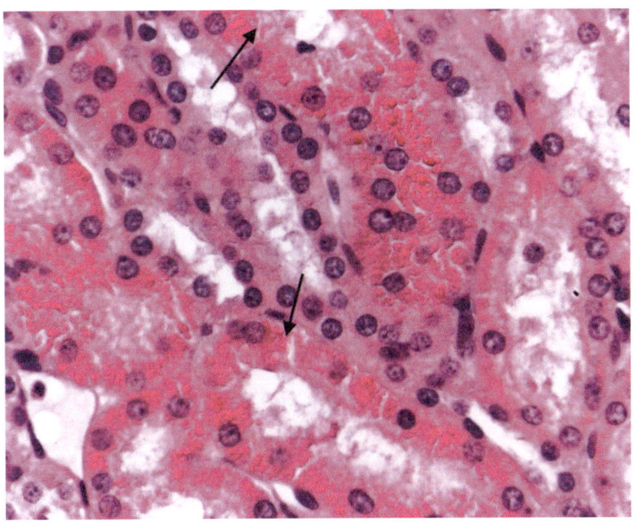

**Figure 5-22.** Intracytoplasmic eosinophilic inclusions (*arrows*), PCT, in a female dog treated with a novel pharmaceutical agent. H&E.

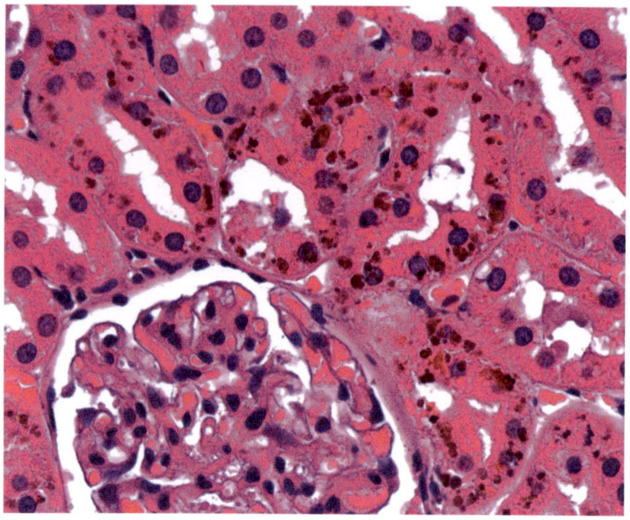

**Figure 5-23.** Brown pigment in tubular epithelium. Pigmented macrophages in the interstitium, in a rat treated with an agrochemical agent. H&E.

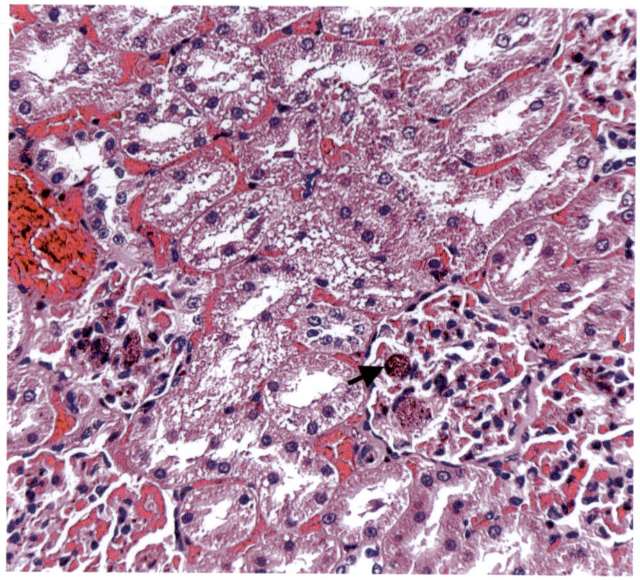

**Figure 5-24.** Pigmented cells in glomeruli (*arrow*), rat treated with Fe-chelating agent. H&E.

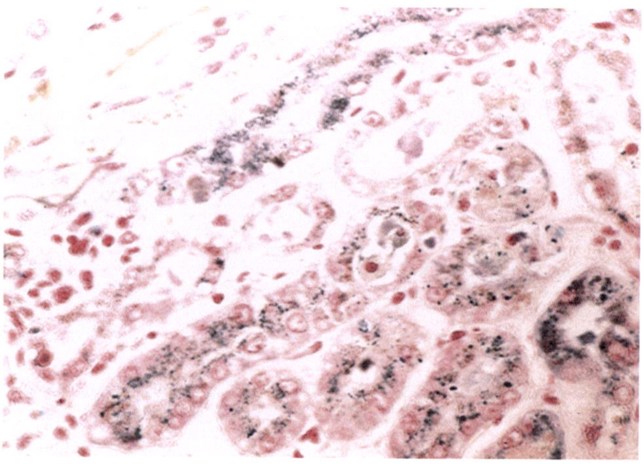

**Figure 5-25.** Copper-containing pigment in renal cortical tubules, in a sheep, shows evidence of copper toxicity. Rubeanic acid.

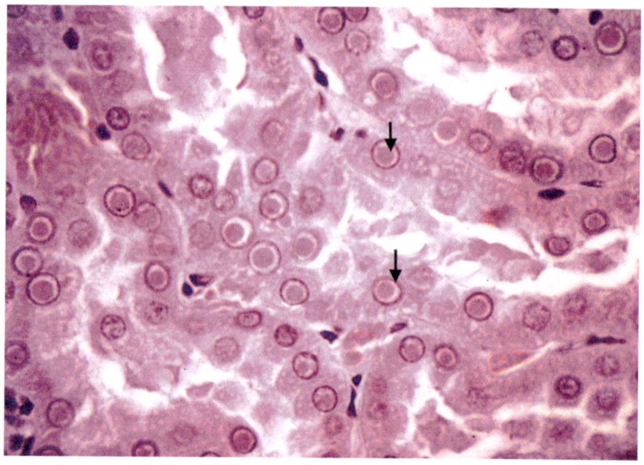

**Figure 5-26.** Intranuclear eosinophilic inclusions (*arrows*) in PCT, in a rat treated with a novel pharmaceutical agent. H&E.

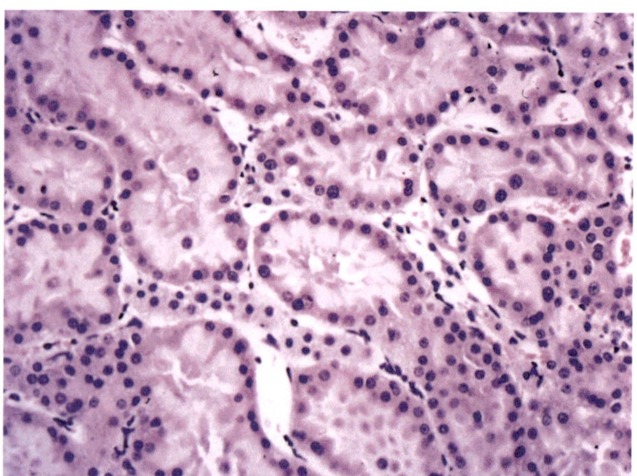

**Figure 5-27.** Hypertrophy of tubular epithelium, pars recta, in a rat treated with an agrochemical agent. Cells are enlarged and tall, almost occluding the lumen. H&E.

Tubular dilation is induced by diuretic agents like furosemide (Figs. 5.28 and 5.29). Degeneration and necrosis are often accompanied by tubular basophilia and dilation. Obstructive lesions in CDs cause dilation of the nephron anterior to the blockage. Sugar alcohols cause tubular dilation in dogs, and lithium causes similar changes in rodents. Lithium also causes hypertrophy of the CDs. Hypertrophy of the CD is seen as a result of treatment with certain diuretic agents and increased intake of sodium chloride. Corticosteroids, when given to pregnant rats, result in cystic dilation of medullary tubules in the offspring owing to defective development of CDs (Fig. 5.30).

Crystalline nephropathy is caused by agents that precipitate crystalline deposits in the CDs, producing an obstructive nephropathy (Fig. 5.31). In addition to causing obstruction, the crystals can cause inflammation locally (Fig. 5.32). The sections of the nephron anterior to the blockage show dilation, casts, and epithelial damage. The change is often seen with a linear distribution leaving sections of renal parenchyma unaffected (Fig. 5.33). The affected areas sometimes show interstitial inflammation. Purine analogues like allopurinol, quinolone antibiotics, acyclovir, methoxyflurane, and sulphonamides are among the agents that evoke this type of nephropathy [26].

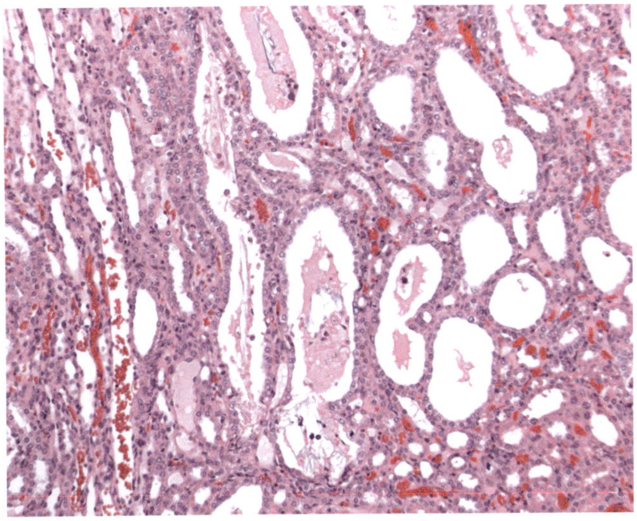

**Figure 5-28.** Tubular dilation and casts, collecting ducts, in a rat treated with an antibacterial agent. H&E.

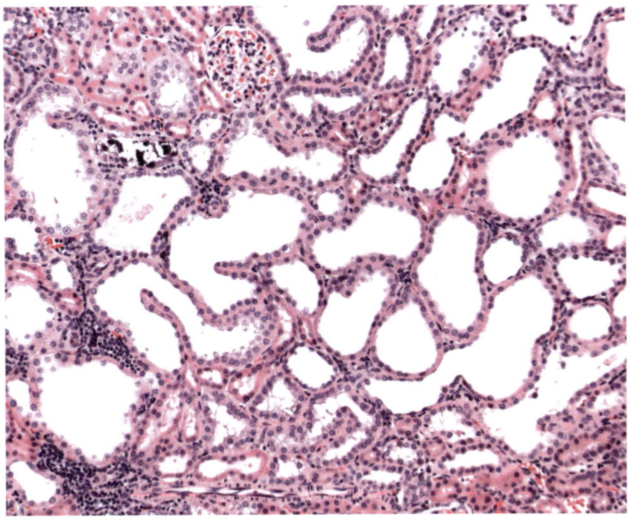

**Figure 5-29.** Tubular dilation, cortex, in a rat. Note interstitial inflammation and mineralisation, multifocal. H&E.

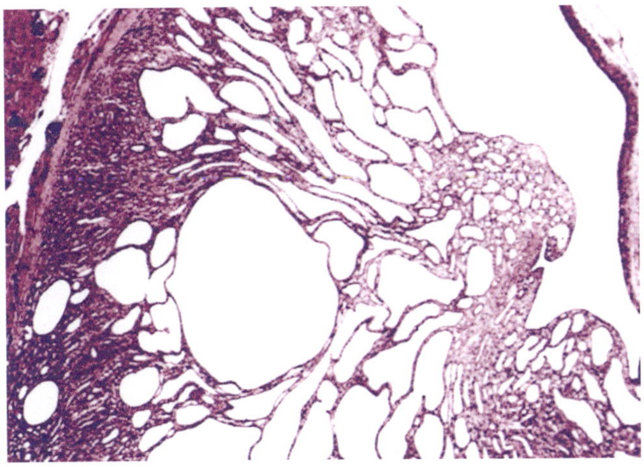

**Figure 5-30.** Cystic dilation of tubules, inner cortex and medulla, in a rat from a reproductive study. H&E.

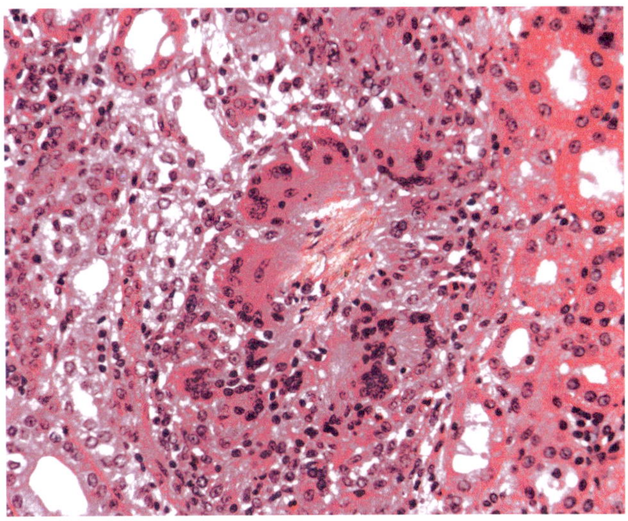

**Figure 5-31.** Crystalline nephropathy, in a dog treated with an antibacterial agent. Note crystals in dilated collecting ducts, some with inflammatory cells and interstitial inflammation. H&E.

Oxalates and other xenobiotics are known to induce crystal deposition in CDs, some of which cause granulomatous inflammation whereas others result in local epithelial hyperplasia of the CD in the renal medulla (Fig. 5.34). Most crystalline deposits are birefringent under polarised light.

Intratubular mineral deposition can be spontaneous in female rodent kidneys in the CD in the outer strip. The change is exaggerated by treatment with xenobiotics. Synthetic diets, acetazolamide, vitamin D, and calcium salts are among the agents that induce mineralisation (Fig. 5.35). Mineralisation can also follow necrosis, cast formation, and crystalline deposits. Parathyroid hyperactivity results in mineralisation, affecting the parenchyma (multifocal) and basement membranes (Fig. 5.36).

On rare occasions, certain carcinogens like aflatoxin, pyrrolizidine alkaloids, and other xenobiotics induce karyomegaly and cytomegaly, affecting the CD and cortical tubular epithelium (Fig. 5.37). The affected cell protrudes into the lumen with hyperchromatic vesicular nuclei (Fig. 5.38).

Regenerative tubular hyperplasia often follows necrosis and cell loss (Fig. 5.39). The affected tubules appear basophilic, sometimes multilayered, and cells have vesicular nuclei (Fig. 5.40). In simple hyperplasia, the tubules demonstrate increased cellularity seen during chronic nephropathy. The epithelium may show minimal folding. The hyperplasia is complex or atypical, when the proliferating epithelium forms papillary ingrowths into the lumen or atypical epithelium proliferates to obliterate the lumen. The important

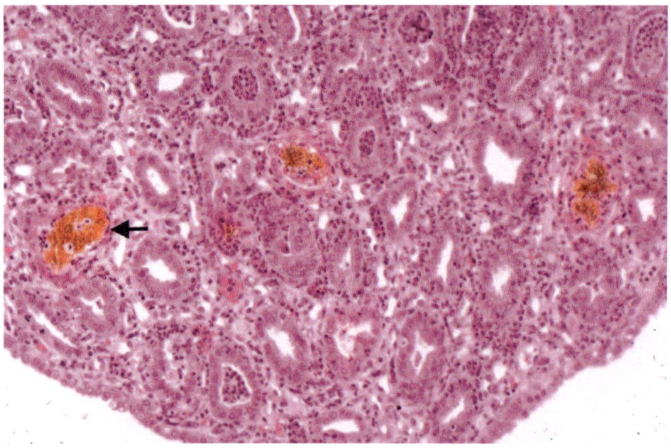

**Figure 5-32.** Pigmented crystals in collecting ducts (*arrow*), in a monkey. Papillary ducts show hyperplasia and interstitial inflammation. H&E.

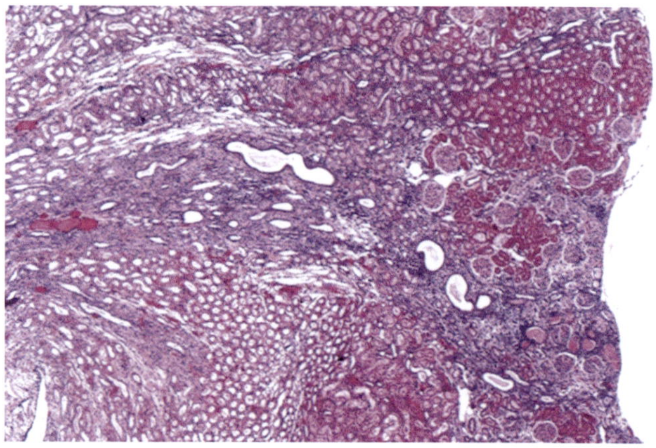

**Figure 5-33.** Linear cortical scar, kidney, in a rat. The scar shows tubular basophilia, dilation, interstitial fibrosis, and inflammation. Adjacent parenchyma remains unaffected. H&E.

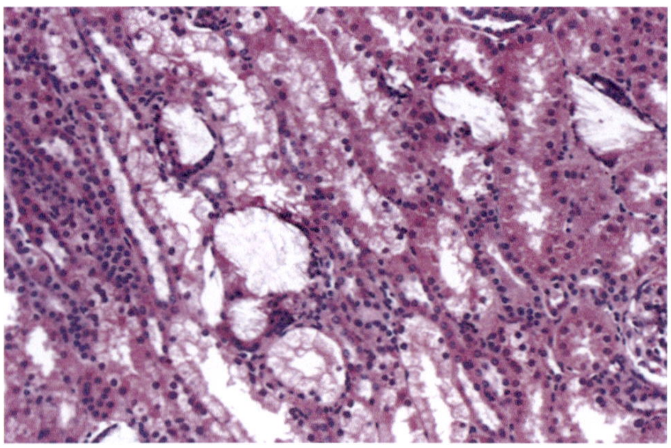

**Figure 5-34.** Tubular vacuolation and crystals, some with giant cell reaction, in a monkey treated with ethylene chloride. H&E.

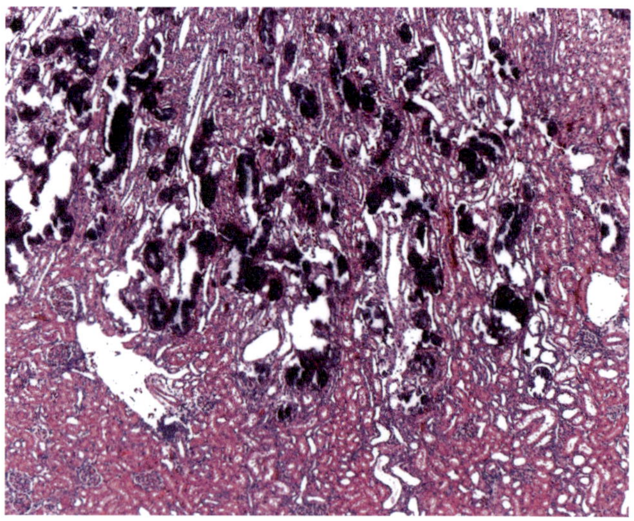

**Figure 5-35.** Mineralisation, marked, inner cortex and medulla, in a rat treated with a vitamin D analogue. H&E.

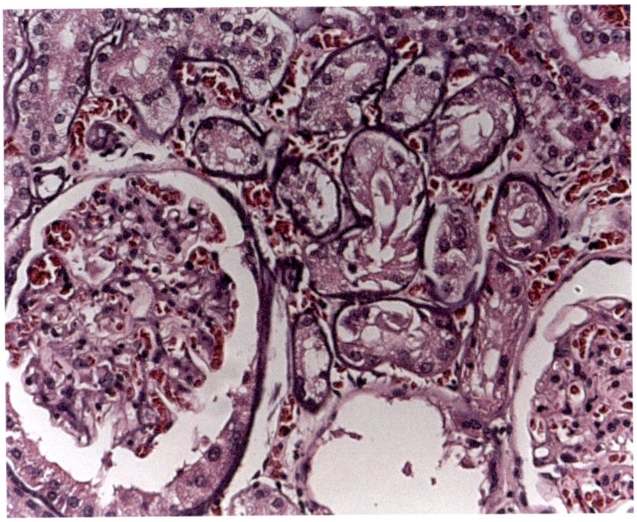

**Figure 5-36.** Mineralisation, basement membranes, cortex, in a rat. H&E.

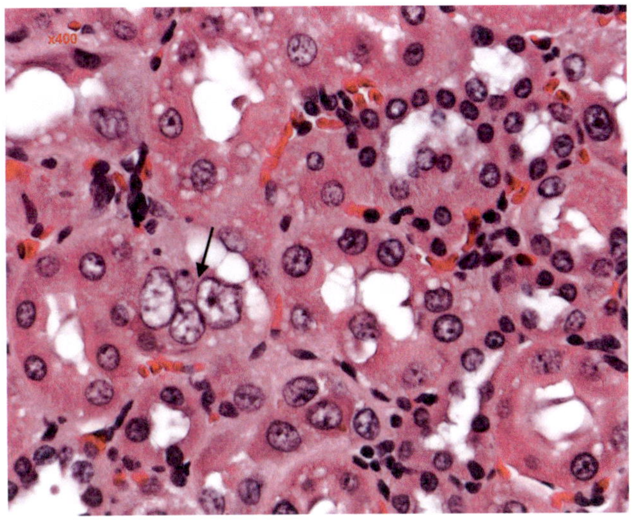



**Figure 5-37.** Cytomegaly and karyomegaly (*arrow*), renal cortex, in a rat treated with an industrial chemical. H&E.

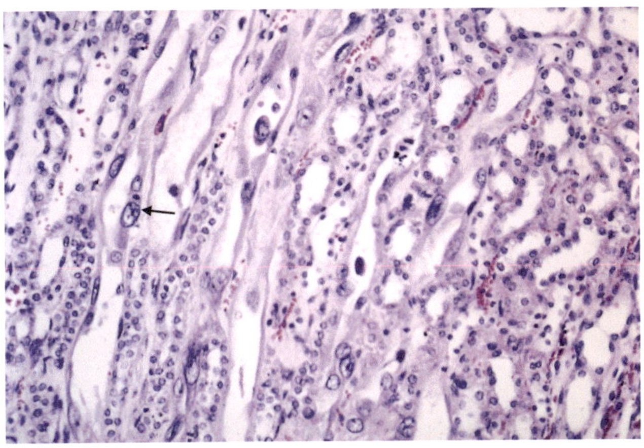

**Figure 5-38.** Cytomegaly and karyomegaly (*arrow*), medullary collecting ducts, in a rat treated with an anti-inflammatory agent (with kind permission from Springer Science + Business Media B.V) [5]. H&E.

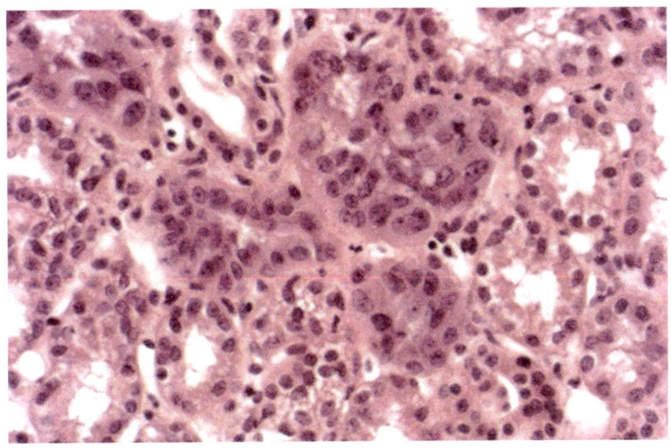

**Figure 5-39.** Regenerative hyperplasia, PCT, in a rat. Note basophilic multilayered epithelium. H&E.

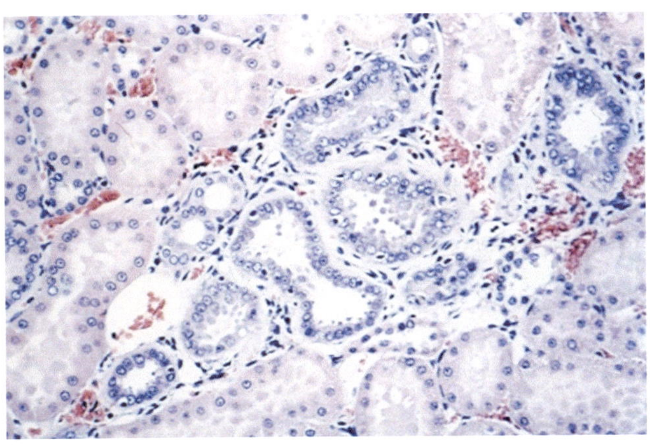

**Figure 5-40.** Regenerative hyperplasia of cortical tubules, in a rat. Note dilated tubules, basophilic epithelium, vesicular nuclei, and focal multilayering. H&E (With kind permission from Springer Science + Business Media B.V [5]).

feature is maintenance of the basement membrane (tubular outline) (Fig. 5.41). On rare occasions, hyperplasia can occur affecting only a localised area of the tubular epithelium (Fig. 5.42). This has been observed in rats treated with a herbicide (personal observation).

Focal tubular phenotypic alteration is seen in chronic studies or in aged animals (Fig. 5.43). This appears as enlarged tubules lined by cells showing altered staining properties such as increased eosinophilia, basophilia, or clear cytoplasm (Figs. 5.44–5.46). The cells are hypertrophic, show invaginations, and can be multilayered. The true nature of these is not clear, but certain xenobiotics are known to induce these altered tubules during chronic treatments.

### 5.1.4 Papilla

Several nonsteroidal anti-inflammatory drugs (NSAIDs), analgesics, and some agrochemicals are known to induce renal papillary necrosis (RPN) in experimental animals (Fig. 5.47) [27, 28]. RPN is the acute necrosis of the renal papillary matrix, interstitial cells and vessels, and papillary tubules (Figs. 5.48 and 5.49). The changes initially develop in the papillary tip as foci of interstitial degeneration and appear as pale pink foci of hyalinisation (Fig. 5.50). The lesions extend to involve blood vessels and CDs, ending in necrosis of the entire papillary tip. A haemorrhagic zone separates the healthy papilla from the necrotic zone; inflammation is not often seen.

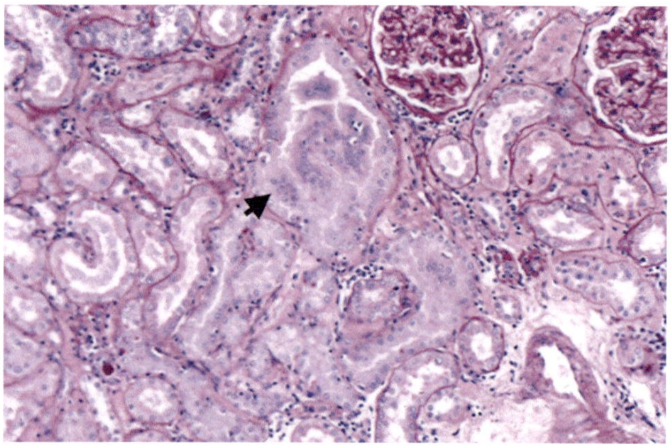

**Figure 5-41.** Atypical hyperplasia, renal cortex, in a rat. Note intratubular papillary proliferation within a dilated tubule (*arrow*) and intact basement membrane. PAS (With kind permission from Springer Science+Business Media B.V [5]).

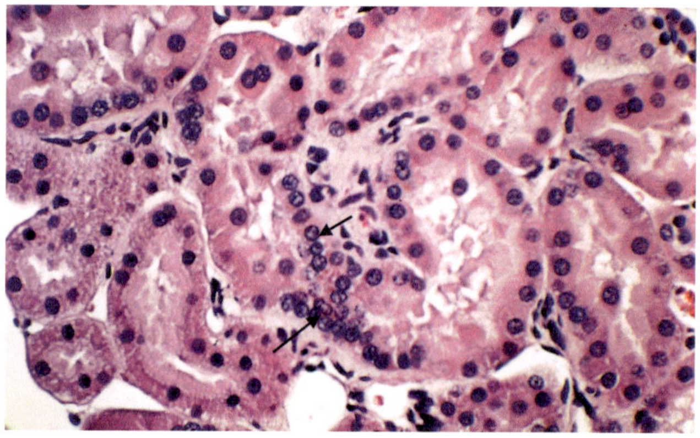

**Figure 5-42.** Tubular hyperplasia, intratubular, partial, pars recta, in a rat treated with an herbicide. Note area of nuclear crowding and increased basophilia (*arrows*). H&E.

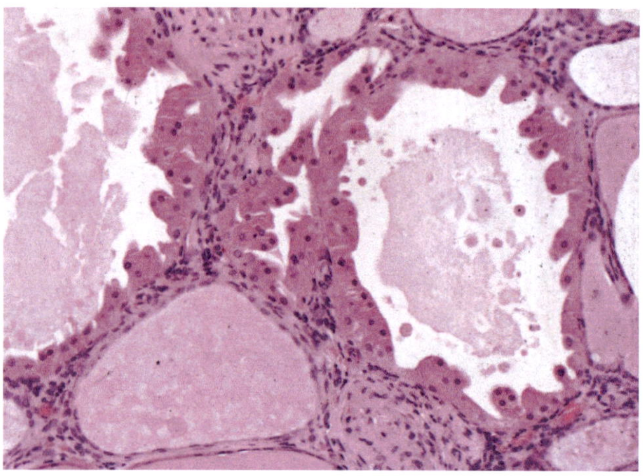

**Figure 5-43.** Tubular eosinophilia and hypertrophy, in a rat. Note enlarged, dilated tubule lined by hypertrophic eosinophilic epithelium. H&E (With kind permission from Springer Science+Business Media B.V [5]).

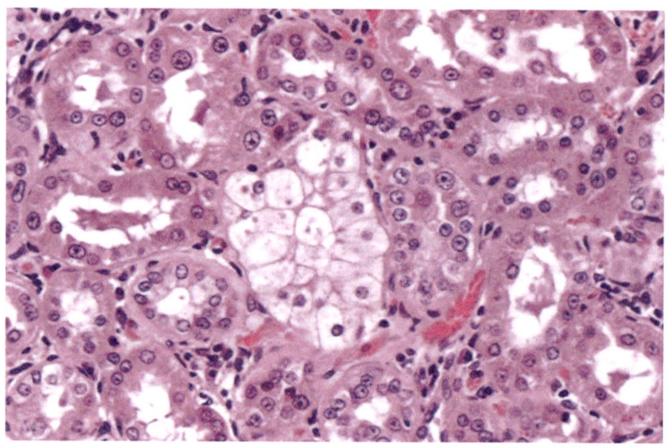

**Figure 5-44.** Clear tubule, renal cortex, in a rat. Note tubule lined by enlarged cells with clear cytoplasm. H&E (With kind permission from Springer Science+Business Media B.V [5]).

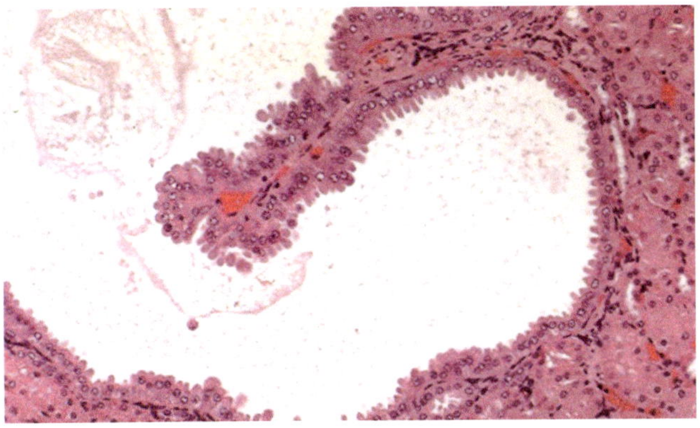

**Figure 5-45.** Cystic hyperplastic tubule, cortex, in a rat. Cystic tubule lined by eosinophilic cells shows papillary ingrowth. H&E.

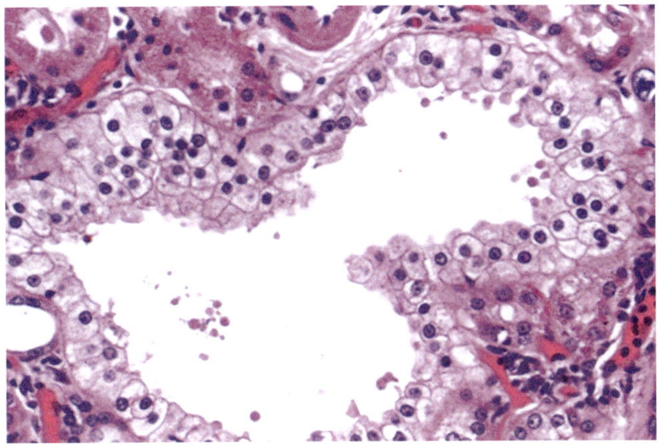

**Figure 5-46.** Clear tubule, renal cortex, in a rat. Note enlarged tubule lined by clear cells and multilayering. H&E (With kind permission from Springer Science + Business Media B.V [5]).

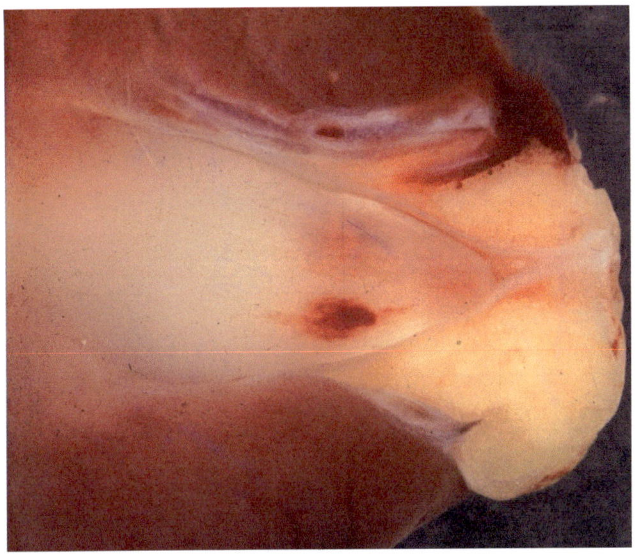

**Figure 5-47.** Renal papillary necrosis, in a rat treated with a nonsteroidal anti-inflammatory agent. Note pale and haemorrhagic areas in the papillary tip.

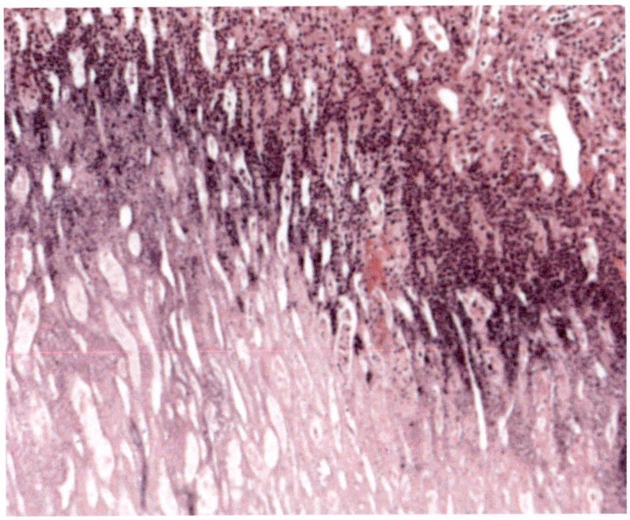

**Figure 5-48.** Renal papillary necrosis (RPN), area of papillary necrosis, in a rat treated with a nonsteroidal anti-inflammatory drug (NSAID). Necrotic area is separated by an inflammatory zone. H&E.

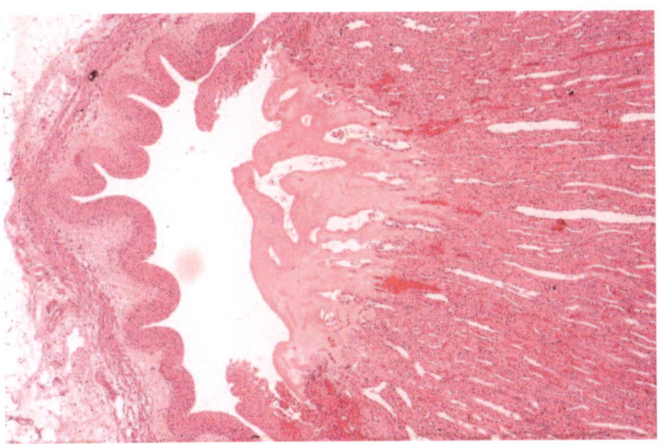

**Figure 5-49.** RPN, in a monkey treated with an NSAID. Note scanty inflammatory cell infiltration. H&E.

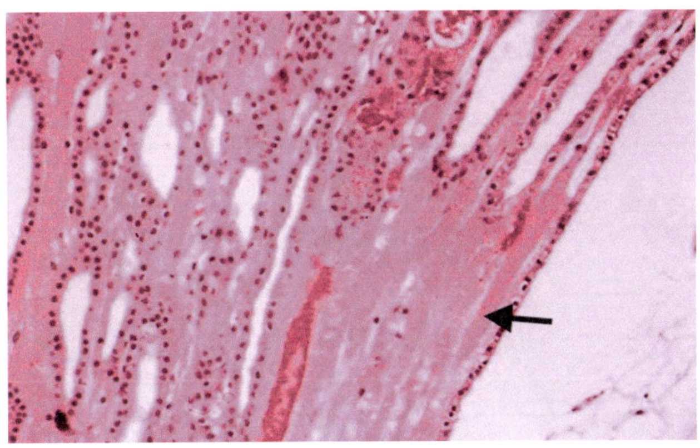

**Figure 5-50.** RPN, early, in a rat treated with an NSAID. A small area in renal papilla shows hyalinisation and early degeneration (*arrow*). H&E.

Alcian blue staining is reduced owing to loss of glycosaminoglycans. Interstitial degeneration, lipid deposition, and degeneration of capillary endothelium occur. 2-Bromo-ethamine hydrobromide, dapsone, cyclophosphamide, and aspirin are among the agents that produce RPN. In some cases, the necrotic zone breaks off. Repair by regeneration of the papillary epithelium and/or scarring occurs. The papillary tip can appear irregular owing to regenerative hyperplasia of the epithelium (Fig. 5.51).

Agents like NSAIDs and saccharin induce papillary epithelial hyperplasia (Figs. 5.52 and 5.53). Vacuolation and intracytoplasmic inclusions are induced by certain xenobiotics such as carbonic anhydrase inhibitors (Fig. 5.54) [29]. Intracytoplasmic eosinophilic granules have been seen in the papillary ducts of rats treated with an industrial chemical (Fig. 5.55).

Renal pelvic dilation can be induced by certain NSAIDs during prolonged treatment (Fig. 5.56). Treatment of dogs with corticosteroids produced mild thickening of epithelium of renal pelvis. This was not a true hyperplasia, because there was no change in the basal layers but a slight increase in cellularity of the superficial layers, the cells displaying small pyknotic nuclei. It appears that there is deficient cell deletion from the surface rather than proliferation. Submucosal inflammation and granulomata have been seen in the pelvis of rats treated with a pharmaceutical intermediary (Fig. 5.57).

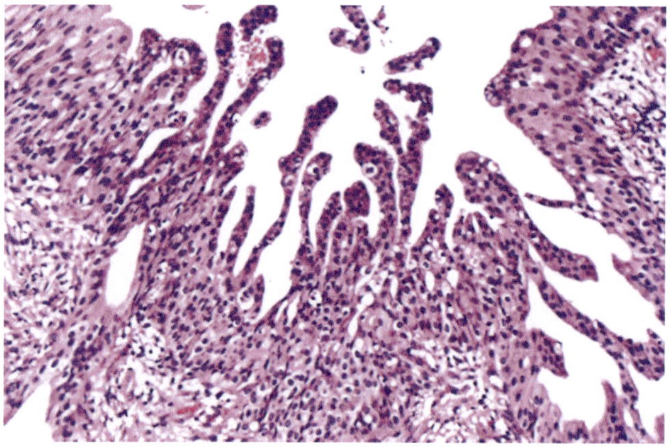

**FIGURE 5-51.** Papillary hyperplasia, in a monkey treated with an NSAID. Note villous proliferation of papillary epithelium. H&E.

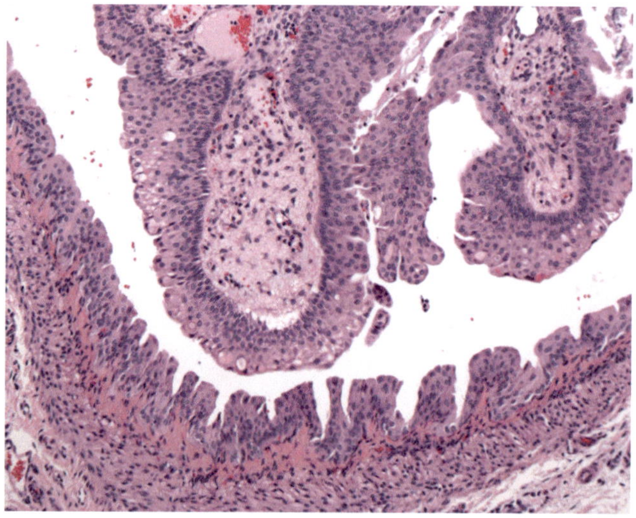

**FIGURE 5-52.** Epithelial hyperplasia, papilla and pelvis, in a pig treated with an antibacterial agent. H&E.

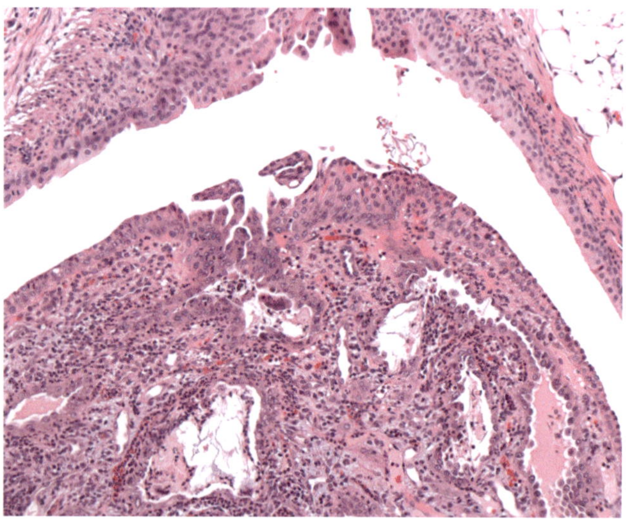

**FIGURE 5-53.** Epithelial hyperplasia and inflammation, papilla and pelvis, in a pig treated with an antibacterial agent. Note crystals in papillary ducts and interstitial inflammation. H&E.

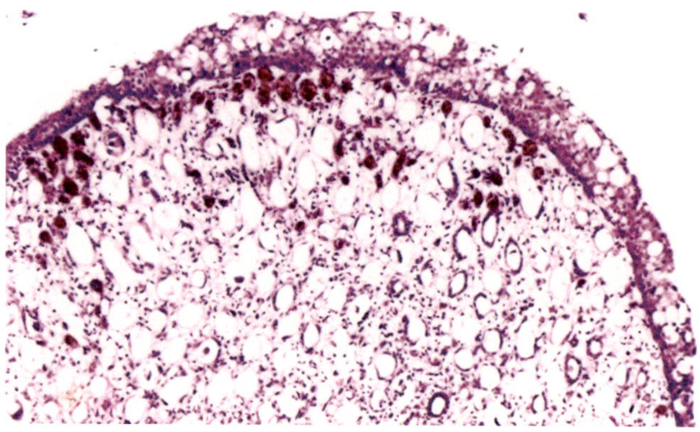

**FIGURE 5-54.** Vacuolation, papillary epithelium, in a rat. H&E (With kind permission from Springer Science + Business Media B.V [5]).

## 5.1.5 Vascular Changes

Systemic responses such as atherosclerosis can affect renal vessels, as noticed in monkeys fed on a high-cholesterol diet. Hypervitaminosis D and parathormone excess result in metastatic calcification of renal vessels and basement membranes. Renal arteriolar hypertrophy, occlusive thickening, and fibrinoid necrosis are seen in renal arterioles of hypertensive rats. Fibrinoid necrosis is induced in rats treated with cyclosporine. Vasculitis is seen in the renal vessels of rats treated with vasodilating antihypertensive agents, phosphodiesterase inhibitors, and daunomycin (Figs. 5.58 and 5.59). Thrombosis and infarction are induced by serotonin. A novel hypolipidaemic agent has resulted in thrombosis of the arcuate veins in monkeys.

Angiotensin-converting enzyme (ACE) inhibitors cause hyperplasia of the renin-producing cells of the juxtaglomerular apparatus (Figs. 5.60 and 5.61) [30, 31]. The afferent arterioles of the glomeruli become hyperplastic. This change can affect all laboratory species but is reversible [10, 30, 31]. In prolonged treatment, the lesion can become nodular in mice owing to extreme hyperplasia (Fig. 5.62). In ACE inhibitor toxicity, the renal parenchyma also reveals basophilic atrophic tubules with thickened basement membrane, peritubular fibrosis, and interstitial lymphocytic infiltration (Fig. 5.63).

Interstitial nephritis is induced by chronic treatment with sulphonamides, allopurinol, cimetidine, and rifamycin. Interstitial fibrosis and chronic inflammation can be partly mediated by immune responses. Interstitial fibrosis is seen in treatment with cisplatin and oestrogens in dogs.

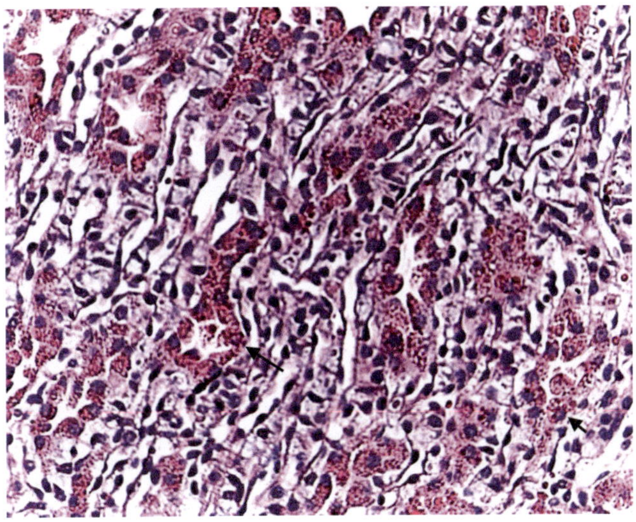

**Figure 5-55.** Intracytoplasmic eosinophilic granular inclusions, papillary ducts (*arrow*), in a rat treated with an industrial chemical. H&E.

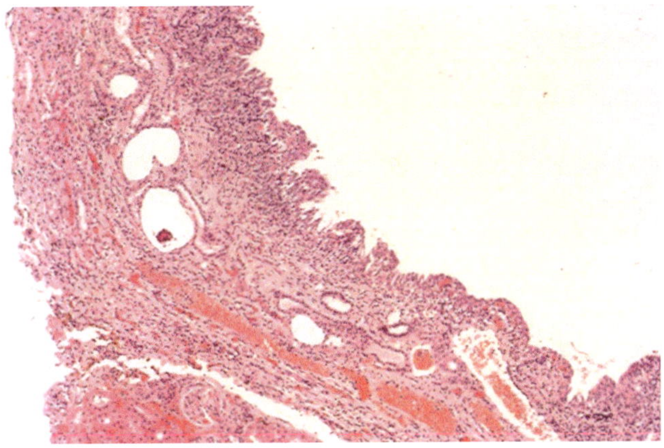

**Figure 5-56.** Pyelitis and pelvic dilation, in a rat treated with an agrochemical agent. H&E.

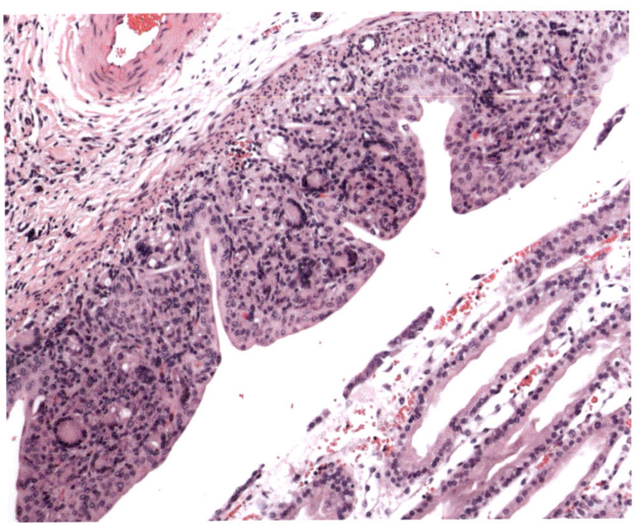

**Figure 5-57.** Pelvic inflammation and hyperplasia, in a rat treated with an industrial chemical. Note subepithelial granulomatous inflammation with giant cells. H&E.

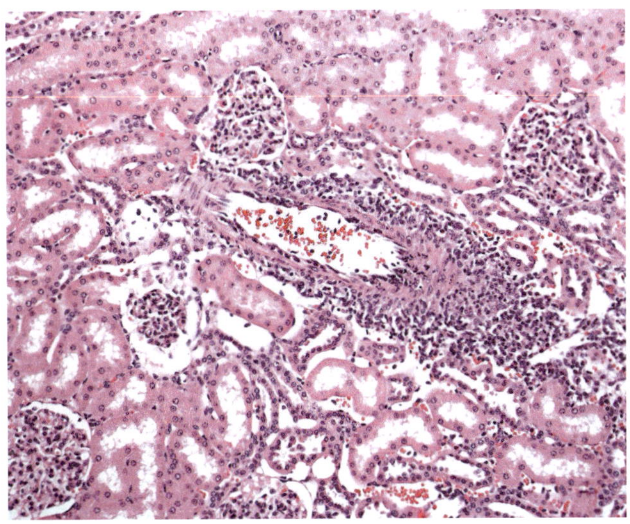

**Figure 5-58.** Vasculitis, renal cortex, in a monkey treated with a novel immunomodulator. H&E.

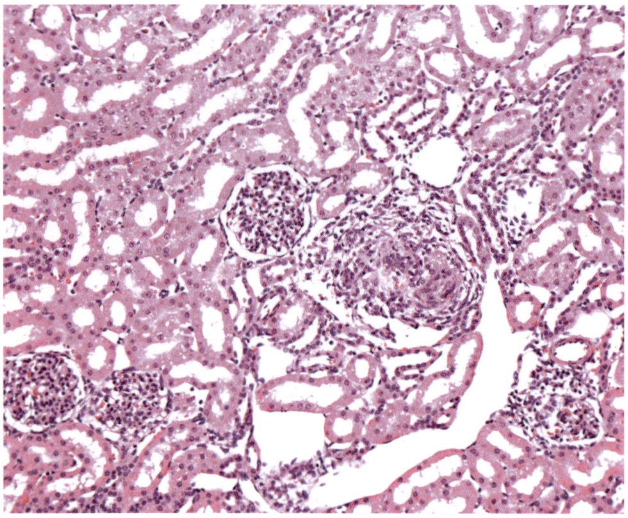

**Figure 5-59.** Vasculitis, renal cortex, in a rat treated with a phosphodiesterase-4 (PDE-4) inhibitor. H&E.

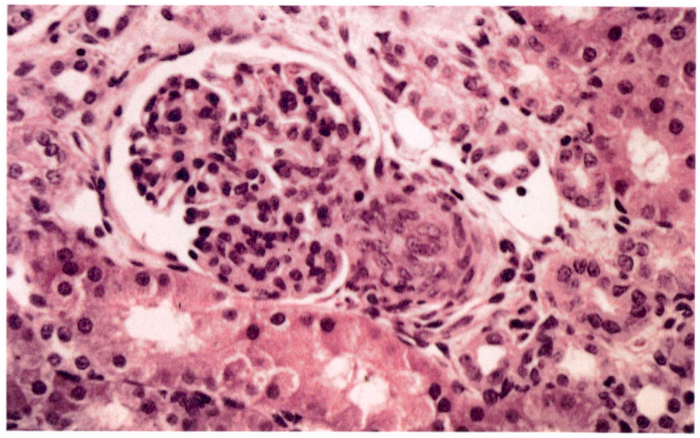

**Figure 5-60.** Arterial hypertrophy, afferent arteriole, renal corpuscle, in a rat treated with an angiotensin-converting enzyme (ACE) inhibitor. H&E.

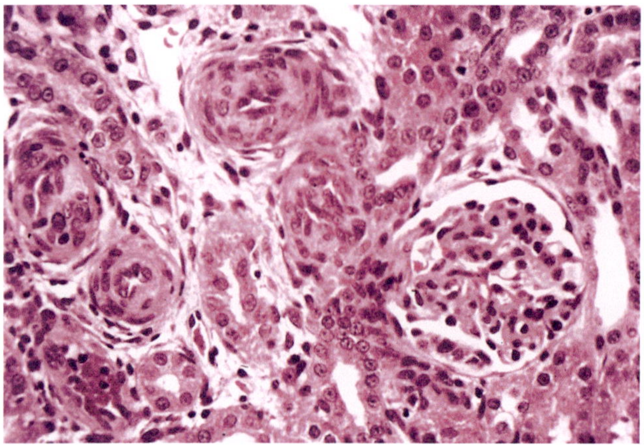

**Figure 5-61.** Arterial hypertrophy, renal cortex, in a rat treated with an ACE inhibitor. Multiple hypertrophic arterioles are seen in the cortex. H&E (With kind permission from Springer Science+Business Media B.V [5]).

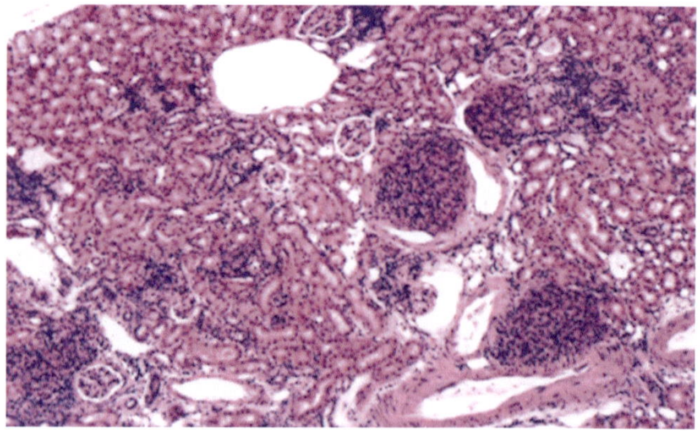

**Figure 5-62.** Arteriolar hypertrophy, nodular, renal cortex, in a mouse treated long term with an ACE inhibitor. H&E.

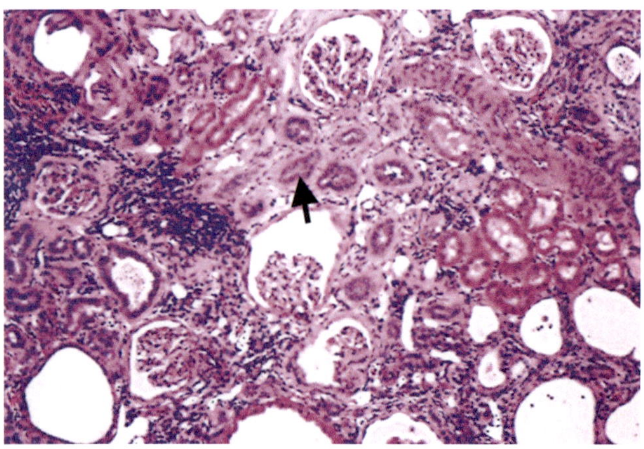

**Figure 5-63.** Interstitial and peritubular fibrosis (*arrow*) and interstitial inflammation, basophilic and dilated tubules, in a mouse treated long term with an ACE inhibitor. H&E.

## 5.1.6 Tumours

Renal adenomas and adenocarcinomas are induced by genotoxic agents like dimethylnitrosamine (DMN), lead salts, and aflatoxin (Figs. 5.64 and 5.65). Renal adenomas are induced in male rats by chronic exposure to hydrocarbon derivatives. The mechanisms of carcinogenesis have been surveyed [32], and guides for the classification and interpretation of renal hyperplasias and tumours in rodents are available [1, 12]. In rats, a type of tubular tumour of suspected familial origin is reported [33, 34]. These have a characteristic phenotype with a lobulated appearance and cells with amphophilic, vacuolated cytoplasm. A continuum of hyperplasias, adenomas, and carcinomas occur with this phenotype. It is recommended to interpret this type of tumour separately from other renal tumours for safety assessment.

Nephroblastomas are induced in rats by ethyl nitrosourea, and renal mesenchymal tumours are induced by DMN and cycasin [35–37]. Renal pelvic tumours (transitional cell carcinomas) are induced by phenacetin and phenazone in rats [38].

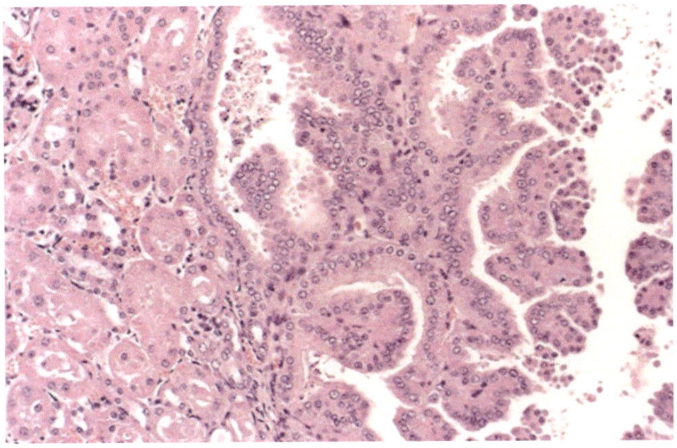

**Figure 5-64.** Renal tubular adenoma, in a mouse.

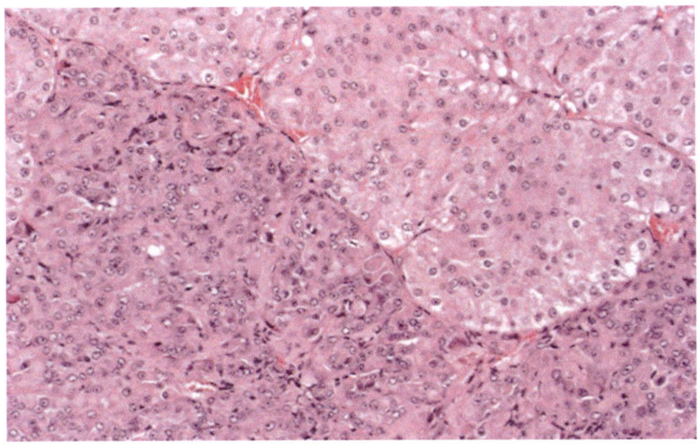

**Figure 5-65.** Renal tubular carcinoma, in a rat. Neoplastic cells are arranged in a trabecular pattern, and solid sheets of more basophilic cells are also present. H&E.

## 5.2 Urinary Bladder

Induced changes of the urinary bladder are few owing to the bladder's limited responses to injury; the urinary bladder is a rare target organ in toxicity studies. Proper fixation of the bladder mucosa by careful distension with fixatives to avoid folds and an artefactual appearance of thickening of the mucosa is recommended. The changes encountered are:

- Mucosal necrosis, erosion, ulceration
- Mucosal hyperplasia
- Calculi
- Vascular changes
- Tumours

A number of chemicals can cause injury to mucosa, resulting in necrosis, inflammation, haemorrhage, and regenerative hyperplasia. The affected epithelium sometimes reveals intracytoplasmic erythrocytes. Chemicals like methyl methanesulphonate, ethylsulphanyl-naphthoate, sulphonamide, and cyclophosphamide are cytotoxic. Urothelial hyperplasia can be focal or diffuse and can be simple, papillary, or nodular (Figs. 5.66 and 5.67). It sometimes shows focal squamous metaplasia and can be associated with inflammation (Figs. 5.68 and 5.69). Most of the hyperplasias are reversible on stoppage of exposure to the chemical in question. Some agents produce hyperplasia without necrosis, such as phenacetin, saccharine, and vitamin A deficiency. Certain peroxisome proliferator-activated receptor agonists (antidiabetic agents) and Raf kinase

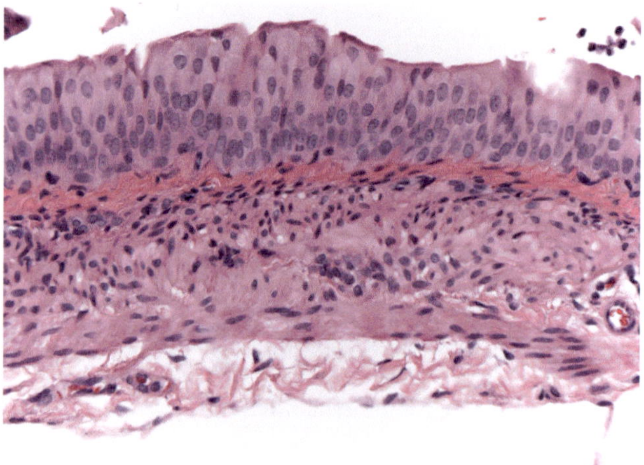

**FIGURE 5-66.** Urothelial hyperplasia, urinary bladder, in a rat. H&E.

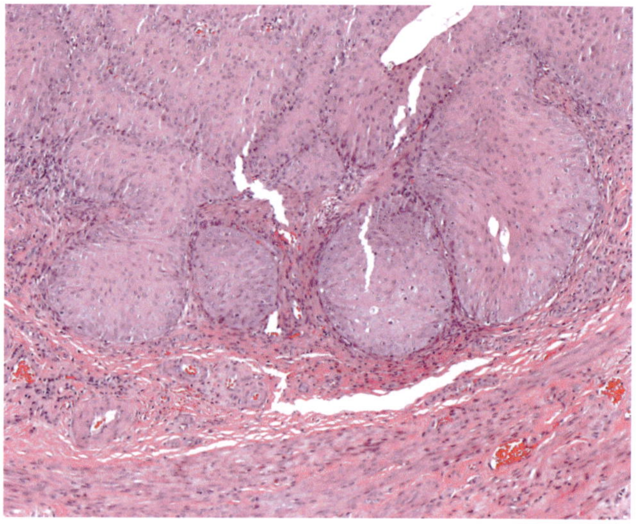

**FIGURE 5-67.** Nodular hyperplasia, urinary bladder, in a rat treated with a peroxisome proliferator-activated receptor (PPAR) agonist. H&E.

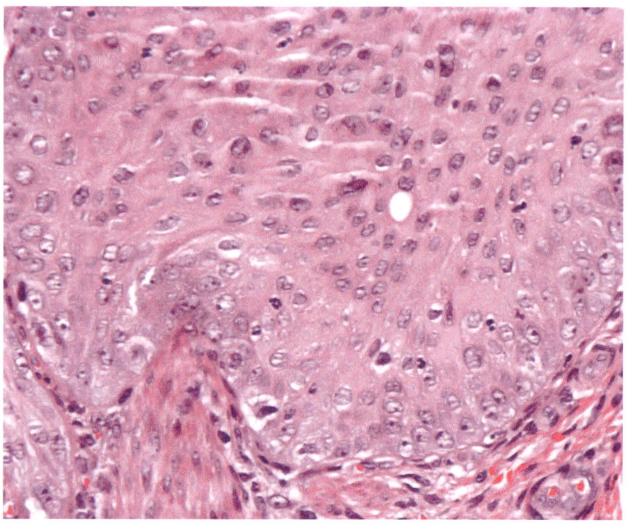

**FIGURE 5-68.** Squamous metaplasia, urinary bladder, in a rat. H&E.

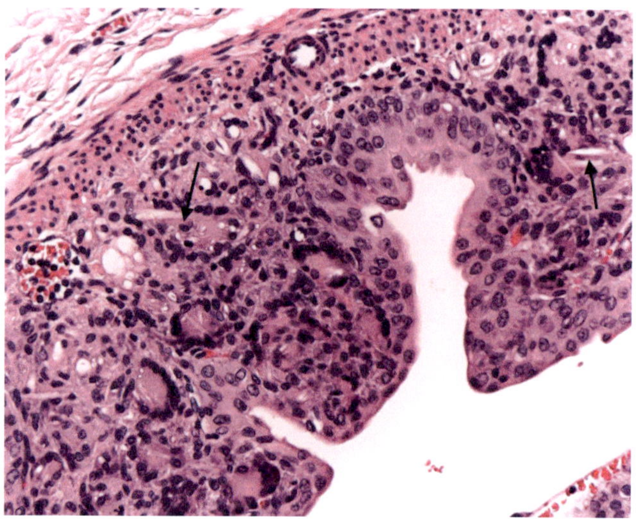

**FIGURE 5-69.** Granulomatous inflammation (*arrow*) and urothelial hyperplasia, urinary bladder, in a rat treated with an industrial chemical. H&E.

inhibitors cause bladder hyperplasia and neoplasia in rodents [39–41]. Some of these agents result in epithelial vacuolation, but not hyperplasia, in the urinary bladder of monkeys [42]. Acetazolamide results in inflammation and hyperplasia. Mechanical irritation caused by calculi, crystals, or foreign bodies can produce urothelial hyperplasia and neoplasia in rodents. Thinning of the bladder epithelium or atrophy has been seen in dogs treated with high doses of corticosteroids. Bladder calculi are induced by carbonic anhydrase inhibitors [43], sulphonamides, agents that alter urinary pH, and imbalance of dietary calcium, potassium, or magnesium. Calculi consist of calcium phosphate, magnesium phosphate, and/or calcium oxalate. They are often mixtures.

Administration of a psychoactive agent to mice over a long period produced focal subepithelial angiectasis, angiomatous hyperplasia, and angiomatous tumours of the bladder mucosa (Figs. 5.70 and 5.71).

Some agents cause persistent hyperplasia over a period which becomes irreversible hyperplasia, progressing to preneoplasia and tumours. Tumours appear as papillomas, urothelial carcinomas, squamous cell carcinomas, or even as combinations. PPAR agonists and saccharine are tumorigenic in rodents (Figs. 5.72 and 5.73).

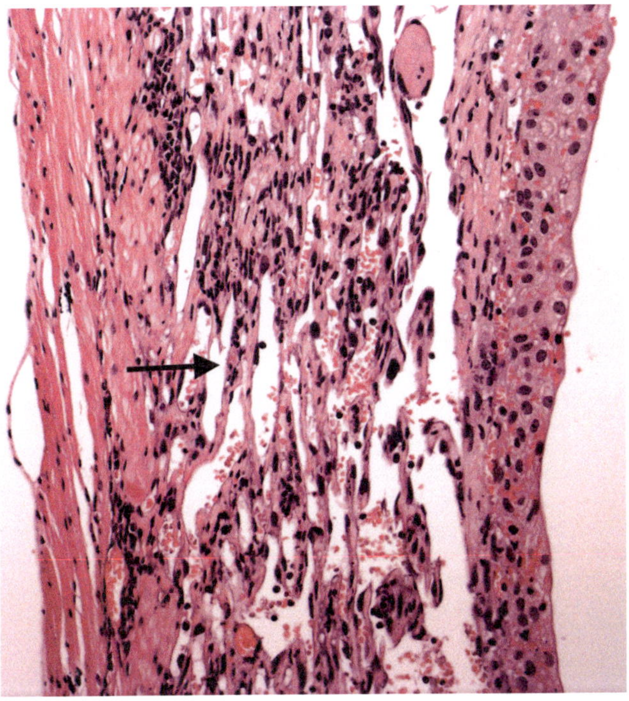

**Figure 5-70.** Angiomatous hyperplasia (*arrow*), submucosa, urinary bladder, in a mouse treated with a psychoactive agent. H&E.

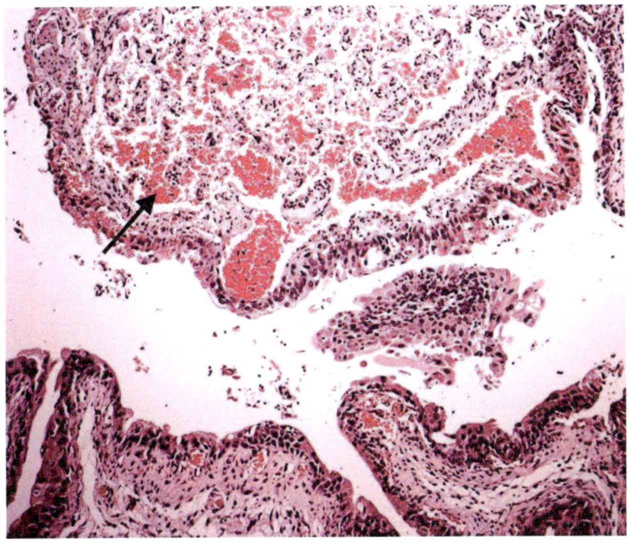

**Figure 5-71.** Haemangioma (*arrow*), urinary bladder, in a mouse treated with a psychoactive agent. H&E.

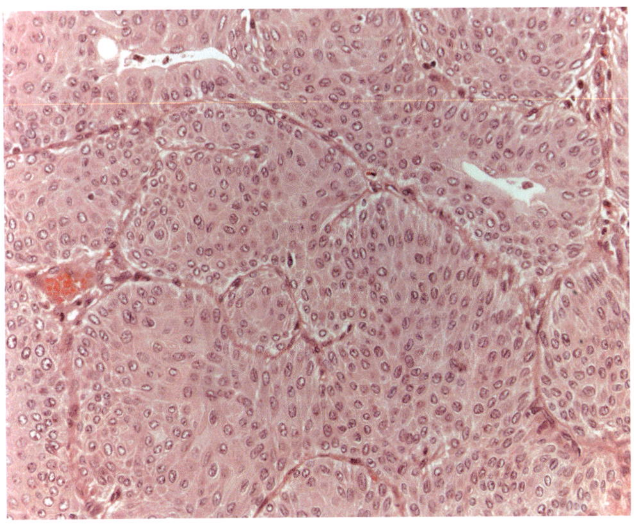

**Figure 5-72.** Urothelial carcinoma, urinary bladder, in a rat. Atypical neoplastic cells are arranged in groups surrounded by basement membrane. H&E.

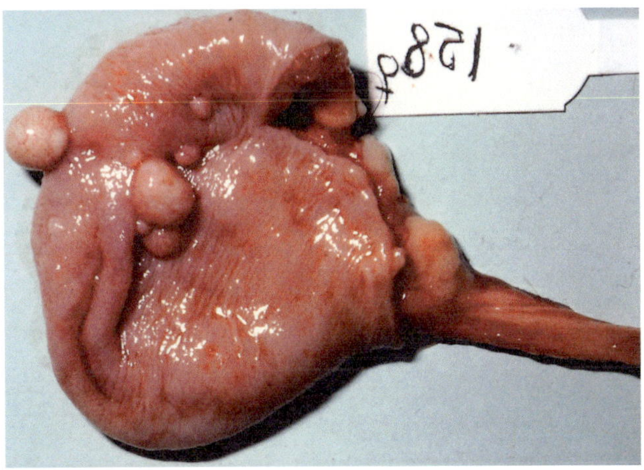

**Figure 5-73.** Carcinoma, urinary bladder, in a dog. H&E.

# References


1. Frazier KS, Seely JC, Hard GC, Betton G, Burnett R, Nakatsuji S, et al. Proliferative and nonproliferative lesions of the rat and mouse urinary system. Toxicol Pathol. 2012;40:14S–86.
2. Ryan GB, Karnovsky MJ. An ultrastructural study of the mechanisms of proteinuria in aminonucleoside nephrosis. Kidney Int. 1975;8:219–32.
3. Weening JJ, Rennke HG. Glomerular permeability and polyanion in adriamycin nephrosis in the rat. Kidney Int. 1983;24:152–9.
4. Tucker MJ. Some effects of prolonged administration of a progestogen to dogs. Proc Eur Soc Study Drug Toxic. 1971;12: 228–38.
5. Gopinath C, Prentice DE, Lewis DJ. The urinary system. In: Atlas of experimental toxicological pathology. Lancaster: MTP Press Ltd; 1987. p. 77.
6. Mazue G, Newman AJ, Scampini G, Della TP, Hard GC, Iatropoulos MJ, et al. The histopathology of kidney changes in rats and monkeys following intravenous administration of massive doses of FCE 26184, human basic fibroblast growth factor. Toxicol Pathol. 1993;21:490–501.
7. Robinson CJ, Egoron I, Balazs T. Strain differences in the induction of antinuclear antibodies by mercuric chloride, gold sodium thiomaleate and D-penicillamine in inbred mice. Fed Proc. 1983;42:1213.
8. Robinson CJ, Abraham AA, Balazs T. Induction of anti-nuclear antibodies by mercuric chloride in mice. Clin Exp Immunol. 1984;58:300–6.
9. Wright NG, Nash AS. Experimental ampicillin glomerulonephropath. J Comp Pathol. 1984;94:357–61.
10. Crabtree C. The structure of Bowman's capsule and castrate and testosterone treated mice as an index of hormonal effect on the renal cortex. Endocrinology. 1941;29:197–203.
11. Greaves P. Urinary tract. In: Histopathology of preclinical toxicity studies. Amsterdam: Academic; 2007. p. 570.
12. Hard GC, Seely JC. Recommendations for the interpretation of renal tubule proliferative lesions occurring in rat kidneys with advanced chronic progressive nephropathy (CPN). Toxicol Pathol. 2005;33:641–9.
13. Hard GC, Seely JC. Histological investigation of diagnostically challenging tubule profiles in advanced chronic progressive nephropathy (CPN) in the Fischer 344 rat. Toxicol Pathol. 2006;34:941–8.
14. Hard GC, Betz LJ, Seely JC. Association of advanced chronic progressive nephropathy (CPN) with renal tubule tumors and precursor hyperplasia in control F344 rats from two-year carcinogenicity studies. Toxicol Pathol. 2012;40:473–81.
15. Travlos GS, Hard GC, Betz LJ, Kissling GE. Chronic progressive nephropathy in male F344 rats in 90-day toxicity studies: its occurrence and association with renal tubule tumors in subsequent 2-year bioassays. Toxicol Pathol. 2011;39:381–9.
16. Hard GC, Whysner J, English JC, Zang E, Williams GM. Relationship of hydroquinone-associated rat renal tumors with spontaneous chronic progressive nephropathy. Toxicol Pathol. 1997;25:132–43.
17. Hard GC, Banton MI, Bretzlaff RS, Dekant W, Fowles JR, Mallett AK, et al. Consideration of rat chronic progressive nephropathy in regulatory evaluations for carcinogenicity. Toxicol Sci. 2013;132:268–75.
18. Hard GC, Khan KN. A contemporary overview of chronic progressive nephropathy in the laboratory rat, and its significance for human risk assessment. Toxicol Pathol. 2004;32:171–80.
19. Wold JS. Cephalosporin toxicity. In: Hook JB, editor. Toxicology of the kidney. New York: Raven; 1981. p. 251–66.
20. Bulger RE. Renal damage caused by heavy metals. Toxicol Pathol. 1986;14:58–65.
21. Hottendorf GH, Williams PD. Aminoglycoside nephrotoxicity. Toxicol Pathol. 1986;14:66–72.
22. Mihatsch MJ, Ryffel B, Hermle M, Brunner FP, Thiel G. Morphology of cyclosporine nephrotoxicity in the rat. Clin Nephrol. 1986;25 Suppl 1:S2–8.
23. Phillips RD, Cockrell BY. Kidney structural changes in rats following inhalation exposure to C10-C11 isoparaffinic solvent. Toxicology. 1984;33:261–73.
24. Hard GC. Some aids to histological recognition of hyaline droplet nephropathy in ninety-day toxicity studies. Toxicol Pathol. 2008;36:1014–7.
25. Alden CL. A review of unique male rat hydrocarbon nephropathy. Toxicol Pathol. 1986;14:109–11.
26. Tucker Jr WE, Macklin AW, Szot RJ, Johnston RE, Elion GB, de Miranda P, et al. Preclinical toxicology studies with acyclovir: acute and subchronic tests. Fundam Appl Toxicol. 1983;3:573–8.
27. Bach PH, Bridges JW. Chemically induced renal papillary necrosis and upper urothelial carcinoma. Part 1. Crit Rev Toxicol. 1985;15:217–329.
28. Bach PH, Bridges JW. Chemically induced renal papillary necrosis and upper urothelial carcinoma. Part 2. CRC Crit Rev Toxicol. 1985;15:331–441.
29. Owen RA, Durand-Cavagna G, Molon-Noblot S, Boussiquet-Leroux C, Berry PH, Tonkonoh N, et al. Renal papillary cytoplasmic granularity and potassium depletion induced by carbonic anhydrase inhibitors in rats. Toxicol Pathol. 1993;21:449–55.
30. Owen RA, Molon-Noblot S, Hubert MF, Siegl PK, Eydelloth RS, Keenan KP. Juxtaglomerular cell hypertrophy and hyperplasia induced in rhesus monkeys by angiotensin II receptor antagonists. Lab Invest. 1994;71:543–51.
31. Owen RA, Molon-Noblot S, Hubert MF, Kindt MV, Keenan KP, Eydelloth RS. The morphology of juxtaglomerular cell hyperplasia and hypertrophy in normotensive rats and monkeys given an angiotensin II receptor antagonist. Toxicol Pathol. 1994; 22:606–19.
32. Hard GC. Mechanisms of chemically induced renal carcinogenesis in the laboratory rodent. Toxicol Pathol. 1998;26:104–12.
33. Hard GC, Seely JC, Kissling GE, Betz LJ. Spontaneous occurrence of a distinctive renal tubule tumor phenotype in rat carcinogenicity studies conducted by the national toxicology program. Toxicol Pathol. 2008;36:388–96.
34. Hall WC, Elder B, Walker CL, Cai SL, Peters DG, Goodman DG, et al. Spontaneous renal tubular hyperplastic and neoplastic lesions in three Sprague–Dawley rats from a 90-day toxicity study. Toxicol Pathol. 2007;35:233–41.
35. Driver HE, White IN, Butler WH. Dose–response relationships in chemical carcinogenesis: renal mesenchymal tumours induced in the rat by single dose dimethylnitrosamine. Br J Exp Pathol. 1987;68:133–43.
36. Hard GC. Experimental models for the sequential analysis of chemically-induced renal carcinogenesis. Toxicol Pathol. 1986;14:112–22.
37. Hara H, Miyao M, Moriki T, Kutsukake F, Yamane T. Histological and ultrastructural studies of nephroblastoma in rats induced transplacentally by ethylnitrosourea. Acta Pathol Jpn. 1982; 32:385–98.
38. Johansson SL. Carcinogenicity of analgesics: long-term treatment of Sprague–Dawley rats with phenacetin, phenazone, caffeine and paracetamol (acetaminophen). Int J Cancer. 1981;27:521–9.

39. Wisler JA, Afshari C, Fielden M, Zimmermann C, Taylor S, Carnahan J, et al. Raf inhibition causes extensive multiple tissue hyperplasia and urinary bladder neoplasia in the rat. Toxicol Pathol. 2011;39:809–22.

40. El Hage H. Preclinical and clinical safety assessments for PPAR agonists. Rockville: Center for Drug Evaluation and Research, FDA; 2004.

41. Yki-Yarvinen H. Drug therapy, thiazolidinediones. N Engl J Med. 2004;351:1106–18.

42. Hardisty JF, Anderson DC, Brodie S, Cline JM, Hahn FF, Kolenda-Roberts H, et al. Histopathology of the urinary bladders of cynomolgus monkeys treated with PPAR agonists. Toxicol Pathol. 2008;36:769–76.

43. Molon-Noblot S, Boussiquet-Leroux C, Owen RA, Irisarri E, Durand-Cavagna G, Peter CP, et al. Rat urinary bladder hyperplasia induced by oral administration of carbonic anhydrase inhibitors. Toxicol Pathol. 1992;20:93–102.

# 6 The Male Reproductive System

Toxicologic assessment of the male reproductive system has gained increasing importance over the past two decades because of potential effects on human fertility. This chapter outlines best practice for histopathological assessment of the male reproductive tract and describes common induced lesions seen in male reproductive organs in safety assessment studies, with examples of causative agents and brief outlines of their mechanisms.

The potential for chemicals to adversely affect male reproductive function in humans became very apparent in the 1970s when the adverse effects of chemicals such as dibromochloropropane and lead on the testes and on the fertility of occupationally exposed workers were demonstrated. Over the past few decades, the focus of concern has moved to the potential of environmental endocrine disrupting chemicals to affect development and function of the male reproductive tract following in utero and postnatal exposure. In addition, many classes of pharmaceuticals (e.g. anticancer agents) are associated with male reproductive tract toxicity. The need for the pathologist to be able to detect early and subtle effects on spermatogenesis has become essential, not just for pharmaceuticals but for agrochemicals and industrial chemicals. In addition, drugs intended for paediatric use must be assessed for potential effects on the development of the male reproductive organs through puberty. Specifically designed reproductive study protocols over one or multiple generations are now routinely used for the safety assessment of compounds with the potential to affect organ development and fertility. Depending on the study type and regulatory guidelines, these reproductive protocols generally rely on gross examination of developmental milestones, sperm assessment, and fertility parameters for overall evaluation. Histopathology may or may not be an included endpoint. In fact, the routine 4- and 13-week general toxicity studies are two of the most important study types in which the toxicologic pathologist may identify and characterise reproductive disturbances, but only if the testes are fixed in an appropriate manner and the pathologist is familiar with the features and dynamics of the spermatogenic cycle in the species under study.

Fixatives that provide good cellular detail and minimal artefact in the testes, such as Bouin's or modified Davidson's, are routinely used instead of 10 % neutral buffered formalin (NBF) [1]. Resin-embedded sections provide better cellular detail than routine paraffin-embedded sections and may be used if high resolution is required to detect early changes. In addition, widely accepted best practice guidelines for the assessment of toxicity of the male reproductive tract are available in the literature [2–5].

Interpretation of findings in the male reproductive tract can be complicated by the age of the animals, particularly in large animal studies in which animals are immature at the end of short-term studies. In cynomolgus macaques, maturity in males generally occurs between 4.5 and 6 years of age but this can vary widely and will also be influenced by the body weight of the animal [6–9]. In routine safety assessment studies, males are often still juvenile or sexually immature at the end of study, and spermatogenesis may not even have begun. Similarly, in beagles, sexual maturity occurs in the male between 7 and 10 months of age but may not be complete until 12 months of age. Again there is significant variability between animals from a single supplier and also between supplier and strain [10, 11] (e.g. Marshall beagles mature later than Harlan beagles) [12]. Variations between strains and suppliers should also be considered when interpreting possible

C. Gopinath, V. Mowat, *Atlas of Toxicological Pathology*,
DOI 10.1007/978-1-62703-998-7_6, © Springer Science+Business Media New York 2014

treatment effects in rats, as there can be minor differences between Han Wistar rats and Sprague–Dawley rats and measurements of sexual maturity can continue to increase up until 12 weeks of age [13].

If dogs are placed on study when young (generally 5–6 months), they will usually be immature or just starting to mature at the end of a 2- or 4-week study, which precludes evaluation of testicular toxicity. At the end of a 13-week study, they will generally be of appearances ranging from maturing, on the cusp of maturity, to fully mature, with wide variation between animals. Peripubertal dogs exhibit a wide range of lesions that are similar to induced changes. Even in individual dogs, there may be a lack of synchronisation of maturity between testes and prostate due to differential expression of androgen receptors between testis and prostate. During the peripubertal period, spermatogenesis is inefficient and may not begin in all of the tubules at the same time. Large numbers of sloughed germ cells and multinucleate cells are seen in the tubular lumens and the epididymides at this time. Degenerative changes decrease as animals mature [10, 11]. As the morphology seen during the development of spermatogenesis may be similar to that which occurs secondary to treatment with a testicular toxicant (e.g. decreased numbers of elongating spermatids, multinucleate degenerating germ cells), it is difficult and sometimes impossible to distinguish degeneration associated with maturation from degeneration associated with toxicity. To prevent false-positive or false-negative results occurring due to maturation status, it is recommended that dogs should be at least 10 months of age and rats at least 10 weeks of age at the end of any study [2, 14].

Changes in the male reproductive system occur due to a wide variety of direct and indirect mechanisms. Indirect mechanisms are frequently due to hormonal disruption through the hypothalamic–pituitary–gonadal (HPG) axis but may also be due to alterations in fluid resorption in the efferent ducts or vascular compromise.

Finally, effects on fertility due to effects on epididymal sperm may occur in the absence of histopathological changes in the epididymis and testis. These are only detectable in studies designed to assess quantity and quality of sperm and reproductive performance.

## 6.1 Testes

Familiarity with the spermatogenic cycle in different laboratory species is essential for detecting subtle effects and for understanding the aetiology and progression of testicular lesions. The duration of spermatogenesis and the spermatogenic cycle vary among species. It is important that the pathologist is familiar with germ cell development and the stage maps of commonly used laboratory species. The process and stages of spermatogenesis, and their duration in common laboratory species, have been extensively studied and documented by several authors [15–20]. Although the fundamentals of the spermatogenic cycle are similar among species, certain details vary. These can have a significant impact on histopathological changes. The number of stages and their cellular make-up varies among species. The organisation of cell associations along the length of the tubule is linear for most mammalian species, including most species of monkey used in toxicologic studies. Thus, a tubular cross section normally contains only one cell association and the adjoining length of tubule (often the adjacent tubule in a cross section of testis) will generally contain the consecutive stage. In dogs, the lobular arrangement of individual tubules and the length of tubule occupied by a single stage generally mean that many adjacent cross sections contain the same stage. In humans and marmosets, cell associations are arranged in a helical pattern, resulting in a mosaic of cell associations in a single cross section.

The testis is partially protected from toxicity by the blood–tubule barrier, which is mainly formed by the tight junctions between the Sertoli cells, with the capillary endothelial cells and peritubular cells serving as partial barriers. To exert their effects directly on germ cells, testicular toxicants must pass through the Sertoli cells after entering the interstitial fluid via the vascular system. Spermatogonia, however, lie outside this barrier and are exposed to toxicants that enter the interstitial fluid.

Compounds may exert their effects on the testes due to direct toxicity involving one or more cell populations, through hormonal changes or secondary to metabolic changes or deficiencies [21]. Metabolism of xenobiotics may be different between species and strains of rodent, so susceptibility to testicular toxicity can vary quite markedly [22]. Susceptibility also varies frequently with species; for example, certain neurokinin receptor antagonists cause testicular atrophy in beagle dogs but not in rodents [23].

Direct mechanisms include effects on Sertoli cells, Leydig cells, or different groups of germ cells. However, many toxicants that appear to have an effect on a specific germ cell type are now thought to act through the Sertoli cell by disturbing a regulatory or supportive cellular process within the Sertoli cell that is critical to that particular germ cell type [24]. Toxicants can be either the test article or its metabolites, which may be metabolised elsewhere in the body and brought by the haematogenous route or metabolised within the target cell or by an adjacent cell. The Leydig cell is a major source of enzyme metabolism and the Sertoli cell also contains a number of important enzymes, but the germ cells predominantly contain cytoprotective enzymes.

Indirect mechanisms include hormonal disruption to the hypothalamic–pituitary–gonadal axis or locally within the testes, circulatory and fluid balance disturbances, damage to the blood–testis barrier, and nutritional deficiencies. Zinc and vitamin A deficiency may cause impaired spermatogenesis, as can low body weight and reduced food intake [25]. Although the early morphological changes of different testicular toxicants are often cell and stage specific, prolonged exposure to most agents results in a similar end-stage picture, with contracted tubules depleted of most germ cells and lined only by Sertoli cells (Fig. 6.1).

Induced changes seen in the testes are listed below:

- Interstitial oedema
- Inflammation
- Seminiferous tubular dilation
- Sperm retention
- Maturation arrest
- Degeneration of different cell populations/stages
- Seminiferous tubular degeneration
- Tubular atrophy
- Sertoli cell vacuolation/degeneration
- Leydig cell degeneration/atrophy
- Leydig cell hyperplasia/tumours
- Spermatozoal damage

Cadmium damages the testicular blood supply, increasing vascular permeability and causing interstitial oedema. This oedema reduces blood flow, resulting in ischaemic necrosis and inflammation. Induced inflammation in the testis is rare due to the immunological privilege conferred by the blood–testis barrier. When it occurs, inflammation is usually due to agents that have compromised the blood flow, resulting in ischaemic necrosis and breakdown of the Sertoli cell tight junctions that make up the blood–testis barrier (e.g. cadmium, human chorionic gonadotrophin). Intratubular fluid in the seminiferous tubules is produced by the Sertoli cells and is largely resorbed by the rete testis and efferent ducts. Substances that influence fluid production, which is androgen-dependent, can result in reduced fluid production and reduced tubular diameter [4]. Increased intratubular fluid, due to either increased production or accumulation secondary to blockage such as that caused by spermatocoeles, can result in initial seminiferous tubular dilation and increased testis weight. Prolonged fluid accumulation and dilation can lead to tubular atrophy (Fig. 6.2). Tubular contraction, which is mediated by substances that control the peritubular myoid cells, including oxytocin and prostaglandins, is essential for movement of fluid to the rete testis. Blockage in the rete testis, efferent ducts, or epididymis can also result in diffuse seminiferous tubular dilation and atrophy as a secondary consequence (Fig. 6.3) [4, 26]. Several compounds including carbendazim, benomyl, and a leukotriene $A_4$ hydrolase inhibitor cause occlusion of the efferent ductules by granulomatous inflammation. The degree and severity of the secondary testicular changes (tubular dilation and tubular degeneration/atrophy) depend on the number of efferent ducts that are blocked. Although the efferent ducts located in the epididymal fat pads are not usually collected, they may form a grossly visible mass that is sampled at necropsy [26–28]. Oestrogen and endothelin play important roles in fluid resorption in the efferent ducts [29, 30]. Some 5-hydroxytryptamine agonists cause constriction of the vasculature surrounding the extratesticular rete, resulting in impaired fluid resorption from the efferent ducts and rete with consequent dilation of the rete and seminiferous tubules with fluid [31].

Spermatid retention in the rat occurs due to impaired release of mature step-19 spermatids from stage VIII tubules. Although this change can be a primary toxicant-induced effect, it is also caused by reduced testosterone levels because spermatid release is an androgen-dependent process. Boric acid, classically, and a variety of other testicular toxicants including oestradiol 3-benzoate, deoxynivalenol, and 2-bromopropane can induce spermatid retention [32–34]. The change can be quite subtle and difficult to recognise on first examination of the testis, but it is generally accompanied by the presence of small amounts of cell debris in the epididymis. Therefore, if epididymal cell debris is seen with no apparent change in the testes, it can indicate a low level of spermatid retention. In such cases, high-power examination of stage IX–XIII tubules will reveal the presence of retained step-19 spermatids in the lumen of tubules in stages IX to XI or phagocytosed in the basal cytoplasm of Sertoli cells in stage XII/XIII tubules (Figs. 6.4 and 6.5).

In nose-only inhalation studies, degenerative testicular changes are sometimes seen in control rats at a higher incidence than in other types of studies. Changes

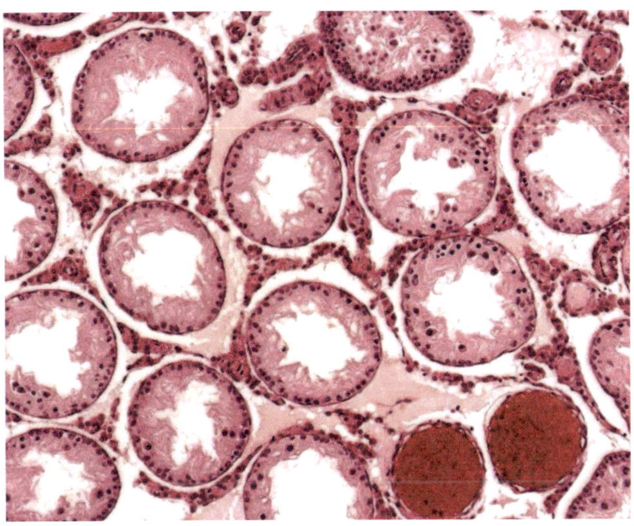

**Figure 6-1.** Diffuse tubular atrophy in the testis of a rat. The seminiferous tubules are markedly atrophic, with only Sertoli cells remaining in most. A few still retain spermatogonia and some pachytene spermatocytes. H&E.

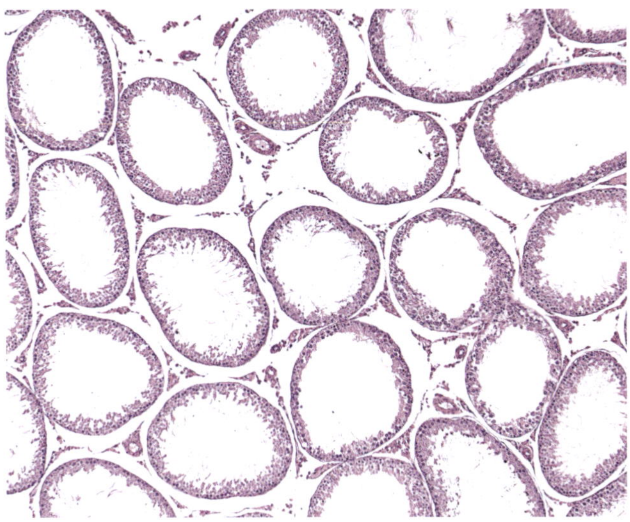

**Figure 6-2.** Tubular dilation in the testis of a rat. Tubules have markedly dilated lumens, with disruption and vacuolation of the seminiferous epithelium in some of them. This change is often secondary to blockage in the efferent ducts. H&E.

are generally of minimal to mild severity, multifocal, and comprise a range of changes including bilateral seminiferous epithelial vacuolation and tubular degeneration characterised by increased degeneration of round and elongate spermatids, with the formation of eosinophilic bodies in the tubular lumen. No particular stage is affected. This phenomenon is considered likely due to stress during the inhalation procedure, due to either heat or immobilisation [35, 36]. In studies of this type, higher incidences of testicular findings in the treated groups have been noted with β-adrenergics and flame retardants, which did not induce testicular toxicity when administered by whole body inhalation exposure. Such apparently treatment-related incidences should be interpreted with caution, if they are not seen with other routes of exposure (Figs. 6.6 and 6.7) [36].

Cell- and stage-specific degeneration of the seminiferous epithelium is best visualised in 2–4-week studies in rodents; in longer-term studies, changes become less specific and involve more cell types. Commonly seen degenerative changes include vacuolation, multinucleated giant cells, and tubular degeneration/atrophy. Multinucleated giant cells are formed by degenerating germ cells, often spermatids, within the seminiferous

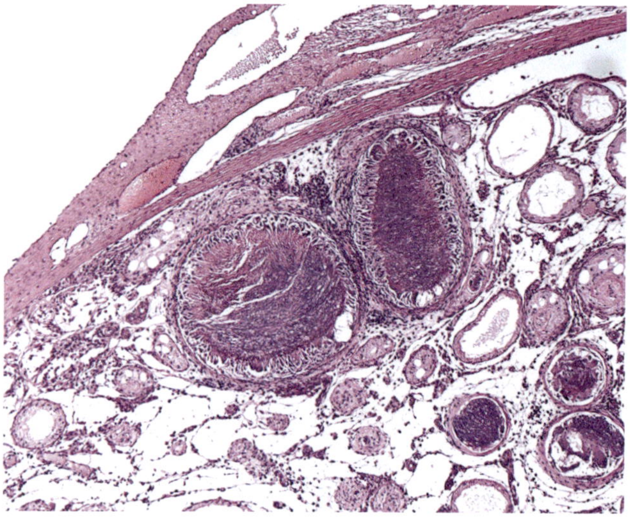

**Figure 6-3.** Spermatocoele in the testes of a rat. Two rete tubules are markedly distended, with accumulation of spermatids in the lumen surrounded by multinucleate foreign-body giant cells. The surrounding tubules are atrophic, some with mineralised contents. H&E.

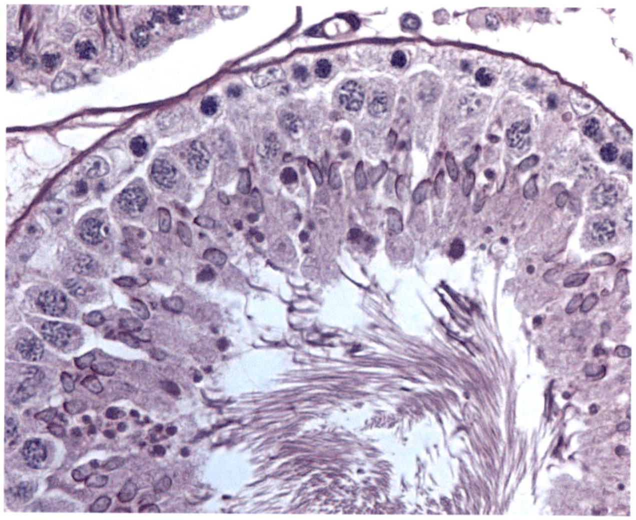

**Figure 6-4.** Spermatid retention in the testis of a rat. This stage IX tubule contains normal elongate spermatids of this stage, overlaid by a population of step-19 spermatids. These retained spermatids should have been released during stage VIII. Periodic acid–Schiff–haematoxylin (PAS/H).

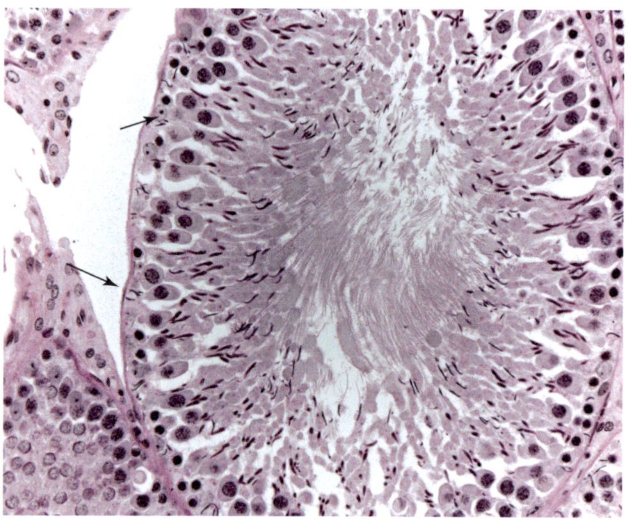

**Figure 6-5.** Phagocytosis of retained spermatids in stage XII tubule of rat testis. There is an entire generation of step-19 spermatids in the lumen of the tubule overlying a normal layer of step-12 spermatids. A few step-19 spermatids lying along the basement membrane of the tubule have been phagocytosed by the Sertoli cells. H&E.

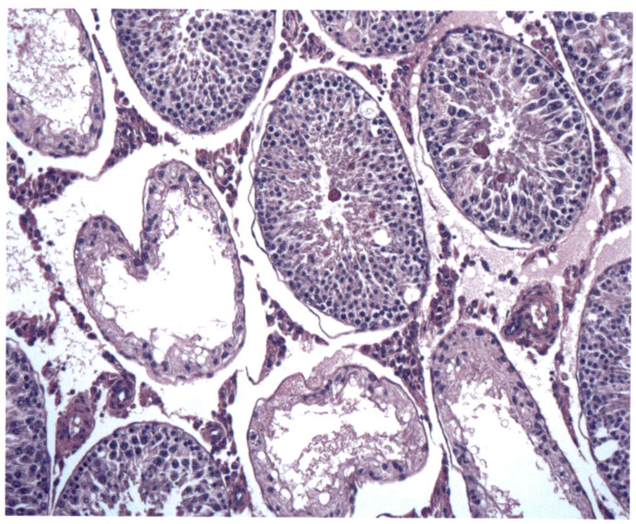

**Figure 6-6.** Vacuolation, germ cell degeneration, and focal seminiferous epithelial atrophy in the testes of a rat. Eosinophilic bodies containing degenerating elongate spermatids are present. This is a control from a snout-only inhalation study; the changes are procedural. H&E.

epithelium, extruded into the tubular lumen and eventually into the epididymal lumen (Fig. 6.8). Vacuolation of the seminiferous epithelium results from a number of degenerative changes, including accumulation of fluid or lipids, as well as from loss of germ cells [37]. Loss of specific cell types or targeting of tubules of a specific stage may be evident (Figs. 6.9–6.13). Reductions in testosterone are initially associated with degeneration of elongate spermatids during and after stage VIII, followed by generalised depletion of all elongating and maturation phase spermatids [4].

Ethylene glycol monomethyl ether, which is used as an industrial solvent, is a well-studied example of a cell- and stage-specific testicular toxicant that targets

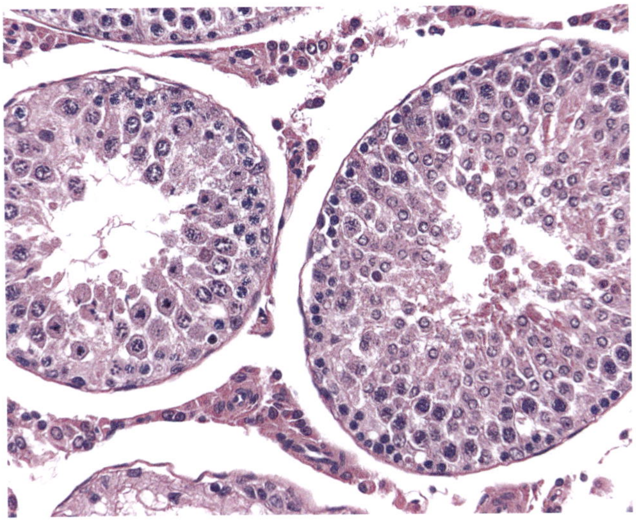

**Figure 6-7.** Higher power of the testes in Fig. 6.6. Depletion of elongate spermatids and dividing spermatocytes (*left*), with partial sloughing of round spermatids (*right*). Eosinophilic bodies containing degenerating spermatids are present in the lumen. H&E.

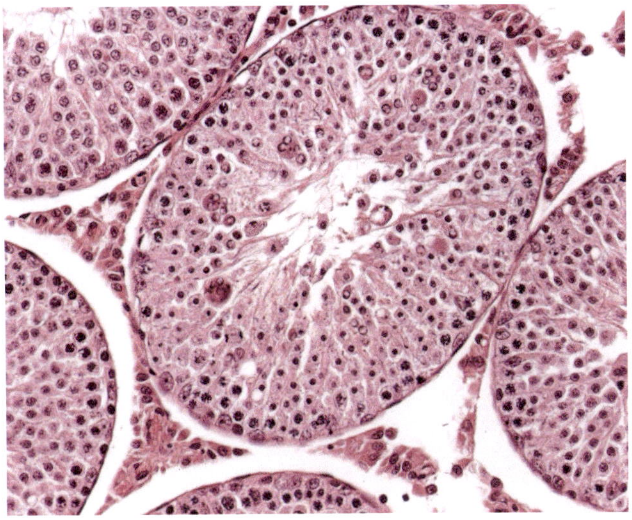

**Figure 6-8.** Testis of a rat, a stage XIV tubule with seminiferous epithelial degeneration. Degeneration of secondary spermatocytes, dividing spermatocytes, and round spermatids is present. Round spermatids are vacuolated, with some coalescing to form multinucleate cells. H&E.

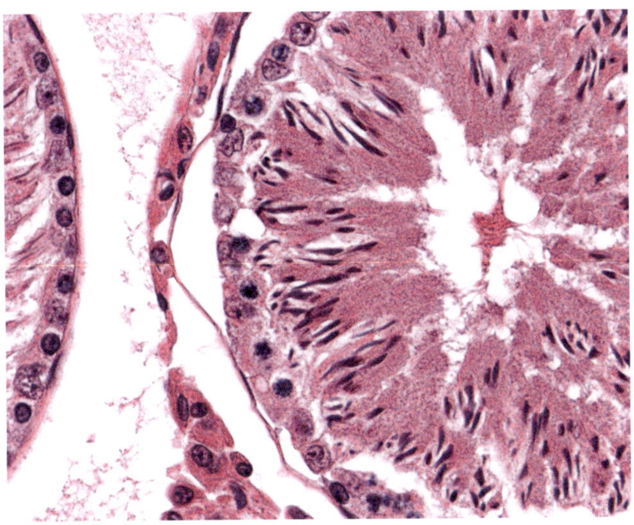

**Figure 6-9.** Stage XII tubule from a rat with complete loss of pachytene spermatocytes and partial depletion of zygotene spermatocytes. A spermatogonium ('type A') is present on the basal membrane. In the stage V tubule (*left*), the basement membrane is lined by many type B spermatogonia but is missing all its pachytene spermatocytes and round spermatids. This is the typical appearance of a testis from a rat that has undergone a short recovery period following 2–4 weeks dosing with a spermatogonial toxicant. H&E.

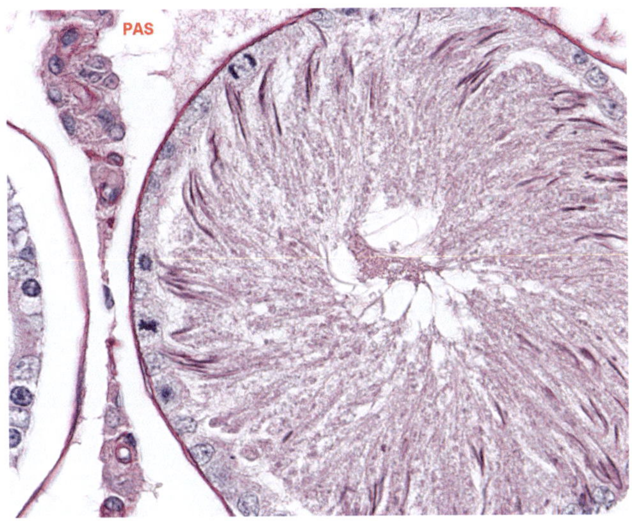


**Figure 6-10.** Stage XIV tubule from a rat recovering from dosing with a spermatogonial toxicant. The tubule has a complete population of step-17 spermatids but is missing all round spermatids and all pachytene spermatocytes. A few intermediate spermatogonia are undergoing mitotic division. Normal spermatogenesis requires at least 8 weeks to become re-established following depletion of spermatogonia. PAS/H.

pachytene spermatocytes. There is varying susceptibility at different stages, dependent on dose and duration of exposure—dividing (stage XIV) and early pachytene (stages I–II) are more susceptible than late pachytene (stages VIII–XIII), which are more susceptible than mid-pachytene (stages III–VII) [38]. Spermatogonia, which are often targeted by anticancer agents, also show differential susceptibility with the rapidly dividing differentiating spermatogonial population being more sensitive than the slowly dividing stem cell spermatogonial pool.

Detection of testicular toxicants in dogs poses several challenges. Familiarity with the differences between peripubertal changes associated with age versus common background lesions seen in adult animals is essential. Focal hypoplasia of seminiferous tubules is a common background finding in dogs of any age (Fig. 6.14). Degenerating spermatids and large numbers of multinucleate giant cells are common in peripubertal dogs and can mimic toxicity (Fig. 6.15).

Hypospermatogenesis is seen as a common background lesion indicative of general inefficiency of

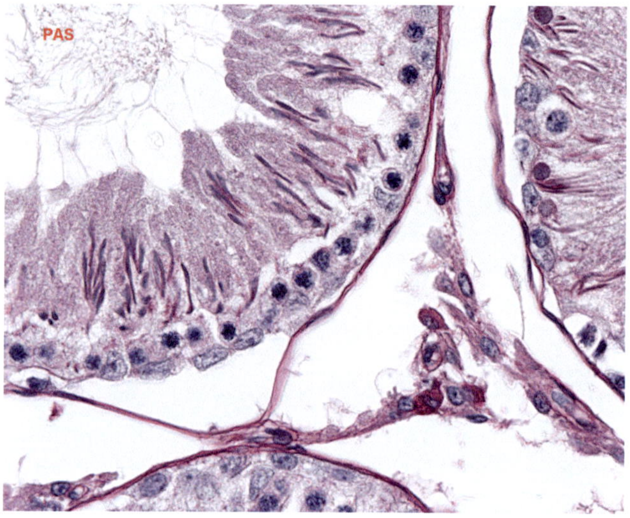


**Figure 6-11.** Stage XII tubule from a rat with complete loss of pachytene spermatocytes and partial depletion of zygotene spermatocytes. PAS/H.

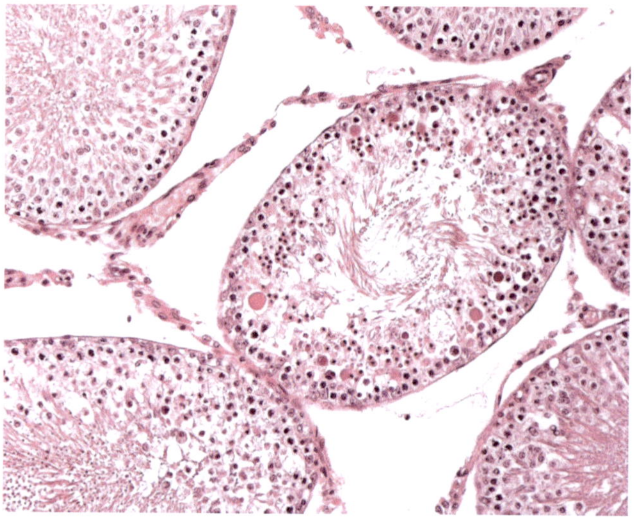

**Figure 6-12.** Tubular degeneration in a rat testis. Spermatogonia, spermatocytes, and round spermatids are degenerating in the central stage VII tubule, whereas elongate spermatids appear less affected. H&E.

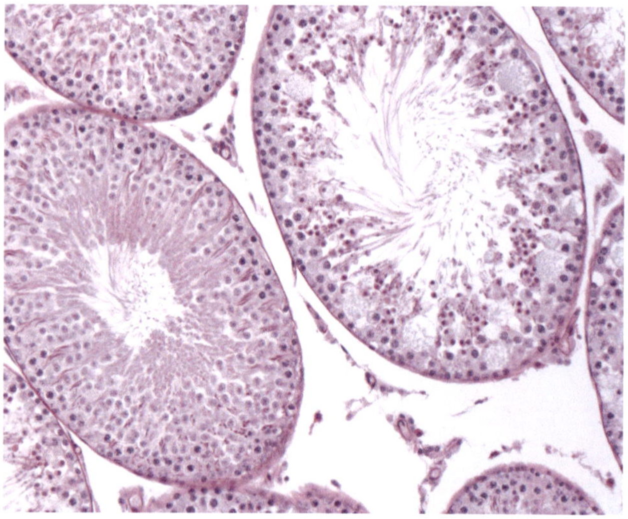

**Figure 6-13.** Tubular degeneration in a rat testis. Round spermatids have largely been lost in the stage IV tubule (*right*), with degeneration of germ cells and pachytene spermatocytes evident. The tubules (*left*) appear unaffected. PAS/H.

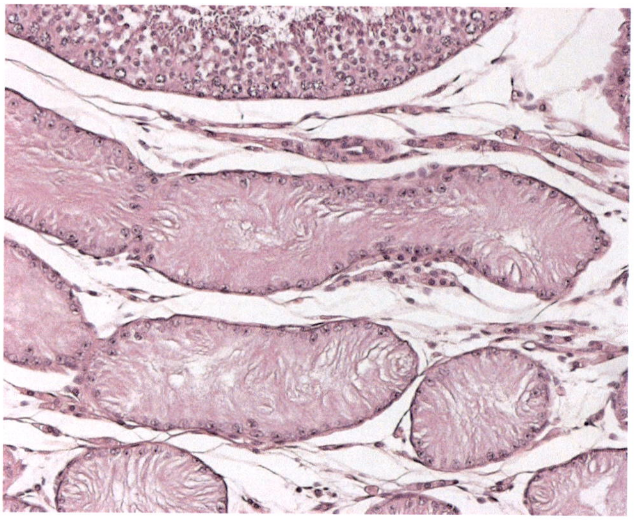

**Figure 6-14.** Focal hypoplasia in the testis of a dog. The tubules appear inactive and are lined by Sertoli cells with no evidence of spermatogenesis. This is a common background finding in young and adult dogs and likely represents areas of tubules where migration of germ cells failed during development. Completely atrophic tubules have a similar appearance. H&E.

canine spermatogenesis, but it can also be a test article-related change caused by intermittent or partial inhibition of spermatogonial division and differentiation. An apparent dose relationship in decreased maturation status of dogs at the end of a study can indicate delayed maturity, but this diagnosis is made difficult by the small group numbers and the variable ages at which dogs reach maturity (Fig. 6.16).

Seminiferous tubular degeneration is sometimes mediated by direct toxicity to the Sertoli cells, often through effects on cytoskeletal components. Several testicular toxicants such as phthalate esters and DNB (1, 3 dinitrobenzene) exert their effects on spermatogenesis via the Sertoli cells [39]. Initially, vacuolation and rarefaction of the Sertoli cells are seen histologically followed by loss of contact between the Sertoli and germ cells, which are then exfoliated into the lumen (Fig. 6.17).

Ultrastructurally, vacuolation or rarefaction of smooth endoplasmic reticulum is seen as an early event with phthalates [40]. Vacuolation of Sertoli cells is also seen in phospholipidosis, presumably due to the cell's phagocytic role (Fig. 6.18). Compounds such as 2–5 hexanedione, colchicines, carbendazim, and vinblastine exert their effect on Sertoli cells by disruption of microtubules, causing loss of cytoskeletal support that results in breakdown of the linkage of the Sertoli cells with germ cells [39, 41]. The loss of connection results in the affected cells moving away from the basement membrane and towards the lumen. With DNB, early changes in the Sertoli cell are followed by pachytene spermatocyte degeneration and phagocytosis by Sertoli cells [42].

Leydig cell toxicity generally manifests morphologically as atrophy of interstitial cells, due to direct or indirect (through decreased LH) inhibition of testosterone biosynthesis resulting in a reduction in testosterone levels. Oestradiol benzoate inhibits spermatogenesis and produces Leydig cell atrophy in the rat (Fig. 6.19a, b). A few compounds such as ethane dimethanesulphonate (EDS) are cytotoxic and result in destruction of the Leydig cell population. Ultrastructural changes seen with EDS include karyopyknosis, cytoplasmic vesiculation, and accumulation of lipid inclusions and large lipofuscin granules [43].

Normal Leydig cell populations vary widely between different species in quantity and behaviour. In mini-pigs, the interstitium is almost filled with Leydig cells, whereas in rodents, the population of these cells is much smaller. A wide range of compound classes, including antiandrogens, dopamine agonists, and peroxisome proliferators, induce Leydig cell hyperplasia and tumours in rats but not in other species. These tumours are generally considered to develop due to rat-specific mechanisms and are therefore not relevant to humans.

A variety of compound classes are associated with Leydig cell tumour induction in rats, generally by either inhibition of steroid synthesis or blockage of androgen receptors (e.g. testosterone biosynthesis inhibitors block conversion of 17-hydroxy progesterone to androstenedione). These eventually result in reduced testosterone levels, increased stimulation of Leydig cells, and lack of feedback inhibition via the hypothalamic–pituitary axis, leading to Leydig cell hyperplasia and adenomas and, rarely, carcinomas. Rats are particularly sensitive to this mechanism due to their high LH levels and the presence of LHRH receptors on the Leydig cells. Prenatal exposure to phthalates in rats induces atypical Leydig cell hyperplasia in adults due to reduced testosterone levels [44, 45].

HMG-CoA reductase inhibitors block cholesterol synthesis. Drugs that modify dopamine pathways eventually affect luteinizing hormone levels and result in tumours. Prolactin inhibitors also induce Leydig cell hyperplasia as prolactin regulates LH receptors on the Leydig cell. Several peroxisome proliferators, including clofibrate, induce Leydig cell tumours in rats, possibly through reduced

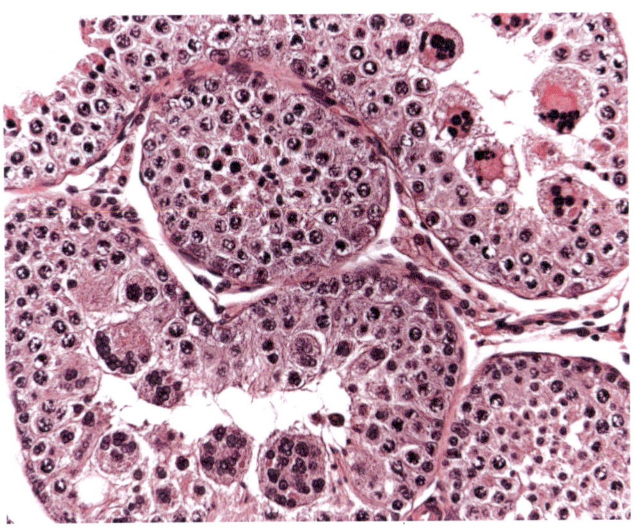

**Figure 6-15.** Testis from a dog on a short-term study. Several multinucleate giant cells, containing coalescing round spermatids, are present in the tubular lumens. Background changes in dogs of this age can mimic testicular toxicity, complicating interpretation. H&E.

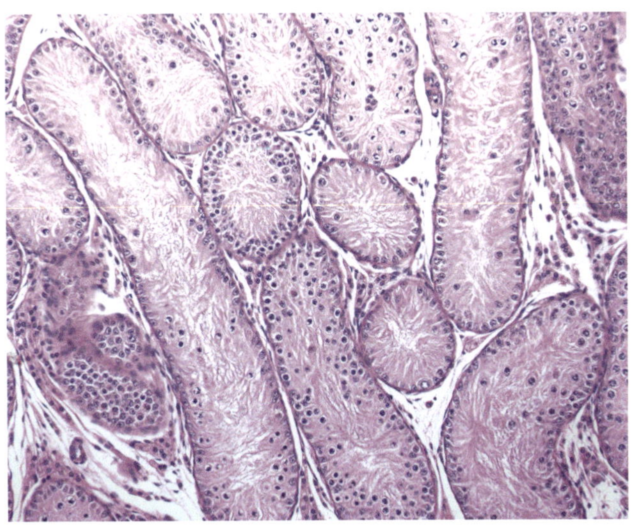

**Figure 6-16.** Delayed maturity in a dog from a 13-week study. The morphology is more typical of a 6–7-month-old dog than an 8–9-month-old dog. Tubules are lined largely by Sertoli cells and have poorly developed lumens. Germ cells of different types are present in some tubules, but spermatogenesis is not apparent. This highlights the difficulties of interpreting findings in nonadult dogs. H&E.

testosterone or increased oestrogen levels. Calcium channel blockers such as isradipine can also cause Leydig cell tumours. Cadmium induces tumours secondary to testicular necrosis. It causes destruction of Leydig cells and also induces interstitial cell tumours, through either DNA damage or disruption of DNA repair [46].

In rats, Leydig cell hyperplasia and tumours are expansile (Fig. 6.20). Leydig cell tumours are generally benign in rodents although they may grow very large, causing compression of the surrounding seminiferous tubules and often obliteration of the normal testicular structures.

In mice, Leydig cell hyperplasia and tumours are generally associated with high oestrogen levels. Tamoxifen causes Leydig cell tumours in mice but not in rats, possibly through a direct oestrogenic effect. The morphology of Leydig cell hyperplasia in mice differs from rats as hyperplasia often infiltrates between seminiferous tubules rather than expanding and compressing them (Fig. 6.21). Benign and malignant Leydig cell tumours in rodents are morphologically similar, with malignancy being diagnosed based on invasive or metastatic behaviour (Figs. 6.22 and 6.23a, b).

Compounds that directly affect spermatozoa generally do so by interfering with their high-energy requirements at different levels. Compounds that reduce ATP levels impair motility (e.g. α-chlorohydrin). Compounds can also interfere with the complex maturation of sperm as they pass through the epididymis, or can cause oxidative damage to the sperm, especially if the chemical gains access to the seminal fluid.

In juvenile studies, or studies on immature animals, treated groups can display delayed development or maturity when compared with the controls, although there is no overt evidence of toxicity.

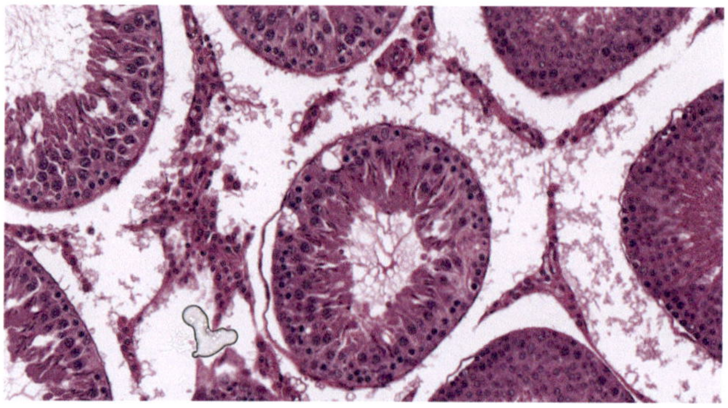

**Figure 6-17.** Sertoli cell vacuolation in a rat testis. Large and small vacuoles are present in a few Sertoli cells in the central stage XI tubule, with focal loss of pachytene spermatocytes (*right*). The tubule is otherwise normal. H&E.

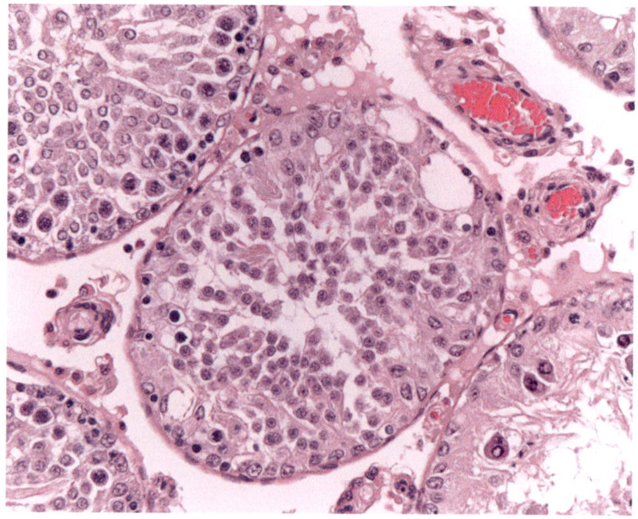

**Figure 6-18.** Sertoli cell vacuolation and seminiferous tubular degeneration of a rat testis, from a long-term study with a phospholipidotic. Sertoli cell cytoplasm is vacuolated and disorganised with large vacuoles distending some cells. Pachytene spermatocytes are largely absent with a few degenerating cells remaining. Round spermatids are exfoliating into the lumen. H&E.

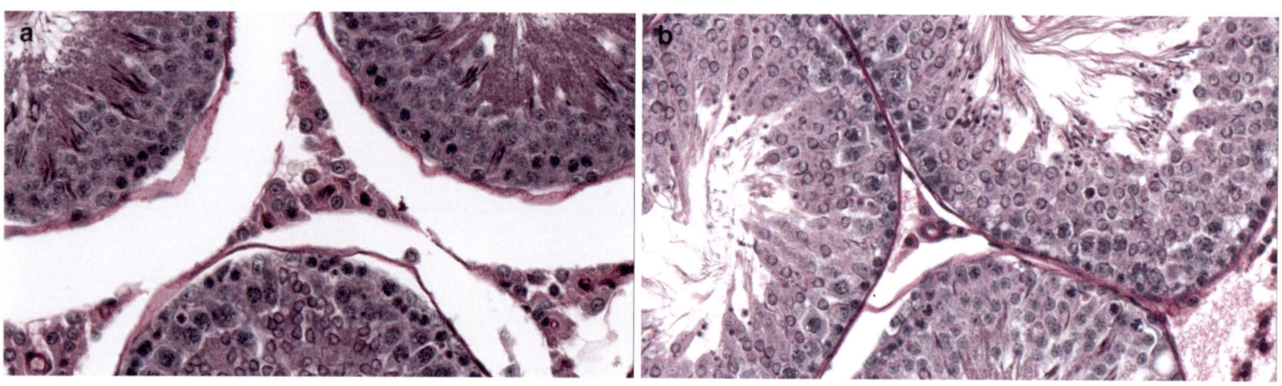

**Figure 6-19.** (**a**) A control with a normal population of Leydig cells. (**b**) Leydig cell atrophy in the testis of a rat. Leydig cells are almost completely absent from the interstitial spaces, with only occasional cells remaining. Decreased numbers of step-19 spermatids and spermatid retention in the basal cytoplasm of the stage VII/IX tubules at the top are also characteristic of low testosterone levels.

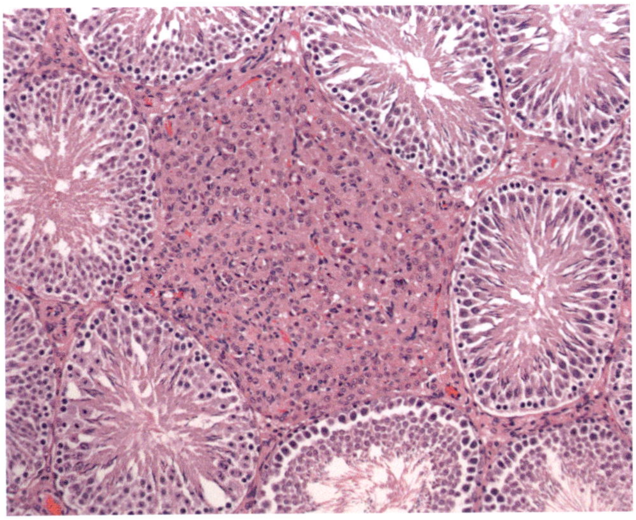

**Figure 6-20.** Leydig cell hyperplasia in a rat testis. The lesion is focal, causing slight compression of the surrounding tubules. H&E.

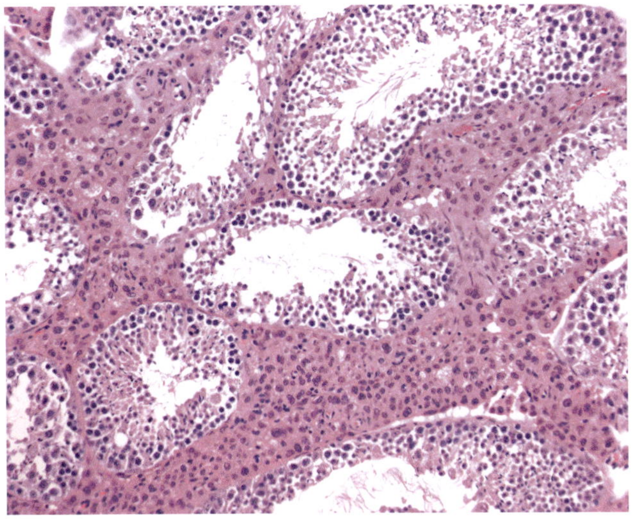

**Figure 6-21.** Leydig cell hyperplasia in a mouse testis. Proliferating Leydig cells are infiltrating diffusely around the seminiferous tubules, which appear largely normal. H&E.

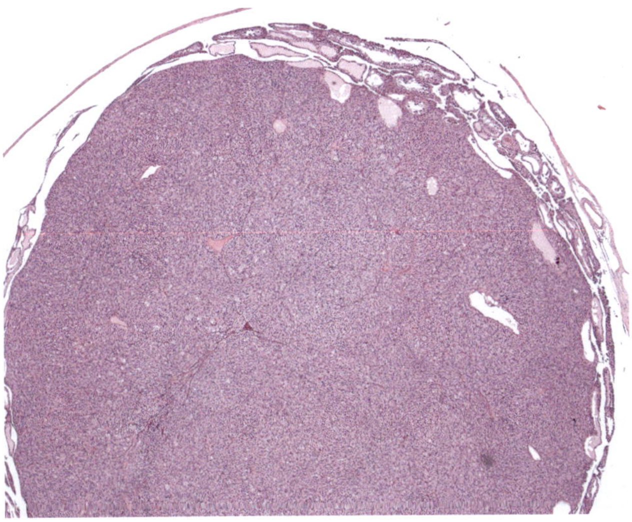

**Figure 6-22.** Leydig cell adenoma in the testis of a mouse. The tumour consists of sheets and packets of pale eosinophilic cells and has replaced most of the normal testicular structures, with a few atrophic tubules present at the periphery. These are often associated with increased oestrogen in mice. H&E.

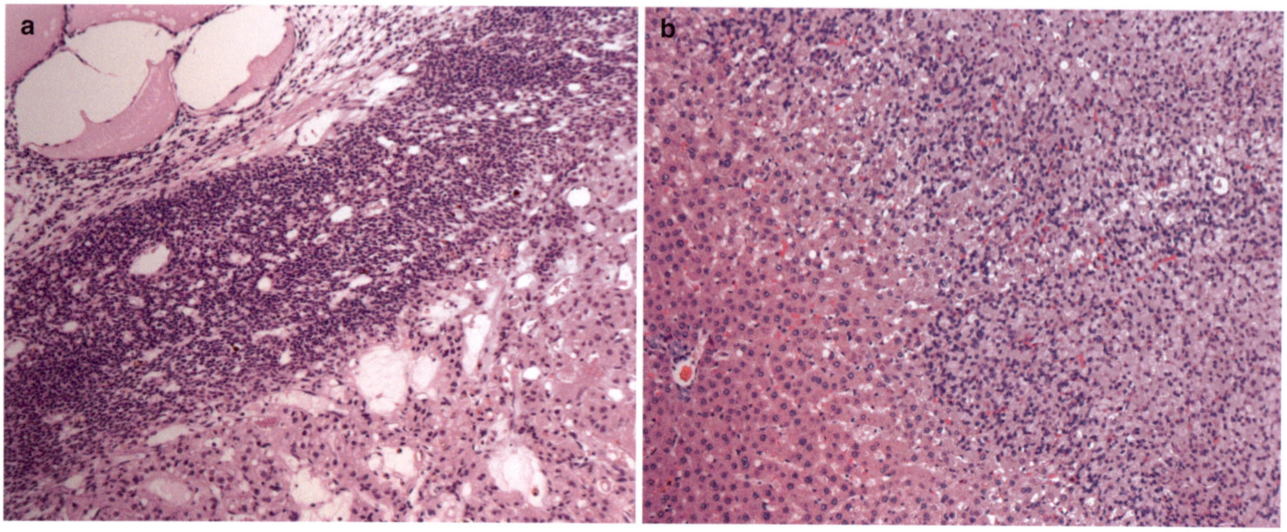

**Figure 6-23.** (**a**) Leydig cell carcinoma in the testis of a rat. The tumour comprises two cell populations, one of small basophilic cells with scanty cytoplasm and the other of large pale cells with round nuclei and eosinophilic vacuolated cytoplasm. (**b**) Metastasis from the same tumour in the liver. Metastatic cells are well differentiated but invasive. H&E.

## 6.2 Epididymis

Changes seen in the epididymis are often secondary to testicular toxicity (e.g. reduced sperm content and increased cellular debris). However, the epididymis itself can be a target for xenobiotics, and because of its role in sperm maturation, epididymal toxicity can impair fertility with or without detectable histopathological changes. Effects on the epididymis can be exerted through direct or indirect toxicity by a variety of mechanisms [28]. Reductions in hormonal levels are probably the commonest mechanism of indirect toxicity:

- Reduced sperm/absence of sperm
- Increased cellular debris
- Epididymal atrophy
- Sperm granulomas
- Epithelial vacuolation/inclusions
- Epithelial apoptosis
- Epithelial hyperplasia

Reduction or absence of sperm and increased cellular debris in the epididymides are generally secondary to testicular pathology (Fig. 6.24). However, oxidative DNA damage of epididymal sperm due to inflammatory cell products caused by toxicants such as methyl chloride has been demonstrated.

Epididymal atrophy often accompanies testicular atrophy due to reduced sperm and fluid output from the testis. Since epididymal function is androgen-dependent, decreased testosterone levels or administration of anti-androgens will also result in apoptosis and atrophy of the tissue. Epididymal atrophy is also common in older rats as a spontaneous finding, accompanying testicular atrophy. Cribriform change, often seen in atrophic epididymides, has sometimes been considered a form of hyperplasia but is more likely caused by piling up of the epithelium following contraction of the lumen (Fig. 6.25) [47].

Several different compound classes produce sperm granulomas in different laboratory species by a variety of mechanisms. Methyl chloride, when administered by inhalation, affects specific regions of the epididymal epithelium in rats, resulting in development of sperm granulomas in the proximal cauda [47]. Gossypol targets the epididymal epithelium in young rats, causing cell degeneration and exfoliation [48]. Other compounds (e.g. dibromochloropropane and cadmium) increase capillary permeability, resulting in vascular and epithelial damage and oedema (Fig. 6.26). This leads to formation of spermatocoeles that rupture and form sperm granulomas. Histologically, sperm granulomas appear as areas of sperm surrounded by a granulomatous reaction comprising foreign-body giant cells, histiocytes, and varying degrees of fibrosis (Fig. 6.27). 2-Methylimidazole induces sperm granulomas in mice, specifically in the proximal caput of the epididymis and/or efferent ducts [49]. Phosphodiesterase-4 inhibitors also cause sperm granulomas, subsequent to dilation of the efferent ducts and of the epididymal tubules [50]. L-cysteine in young rats affects maturation and results in tubular rupture, possibly due to impaired duct development or increased fluid due to increased vascular permeability [51, 52]. Drugs affecting the autonomic nervous system and vasodilating antihypertensives are also reported to induce sperm granulomas in rodents. Oxidosqualene cyclase inhibitors have produced sperm granulomas in dogs, presumed to be secondary to epithelial degeneration [53].

Vacuolation of epididymal epithelium occurs with compounds inducing phospholipidosis (Fig. 6.28). Morphologically, fine vacuoles, presumably representing accumulation of phospholipid, are seen in the epithelium, with no evidence of degeneration or necrosis. The entire epididymis may be affected or only specific regions such as the caput. Although endocytic vesicles are a normal finding in the clear cells of the epithelium of the cauda, their incidence appears to be increased by antipsychotic drugs (personal observation) (Fig. 6.29).

Administration of cadmium chloride is associated with impaired secretion of clear cells and increased peritubular interstitial tissue [54]. Ethane dimethanesulphonate (EDS) and chloroethyl methanesulphonate (CMS), both alkylating antitumor agents, cause destruction of clear cells and reduced numbers of sperm in the cauda epididymis through a mechanism unrelated to their Leydig cell toxicity and accompanying reductions in testosterone levels [28]. In rodents, a reduction in testosterone levels is associated with increased apoptosis of epithelial cells, particularly in the caput (Fig. 6.30). Oestrogens reduce androgen levels, changing the composition of epididymal fluid [55]. Oestrogenic treatment is associated with vacuolation and apoptosis of the epididymal epithelium [56].

Epithelial hyperplasia of the epididymis is not a recognised diagnosis in rodents, but it has been recorded in cynomolgus monkeys given epidermal growth factor [57]. Compounds that affect spermatozoal passage through the epididymis, such as α-chlorohydrin, at low doses inhibit the glycolytic pathway, causing reduced motility and fertilising capability of the epididymal sperm. Chlorosugars have a similar mechanism of toxicity.

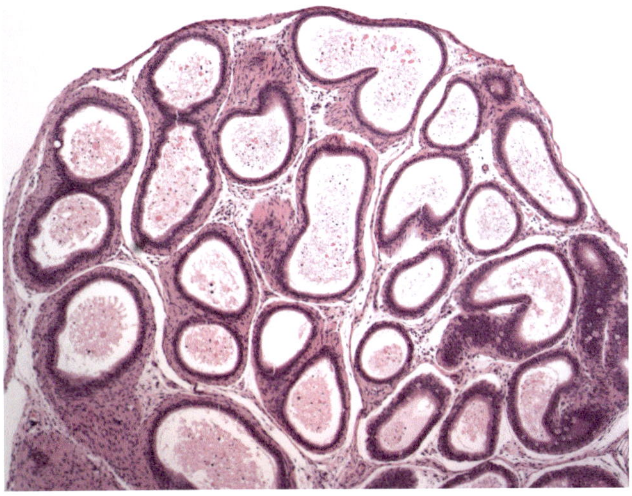

**FIGURE 6-24.** Reduced sperm and cell debris in the cauda epididymis of a rat. The tubules are mildly atrophic and contain cell debris and eosinophilic material. H&E.

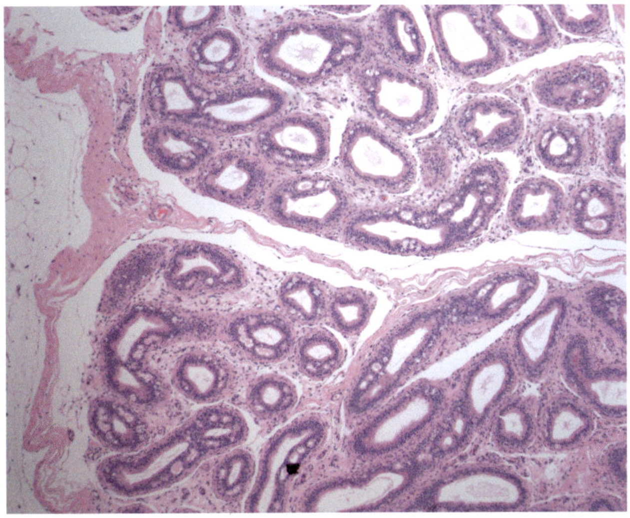

**FIGURE 6-25.** Epididymal atrophy in a mouse, secondary to testicular atrophy. The epididymis is smaller than normal with absence of luminal sperm. Many tubules display reduced lumens with cribriform change and pseudoglandular formation in the epithelium, which should not be mistaken for hyperplasia. H&E.

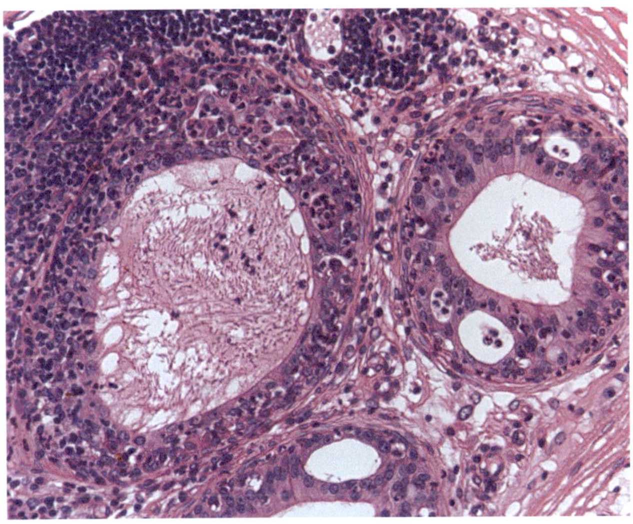

**FIGURE 6-26.** Epithelial inflammation and necrosis in the epididymis, rat. Vesicles and mixed inflammatory cell infiltration are seen in the tubular epithelium. Degeneration of epithelial cells is seen in one tubule.

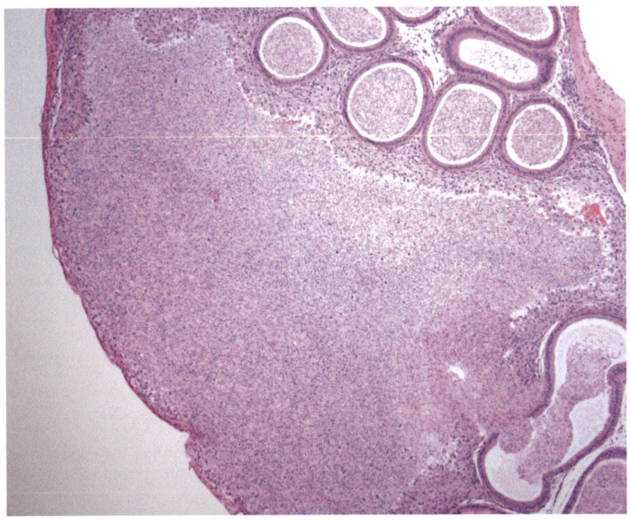

**FIGURE 6-27.** Sperm granuloma in the epididymal corpus of a mouse. Rupture and escape of sperm from a tubule (*right*) is evident. Sperm have elicited a histiocytic reaction. H&E.

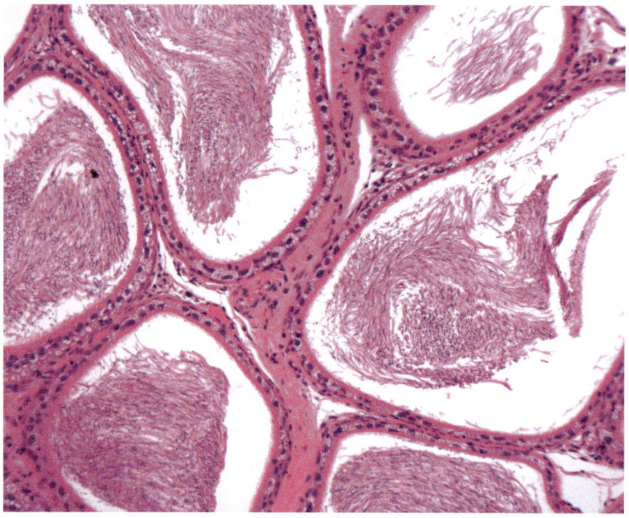

**Figure 6-28.** Vacuolation of the epididymal epithelium in a rat given a phospholipidotic compound. Microvesicular vacuolation of the tubular epithelium in the corpus is present, causing minimal hypertrophy of the cells. H&E.

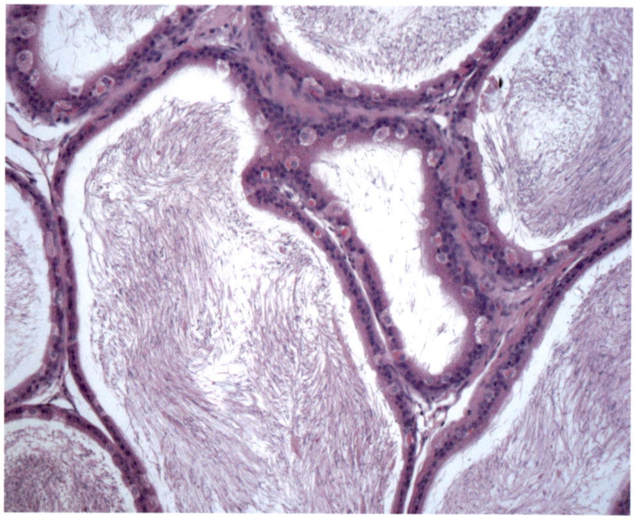

**Figure 6-29.** Increased endocytic vesicles in the clear cells, epididymis of a rat. Small brightly eosinophilic droplets of varying sizes are present in some epithelial cells from the cauda. These vesicles are normal, but their incidence is possibly increased by certain agents. H&E.

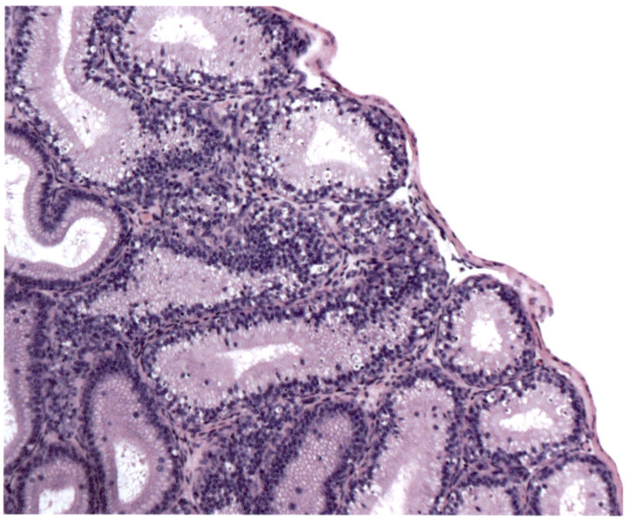

**Figure 6-30.** Single-cell necrosis of the epididymal epithelium in a mouse. Several apoptotic cells are present in the epithelium of the caput. This change is associated with decreased testosterone. Weight loss in mice causes decreased testosterone levels. H&E.

## 6.3 Accessory Sex Glands

### 6.3.1 Seminal Vesicles/Prostate

Induced changes in these organs can be due to direct or indirect toxicity. Indirect toxicity is generally due to hormonal perturbation, often with both seminal vesicles and prostate being affected. Induced changes seen in both organs are given below:

- Inflammation
- Atrophy
- Epithelial hyperplasia
- Squamous metaplasia/squamous cell carcinomas
- Adenoma/adenocarcinoma

Suppurative inflammation of the prostate, sometimes progressing to abscessation, is a common background change in older rats. Prostatic inflammation is induced by a range of compound classes including industrial chemicals and oestradiol (Fig. 6.31) [58, 59]. Inflammation is also induced by prenatal exposure to atrazine, a herbicide, which is associated with delayed prostate development.

Reduced levels of testosterone, due to interference with the HPG axis or steroidogenesis, are a common cause of atrophy of the secondary sex organs in rodents. Inhibition of 5 $\alpha$-reductase, treatment with oestrogens, and anti-androgens classically induce atrophy of the prostate and seminal vesicles [60]. Morphologically, secretory activity of the seminal vesicles is reduced, initially, followed by flattening and inactivity of the epithelium with decreased luminal diameter (Figs. 6.32 and 6.33). A reduction in organ weight is a sensitive indicator of atrophy, which may not be detectable on histologic examination. Synthetic progestogens induce prostatic atrophy in dogs, seen histologically as shrunken, empty acini lined by flattened epithelial cells (Fig. 6.34). Cimetidine and benzodiazepines are associated with reduced prostate weights in dogs; cimetidine is also associated with lower prostate and seminal vesicle weights in rats. Inhibition of testosterone synthesis is presumed to be the causative mechanism for these reductions.

Administration of androgens causes prostatic epithelial hypertrophy and hyperplasia in many laboratory species (Figs. 6.35–6.37). Epidermal growth factor causes epithelial hypertrophy and hyperplasia of the prostate and seminal vesicles in monkeys [57].

Chronic oestrogenic exposure, vitamin A deficiency, prostaglandins, and administration of halogenated hydrocarbons can induce squamous metaplasia of the prostatic and seminal vesicular epithelium in rodents [61]. This change, particularly in the prostate, can become very marked and may progress to squamous cell carcinomas. Nitrosamines induce squamous cell carcinomas of the prostate in rats [62]. Adenomas and adenocarcinomas of the prostate have been induced

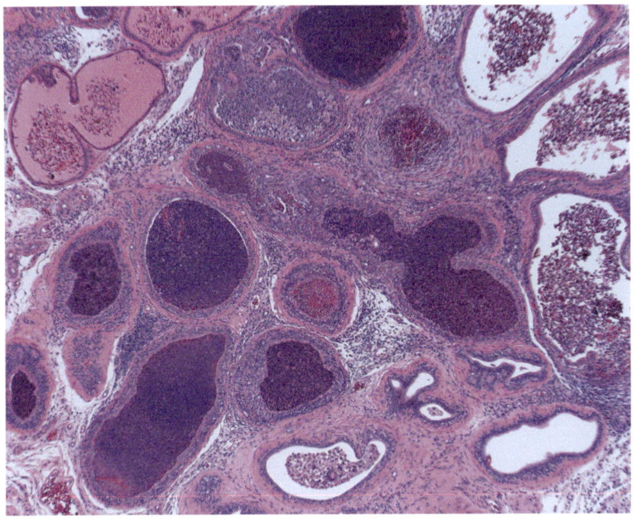

**Figure 6-31.** Purulent inflammation of the prostate in a rat treated with an industrial chemical from a short-term study. The acini are collapsed and contain large numbers of degenerating neutrophils and epithelial debris. Some epithelial degeneration and hyperplasia are evident in some acini. H&E.

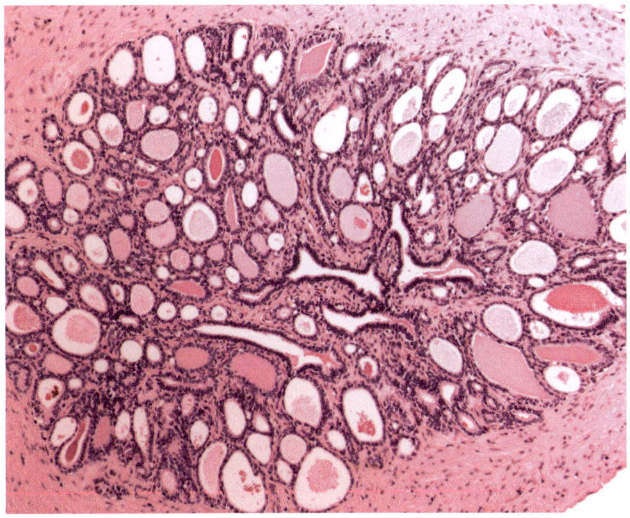

**Figure 6-32.** Atrophy of the seminal vesicles in a rat. The diameter is reduced with absence of luminal secretion. The acini are small with flattened inactive epithelium. Decreased androgenic stimulation is the commonest cause of this change. H&E.

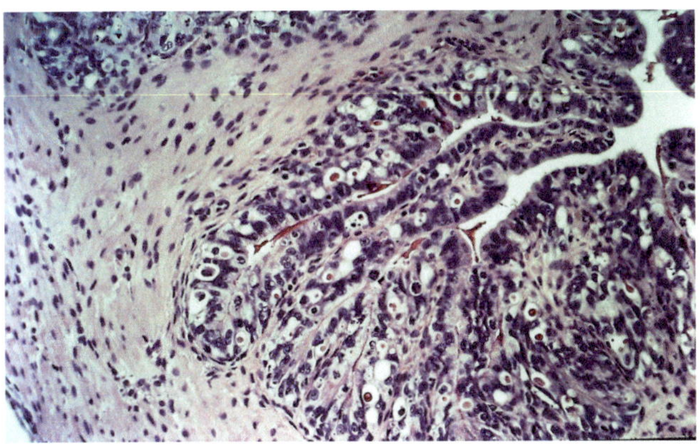

**Figure 6-33.** Atrophy with epithelial single-cell necrosis of the seminal vesicles in a rat. Loss of acini is present. Numerous apoptotic cells are present in the columnar epithelium of the acini and lining the lumen. H&E.

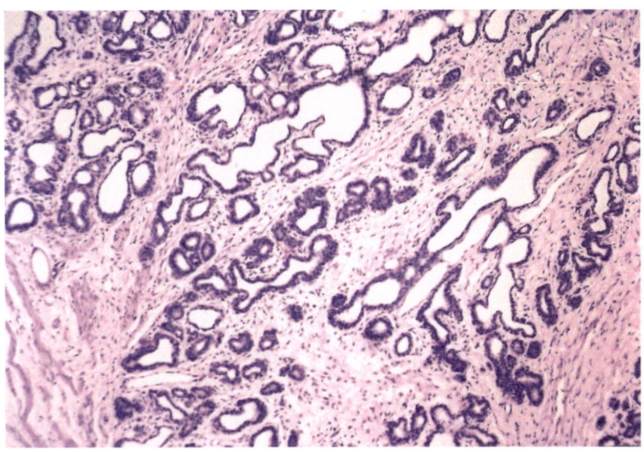

**Figure 6-34.** Atrophy of the prostate in a dog. The acini are greatly reduced in size with flattened epithelium and absence of secretion. H&E.

in rats with a wide range of industrial chemicals including methylcholanthrene, nitrosoureas, and polychlorinated biphenyls [63, 64]. Trifluridine, an antiviral for ophthalmic use, has been reported to induce carcinosarcomas of the prostate in rats [65].

Induced lesions of other accessory sex glands are rare, although a range of background pathology is evident in older rodents. Congestion, haemorrhage, and inflammation of the penis and associated structures often occur as part of the spontaneously occurring urological syndrome in mice (Fig. 6.38). These changes can also be induced.

The preputial gland is a modified sebaceous gland, its counterpart in female rodents being the clitoral gland. Cystic atrophy of the preputial gland is a common age-related change in older rodents, notably rats. Abscesses of the preputial gland are also common as a background finding. Tumours of the preputial gland are seen occasionally as incidental findings and include adenomas and adenocarcinomas, papillomas, and squamous cell carcinomas (Fig. 6.39). A wide range of genotoxic and nongenotoxic test articles induce tumours of these glands in rats including 7, 12-dimethylbenz(a) anthracene, azoxymethane, and testosterone propionate, among many others [66, 67]. Tumours of the preputial and clitoral glands are often induced along with tumours of other organs or sebaceous glands. Ganciclovir, an antiviral, induces tumours of this gland in both sexes in mice [68]. Nalidixic acid also causes a range of tumours in these glands in rats [62].

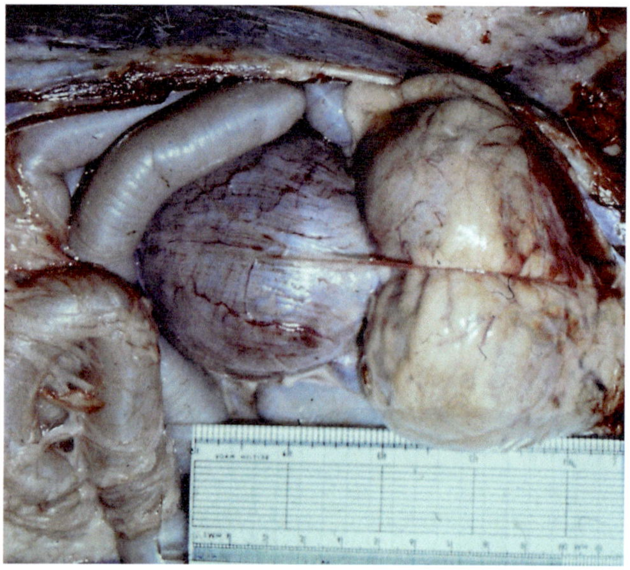

**FIGURE 6-35.** Prostate enlargement in a dog treated with an oestrogenic compound. ((With kind permission from Springer Science + Business Media B.V). H&E.

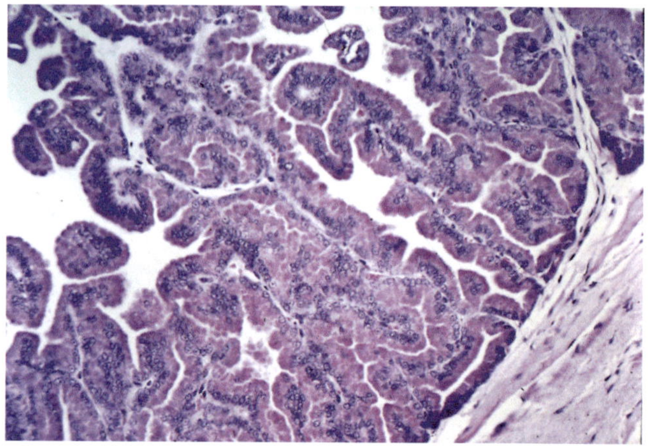

**FIGURE 6-36.** Hypertrophy of the prostate in a dog. Note the complex infolding of the epithelium and dilated lumina. The lining cells are tall columnar. This type of change may be induced by androgenic compounds (With kind permission from Springer Science + Business Media B.V). H&E.

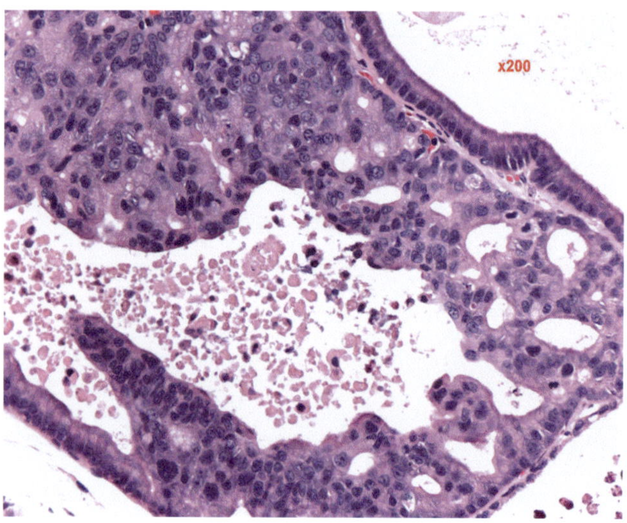


**FIGURE 6-37.** Focal atypical prostatic hyperplasia in a rat. The prostatic epithelium is hypertrophic, with multilayering in several areas. An area of nodular hyperplasia is also present. H&E.

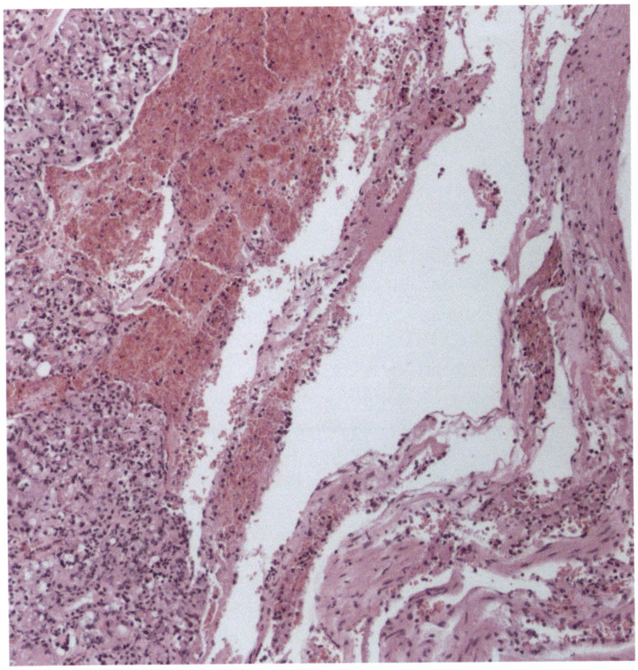

**Figure 6-38.** Congestion, haemorrhage, and inflammation of the urethral gland, corpus cavernosum, and bulbocavernosus muscle are present. This change is often seen spontaneously in mice with urological syndromes associated with urethral blockage but can be induced as well. H&E.

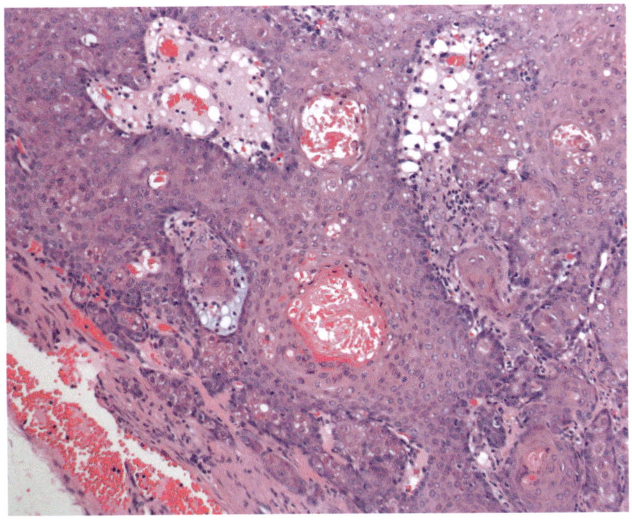

**Figure 6-39.** Squamous cell carcinoma of the preputial gland in a rat from a long-term study. Remnants of the normal gland are present (*left corner*), but the tumour has replaced most of the gland. Tumour cells are moderately differentiated, forming keratin pearls in some areas. H&E.

## References


1. Latendresse JR, Warbrittion AR, Jonassen H, Creasy DM. Fixation of testes and eyes using a modified Davidson's fluid: comparison with Bouin's fluid and conventional Davidson's fluid. Toxicol Pathol. 2002;30:524–33.
2. Lanning LL, Creasy DM, Chapin RE, Mann PC, Barlow NJ, Regan KS, et al. Recommended approaches for the evaluation of testicular and epididymal toxicity. Toxicol Pathol. 2002; 30:507–20.
3. Creasy DM. Histopathology of the male reproductive system II: interpretation. Curr Protoc Toxicol. 2002. Chapter 16:Unit 16.
4. Creasy DM. Pathogenesis of male reproductive toxicity. Toxicol Pathol. 2001;29:64–76.
5. Creasy DM. Evaluation of testicular toxicity in safety evaluation studies: the appropriate use of spermatogenic staging. Toxicol Pathol. 1997;25:119–31.
6. Meyer JK, Fitzsimmons D, Hastings TF, Chellman GJ. Methods for the prediction of breeding success in male cynomolgus monkeys (Macaca fascicularis) used for reproductive toxicology studies. J Am Assoc Lab Anim Sci. 2006;45:31–6.
7. Smedley JV, Bailey SA, Perry RW, O Rourke CM. Methods for predicting sexual maturity in male cynomolgus macaques on the basis of age, body weight, and histologic evaluation of the testes. Contemp Top Lab Anim Sci. 2002;41:18–20.
8. Haruyama E, Ayukawa Y, Kamura K, Mizutamari M, Ooshima Y, Tanimoto A. Morphometric examination for development of reproductive organs in male cynomolgus monkeys. Toxicol Pathol. 2012;40:918–25.
9. Haruyama E, Suda M, Ayukawa Y, Kamura K, Mizutamari M, Ooshima Y, et al. Testicular development in cynomolgus monkeys. Toxicol Pathol. 2012;40:935–42.
10. Rehm S. Spontaneous testicular lesions in purpose-bred beagle dogs. Toxicol Pathol. 2000;28:782–7.
11. Goedken MJ, Kerlin RL, Morton D. Spontaneous and age-related testicular findings in beagle dogs. Toxicol Pathol. 2008;36:465–71.
12. Dorso L, Chanut F, Howroyd P, Burnett R. Variability in weight and histological appearance of the prostate of beagle dogs used in toxicology studies. Toxicol Pathol. 2008;36:917–25.
13. Campion SN, Carvallo FR, Chapin RE, Nowland WS, Beauchamp D, Jamon R, et al. Comparative assessment of the timing of sexual maturation in male Wistar Han and Sprague–Dawley rats. Reprod Toxicol. 2013;38C:16–24.
14. Creasy DM. Reproduction of the rat, primate, dog and pig. In: McInnes EF, editor. Background lesions in laboratory animals: a colour atlas. Edinburgh: Saunders Elsevier; 2012.
15. Clermont Y, Leblond CP, Messier B. Duration of the cycle of the seminal epithelium of the rat. Arch Anat Microsc Morphol Exp. 1959;48(Suppl):37–55.
16. Clermont Y, Leblond CP. Differentiation and renewal of spermatogonia in the monkey, Macacus rhesus. Am J Anat. 1959;104:237–73.
17. Clermont Y, Leblond CP. Spermiogenesis of man, monkey, ram and other mammals as shown by the periodic acid-Schiff technique. Am J Anat. 1955;96:229–53.
18. Clermont Y, Leblond CP. Renewal of spermatogonia in the rat. Am J Anat. 1953;93:475–501.
19. Dreef HC, van Esch E, de Rijk EP. Spermatogenesis in the cynomolgus monkey (Macaca fascicularis): a practical guide for routine morphological staging. Toxicol Pathol. 2007;35: 395–404.

20. Russell LD, Ettlin RA, Sinha-Hikim AP, Clegg ED, editors. Histological and histopathological evaluation of the testis. Clearwater: Cache River Press; 1990.

21. Moss EJ, Thomas LV, Cook MW, Walters DG, Foster PM, Creasy DM, et al. The role of metabolism in 2-methoxyethanol-induced testicular toxicity. Toxicol Appl Pharmacol. 1985;79:480–9.

22. Roberts A, Renwick AG, Ford D, Creasy DM, Gaunt I. The metabolism and testicular toxicity of cyclohexylamine in rats and mice during chronic dietary administration. Toxicol Appl Pharmacol. 1989;98:216–29.

23. Losco PE, Leach MW, Sinha D, Davis P, Schmahai TJ, Nomier A, et al. Administration of an antagonist of neurokinin receptors 1, 2, and 3 results in reproductive tract changes in beagle dogs, but not rats. Toxicol Pathol. 2007;35:310–22.

24. Creasy DM, Chapin RE. Male reproductive system. In: Haschek W, Rousseaux C, editors. Handbook of toxicologic pathology. Philadelphia: Elsevier; 2013.

25. Everds NE, Snyder PW, Bailey L, Bolon B, Creasy DM, Foley GL, et al. Interpreting stress responses during routine toxicity studies: a review of the biology, impact, and assessment. Toxicol Pathol. 2013;41:560–614.

26. La DK, Creasy DM, Hess RA, Baxter E, Pereira ME, Johnson CA, et al. Efferent duct toxicity with secondary testicular changes in rats following administration of a novel leukotriene A(4) hydrolase inhibitor. Toxicol Pathol. 2012;40:705–14.

27. Gotoh Y, Netsu J, Nakai M, Nasu T. Testicular damage after exposure to carbendazim depends on the number of patent efferent ductules. J Vet Med Sci. 1999;61:755–60.

28. Hess RA. Effects of environmental toxicants on the efferent ducts, epididymis and fertility. J Reprod Fertil. 1998;53:247–59.

29. Hess RA, Bunick D, Lee KH, Bahr J, Taylor JA, Korach KS, et al. A role for oestrogens in the male reproductive system. Nature. 1997;390:509–12.

30. Hess RA, Bunick D, Lubahn DB, Zhou Q, Bouma J. Morphologic changes in efferent ductules and epididymis in estrogen receptor-alpha knockout mice. J Androl. 2000;21:107–21.

31. Piner J, Sutherland M, Millar M, Turner K, Newall D, Sharpe RM. Changes in vascular dynamics of the adult rat testis leading to transient accumulation of seminiferous tubule fluid after administration of a novel 5-hydroxytryptamine (5-HT) agonist. Reprod Toxicol. 2002;16:141–50.

32. Son HY, Kim YB, Kang BH, Cho SW, Ha CS, Roh JK. Effects of 2-bromopropane on spermatogenesis in the Sprague–Dawley rat. Reprod Toxicol. 1999;13:179–87.

33. Ikegawa S, Hata J, Nakatomi K, Asaga H, Kaji M, Sugawara S, et al. Collaborative work to determine the optimal administration period and parameters to detect drug effects on male rat fertility—study on estradiol benzoate effects. J Toxicol Sci. 1995;20:251–63.

34. Sprando RL, Collins TF, Black TN, Olejnik N, Rorie JI, Eppley RM, et al. Characterization of the effect of deoxynivalenol on selected male reproductive endpoints. Food Chem Toxicol. 2005;43:623–35.

35. Lee P, Frame SR, Sykes GP, Valentine R. Testicular degeneration and spermatid retention in young male rats. Toxicol Pathol. 1993;21:292–302.

36. Brock WJ, Trochimowicz HJ, Farr CH, Millischer RJ, Rusch GM. Acute, subchronic, and developmental toxicity and genotoxicity of 1,1,1-trifluoroethane (HFC-143a). Fundam Appl Toxicol. 1996;31:200–9.

37. Creasy D, Bube A, de Rijik E, Kandori H, Kuwahara M, Masson R, et al. Proliferative and nonproliferative lesions of the rat and mouse male reproductive system. Toxicol Pathol. 2012;40: 40S–121.

38. Foster PM, Creasy DM, Foster JR, Gray TJ. Testicular toxicity produced by ethylene glycol monomethyl and monoethyl ethers in the rat. Environ Health Perspect. 1984;57:207–17.

39. Moffit JS, Bryant BH, Hall SJ, Boekelheide K. Dose-dependent effects of sertoli cell toxicants 2,5-hexanedione, carbendazim, and mono-(2-ethylhexyl) phthalate in adult rat testis. Toxicol Pathol. 2007;35:719–27.

40. Creasy DM, Foster JR, Foster PM. The morphological development of di-N-pentyl phthalate induced testicular atrophy in the rat. J Pathol. 1983;139:309–21.

41. Russell LD, Malone JP, MacCurdy DS. Effect of the microtubule disrupting agents, colchicine and vinblastine, on seminiferous tubule structure in the rat. Tissue Cell. 1981;13:349–67.

42. Blackburn DM, Gray AJ, Lloyd SC, Sheard CM, Foster PM. A comparison of the effects of the three isomers of dinitrobenzene on the testis in the rat. Toxicol Appl Pharmacol. 1988; 92:54–64.

43. Kerr JB, Knell CM, Abbott M, Donachie K. Ultrastructural analysis of the effect of ethane dimethanesulphonate on the testis of the rat, guinea pig, hamster and mouse. Cell Tissue Res. 1987;249:451–7.

44. Shirai M, Wakui S, Wempe MF, Mutou T, Oyama N, Motohashi M, et al. Male Sprague–Dawley rats exposed to in utero di(n-butyl) phthalate dose dependent and age-related morphological changes in leydig cell smooth endoplasmic reticulum. Toxicol Pathol. 2013;41(7):984–91.

45. Wakui S, Takahashi H, Mutou T, Shirai M, Jutabha P, Anzai N, et al. Atypical Leydig cell hyperplasia in adult rats with low T and high LH induced by prenatal Di(n-butyl) phthalate exposure. Toxicol Pathol. 2013;41:480–6.

46. Waalkes MP, Rehm S, Devor DE. The effects of continuous testosterone exposure on spontaneous and cadmium-induced tumors in the male Fischer (F344/NCr) rat: loss of testicular response. Toxicol Appl Pharmacol. 1997;142:40–6.

47. Foley GL. Overview of male reproductive pathology, Toxicol Pathol. 2001;29:49–63.

48. Chapin RE, White RD, Morgan KT, Bus JS. Studies of lesions induced in the testis and epididymis of F-344 rats by inhaled methyl chloride 1. Toxicol Appl Pharmacol. 1984;76:328–43.

49. de Andrade SF, Oliva SU, Klinefelter GR, De Grava KW. Epididymis-specific pathologic disorders in rats exposed to gossypol from weaning through puberty. Toxicol Pathol. 2006;34: 730–7.

50. Tani Y, Foster PM, Sills RC, Chan PC, Peddada SD, Nyska A. Epididymal sperm granuloma induced by chronic administration of 2-methylimidazole in B6C3F1 mice. Toxicol Pathol. 2005;33:313–9.

51. Heuser A, Mecklenburg L, Ockert D, Kohler M, Kemkowski J. Selective inhibition of PDE4 in Wistar rats can lead to dilatation in testis, efferent ducts, and epididymis and subsequent formation of sperm granulomas. Toxicol Pathol. 2013;41: 615–27.

52. Sawamoto O, Kurisu K, Kuwamura M, Kotani T, Yamate J. Relationship of interstitial edema with L-cysteine-induced sperm granulomas in the pubertal rat epididymis. Exp Toxicol Pathol. 2003;55:121–7.

53. Pyrah IT, Kalinowski A, Jackson D, Davies W, Davis S, Aldridge A, et al. Toxicologic lesions associated with two related inhibitors of oxidosqualene cyclase in the dog and mouse. Toxicol Pathol. 2001;29:174–9.

54. Zschauer A, Hodel C. Drug-induced histological changes in rat seminiferous tubular epithelium. Arch Toxicol. 1980;4:466–70.

55. Jenkins AD, Lechene CP, Howards SS. The effect of estrogen administration in vivo on the elemental composition of the

intraluminal fluids of the seminiferous tubules, rete testis, and epididymis of the rat. J Androl. 1983;4:272–5.

56. Dunn TB, Green AW. Cysts of the epididymis, cancer of the cervix, granular cell myoblastoma, and other lesions after estrogen injection in newborn mice. J Natl Cancer Inst. 1963;31:425–55.

57. Reindel JF, Gough AW, Pilcher GD, Bobrowski WF, Sobocinski GP, de la Iglesia FA. Systemic proliferative changes and clinical signs in cynomolgus monkeys administered a recombinant derivative of human epidermal growth factor. Toxicol Pathol. 2001;29:159–73.

58. Foley GL. Overview of male reproductive pathology. Toxicol Pathol. 2001;29:49–63.

59. Harris MT, Feldberg RS, Lau KM, Lazarus NH, Cochrane DE. Expression of proinflammatory genes during estrogen-induced inflammation of the rat prostate. Prostate. 2000;44:19–25.

60. Hossaini A, Dalgaard M, Vinggaard AM, Pakarinen P, Larsen JJ. Male reproductive effects of octylphenol and estradiol in Fischer and Wistar rats. Reprod Toxicol. 2003;17:607–15.

61. Andersson H, Tisell LE. Morphology of rat prostatic lobes and seminal vesicles after long-term estrogen treatment. Acta Pathol Microbiol Immunol Scand. 1982;90:441–8.

62. Greaves P. Male genital tract. In: Histopathology of preclinical toxicity studies. Philadelphia: Elsevier; 2011.

63. Stoica G, Koestner A. Diverse spectrum of tumors in male Sprague–Dawley rats following single high doses of N-ethyl-N-nitrosourea (ENU). Am J Pathol. 1984;116:319–26.

64. Cooper TP, Barham RE, Ansell JS. Methylcholanthrene-induced adenocarcinoma of the prostate in rat. Surg Forum. 1974;25:546–7.

65. Monarch Pharmaceuticals. Viroptic (trifluridine) 1 % ophthalmic solution prescribing information. Bristol: Monarch Pharmaceuticals Inc.; 2000.

66. Ward JM. Dose response to a single injection of azoxymethane in rats. Induction of tumors in the gastrointestinal tract, auditory sebaceous glands, kidney, liver and preputial gland. Vet Pathol. 1975;12:165–77.

67. Yoshida H. Preputial tumors induced by intragastric intubations of 7,12-dimethylbenz(a)anthracene in gonadectomized female and male rats. J Cancer Res Clin Oncol. 1983;105:299–302.

68. ClinicalTrials.gov. Neonatal CMV Ganciclovir Follow-up study; 2013. Accessible at http://clinicaltrials.gov/ct2/show/NCT00031421.

# 7 The Female Reproductive System

The importance of various morphological features occurring in different species at different stages of oestrous or menstrual cycle is stressed. Other external factors such as age, nutrition, and stress on oestrous cycle are discussed. Induced lesions occurring in ovaries, uterus, cervix, and vagina in different species are included. A few inducible tumours of the female reproductive tract are also illustrated.

## 7.1 Introduction

The reproductive tract of the adult female is subject to cyclical changes that alter the morphology and function at different phases of the oestrous cycle. Considerable interspecies variations exist in these, in both morphology and duration of the phases. A clear knowledge of the normal histology, the changes specific to each of the laboratory animal species, and their background pathology are essential for correct interpretation of the results of any toxicity study [1–5]. Many changes produced during toxicity studies, especially with steroids, mimic morphological changes seen during the oestrous cycle, albeit in different sequences. The changes induced in various parts of the reproductive tract can occur owing to direct toxicity of the test substance or to hormonal mediation. Age plays an important role because it also produces morphological changes. The nutritional status and environmental stress of the animal must be borne in mind because these can influence the oestrous cycle. Imbalance of endogenous hormones or administration of exogenous hormones results in clear morphological changes in the female reproductive tract.

## 7.2 Ovaries

Toxicity can be exerted by direct or indirect means. Direct toxins are those that act directly without hormonal mediation. These are agents or their metabolites that bind with macromolecules within ovarian structures. Others produce their effects through hormonal mediation. These changes can mimic the changes seen during different phases of the cycle, but they occur for a more prolonged interval or appear as if the phase of the cycle is suspended. Ovarian changes induced by different agents are:

- Oocyte degeneration/loss
- Atretic follicles
- Absence of corpora lutea
- Persistent/increase in corpora lutea
- Follicular cysts
- Ovarian atrophy
- Tubular/stromal hyperplasia
- Mesovarian smooth muscle hyperplasia
- Mesothelial hyperplasia
- Ovarian tumours

C. Gopinath, V. Mowat, *Atlas of Toxicological Pathology*,
DOI 10.1007/978-1-62703-998-7_7, 

Ionising radiation and anticancer agents like cyclophosphamide cause oocyte degeneration and loss (Fig. 7.1) [6]. Irradiation produces necrosis of germ cells, initially affecting primordial follicles. Polycyclic aromatic hydrocarbons affect germ cells but spare granulosa cells [7]. Oocyte and follicular counts, employing immunohistochemical markers where necessary, are useful for measuring follicular activity and atresia [8, 9]. Certain anticancer agents that affect cell growth arrest development of follicles, leading to follicular atresia and a decline in follicular count (Fig. 7.2). In rodents, this leads to reduced numbers of corpora lutea (CL). Hormonal agents suspending the oestrous cycle present changes similar to those in anoestrus, resulting in reduced numbers of CL and follicles, arrest of follicular development, and an increase in atretic follicles. Some contraceptive steroids given to dogs result in increased numbers of similar-sized secondary follicles (Fig. 7.3). Hypophysectomy, oral contraceptives, nitrofurantoin, oestrogens, or progestogens can cause degeneration of follicles, leading to ovarian atrophy (Figs. 7.4 and 7.5). Luteinizing hormone–releasing hormone (LHRH) agonists inhibit follicular development. Short-term administration of oestrogens to rodents and agents cause delayed luteolysis resulting in increased numbers and size of CL. Prolactogenic agents such as butyrophenones result in persistent CL and increased numbers of CL in rodents (Figs. 7.6, 7.7 and 7.8) [10]. Some antihistamines also cause increased numbers of CL in rats. Some xenobiotics cause vacuolation of luteal cells along with increased numbers (Fig. 7.9). Certain phosphodiesterase inhibitors produce increased numbers of large CL in mice, probably through a hormone-mediated mechanism [11]. Flutamide given to rats produces increased CL. Ovarian weights and counting of CL are useful in this context. In rats, some aromatase inhibitors are known to cause atresia of antral follicles, increased luteinized follicles, and interstitial cell hyperplasia in the ovaries, accompanied by uterine atrophy and vaginal mucification [12]. Long-term treatment with some oestrogens and dopaminergic agents like bromocriptine results in prolactin inhibition leading to luteolysis, causing formation of follicular cysts. Aromatase inhibitors produce follicular cysts in dogs. Tamoxifen and β-stimulants also produce follicular cysts in rodents (Figs. 7.10 and 7.11) [13, 14]. Follicular cysts appear as

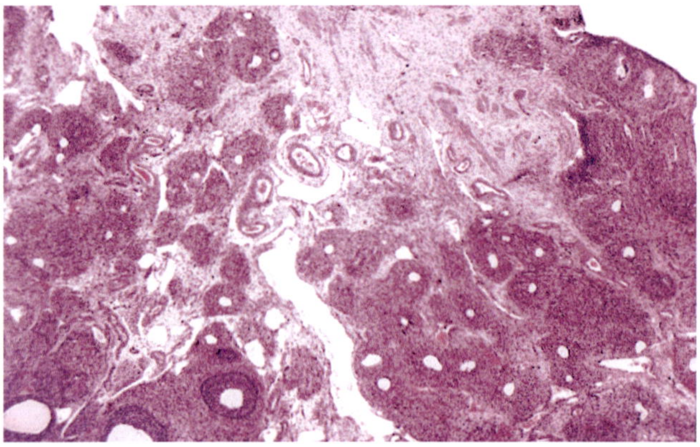

**Figure 7-1.** Loss/degeneration of oocytes/follicles, ovary, in a rat treated with a cytotoxic agent. Haematoxylin and eosin (H&E) (With kind permission from Springer Science + Business Media B.V [45]).

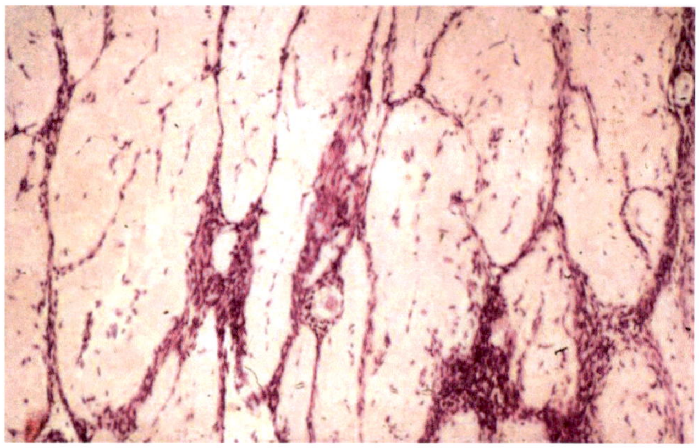

**Figure 7-2.** Atretic follicles, ovary, in a monkey treated long term with a synthetic progestogen. H&E (With kind permission from Springer Science + Business Media B.V [45]).

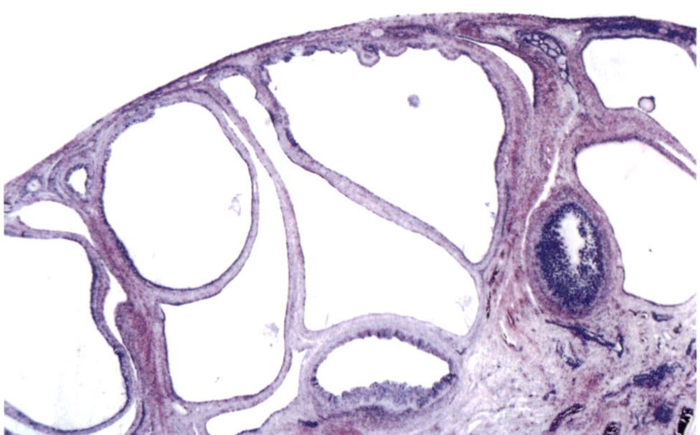

**Figure 7-3.** Simultaneous development of several secondary follicles, ovary, in a dog treated with a sex steroid. H&E.

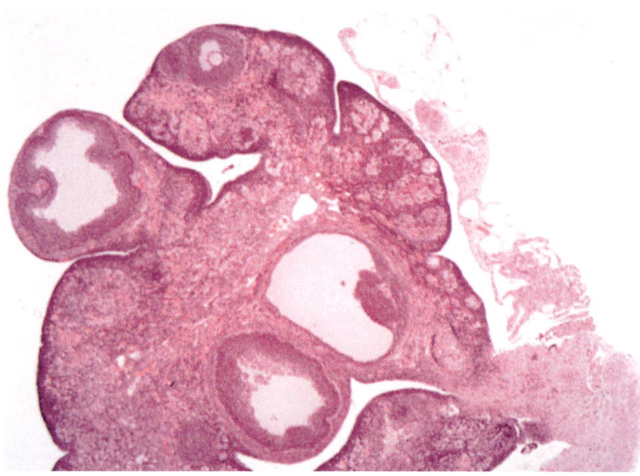

**Figure 7-4.** Atrophy of ovary, in a rat treated long term with a progestogen. Note absent corpora lutea and reduced follicles and stromal proliferation. H&E.

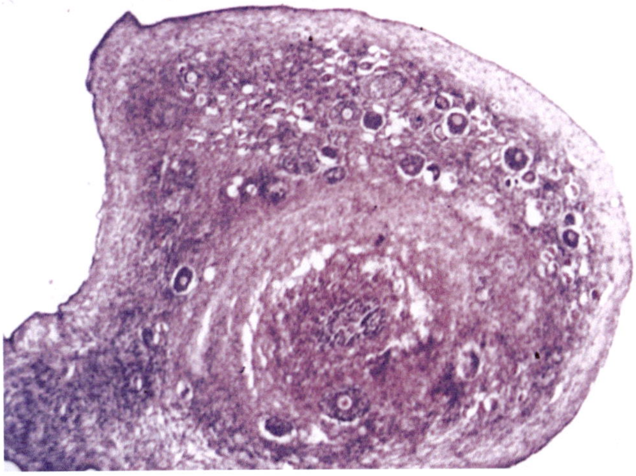

**Figure 7-5.** Atrophy of ovary, in a monkey treated with a progestogen over long periods. Note reduced size, poor follicular development, increased stromal cellularity. H&E.

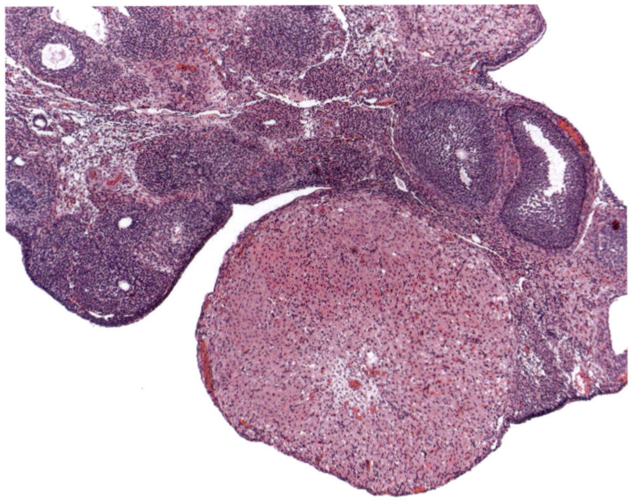

**Figure 7-6.** Persistent and enlarged corpus luteum, ovary, in a rat treated with a hormonal agent. H&E.

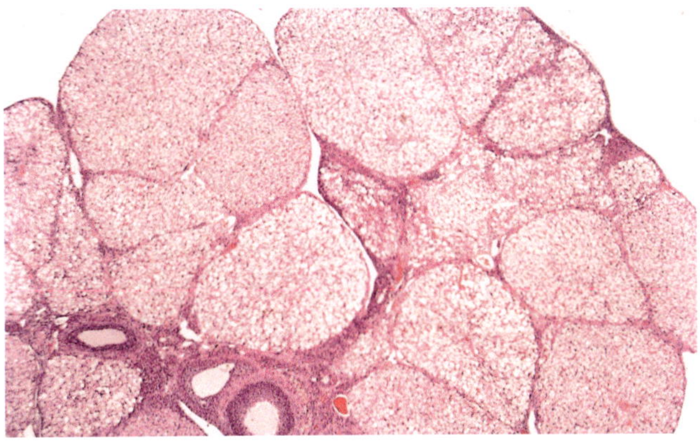

**Figure 7-7.** Increased numbers of corpora lutea, in a rat treated with a neuroleptic agent. H&E.

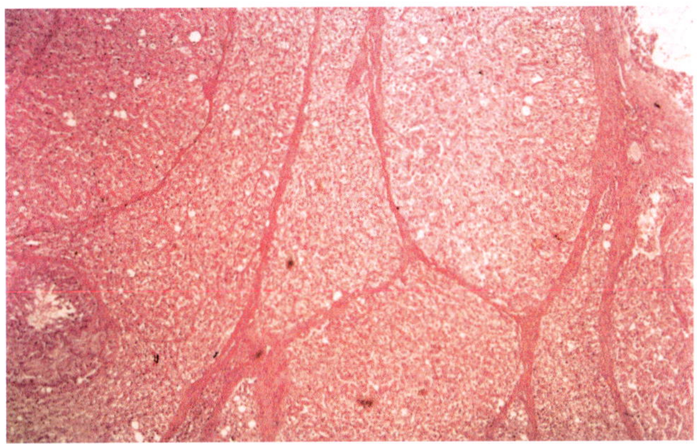

**Figure 7-8.** Increased numbers of corpora lutea and luteinisation of follicles, in a dog treated with an aromatase inhibitor. H&E.

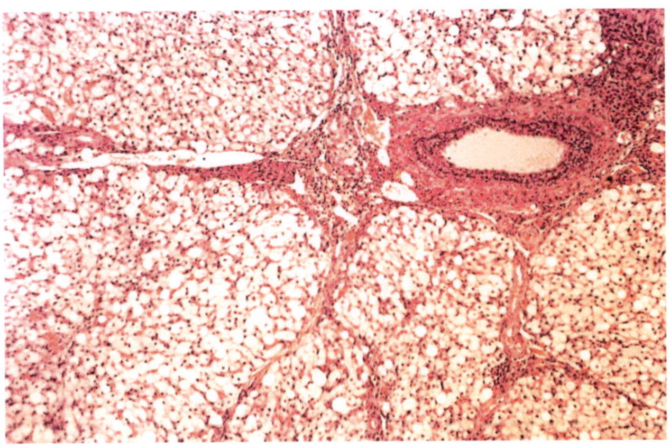

**Figure 7-9.** Increased numbers of corpora lutea with vacuolated luteal cells, in a rat treated with a xenobiotic. H&E.

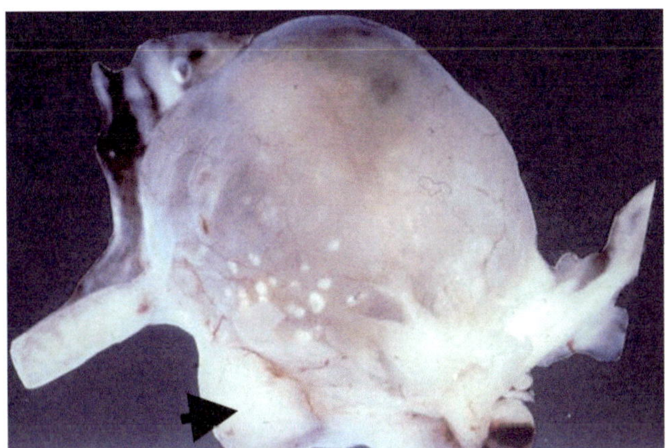

**Figure 7-10.** Cystic follicles, ovary, in a rat treated with a β-adrenergic stimulant. Note the cyst and a nodular white swelling on the ventral aspect (*arrow*), which represents a leiomyoma.

variably sized cysts lined by a thin layer of flattened granulosa cells.

Some agents produce stromal proliferation in the ovaries. Hypophysectomy in rats, growth hormones, and certain agrochemicals produce stromal tubular hyperplasia [15, 16]. The change is gonadotrophin mediated and sometimes appears as Sertoli tubules or Sertoli-like tubular hyperplasia (Fig. 7.12). Anti-androgens, tamoxifen, and nitrofurantoin induce Sertoli cell hyperplasia (Fig. 7.13) [14]. Interstitial cell hyperplasia can be induced in rats treated with certain neuroleptics (Fig. 7.14). Marked luteinisation of different types of follicles and stromal tubules was seen in dogs treated with certain aromatase inhibitors (personal observation) (Figs. 7.15 and 7.16). Synthetic oestrogens like stilboestrol produce mesothelial proliferation of the ovarian serosa in dogs treated for 13–26 weeks. The ovarian serosa revealed florid villous and papillary hyperplasia resembling mesothelioma (Fig. 7.17) [17]. Rhesus monkeys treated with synthetic oestrogens sometimes show increased incidence of ovarian endometriosis, in which islands of endometrial tissue appear on the serosal surface of the ovary (Fig. 7.18).

The mesovarian suspensory ligament adjacent to the ovaries shows smooth muscle hyperplasia in rats treated with a number of β-adrenergic stimulants (Fig. 7.19). The change is a receptor-mediated, species-specific, and site-specific change occurring as a result of exaggerated pharmacological activity. The change can be blocked by co-administration of β-blockers [18].

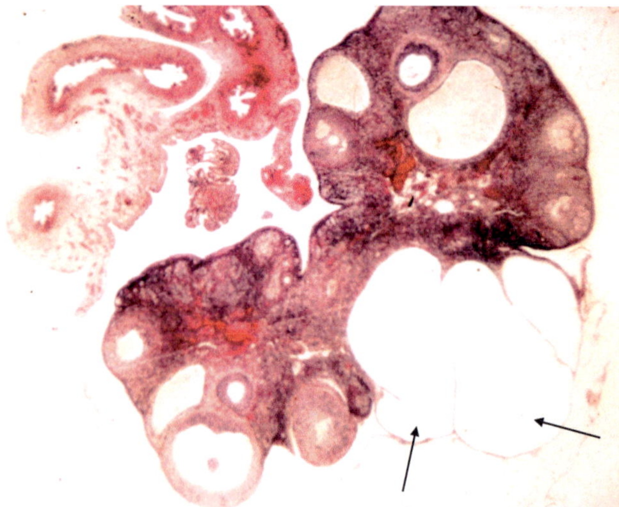

**Figure 7-11.** Cystic follicles (*arrows*), in a rat treated with a β-stimulant drug. H&E (With kind permission from Springer Science + Business Media B.V [45]).

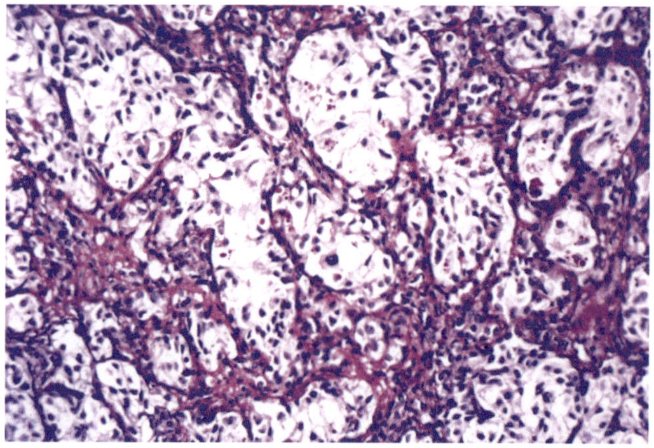

**Figure 7-12.** Sertoliform tubular hyperplasia, ovarian stroma, in a rat. H&E.

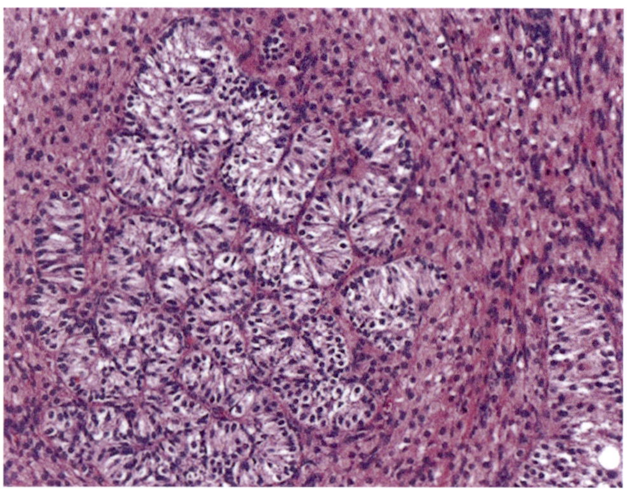

**Figure 7-13.** Tubular hyperplasia (Sertoli tubules), ovarian stroma, in a dog. H&E.

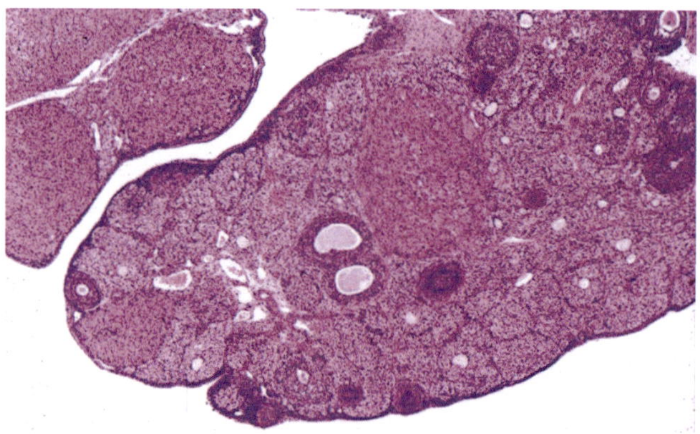

**Figure 7-14.** Interstitial gland hyperplasia, ovarian stroma, in a rat treated with a neuroleptic agent. H&E.

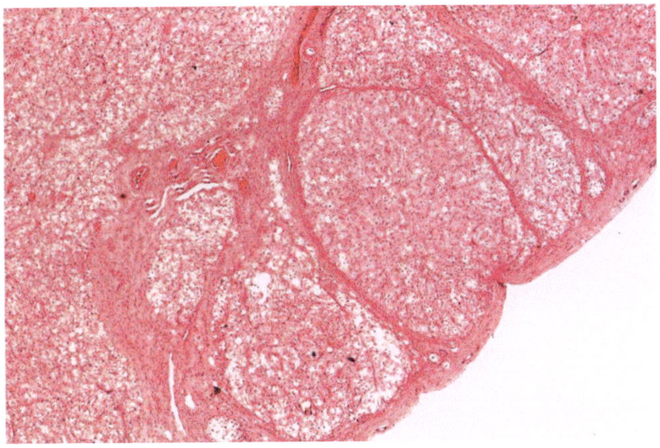

**Figure 7-15.** Marked luteinisation of ovarian stroma, follicles, ovary, in a dog treated with an aromatase inhibitor. H&E.

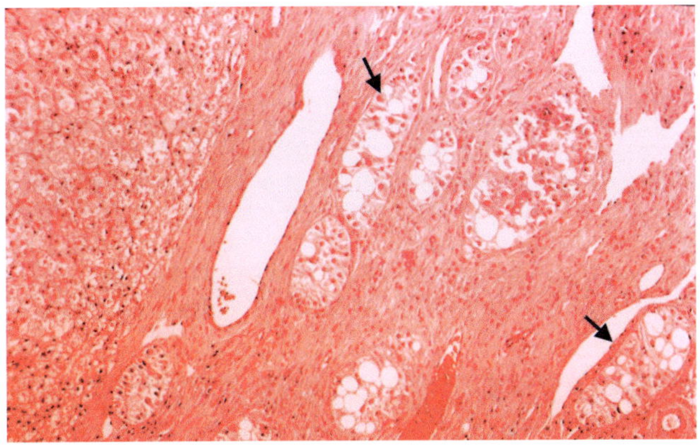

**Figure 7-16.** Luteinisation involving primary follicles and tubules of ovarian stroma (*arrows*), ovary, in a dog treated with an aromatase inhibitor. H&E.

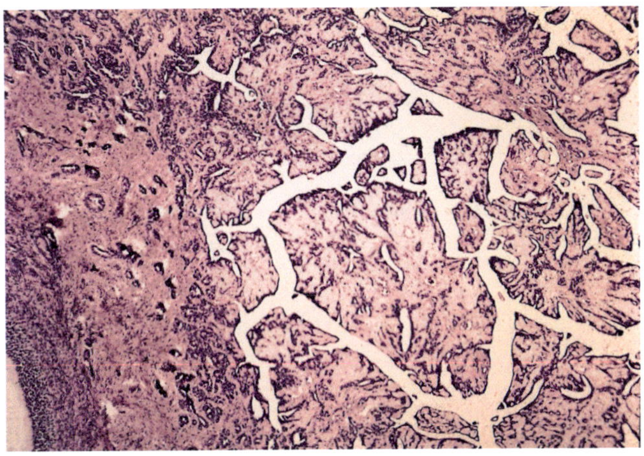

**Figure 7-17.** Mesothelial proliferation, papillary, ovarian serosa, in a dog treated with a synthetic oestrogen. H&E (With kind permission from Springer Science + Business Media B.V [45]).

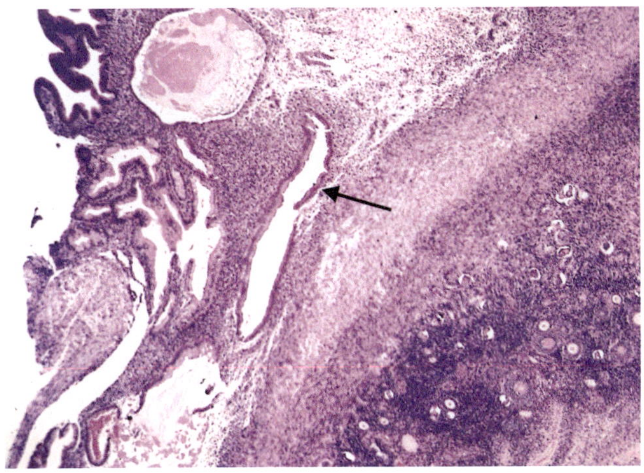

**Figure 7-18.** Endometriosis, ovarian serosa (*arrow*), in a monkey. H&E.

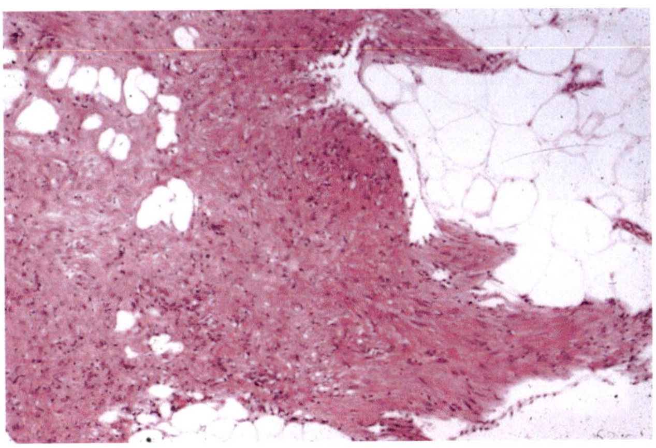

**Figure 7-19.** Smooth muscle hyperplasia, suspensory ligament, ovary, in a rat treated with a β-adrenergic stimulant. H&E.

## 7.2.1 Ovarian Tumours

Rats treated for a long period with several β-adrenergic stimulants develop leiomyomas of the suspensory ligaments or ovaries (Figs. 7.20, 7.21 and 7.22) [18]. These tumours are an extension of the receptor-mediated smooth muscle hyperplasia produced by exaggerated pharmacological activity. The change is species specific and is of no relevance to human safety.

Agents producing damage to the ovarian cortex result in compensatory gonadotrophin-mediated hyperstimulation, which in turn produces granulosa cell or other sex cord–stromal tumours by nongenotoxic mechanisms in rodents (Figs. 7.23 and 7.24) [19]. Raloxifene, an oestrogen receptor modulator, caused granulosa cell hyperplasia in rats, with an isolated occurrence of granulosa cell tumour [19]. The section deals only with some examples of inducible ovarian tumours in rodents.

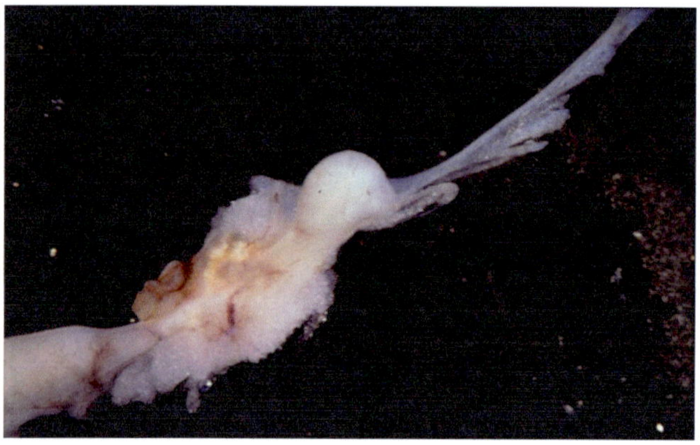

**Figure 7-20.** Ovarian leiomyoma, suspensory ligament, in a rat treated with a β-adrenergic stimulant.

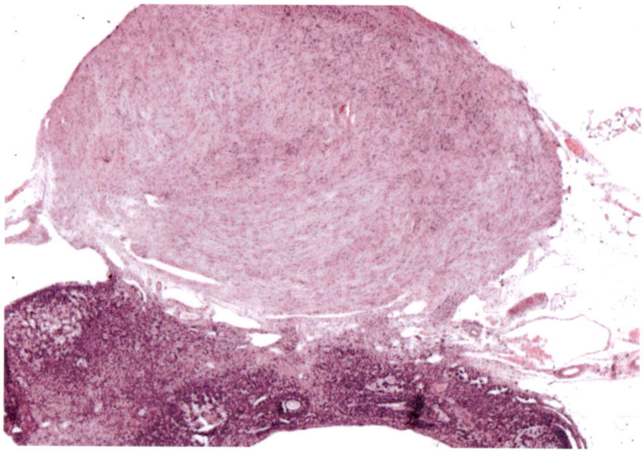

**Figure 7-21.** Ovarian leiomyoma, in a rat treated with a β-stimulant. Note a well-circumscribed growth consisting of bundles of smooth muscle cells. H&E.

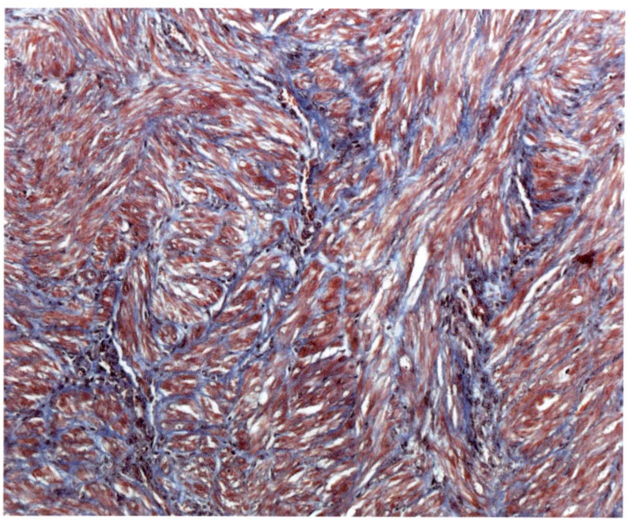

**Figure 7-22.** Ovarian leiomyoma, in a rat treated with a β-stimulant. Note the criss-crossing bundles of smooth muscle cells separated with collagen fibres. Masson's trichrome.

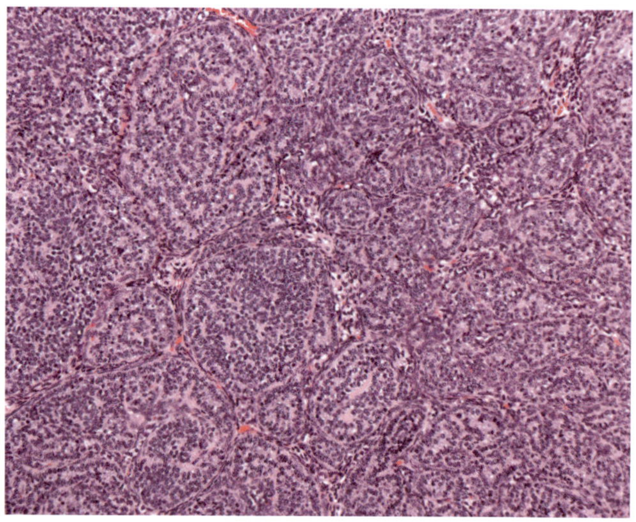

**Figure 7-23.** Granulosa cell tumour, in a mouse. Note the follicular pattern consisting mainly of granulosa cells. H&E.

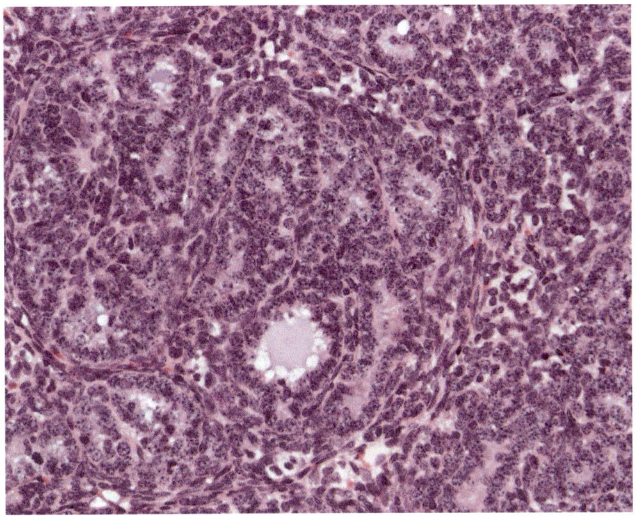

**Figure 7-24.** Granulosa cell tumour, ovary, in a mouse. Note the granulosa cells arranged in differing patterns. Tumour cell nuclei have stippled chromatin. H&E.

## 7.3 Uterus

As with the ovaries, many hormonally mediated changes occurring in the uterus mimic changes similar to those occurring during various phases of the oestrous cycle. The induced changes seen in the uterus are:

- Luminal dilation
- Squamous metaplasia
- Endometrial hyperplasia
- Endometritis
- Uterine atrophy
- Endometriosis
- Adenomyosis
- Decidualisation
- Myometrial hypertrophy
- Mesothelial hyperplasia
- Uterine tumours

Persistent dilation of the uterine lumen is pathologic and can be a sign of hyperoestrogenism. Oestrogens and vitamin A deficiency cause squamous metaplasia of the lining cells and of the glands (Fig. 7.25). Prolonged oestrogen treatment in monkeys results in squamous metaplasia of uterine glands (Fig. 7.26). Endometrial hyperplasia, characterised by increased mucosal thickening, excessive folding, and increase in glands, can be produced in laboratory animals by treatment with oestrogens (Fig. 7.27). In rhesus monkeys, oestrogen treatment causes endometrial hyperplasia, sometimes accompanied by polyps or adenomyosis [20]. Progestogens produce marked endometrial hyperplasia in dogs (Figs. 7.28 and 7.29). If prolonged, cystic endometrial hyperplasia develops. It can result in excessive mucus production in the gland and papillary ingrowths into the lumen in treated dogs (Fig. 7.30) [21, 22]. The lining epithelium becomes hypertrophic and vacuolated in progesterone-treated dogs. In dogs, this has morphological similarities with pseudopregnancy. On some occasions, the endometrial hyperplasia progresses into mucometra and endometritis (Figs. 7.31 and 7.32). Bromocriptine in rats also produces these results owing to the dopaminergic action of the drug. Dopamine blocks prolactin, which in turn results in luteolysis in rodents and consequent hyperoestrogenism [14]. Persistent hyperoestrogenism in rats produces endometrial hyperplasia, endometritis, and endometrial tumours [23].

Certain oestrogens have produced extensive myometrial hypertrophy in dogs. β-Stimulants given long term to mice induce myometrial hypertrophy/hyperplasia. The uterine wall becomes markedly thickened. Diethylstilboestrol given to dogs produces mesothelial hyperplasia of the uterine serosa (Fig. 7.33) [24]. Application of intrauterine devices such as progesterone rings results in the formation of decidual plaques in the endometrium of treated monkeys (Fig. 7.34). The plaques appear as islands of epithelioid cells with abundant eosinophilic cytoplasm in the superficial stroma [25]. Prolonged treatment of monkeys with synthetic progestogens also induces such lesions. Administration of synthetic growth hormone to young female rats produces a florid decidualisation of the uterine horns extending deep into the uterine walls (Fig. 7.35). Recently, extensive multifocal decidualisation of the uterus was induced in rats given a central nervous system agent that disturbs the hormonal balance (Figs. 7.36 and 7.37).

Endometriosis is a condition in which islands of endometrium (both glands and stroma) appear ectopically, usually confined to the pelvic cavity (serosa of uterus, ovaries, intestines, urinary bladder, and mesentery) (Fig. 7.38). This can be seen spontaneously in rhesus monkeys and mice. Oestrogen treatment exaggerates endometriosis in monkeys and induces it in rabbits. Adenomyosis is reported in mice when hyperplastic endometrial glands appear within hyperplastic/hypertrophic myometrial elements; the condition is increased in severity and incidence in mice by treatment with oestrogens and during prolactinaemia (Fig. 7.39) [26, 27]. In mice, this change mimics adenocarcinoma of the endometrium; differential diagnosis is important. In

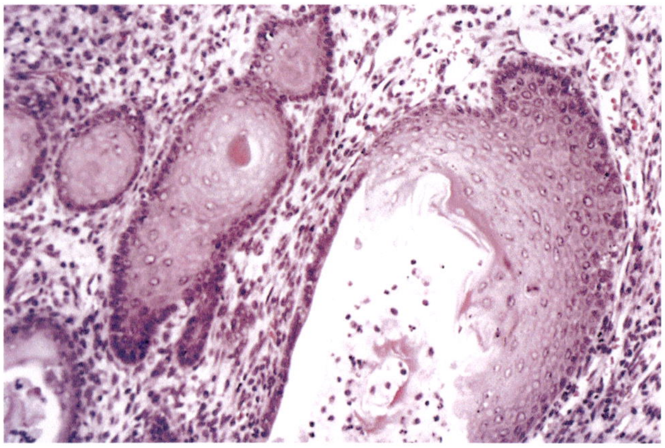

**Figure 7-25.** Squamous metaplasia, endometrial glands, in a rat treated with oestrogen. H&E.

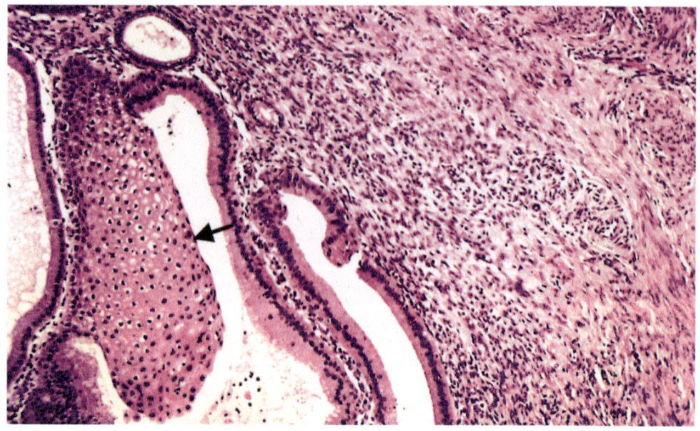

**Figure 7-26.** Squamous metaplasia, endometrial glands (*arrow*), in a monkey treated with oestrogen. H&E (With kind permission from Springer Science + Business Media B.V [45]).

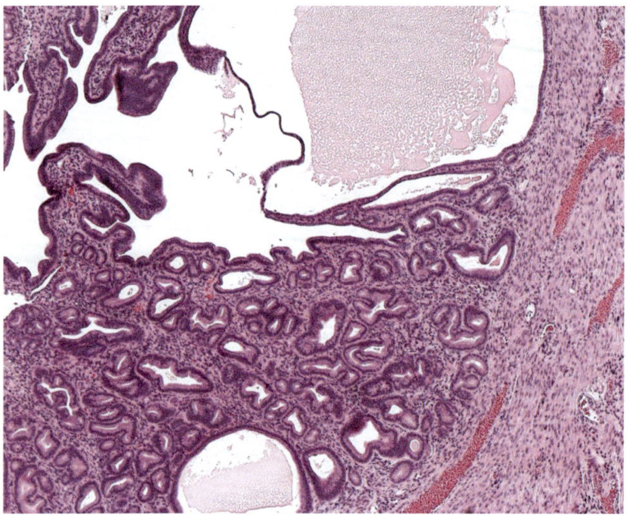

**Figure 7-27.** Endometrial hyperplasia, in a rat treated with a synthetic progestogen. H&E.

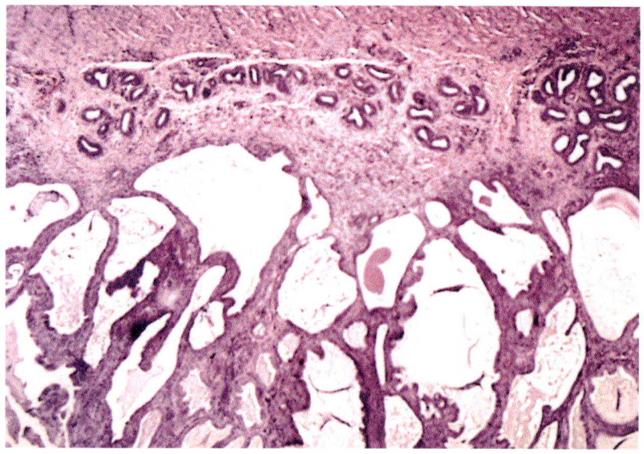

**Figure 7-28.** Endometrial hyperplasia, in a dog treated with a progestogen. H&E (With kind permission from Springer Science + Business Media B.V [45]).

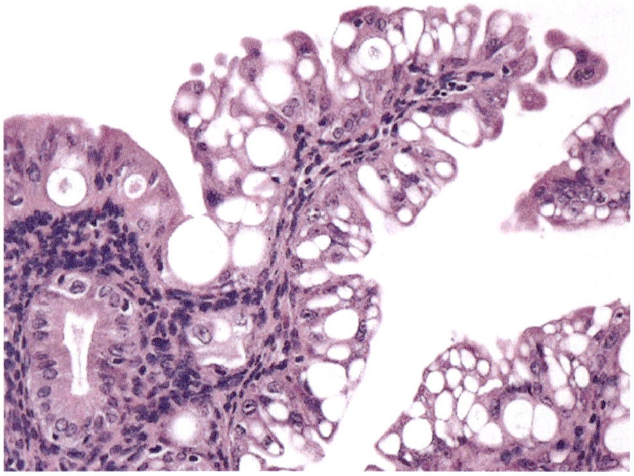

**Figure 7-29.** Hypertrophy and vacuolation of lining epithelium, in progestogen-induced endometrial hyperplasia, in a dog. H&E.

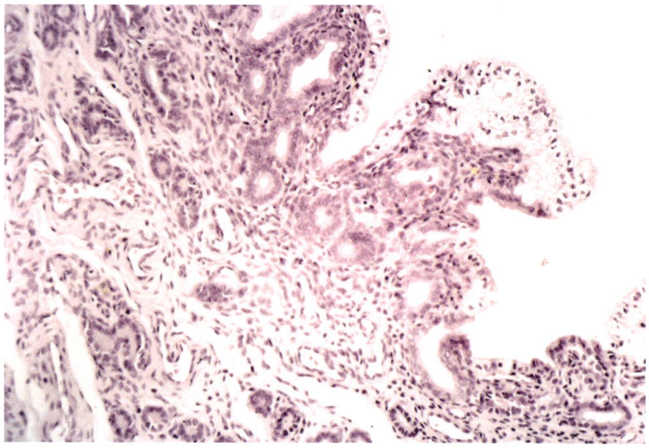

**Figure 7-30.** Papillary projection with fine vacuolation of epithelium in endometrial hyperplasia, in a dog treated with a progestogen. H&E.

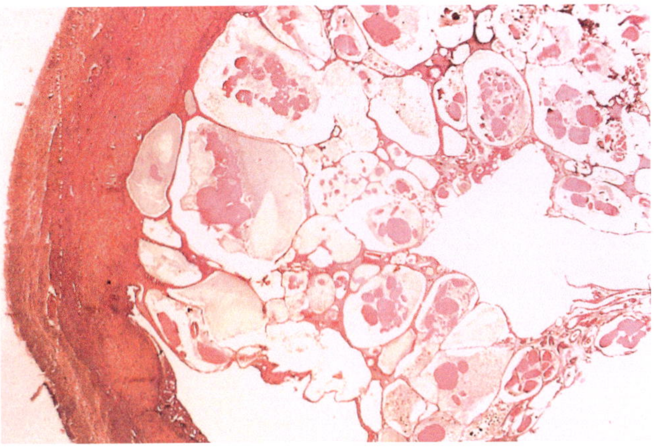

**Figure 7-31.** Mucometra, in a dog treated with a progestogen. Note cystic glands distended with mucous secretion. H&E.

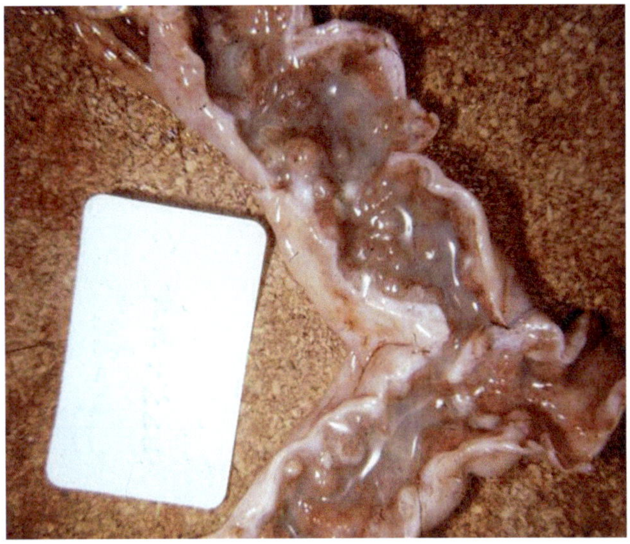

**Figure 7-32.** Pyometra, uterine horns, in a rat. Note the thickening and discoloration of the endometrium.

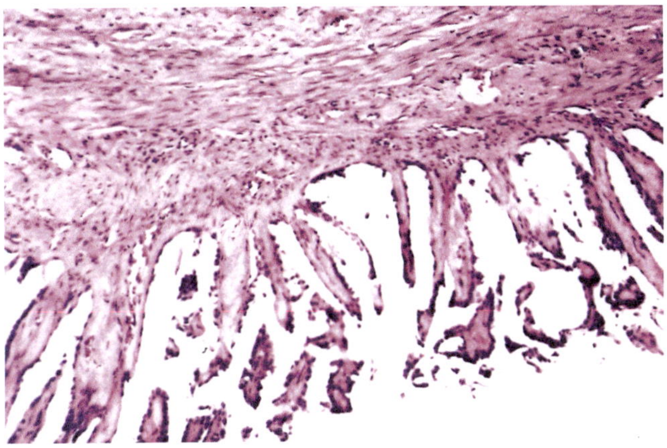

**Figure 7-33.** Mesothelial proliferation, uterine serosa, in a dog treated with a synthetic oestrogen. Note the villous proliferation of serous surface. H&E.

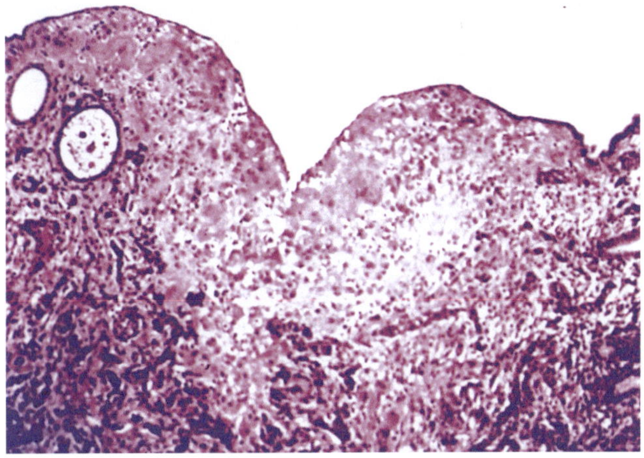

**Figure 7-34.** Decidual plaque, endometrium, in a monkey treated with a progestogen. Note eosinophilic decidual cells adjacent to the lumen. H&E.

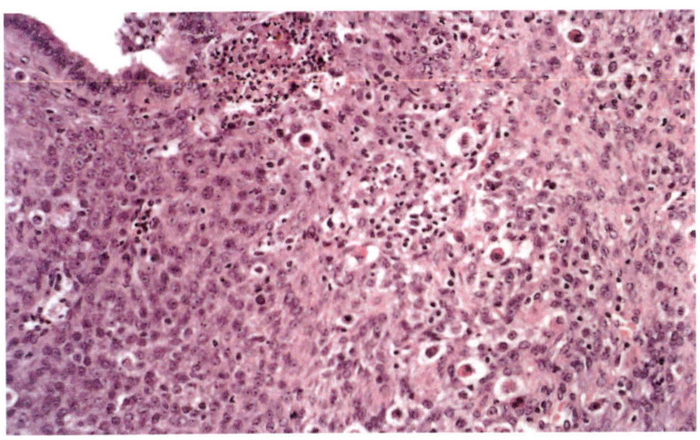

**Figure 7-35.** Decidualisation, endometrium, in a rat. H&E.

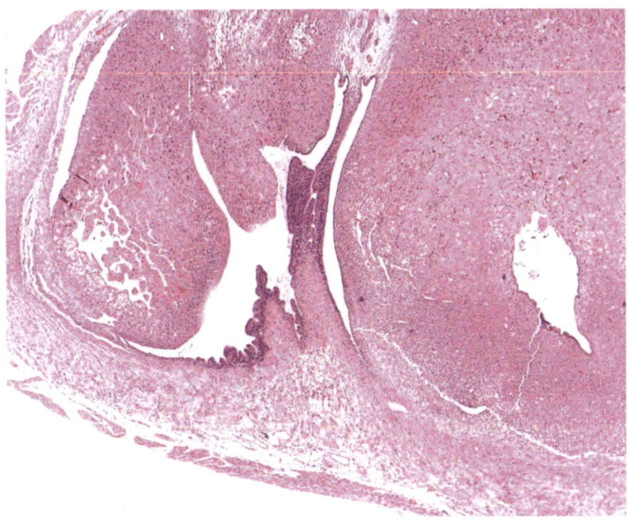

**Figure 7-36.** Multifocal decidualisation, endometrium, in a rat treated with a hormonal agent. H&E.

adenomyosis, the glands are regular and do not reveal any atypia. Adenomyosis is induced in rabbits with oestrogens.

Prolonged treatment of laboratory animals with contraceptive steroids results in gonadotrophic inhibition and uterine atrophy (Figs. 7.40 and 7.41). Delayed maturity in female beagle dogs has been recorded with neurokinin receptor antagonists [28], manifesting as inactive ovaries and uteri. Neuroleptics like butyrophenones and the antioestrogenic tamoxifen produce uterine atrophy. Reduction of size and weight occurs with poorly formed endometrial glands, the stroma appears compact and dark, and the myometrium appears thin and compact with hyperchromatic cells with little cytoplasm. The uterine lumen and its diameter are markedly reduced.

The endometrium showed treatment-related angiomatous hyperplasia and angiectasis, with some vessels displaying thrombi in mice treated long term with a psychoactive drug (Fig. 7.42). Endometrial haemorrhage is observed in dogs treated with certain oestrogens (Fig. 7.43).

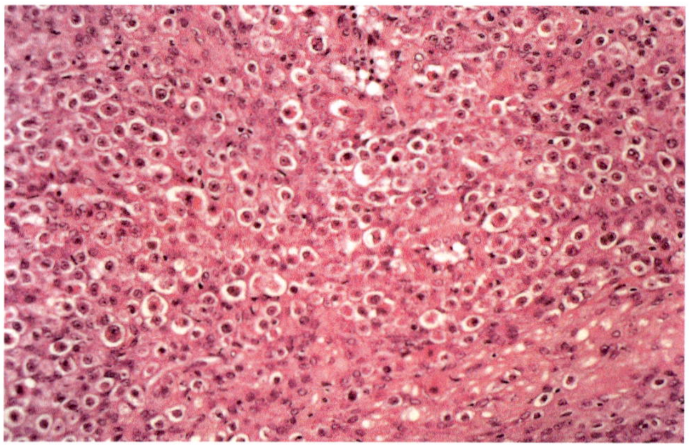

**Figure 7-37.** Decidualisation, endometrium, in a rat treated with a hormonal agent. Note the large decidual cells. H&E.

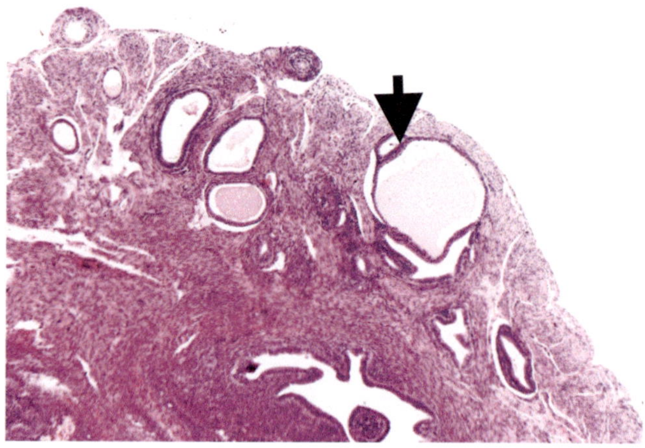

**Figure 7-38.** Endometriosis (*arrow*), uterine wall, in a rat. Note islands of endometrium with glands in myometrium and the serosa. H&E.

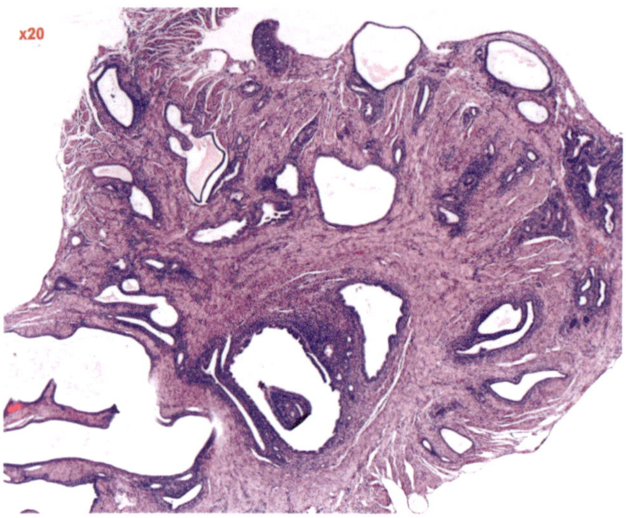


**Figure 7-39.** Adenomyosis, uterus, in a mouse. Note endometrial glands in muscular and serosal layers. Also note hyperplastic myometrium. H&E.

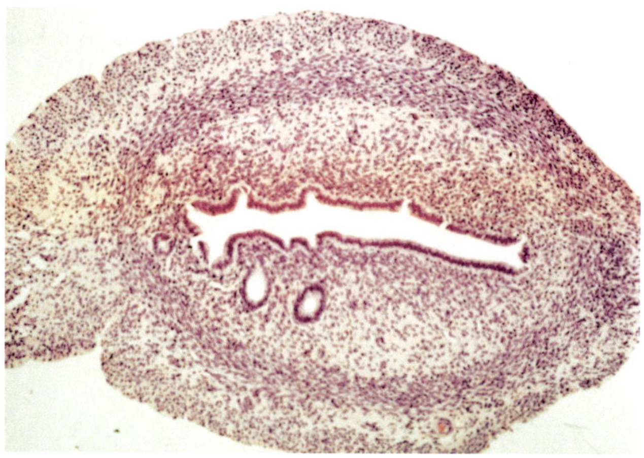

**Figure 7-40.** Atrophy, uterus, in a rat treated with a neuroleptic agent. Note reduced size and diameter of the uterine horn. Sparse endometrial glands. H&E.

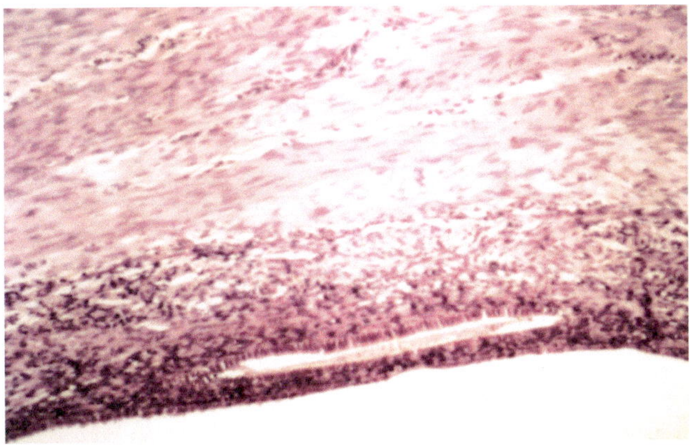

**Figure 7-41.** Atrophy, uterus, in a monkey treated long term with progestogen. Note thin endometrium with reduced numbers of glands and compact stroma. H&E.

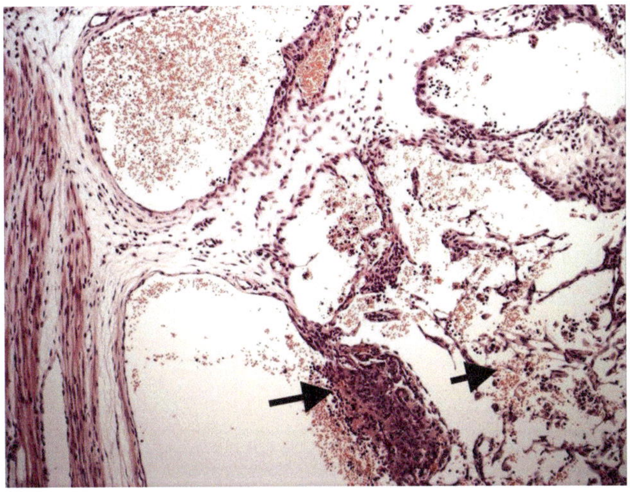

**Figure 7-42.** Angiectasis and angiomatous hyperplasia (*arrows*), endometrium, in a mouse treated with a psychoactive agent. H&E.

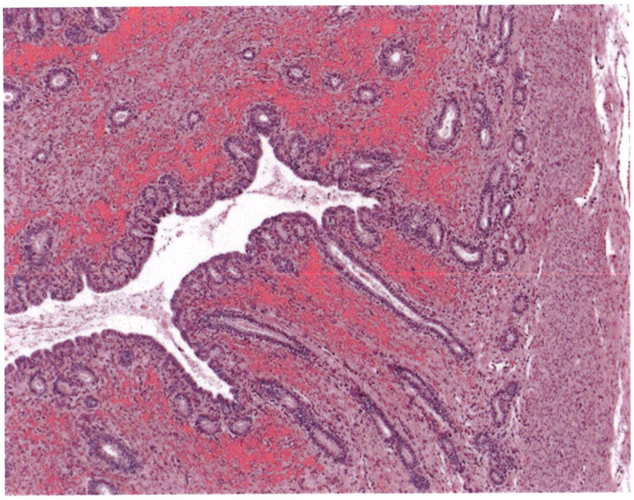

**Figure 7-43.** Endometrial haemorrhage, in a dog treated with an oestrogen. H&E.

## 7.3.1 Uterine Tumours

Long-term treatment of rodents with contraceptive steroids increases the incidence of endometrial polyps and endometrial stromal cell sarcomas (Fig. 7.44) [29]. Pergolide in rats and norethindrone in mice in carcinogenicity studies produce endometrial stromal cell sarcomas. The incidence of endometrial adenocarcinomas is increased in rodent carcinogenicity studies with oestrogens at high dosages (Fig. 7.45). Secondary hyperoestrogenism, as with the dopaminergic agents like bromocriptine and pergolide, also produces similar effects. Prolactin inhibition by dopaminergic agents results in luteolysis in rats resulting in hyperoestrogenism, endometrial hyperplasia, and tumours [30]. Another suggested mechanism includes induction of cytochrome P450 enzymes in the rat liver, which interfere with hydroxylation of oestrogens and result in uterine adenocarcinomas [31]. Mice treated with high doses of many β-adrenergic agents develop smooth muscle tumours of the myometrium (Figs. 7.46 and 7.47). Many β-adrenergic receptor stimulants given to mice for long periods produce receptor-mediated smooth muscle cell hyperplasia and tumours of myometrium [32–34].

A carcinogenicity study in mice with a psychoactive agent produced increased incidences of angiectasis, angiomatous hyperplasia, and haemangiomas of the uterus by nongenotoxic mechanisms (Fig. 7.48).

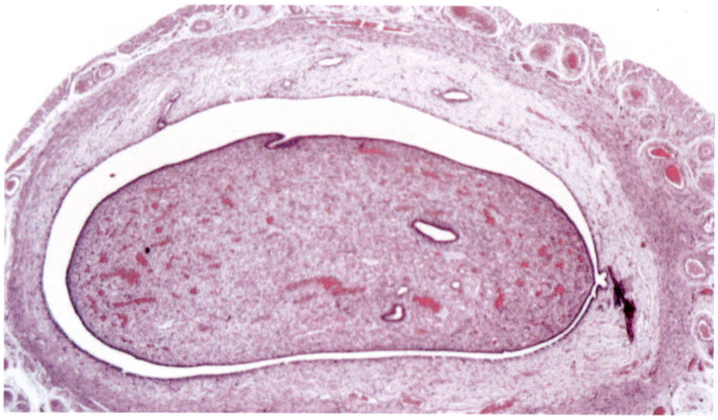

**FIGURE 7-44.** Endometrial polyp, in a rat. H&E.

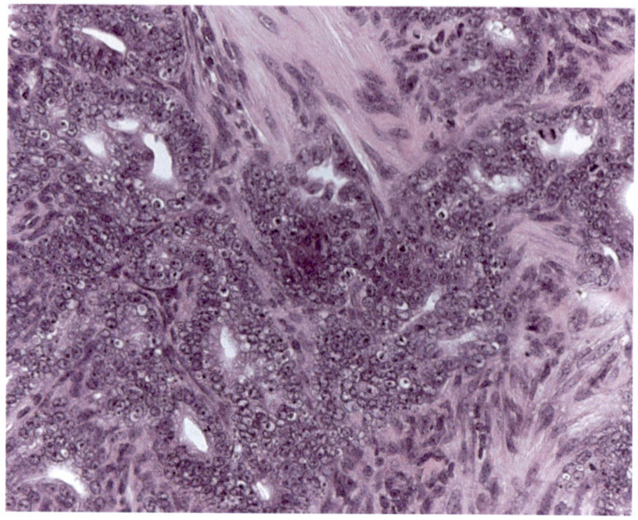

**FIGURE 7-45.** Endometrial adenocarcinoma, uterus, in a rat treated with a dopaminergic agent. Note neoplastic glandular structures invading the myometrium. H&E.

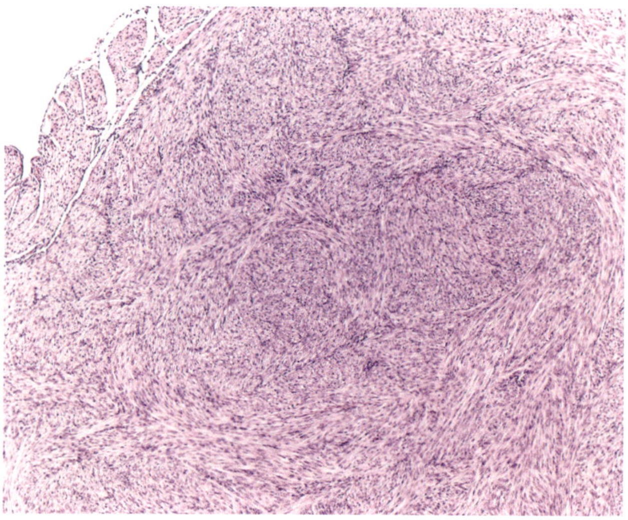

**FIGURE 7-46.** Leiomyoma, uterus, in a mouse treated with a β-adrenergic agent. H&E.

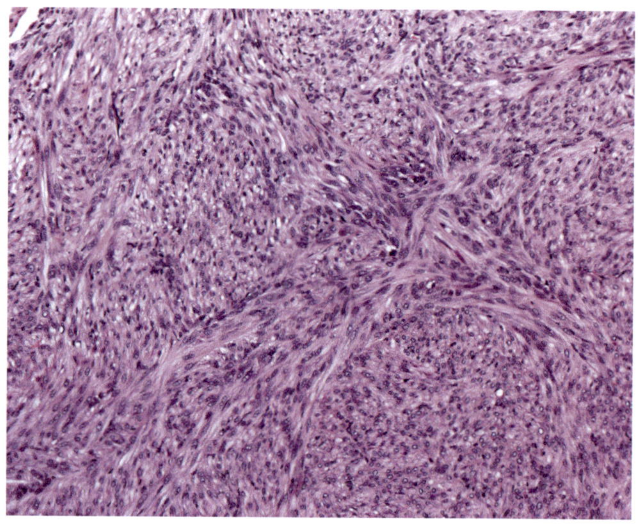

**FIGURE 7-47.** Leiomyoma, uterus, in a mouse. Note criss-crossing bundles of smooth muscle cells forming the tumour. H&E.

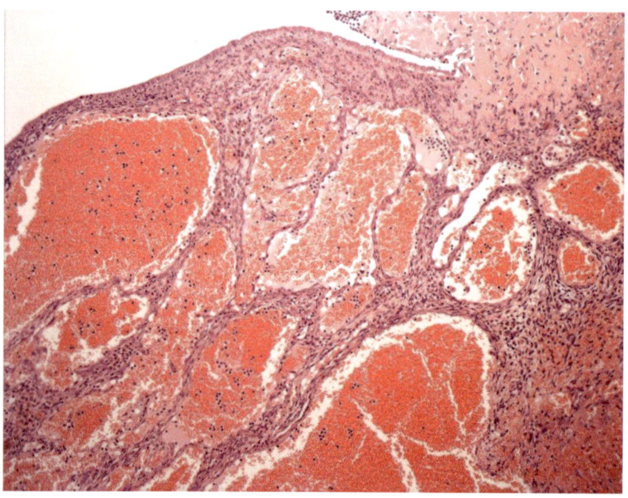

**FIGURE 7-48.** Haemangioma, uterus, in a mouse treated with a psychoactive agent. Note numerous vascular channels lined by proliferating endothelial cells replacing normal structures. H&E.

## 7.4 Vagina and Cervix

Sex hormones induce epithelial changes in the vaginal cervical mucosa. Oestrogens and oestrogen receptor modulators cause hyperplasia and hyperkeratosis, sometimes along with oedema of the subepithelial layer (Fig. 7.49) [35]. The affected mucosa appears thick and leathery with many longitudinal folds in larger laboratory animals. Vaginal keratinisation is used as a measure of oestrogenicity in oophorectomised rats. Progestogens produce mucification, the vaginal epithelium comprising columnar cells and cells containing mucus (Fig. 7.50). Prolonged treatment with sex steroids results in atrophy of the mucosa, which appears thin (1–2 layers) (Figs. 7.51 and 7.52) [36, 37]. Progestogen treatment in monkeys and dogs causes mucoid distension of the endocervix.

Rabbits are used regularly to test irritancy of drugs developed to be administered per vagina [38]. Rabbits are selected owing to their sensitivity and the similarity of their responses when compared with humans. Macroscopic changes such as hyperaemia, haemorrhage, erosion, and ulceration are noted and graded. Microscopically, inflammation, oedema, erosion, ulceration, atrophy, and hyperplasia are noted and graded for evaluation of irritancy potential.

### 7.4.1 Vaginal and Cervical Tumours

An antiviral agent, zidovudine, produced vaginal carcinomas in rats [14].

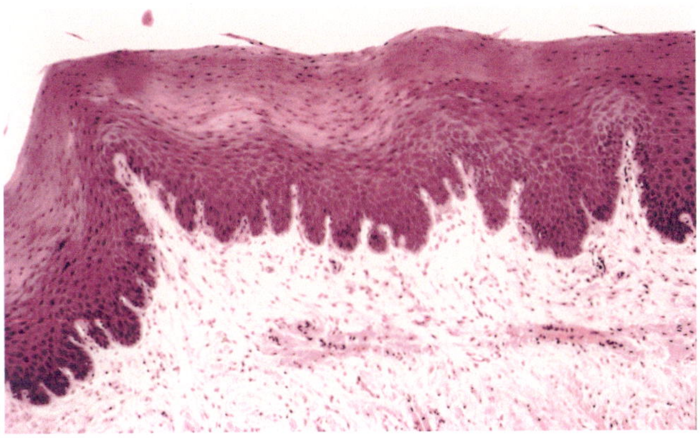

**Figure 7-49.** Thick squamous epithelium with hyperkeratosis, vagina, in a dog treated with an oestrogen. H&E.

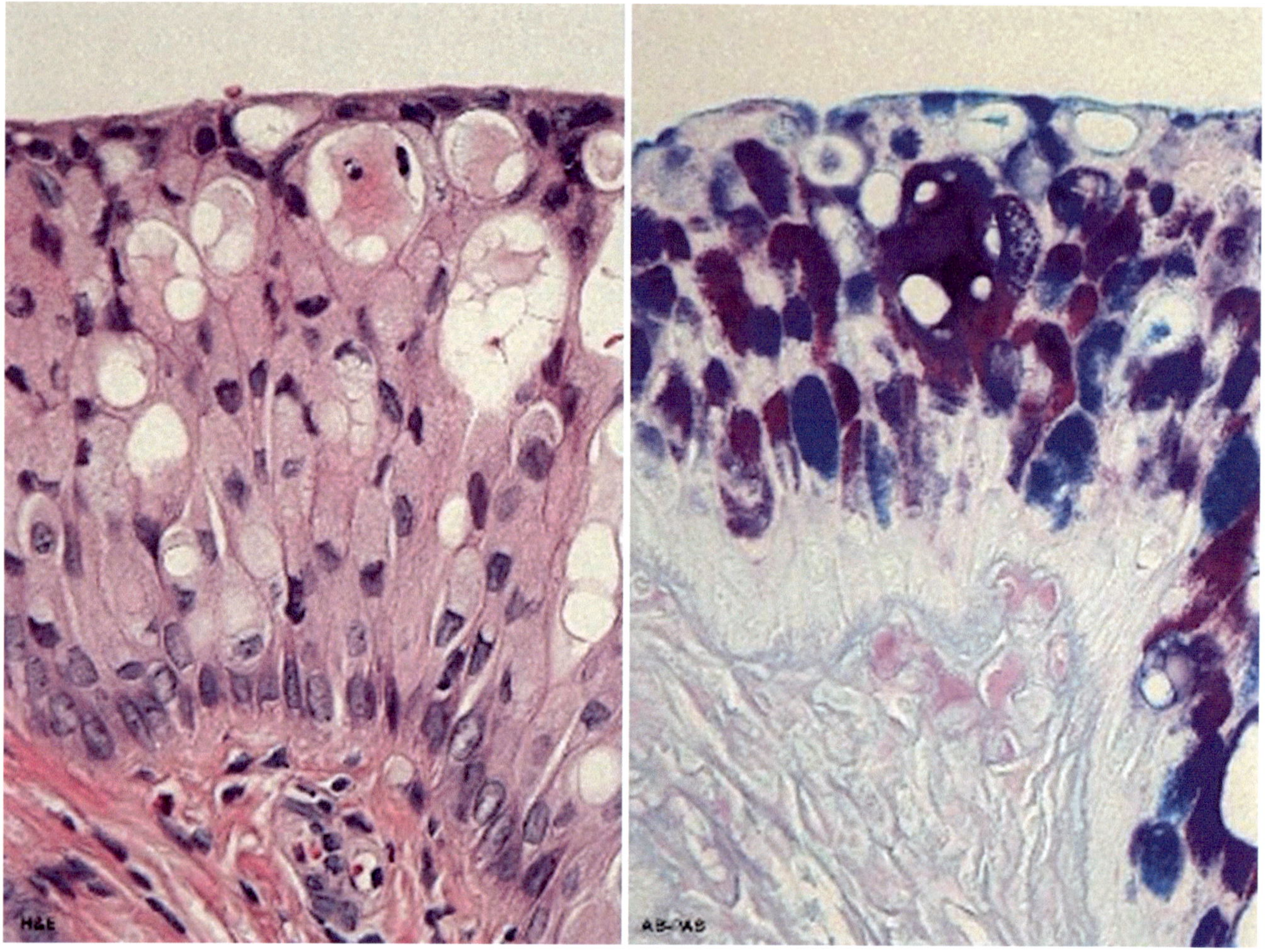


**Figure 7-50.** Mucification, vaginal epithelium, in a rat treated with a progestogen. Note the superficial layer of columnar cells distended with mucin. H&E and periodic acid–Schiff (PAS)/Alcian blue.

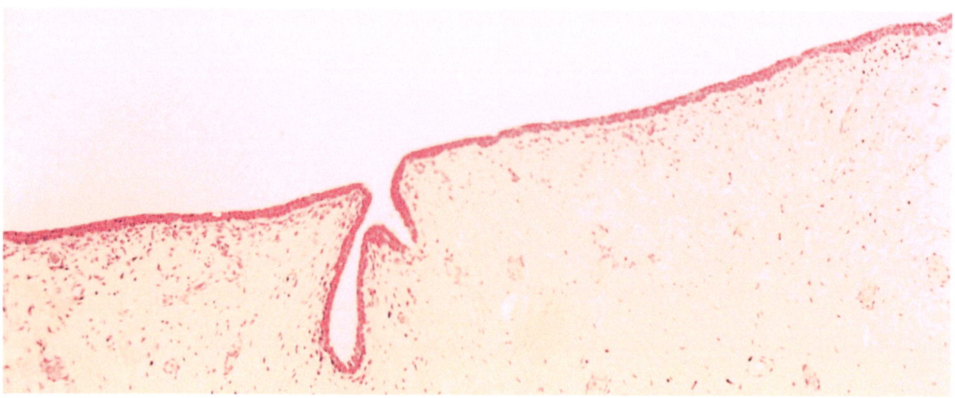

**Figure 7-51.** Atrophy of vaginal epithelium, in a dog treated with a progestogen. Note one or two layers of cuboidal epithelium. H&E.

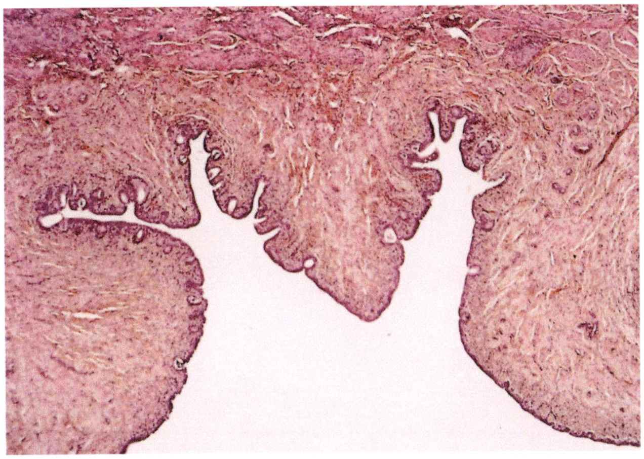

**FIGURE 7-52.** Atrophy of vaginal epithelium, in a monkey treated with a progestogen. Epithelium is lined by a single layer of cuboidal cells. H&E.

## 7.5 Mammary Gland

The mammary gland in females, especially dogs, undergoes profound morphological changes during the oestrous cycle [39, 40]. The changes seen in different phases of the oestrous cycle of dogs can mimic hormone-induced changes. Mammary gland changes are summarised as follows:

- Glandular development
- Acinar/ductular hyperplasia
- Enhanced secretion
- Ductular/acinar dilation
- Hyperplastic nodules and tumours

Many hormones have stimulatory or inhibitory effects on the mammary gland. Progestational and oestrogenic compounds (contraceptive steroids) result in development and hyperplasia of mammary glands in different species of laboratory animals. Oestrogens produce ductular hyperplasia in mice, dogs, and primates [41]. Growth hormone induces ductular dilation and hyperplasia in primates (Figs. 7.53, 7.54 and 7.55). Progesterone, progestogens, and combinations with oestrogens result in marked mammary hyperplasia in dogs and rodents (Figs. 7.56 and 7.57). Mammary glands in male rats have a different morphology with acini lined by larger and more solid cells with indistinct lumen (Fig. 7.58). Hormonal treatments including growth hormone can result in feminisation and hyperplasia of male mammary glands in rodents (Figs. 7.59 and 7.60).

Prolonged treatment with progestogens to dogs produces nodular hyperplasia and tumours including mixed mammary tumours and adenocarcinomas [42]. In dogs, mammary tumorigenesis is mediated through growth hormone. This hormonal pathway is unique to dogs and not applicable to humans [23]. The hyperplastic nodules and tumours in dogs may contain acinar, ductular, and stromal elements. Contraceptive steroids in long-term studies in rodents can result in increased incidences of benign and malignant mammary tumours.

Neuroleptic agents (dopamine antagonistic) given to rodents result in acinar development, increased secretory activity, hyperplasia, and mammary tumours in rodents; this is mediated by prolactin (Figs. 7.61, 7.62, 7.63, 7.64, 7.65 and 7.66) [43]. Dopaminergic agents, conversely, result in inhibition of mammary gland activity and lactation [44].

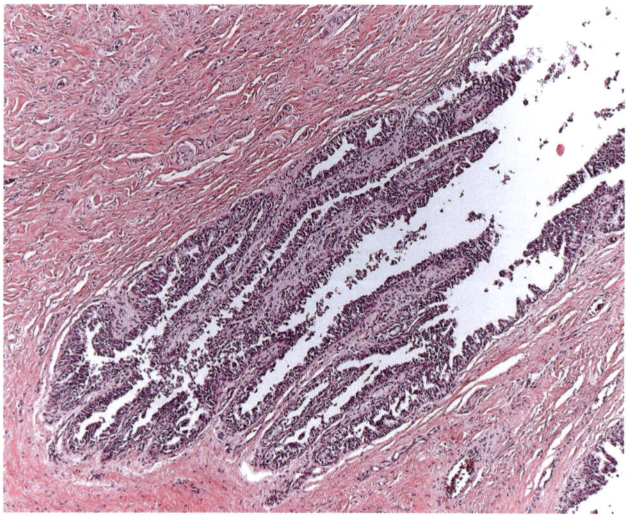

**Figure 7-53.** Ductular hyperplasia and dilation, mammary gland, in a monkey treated with growth hormone. H&E.

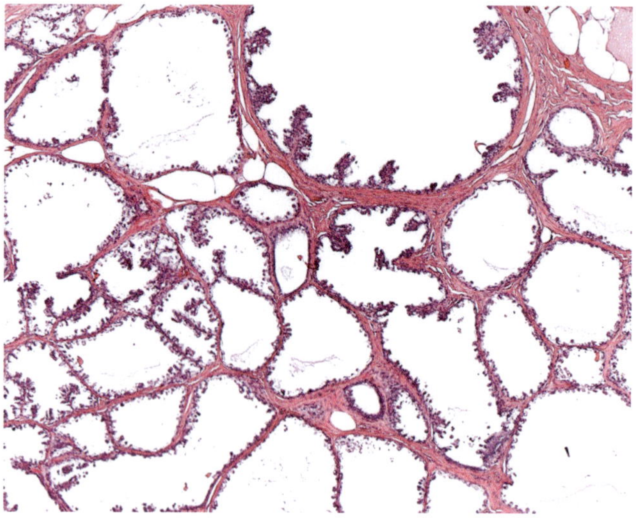

**Figure 7-54.** Acinar/ductular dilation, mammary gland, in a monkey treated with a hormonal agent. H&E.

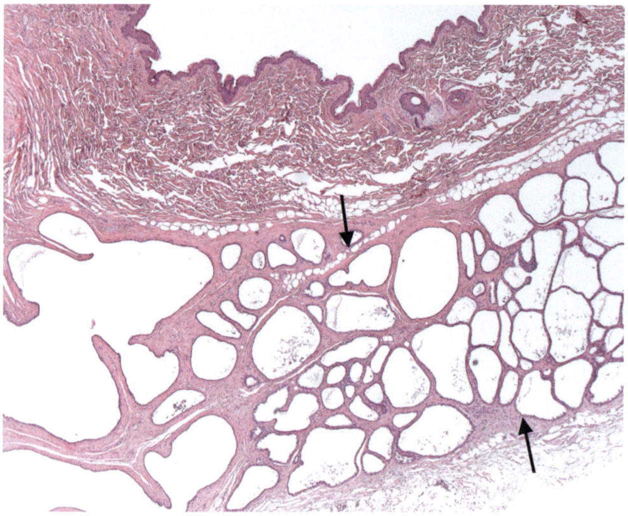

**Figure 7-55.** Acinar dilation and hyperplasia (*arrows*), mammary gland, in a monkey treated with a hormonal agent. H&E.

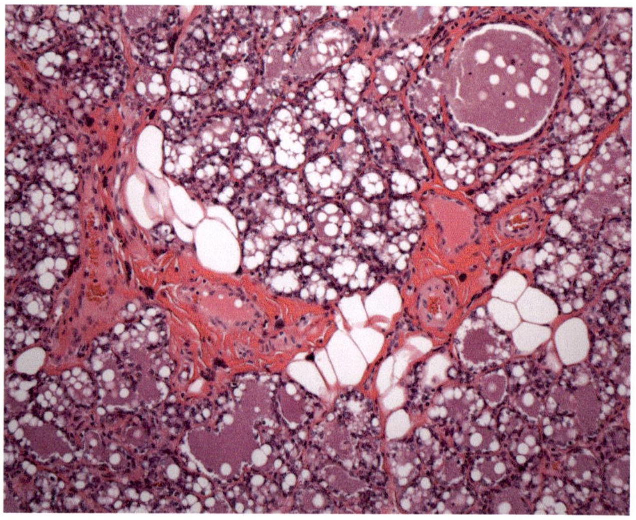

**Figure 7-56.** Lobular hyperplasia, mammary gland, in a rat treated with a neuroleptic agent. H&E.

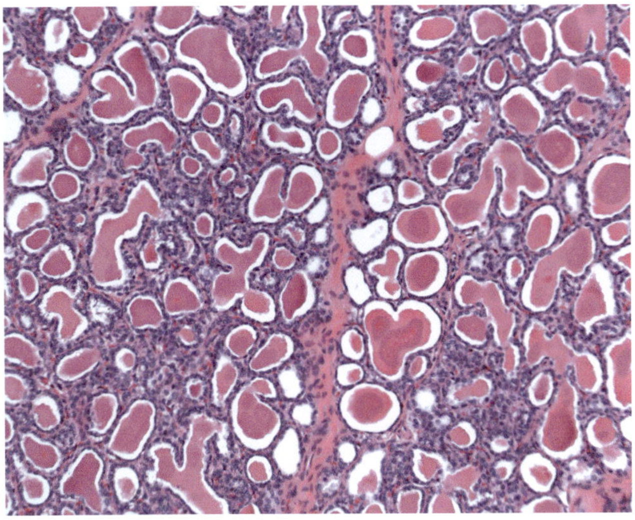

**Figure 7-57.** Marked mammary development, acini with secretion, in a dog treated with a hormonal agent. H&E.

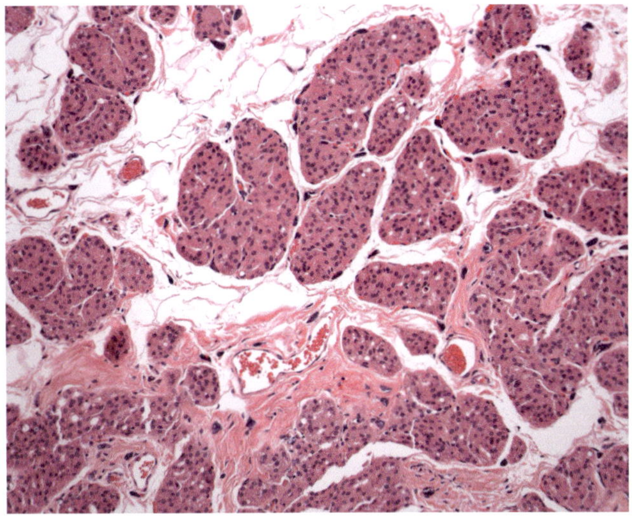

**Figure 7-58.** Mammary gland, normal, in a male rat. Note acini lined by pyramidal cells with little lumen, acini appearing solid. H&E.

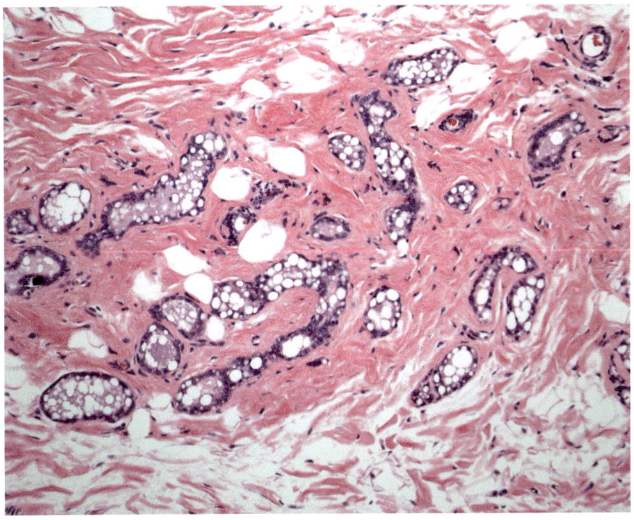

**Figure 7-59.** Feminisation of male mammary acini with increase in stromal collagen, in a rat treated with a hormonal agent. H&E.

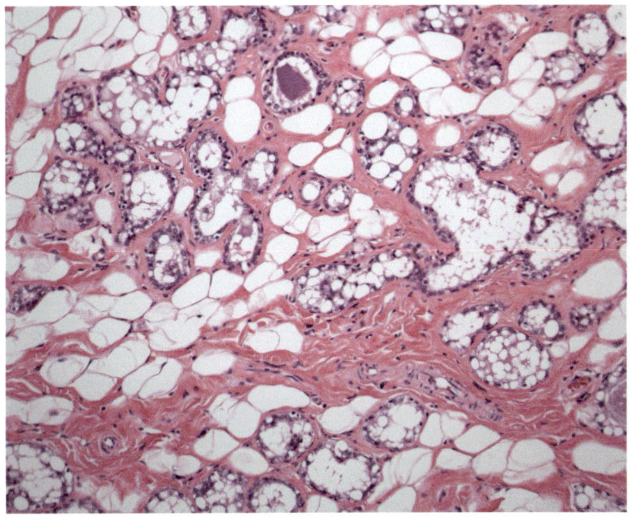

**Figure 7-60.** Feminisation of male mammary acini and lobular hyperplasia, in a rat treated with a hormonal agent. Acini are distended and similar to female mammary gland. H&E.

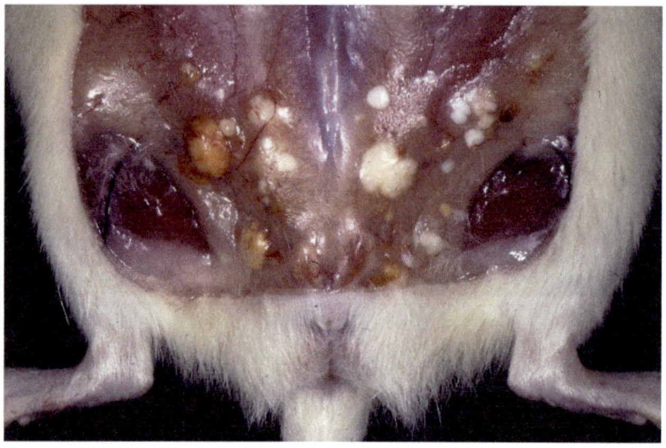

**Figure 7-61.** Distended mammary gland with secretion, in a rat treated with a prolactogenic agent. H&E.

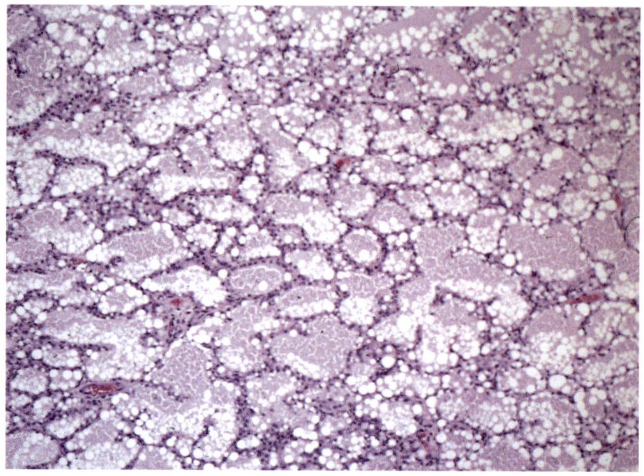

**Figure 7-62.** Mammary adenoma, in a rat. Note sheets of acini with loss of normal architecture such as central ducts. H&E.

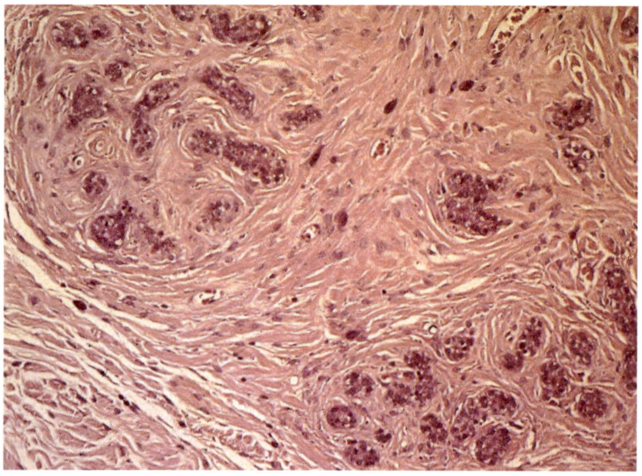

**Figure 7-63.** Mammary fibroadenoma, in a rat. Note almost equal proportion of acinar and fibrous stromal participation. H&E.

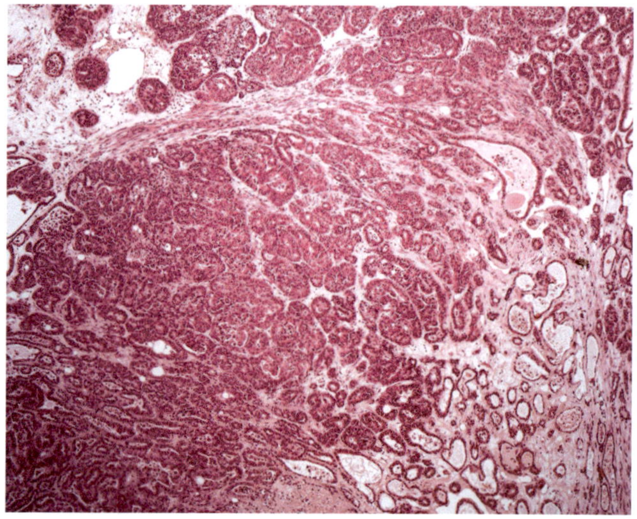

**Figure 7-64.** Mammary adenocarcinoma, in a mouse. Irregular acini lined by multilayered neoplastic cells. H&E.

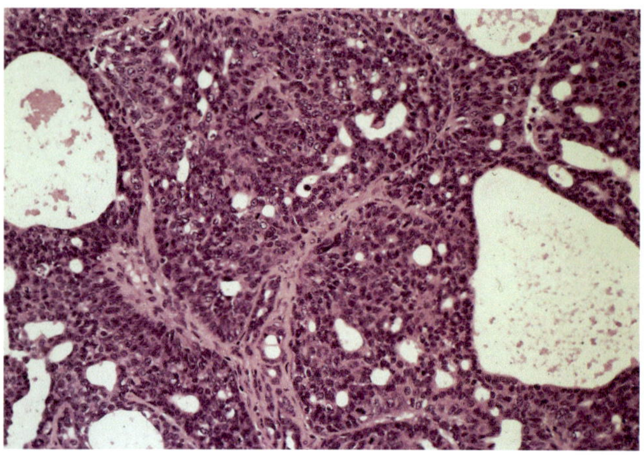

**Figure 7-65.** Mammary adenocarcinoma, in a rat. Note solid lobular pattern and basophilic tumour cells filling up acinar spaces. H&E.

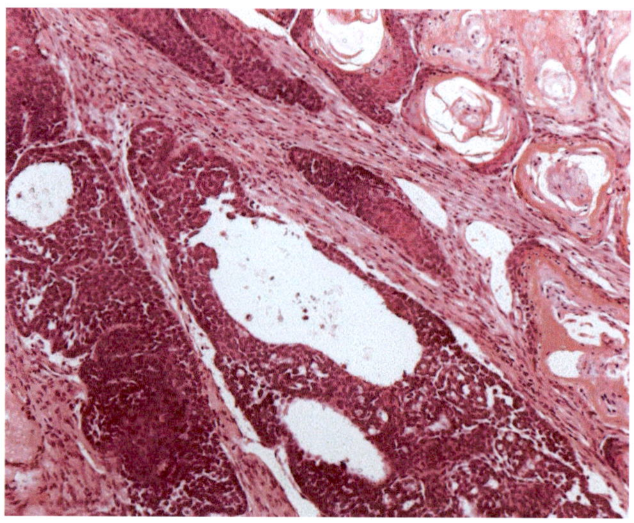

**Figure 7-66.** Mammary adenoacanthoma, in a mouse. Note adenocarcinoma pattern along with keratinising squamous elements within the tumour. H&E.

# References


1. Westwood FR. The female rat reproductive cycle: a practical histological guide to staging. Toxicol Pathol. 2008;36:375–84.
2. Van Esch E, Cline JM, Buse E, Weinbauer GF. The macaque endometrium, with special reference to the cynomolgus monkey (*Macaca fascicularis*). Toxicol Pathol. 2008;36: 67S–100.
3. Gopinath C. Toxicology and pathology of female reproductive tract. Cell Biol Toxicol. 2013;29:131–41.
4. Buse E, Zöller M, Van Esch E. The macaque ovary, with special reference to the cynomolgus macaque (*Macaca fascicularis*). Toxicol Pathol. 2008;36:24S–66.
5. Chandra SA, Adler RR. Frequency of different estrous stages in purpose-bred beagles: a retrospective study. Toxicol Pathol. 2008;36:944–9.
6. Shiromizu K, Thorgeirsson SS, Mattison DR. Effect of cyclophosphamide on oocyte and follicle number in Sprague-Dawley rats, C57BL/6N and DBA/2N mice. Pediatr Pharmacol. 1984;4:213–21.
7. Mattison DR. Morphology of oocyte and follicle destruction by polycyclic aromatic hydrocarbons in mice. Toxicol Appl Pharmacol. 1980;53:249–59.
8. Regan KS, Cline JM, Creasy D, Davis B, Foley GL, Lanning L, et al. STP position paper: ovarian follicular counting in the assessment of rodent reproductive toxicity. Toxicol Pathol. 2005;33:409–12.
9. Muskhelishvili L, Wingard SK, Latendresse JR. Proliferating cell nuclear antigen—a marker for ovarian follicle counts. Toxicol Pathol. 2005;33:365–8.
10. de Baker SBC, Tucker M. Changes in the reproductive organs of rats and dog treated with butyrophenones and related compounds. In: de Baker SBC, Boisser JR, Koll W, editors. Toxicology & side effects of psychotropic drugs, vol. 9. Amsterdam: Excerpta Medica; 1968. p. 113.
11. Losco PE, Poulet FM, Kaminska-McNamara GZ, Klein MF. Myocardial and reproductive system toxicity of SCH 351591, a selective phosphodiesterase-4 inhibitor, in CD-1 mice. Toxicol Pathol. 2010;38:568–82.
12. Mirsky ML, Sivaraman L, Houle C, Potter DM, Chapin RE, Cappon GD. Histologic and cytologic detection of endocrine and reproductive tract effects of exemestane in female rats treated for up to twenty-eight days. Toxicol Pathol. 2011;39:589–605.
13. Nelson LW, Kelly WA, Weikel Jr JH. Mesovarial leiomyomas in rats in a chronic toxicity study of mesuprine hydrochloride. Toxicol Appl Pharmacol. 1972;23:731–7.
14. Greaves P. Female genital tract in histopathology of preclinical toxicity studies. 4th Edn. Amsterdam, Academic Press: 2012. p. 667–723.
15. Arias M, Aschheim P. Hypophysectomy and ageing: primary or secondary ovarian senescence. Experientia. 1974;30:213.
16. Moon HD, Simpson LE, Li CH, Evans HM. Neoplasms in rats treated with pituitary growth hormone III. Reproductive organs. Cancer Res. 1950;10:549–66.
17. Owen NV, Pierce EC, Anderson RC. Papillomatous growths on internal genitalia of bitches administered the synthetic estrogen trans-4,4′-dimethyl-′,-diethylstilbene. Toxicol Appl Pharmacol. 1972;21:582–5.
18. Gopinath C, Gibson WA. Mesovarian leiomyomas in the rat. Environ Health Perspect. 1987;73:107–13.
19. Long GG, Cohen IR, Gries CL, Young JK, Francis PC, Capen CC. Proliferative lesions of ovarian granulosa cells and reversible hormonal changes induced in rats by a selective estrogen receptor modulator. Toxicol Pathol. 2001;29:403–10.
20. Baskin GB, Smith SM, Marx PA. Endometrial hyperplasia, polyps, and adenomyosis associated with unopposed estrogen in rhesus monkeys (*Macaca mulatta*). Vet Pathol. 2002;39:572–5.
21. Anderson RK, Gilmore CE, Schnelle GB. Utero-ovarian disorders associated with use of medroxyprogesterone in dogs. J Am Vet Med Assoc. 1965;146:1311–6.
22. Nelson LW, Kelly WA. Progestogen-related gross and microscopic changes in female beagles. Vet Pathol. 1976;13:143–56.
23. Gopinath C. Comparative endocrine carcinogenesis. In: Harvey PW, Rush KC, Cockburn A, editors. Endocrine and hormonal toxicology. Chichester: Wiley; 1999. p. 156.
24. O'Shea JD, Jabara AG. Proliferative lesions of serous membranes in ovariectomised female and entire male dogs after stilboestrol administration. Vet Pathol. 1971;8:81–90.
25. Wadsworth PF, Heywood R, Allen DG, Sortwell RJ, Walton RM. Treatment of rhesus monkeys (*Macaca mulatta*) with intrauterine devices loaded with levonorgestrel. Contraception. 1979; 20:177–84.
26. Huseby RA, Thurlow S. Effects of prenatal exposure of mice to "low-dose" diethylstilbestrol and the development of adenomyosis associated with evidence of hyperprolactinemia. Am J Obstet Gynecol. 1982;144:939–49.
27. Mori T, Nagasawa H. Mechanisms of development of prolactin-induced adenomyosis in mice. Acta Anat (Basel). 1983;116: 46–54.
28. Losco PE, Leach MW, Sinha D, Davis P, Schmahai TJ, Nomier A, et al. Administration of an antagonist of neurokinin receptors 1, 2, and 3 results in reproductive tract changes in beagle dogs, but not rats. Toxicol Pathol. 2007;35:310–22.
29. Lipschutz A, Iglesias R, Panasevich VI, Salinas S. Pathological changes induced in the uterus of mice with prolonged administration of progesterone and 19-nor-contraceptives. Br J Cancer. 1967;21:160–5.
30. Annon. PERMAX (pergolide mesylate) prescribing information. Auckland: Eli Lilly; 2005.
31. Yoshida M, Katashima J, Ando T, Tanaka T, Uematsu F, Nakae D, et al. Dietary indole-3-carbinol promotes endometrial adenocarcinoma development in rats initiated with N-ethyl-N′-nitro-N-nitrosoguanidine, with induction of cytochrome P450s in the liver and consequent modulation of estrogen metabolism. Carcinogenesis. 2004;25:2257–64.
32. Gibson JP, Sells DM, Cheng HC, Yuk L. Induction of uterine leiomyomas in mice by medroxalol and prevention by propranolol. Toxicol Pathol. 1987;15:468–73.
33. Lewis DJ, Gopinath C. The female reproductive system. In: Turton J, Hooson J, editors. Target organ pathology. London: Taylor & Francis; 1998. p. 407.
34. Sells DM, Gibson JP. Carcinogenicity studies with medroxalol hydrochloride in rats and mice. Toxicol Pathol. 1987;15:457–67.
35. Rehm S, Solleveld HA, Portelli ST, Wier PJ. Histologic changes in ovary, uterus, vagina, and mammary gland of mature beagle dogs treated with the SERM idoxifene. Birth Defects Res B Dev Reprod Toxicol. 2007;80:225–32.
36. Wadsworth PF, Heywood R, Allen DG, Hossack DJ, Sortwell RJ, Walton RM. Treatment of rhesus monkeys (*Macaca mulatta*) with intravaginal rings impregnated with either progesterone or norethisterone. Contraception. 1979;20:339–51.
37. Wadsworth PF, Heywood R, Allen DG, Hossack DJ, Sortwell RJ, Walton RM. Treatment of rhesus monkeys (*Macaca mulatta*)

with intravaginal rings loaded with levonorgestrel. Contraception. 1979;20:559–67.

38. Eckstein P, Jackson MC, Millman N, Sobrero AJ. Comparison of vaginal tolerance tests of spermicidal preparations in rabbits and monkeys. J Reprod Fertil. 1969;20:85–93.

39. Cline JM, Wood CE. The mammary glands of macaques. Toxicol Pathol. 2008;36:130S–41.

40. Chandra SA, Mark CJ, Adler RR. Cyclic morphological changes in the beagle mammary gland. Toxicol Pathol. 2010;38: 969–83.

41. Heywood R, Wardsworth PF. The experimental toxicology of estrogens. In: Chaudhury RR, editor. Pharmacology of estrogens. International encyclopedia of pharmacology and therapeutics, Sect. 106. New York: Pergamon; 1981. p. 68.

42. Nelson LW, Weikel Jr JH, Leno FE. Mammary nodules in dogs during four years treatment with megestrol acetate of chlormadinone acetate. J Natl Cancer Inst. 1973;51:1303–11.

43. Horowski R, Graf KJ. Neuroendocrine effects of neuropsychotropic drugs and their possible influence on toxic reactions in animals and man. Arch Toxicol Suppl. 1979;2:93.

44. Graf KJ, Freidreich E, Matties S, Hassman SH. Homologous radioimmunoassay for canine prolactin and its application in various physiological states. J Endocrinol. 1977;75:93–103.

45. Gopinath C, Prentice DE, Lewis DJ. The reproductive system. In: Atlas of experimental toxicological pathology. Lancaster: MTP Press Ltd; 1987. p. 91–103.

# 8 The Endocrine System

Induced lesions affecting major endocrine glands are illustrated. This chapter is subdivided into lesions affecting the adrenal, thyroid, parathyroid, and pituitary glands and pancreatic islets. Interrelationships with other endocrine and nonendocrine organs are described. A few induced tumours of the endocrine glands are included, and their relative importance to human safety is discussed.

## 8.1 Introduction

Direct toxic effects are rare in most of the endocrine glands, the exception being the adrenal glands. The changes encountered are due mostly to the disturbance of feedback mechanisms of hormones. Diffuse endocrine cells distributed in nonendocrine tissues and those in the reproductive system are not included in this chapter. The older staining methods using various dyes have been replaced by immunohistochemistry for studying the pituitary, thyroid, and islet cells.

## 8.2 Adrenal Glands

Functionally, the adrenal medulla and cortex are two separate organs put together, the commonality being the blood supply. The adrenal glands are vulnerable to toxicity because of their relatively high blood supply; their high lipid content, which makes them liable to storage of lipophilic toxicants; free radical generation during steroid synthesis; their role in bioactivation; the presence of cytochrome P450 enzymes; and being a substrate for lipid peroxidation and changes due to hormonal feedback [1]. The toxic agents exert their effects directly or after metabolic activation. Many xenobiotics are metabolised by enzyme systems, and toxic radicals are produced locally. Toxicity by carbon tetrachloride, chloroform, and 1-(O-chlorophenyl)-1-(p-chlorophenyl)-2,2-dichloroethane (DDD) is through metabolic biotransformation. The induced lesions of the adrenal gland are summarised below:

- Cortex
  - Zona glomerulosa
  - Hypertrophy
  - Atrophy
  - Degeneration/necrosis
  - Z. fasciculata/reticularis
  - Hypertrophy
  - Atrophy
  - Vacuolation
  - Necrosis
  - Inflammation

C. Gopinath, V. Mowat, *Atlas of Toxicological Pathology*,
DOI 10.1007/978-1-62703-998-7_8, © Springer Science+Business Media New York 2014

- Inclusions
- Brown degeneration
- Cystic degeneration
- Hyperplasia
- Tumours
- Medulla
  - Vacuolation
  - Necrosis
  - Atrophy
  - Hyperplasia and tumours

## 8.2.1 Lesions of the Adrenal Cortex

The zona (z.) glomerulosa is the least affected zone in toxicity studies. Diuretics like furosemide cause hypertrophy; the affected cells appear larger, with pale cytoplasm. Sodium deficiency and potassium administration cause hypertrophy of the z. glomerulosa. Spironolactone antagonises aldosterone and results in hypertrophy of the cells along with formation of intracytoplasmic inclusions (spironolactone bodies) in patients and in some experimental animals [2]. In dogs, this produces multifocal enlargement and a convoluted appearance of the z. glomerulosa (Fig. 8.1). This is sometimes accompanied by hyperplasia in dogs (focal multilayering and crowding of nuclei) (Fig. 8.2). This change was seen in a dog study associated with polyuria (personal observation). Calcium channel blockers induce focal or diffuse hypertrophy in rats (Figs. 8.3 and 8.4). Prolactin has a trophic effect on the z. glomerulosa.

Increases in the Na/K ratio, sulphated mucopolysaccharides, timolol maleate, and captopril result in atrophy of the z. glomerulosa [3, 4]. Some of these agents suppress renin release, inhibit angiotensin-converting enzyme, and result in atrophy. Somatostatin also induces

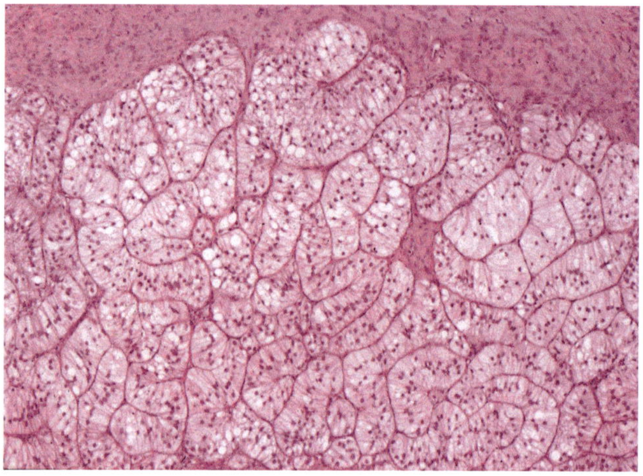

**Figure 8-1.** Focal hypertrophy, z. glomerulosa, in a dog treated with a diuretic. Note focal enlargement and convoluted appearance of cells in the z. glomerulosa. Haematoxylin and eosin (H&E) (With kind permission from Springer Science + Business Media B.V [39]).

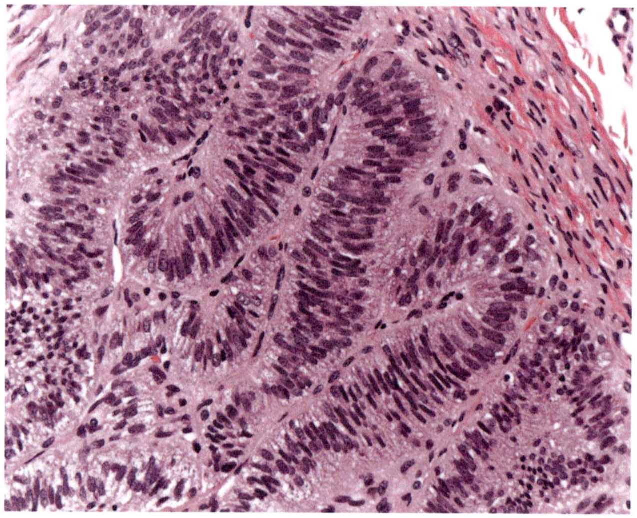

**Figure 8-2.** Hypertrophy/hyperplasia, z. glomerulosa, in a dog treated with a thyromimetic agent. Cells are more basophilic and reveal nuclear crowding. H&E.

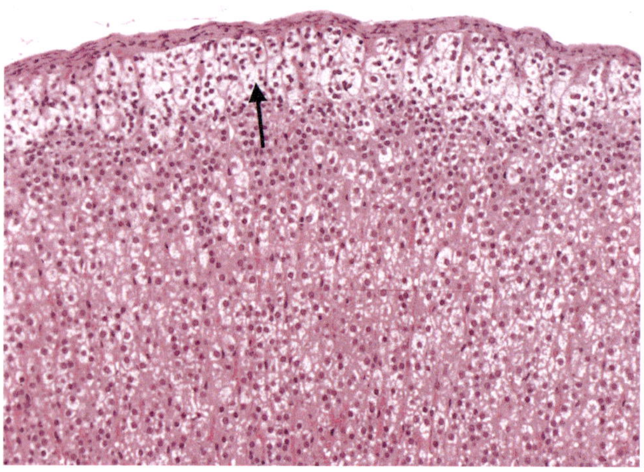

**Figure 8-3.** Diffuse hypertrophy (*arrow*), z. glomerulosa, in a rat treated with a calcium channel blocker. H&E.

atrophy and inhibits aldosterone. Hexadimethrine induces acute degeneration of the z. glomerulosa, mediated through histamine [5]. Administration of adrenocorticotropic hormone (ACTH) causes the cells of the z. glomerulosa to appear less distinct, possibly owing to hypertrophy or expansion of the z. fasciculata.

The z. fasciculata is the largest section of the adrenal cortex and is responsible for the production of corticosteroids or cortisol, depending on the species. Nonspecific stress causes increases in adrenal weight and hypertrophy of the z. fasciculata and reticularis in response to ACTH release (Fig. 8.5). Cortical width increases and cells appear less rarefied owing to decreased steroids or lipid, appearing more eosinophilic. Acute stress responses are driven by glucocorticoids and catecholamine. The responses provide glucose and maintain vascular reactivity. Soon corticoids damp down immunity and switch off stress responses by feedback mechanisms. Inhibitors of steroid synthesis and estrogens cause ACTH release and hypertrophy of the z. fasciculata and reticularis. Hypolipidaemic agents such as lovastatin cause hypertrophy of the z. fasciculata (Fig. 8.6). Adrenal weight is a sensitive indicator of hypertrophy.

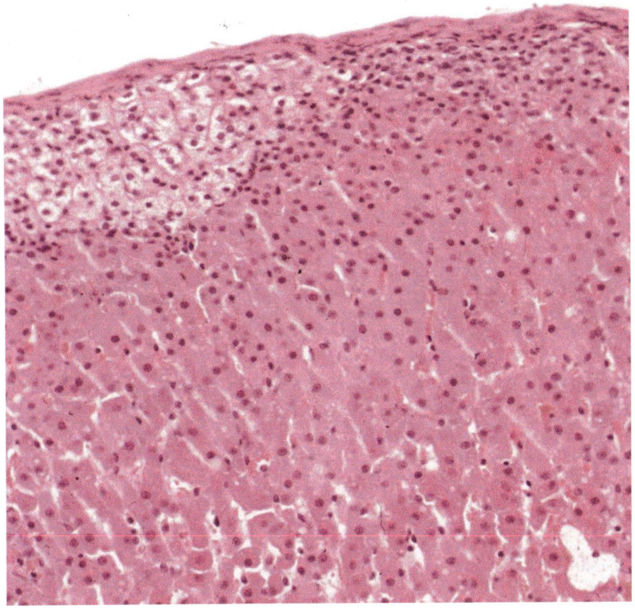

**Figure 8-4.** Focal hypertrophy, z. glomerulosa, in a rat. H&E.

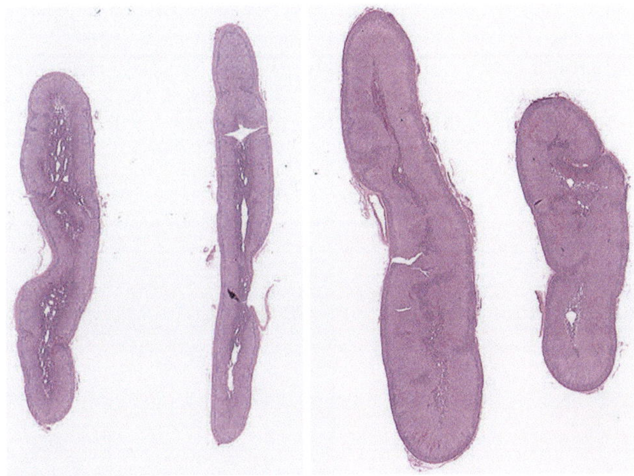

**Figure 8-5.** Cortical hypertrophy with an increase in cortical width in a rat. H&E.

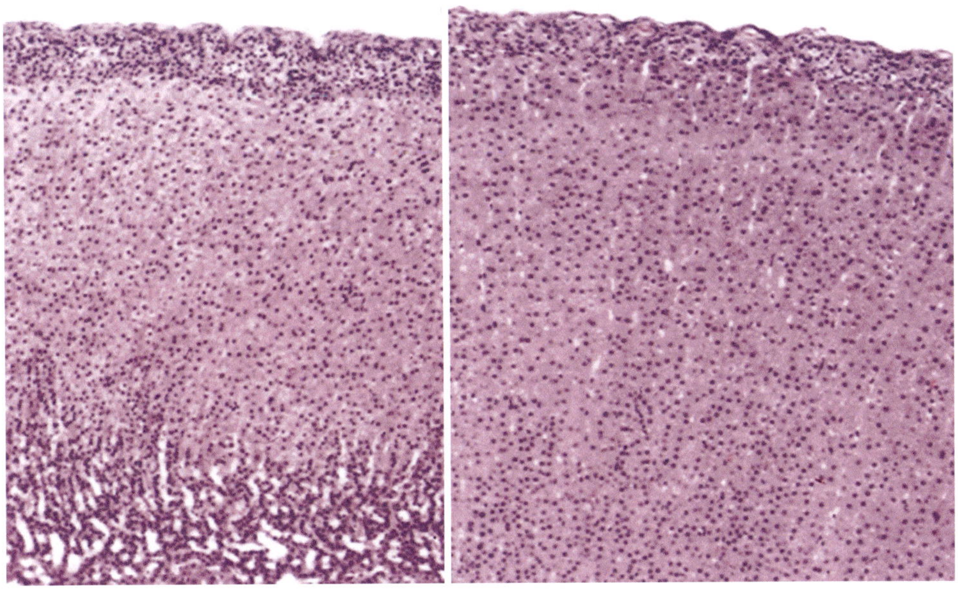

**Figure 8-6.** Cortical hypertrophy, mainly z. fasciculata, in a rat. Enlarged cells and increased width of z. fasciculata. H&E (With kind permission from Springer Science + Business Media B.V [39]).

Corticosteroids, on the other hand, inhibit ACTH and cause regression of the z. fasciculata, leading to atrophy. Cells of the z. fasciculata show apoptosis and loss. Hypophysectomy, glucocorticoids, and progestogens result in adrenal cortical atrophy in treated animals (Figs. 8.7 and 8.8) [6, 7]. Pigment-laden macrophages appear in the atrophic zone. Withdrawal of treatment or administration of ACTH leads to remarkable recovery.

Carbon tetrachloride causes necrosis in the inner zone of the z. fasciculata. This effect is mediated by cytochrome P450 enzymes, which are in greater concentration in the cells of the inner cortex. Acrylonitrile, cysteamine, pyrazole, thioacetamide, and dimethylbenzanthracene are among the necrogenic agents [8, 9]. Hexadimethrine induces infarct-like lesions in the z. fasciculata (Fig. 8.9) [10]. Haemorrhagic necrosis of the adrenal cortex is occasionally seen (Fig. 8.10). Retrograde embolism by medullary cells is thought to cause this type of necrosis. Vitamin B deficiency also causes haemorrhagic necrosis in rats. Bilateral total cortical necrosis is fatal in experimental animals (Fig. 8.11).

Vacuolar degeneration of the z. fasciculata is a common toxic response to a number of xenobiotics. It must be understood that steroids are abundant in normal cortical cells, but neutral fat is an indication of degeneration. Aminoglutethimide inhibits steroidogenesis and results in lipidosis [2]. Chloroform, carbon tetrachloride, and methanol cause fatty vacuolation of the z. fasciculata. The vacuolation can be focal or diffuse, can occur in the inner or outer zone, or can appear scattered in the zone (Figs. 8.12–8.15). O,P'DDD (2,2-bis(2-chlorophenyl-4-chlorophenyl)-1,1-dichloroethane) produces marked diffuse vacuolar degeneration (Fig. 8.16) [10, 11]. Antimycotic agents such as ketoconazole and clotrimazole cause lipidosis in rats and dogs [12]. Vacuolar degeneration coexists with lipid-laden macrophages. In prolonged treatment, a multifocal lipoid hyperplasia ensues. A unique distribution of lipidosis is characterised by the

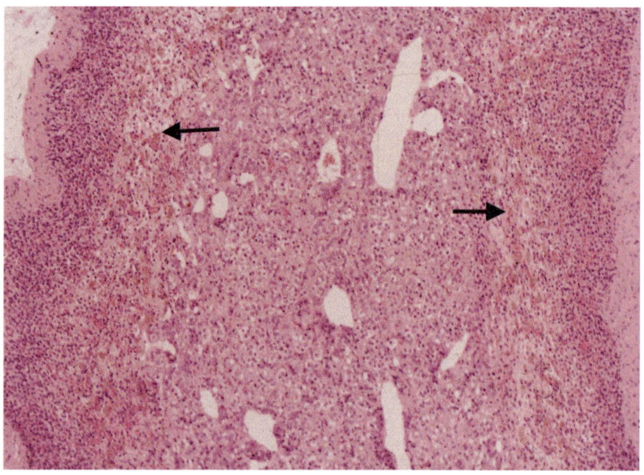

**FIGURE 8-7.** Cortical atrophy, mainly z. fasciculata (*arrows*), in a rat treated with a corticosteroid. Reduced cortical width. H&E.

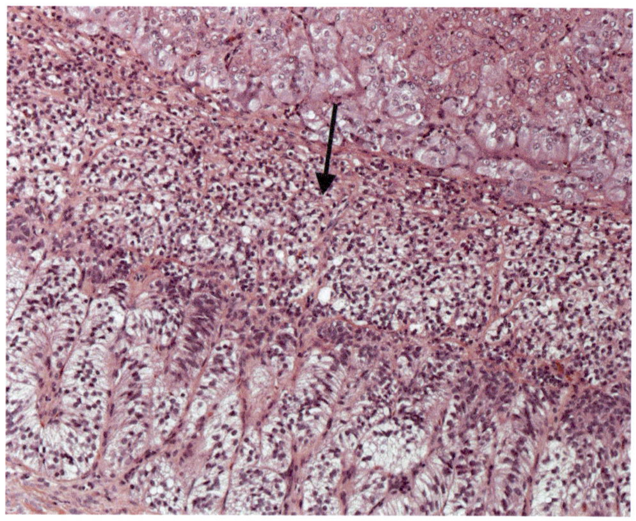

**FIGURE 8-8.** Cortical atrophy, z. fasciculata (*arrow*), in a dog treated with a corticosteroid. H&E.

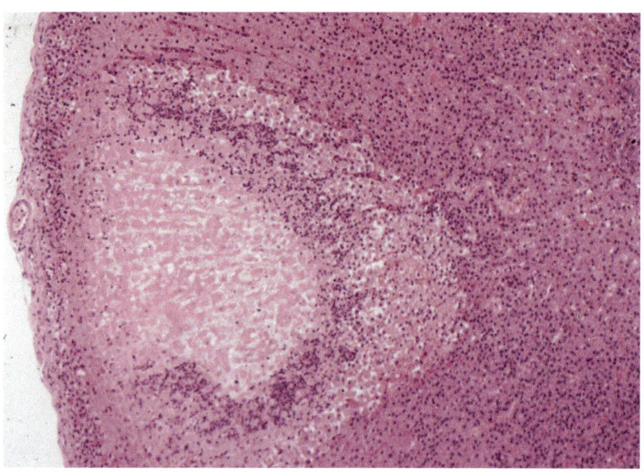

**FIGURE 8-9.** A wedge-shaped area of cortical necrosis in a rat. H&E (With kind permission from Springer Science+Business Media B.V [39]).

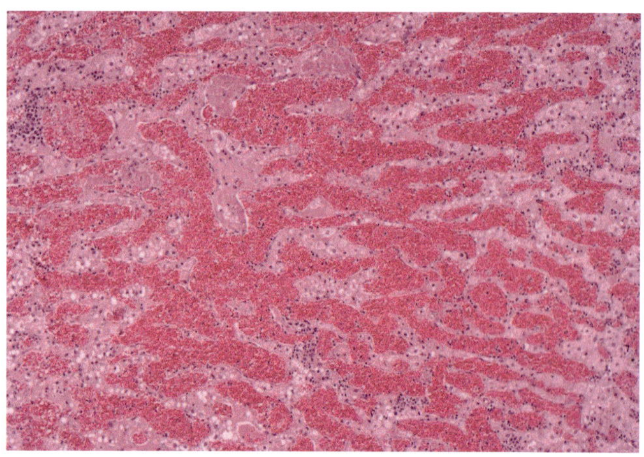

**FIGURE 8-10.** Diffuse cortical necrosis with marked congestion in a rat. H&E.

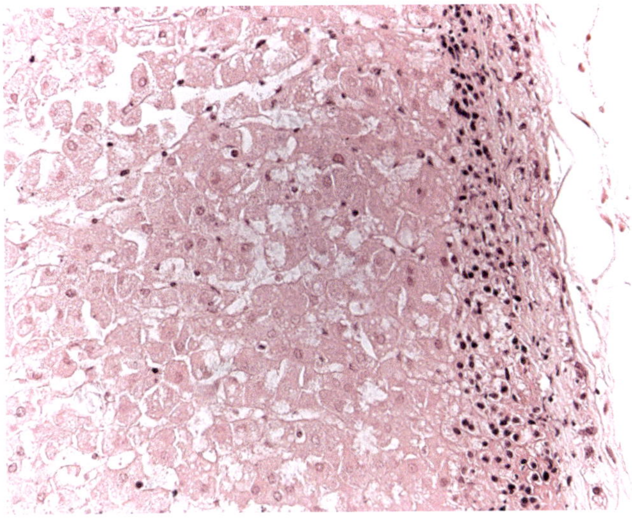

**Figure 8-11.** Diffuse necrosis, z. fasciculata, in a rat. H&E.

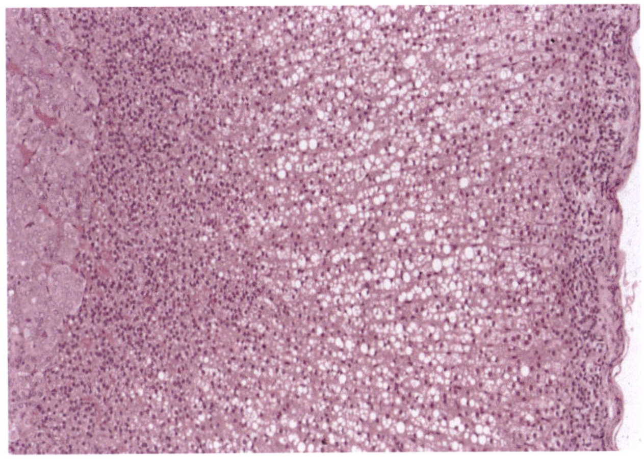

**Figure 8-12.** Cortical vacuolation, z. fasciculata, in a rat. H&E.

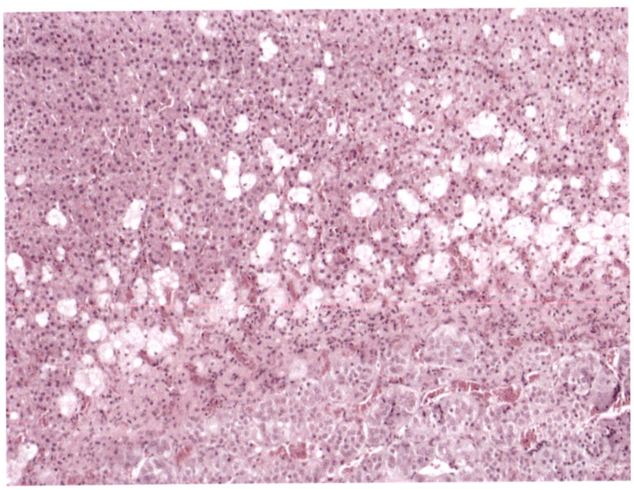

**Figure 8-13.** Vacuolation in the inner adrenal cortex in a rat. H&E.

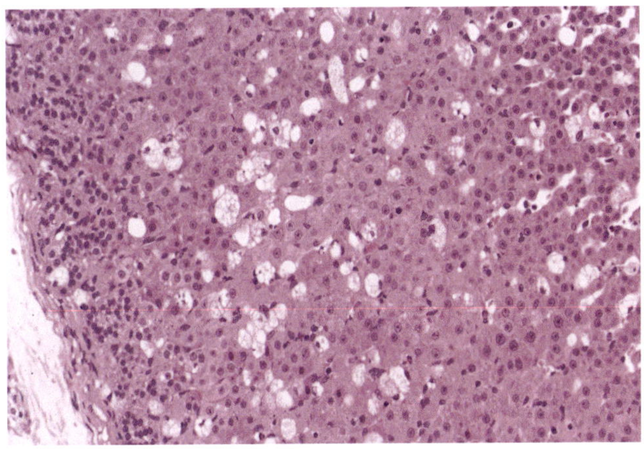

**Figure 8-14.** Vacuolation of scattered cells, z. fasciculata, in a rat. H&E.

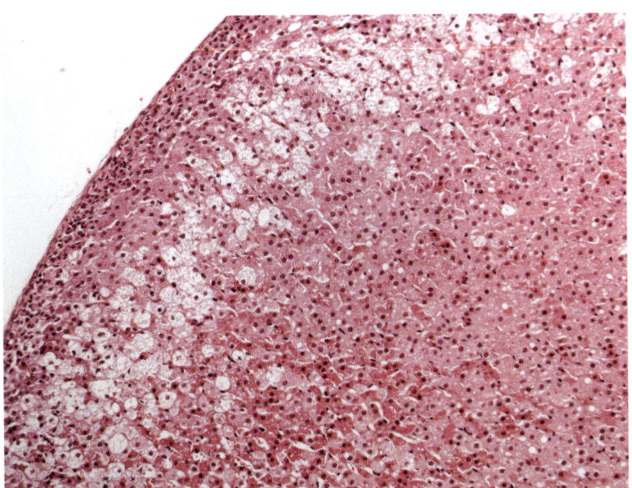

**Figure 8-15.** Vacuolation in the outer adrenal cortex in a rat. H&E.

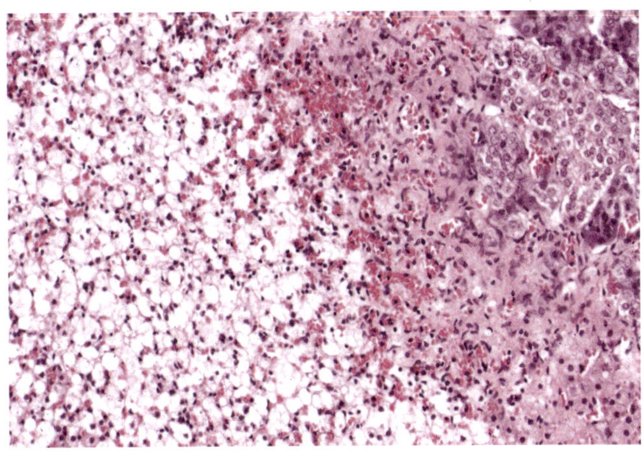

**Figure 8-16.** Marked diffuse vacuolation in a dog treated with an industrial chemical. H&E (With kind permission from Springer Science + Business Media B.V [39]).

presence of a band of vacuolated degenerative or necrotic cells in the z. fasciculata, with the remaining cells unaffected other than by minimal hypertrophy. This change is produced by a certain antimycotic agent when given to primates (personal observation) (Figs. 8.17 and 8.18).

Haemorrhagic cystic degeneration is a spontaneous change in ageing female rats. The change can be exacerbated in rats by treatment with estrogens (Fig. 8.19). In brown degeneration, pigmented macrophages appear in the adrenal cortex, usually in association with cellular degeneration. Synthetic estrogens, propylthiouracil, and ketoconazole cause deposition of ceroid pigment in the adrenal cortex. Intracytoplasmic eosinophilic inclusions are noted in cortical cells during starvation and in treatment with aminoglutethimide, agrochemicals, and some steroids (Fig. 8.20). Pigmentation was seen in the outer cortex of the adrenals of rats treated with an iron-chelating agent (Fig. 8.21).

Focal inflammation of the adrenal cortex has been reported in monkeys treated with synthetic thyroid hormones (Figs. 8.22 and 8.23) [13]. The inflammatory cell foci are associated with single-cell necrosis. The lesion is thought to result from a hypersensitivity response. Sinusoidal cell vacuolation was noted in monkeys treated with an antineoplastic agent.

Focal cortical hyperplasia is produced by prolonged treatment with necrogenic agents, as a regenerative response in rats (Fig. 8.24). Lipoid hyperplasia is produced by inhibitors of steroid synthesis, including agents such as aminoglutethimide, aniline, and amphinone [14].

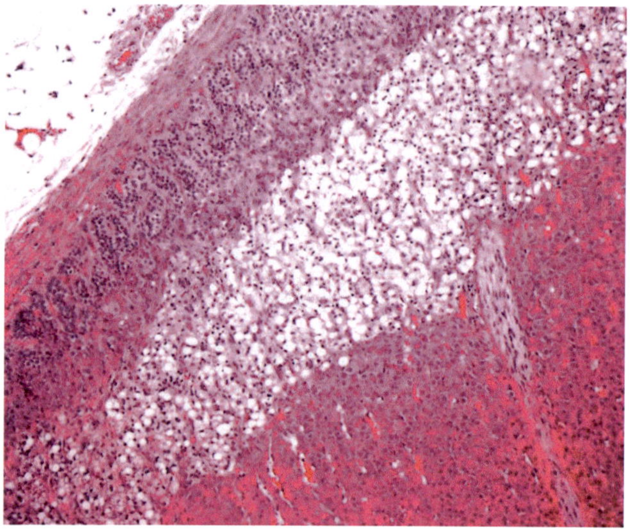

**Figure 8-17.** A central band of vacuolar degeneration, z. fasciculata, in a monkey treated with an antifungal agent. H&E.

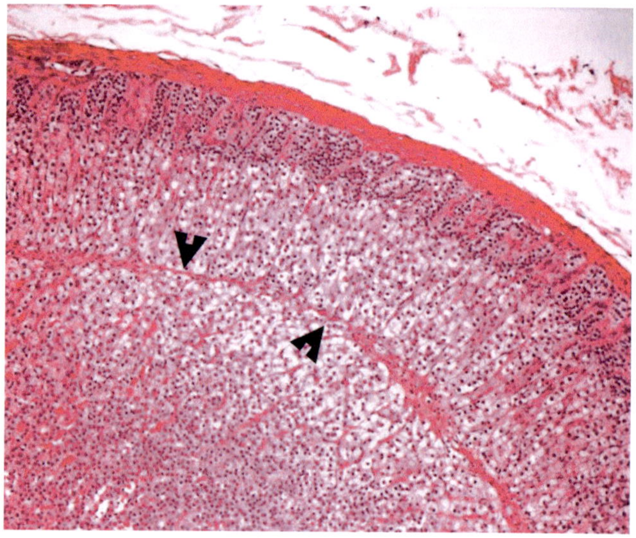

**Figure 8-18.** A thin cortical band of fibrosis (*arrowheads*) in the z. fasciculata of a monkey. H&E.

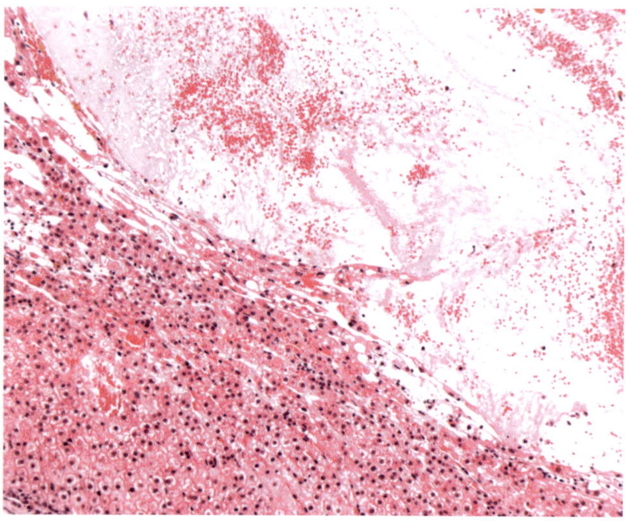

**Figure 8-19.** Cystic degeneration of the cortex in a rat. Large cystic area with loss of cells and haemorrhage. H&E.

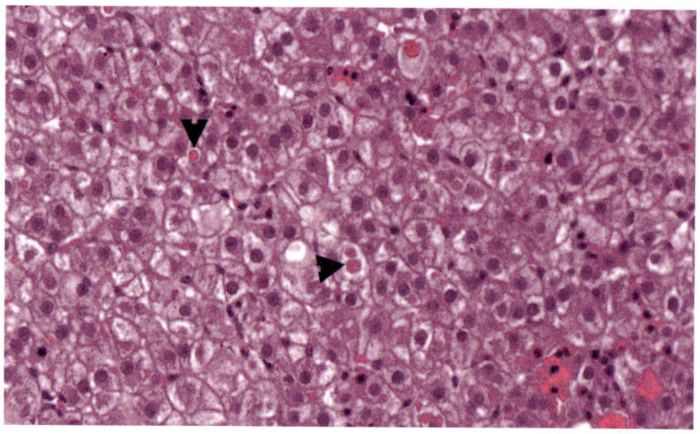

**Figure 8-20.** Intracytoplasmic eosinophilic inclusions (*arrowheads*) in adrenal cortical cells of a rat treated with an agrochemical agent. H&E (With kind permission from Springer Science + Business Media B.V [39]).

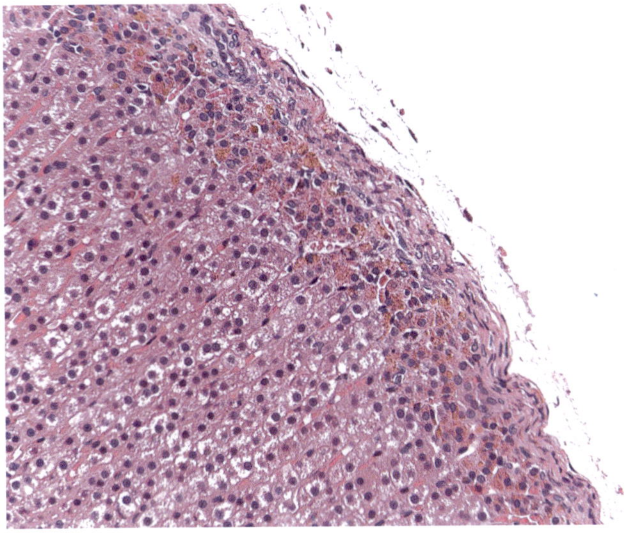

**Figure 8-21.** Pigmentation of the adrenal cortex in a rat treated with an iron-chelating agent. H&E.

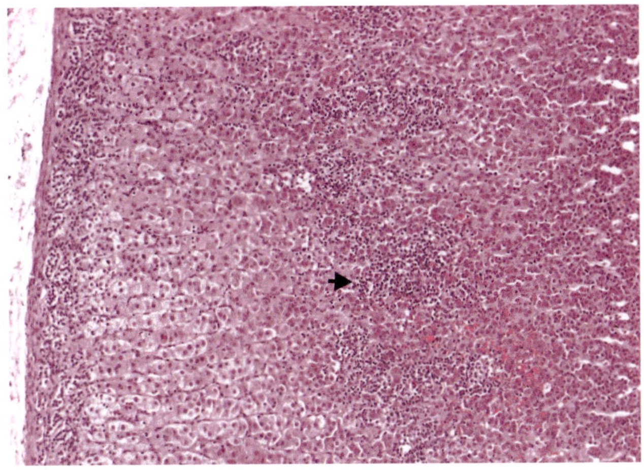

**Figure 8-22.** Focal inflammation of the adrenal cortex (*arrowhead*) in a monkey treated with a synthetic hormone. H&E.

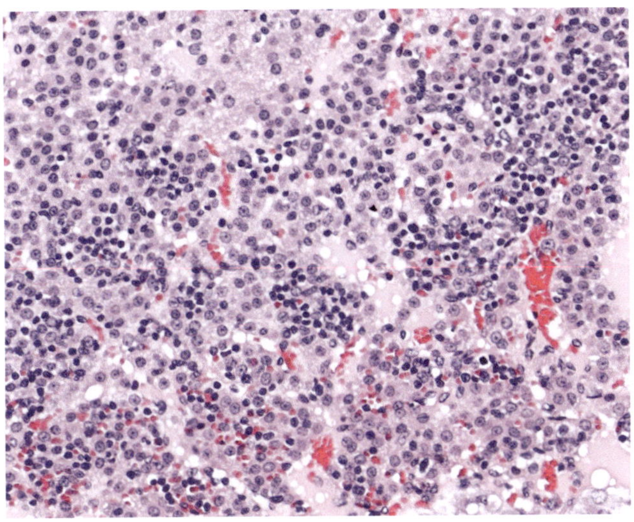

**Figure 8-23.** Focal lymphoid inflammation of the adrenal cortex of a rat treated with a novel pharmaceutical agent. H&E.

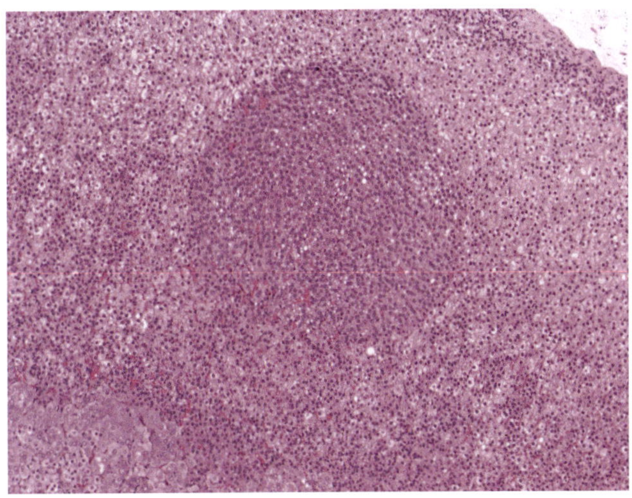

**Figure 8-24.** Focal hyperplasia of the adrenal cortex in a rat. The hyperplastic cells are basophilic and small. H&E.

Treatment with estrogens, urethane, erythropoietin, or aflatoxin resulted in focal hyperplasia and cortical tumours in rodents during carcinogenicity studies (Figs. 8.25–8.28).

## 8.2.2 Lesions of the Adrenal Medulla

Cysteamine hydrochloride, acrylonitrile, and pyrazole produce focal necrosis in the medulla [10]. Necrosis is associated with loss of cells and inflammation. Fibrosis and atrophy follow necrotic lesions (Figs. 8.29 and 8.30). Intracytoplasmic eosinophilic inclusions are seen in monkeys treated with polychlorinated biphenyls. Vacuolation of medullary cells has been reported in monkeys treated with a novel anticancer agent. Triparanol induces phospholipidosis in the medullary cells.

A wide variety of agents, such as nicotine, synthetic retinoids, thiouracil, growth hormone, beta blockers, analgesics, neuroleptics, and a number of sugar alcohols, induce focal hyperplasia of chromocytes in rats and mice [10, 15–17]. The hyperplastic cells appear more basophilic, with vesicular nuclei; on occasions, the cells are smaller (Figs. 8.31 and 8.32). Calcium homeostasis is implicated in the development of proliferative lesions of the adrenal medulla in rodents given high

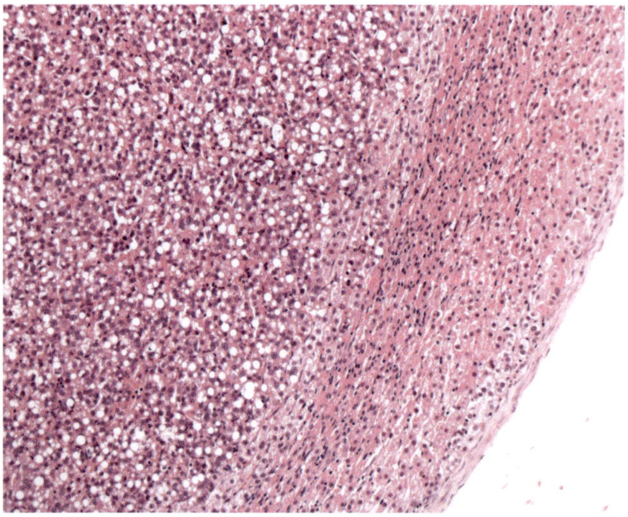

**FIGURE 8-25** Cortical adenoma in a rat. The large, expansive lesion is causing compression in the cortex. H&E.

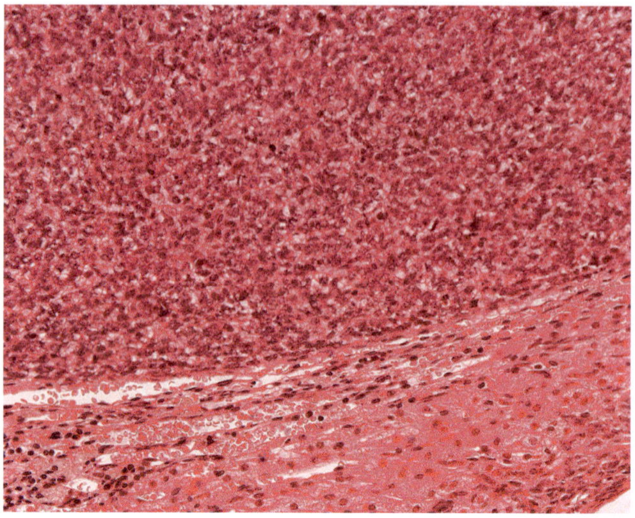

**FIGURE 8-26.** Cortical adenoma of the adrenal gland in a mouse. Fusiform basophilic cells are causing compression. H&E.

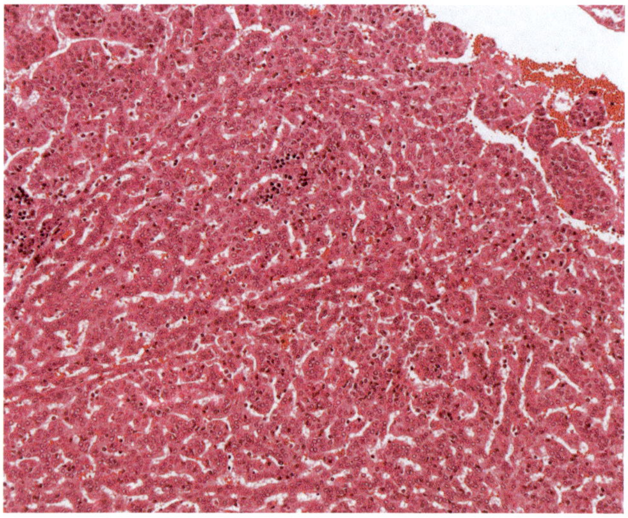

**FIGURE 8-27.** Cortical carcinoma of the adrenal gland in a mouse. Neoplastic cortical cells are arranged in irregular multicellular chords or in a trabecular pattern. H&E.

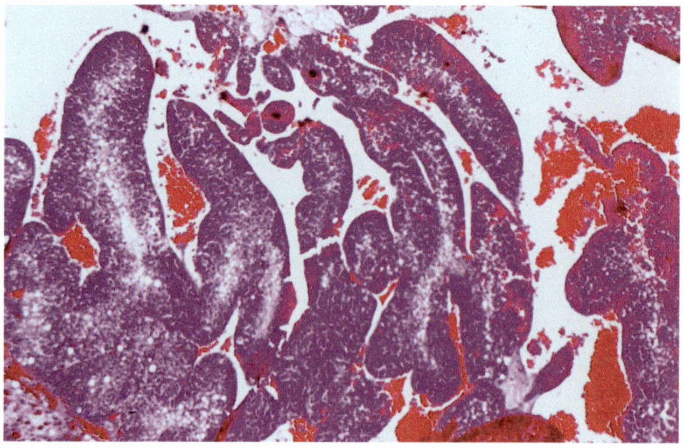

**FIGURE 8-28.** Cortical carcinoma of the adrenal gland in a rat. H&E.

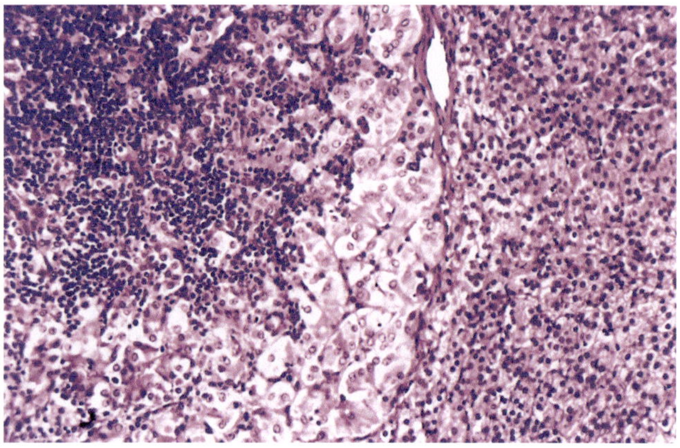

**FIGURE 8-29.** Medullary necrosis and inflammation in a dog treated with a novel pharmaceutical. H&E.

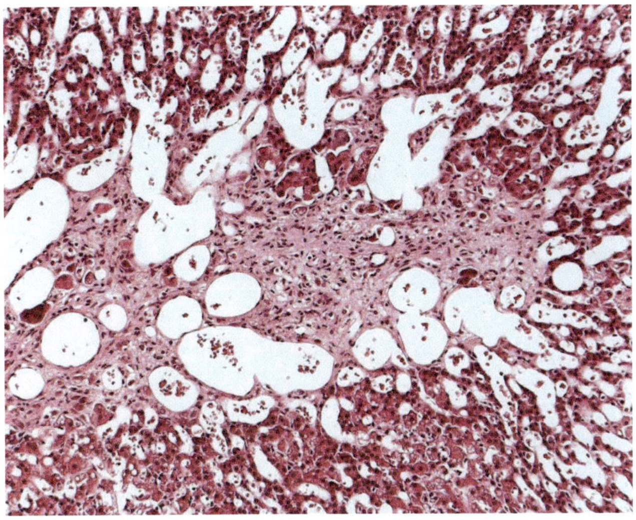

**Figure 8-30.** Medullary atrophy (loss of chromocytes) and fibrosis in a rat treated with a novel pharmaceutical. H&E.

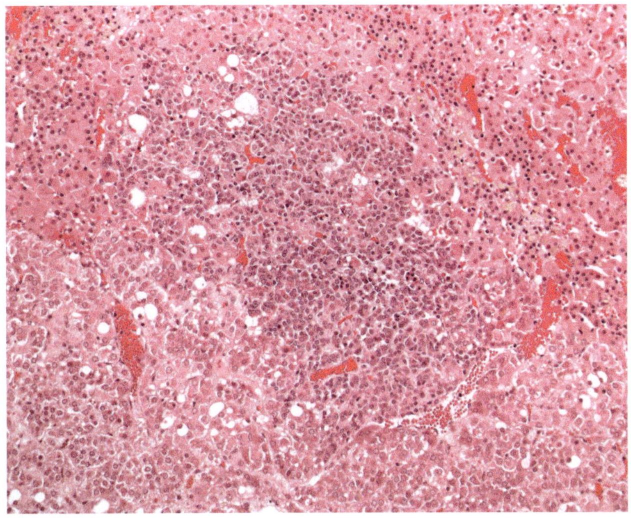

**Figure 8-31.** Medullary hyperplasia in a rat. The hyperplastic cells are small and basophilic. H&E.

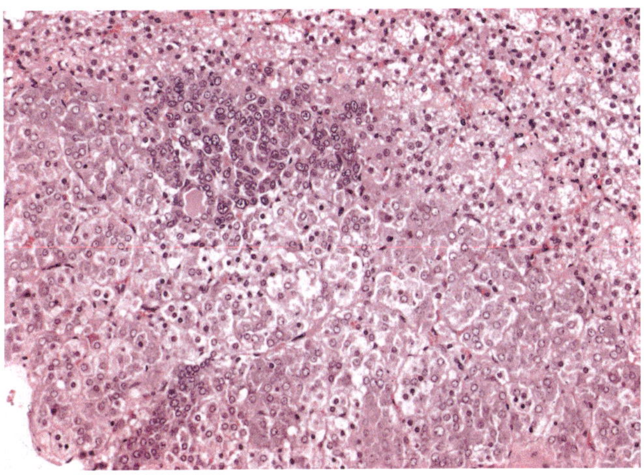

**Figure 8-32.** Focal medullary hyperplasia (a group of basophilic cells) in a rat. H&E (With kind permission from Springer Science + Business Media B.V [39]).

doses of sugar alcohols [15]. In xylitol toxicity, inhibition of catecholamines is suggested as one of the causative mechanisms. Stimulation of the autonomic nervous system and hormonal imbalances are also suggested as causative factors in the production of medullary hyperplasia in rodents. Agents that produce hyperplasia tend to produce tumours in the rodent adrenal medulla. Benign medullary tumours (phaeochromocytomas) in rodents are nonfunctional, even though they stain positive for catecholamines. The tumour cells are arranged in small nests or clusters, with prominent basement membranes surrounding the nests (Figs. 8.33– 8.35). Rats are highly sensitive to growth stimuli: in vitro responses of chromocytes to growth factors have shown rats to be more sensitive than mice, dogs, or humans [18].

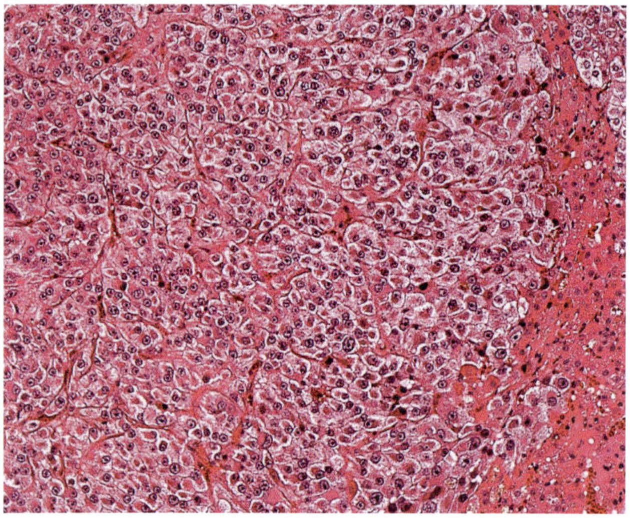

**Figure 8-33.** Phaeochromocytoma of a large-cell type in a rat. Aggregates of chromocytes with abundant cytoplasm are arranged as clumps surrounded by fine strands of connective tissue, causing compression. H&E.

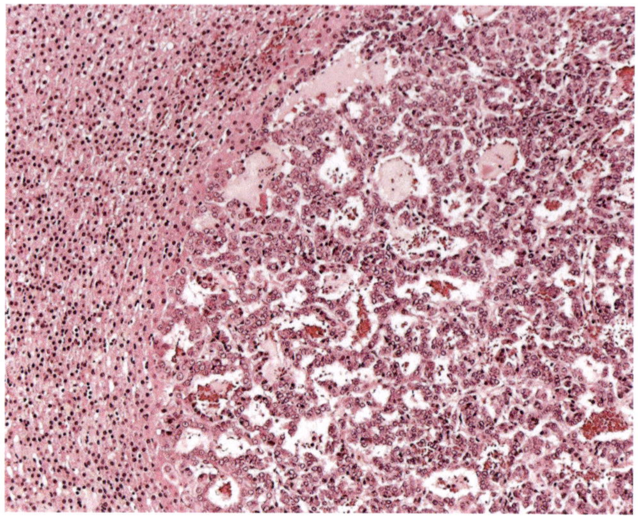

**Figure 8-34.** Phaeochromocytoma (small-cell type) in a rat. H&E.

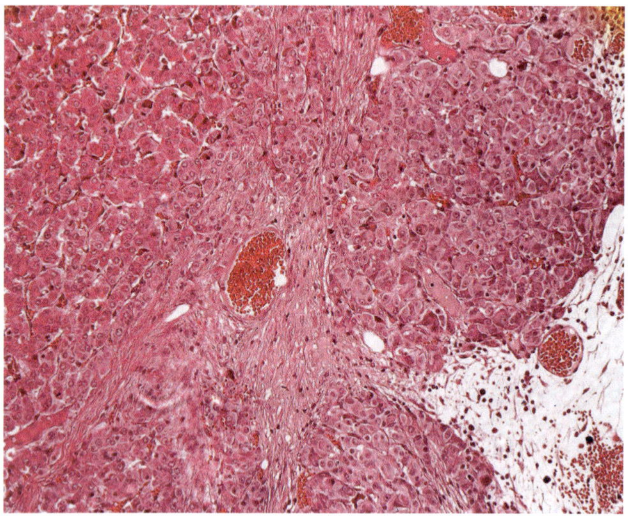

**Figure 8-35.** Malignant phaeochromocytoma in a rat, with evidence of local invasion. H&E.

## 8.3 Thyroid Gland

The thyroid is probably the most commonly affected endocrine gland in toxicity studies. In most cases, the changes noticed in the thyroid gland are hormonally based, and the range of changes is quite small, as given below:

- Induced changes in the thyroid gland
  - Follicular hypertrophy/ hyperplasia
  - Follicular atrophy
  - Follicular pigmentation
  - Chronic thyroiditis
  - Follicular tumours
  - C-cell hyperplasia and tumours

### 8.3.1 Induced Changes in the Thyroid Gland

Age and iodine content in the diet influence follicular morphology. In young rats, the follicular epithelium is comparatively taller; in old rats, the follicle is lined by flat, thin epithelium, and the follicles are more distended with colloid (Figs. 8.36–8.38). Antithyroid agents (goitrogens) induce follicular cell hypertrophy and hyperplasia. Reduction of thyroid hormones (T4 and T3) results in increased secretion of thyroid-stimulating hormone

(TSH), which is trophic to follicular epithelium. Goitrogens like aminotriazole, ethylene nitrosourea, thionamides, propylthiouracil, and lithium act directly on the follicular epithelium, interfering with hormone production at different biochemical loci [19–22]. Iodine deficiency and excess iodine also inhibit hormone production. Iodine transport and incorporation, peroxidation, formation of iodothyronines, synthesis of thyroglobulin, or the release of thyroid hormone are among the various steps that different agents may interfere with. Although the biochemical steps of action vary with different agents, the net results are reduced thyroid hormone levels and consequent TSH release. The morphological effects are TSH-dependent hypertrophy and hyperplasia of follicular cells, especially in rats. Rat follicles are extremely sensitive to TSH. Mice, dogs, and primates also respond, but to higher doses. The stimulated thyroids become larger, with increased weight. Follicles show reduced lumen and colloid and are lined with larger and taller cells (Fig. 8.39). In cases of marked follicular hypertrophy, the whole gland appears more solid because of the reduction of colloid and the increased size of follicular cells. On light microscopy, only hypertrophy is detectable in the early stages, but underlying hyperplasia is evident on morphometric or DNA analysis. If the stimulation is continued over a longer period, the follicular epithelium reveals hyperplasia, evidenced by follicular infolding and nuclear crowding (Figs. 8.40 and

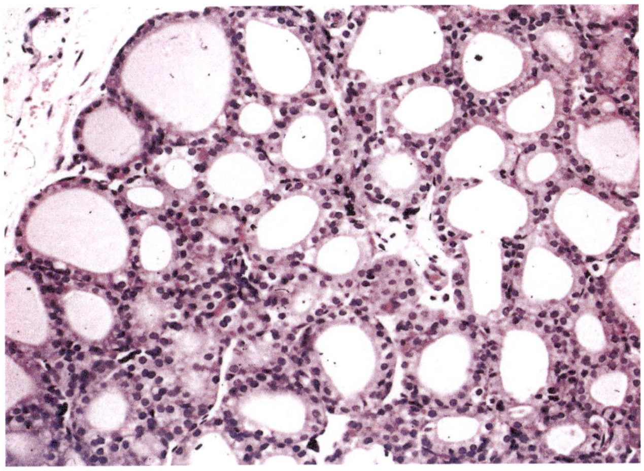

**Figure 8-36.** Normal thyroid in an 8-week-old rat. The epithelium is reasonably tall. H&E.

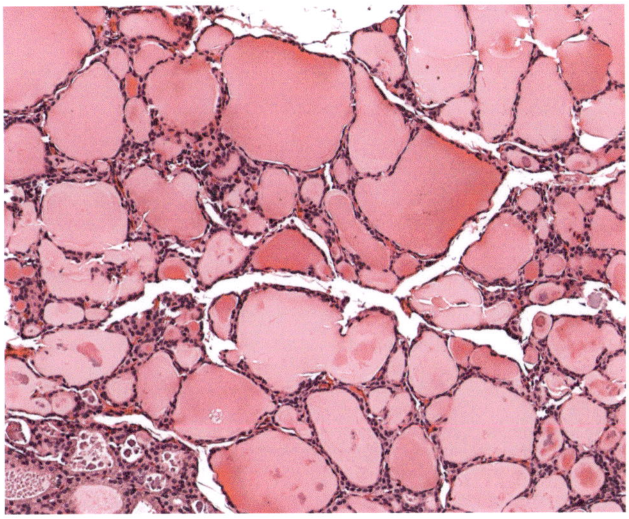

**Figure 8-37.** Normal thyroid in a 70-week-old rat. Follicles are lined with thin epithelium and some colloid concretions. H&E.

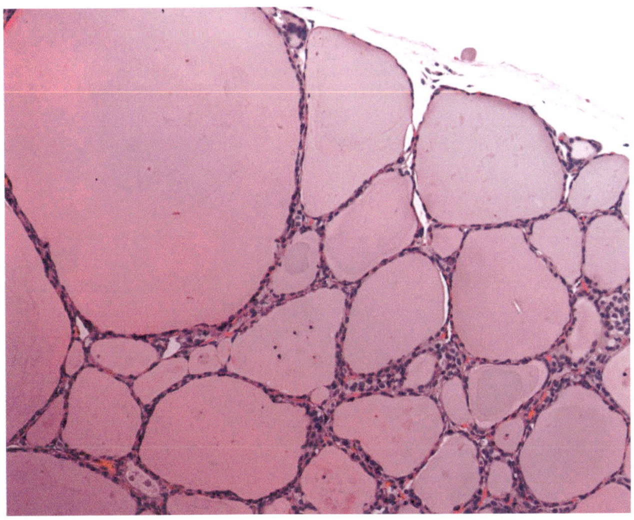

**Figure 8-38.** Normal thyroid in a 100-week-old rat. The peripheral follicles are distended and lined by flat or thin cells. H&E.

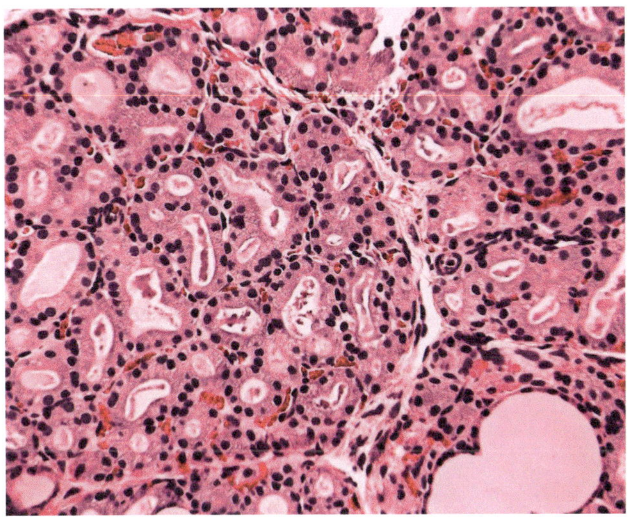

**Figure 8-39.** Follicular hypertrophy/hyperplasia in a rat treated with a goitrogenic chemical. The epithelium is tall, with reduced colloid and reduced follicular lumina. H&E.

8.41). The infolding becomes clearer with prolonged dosing. During long-term studies, the hyperplasia becomes focal and appears as focal follicular cysts and cystic follicular hyperplasia (Figs. 8.42 and 8.43). These foci of cystic follicles show increased basophilia of the lining cells and show papillary ingrowths. As the process is a continuum, it is difficult to clearly differentiate these lesions from early adenomas. In chronic studies where hypertrophy or hyperplasia persists, the colloid shows fragmentation, condensation, concretions, and sometimes mineralisation, as is seen in aged rodents. The hypertrophy and hyperplasia caused by many agents in short-term studies tend to progress into follicular tumours during long-term studies, especially in rats. The sensitivity of the rat is a major factor.

A number of agents cause thyroid follicular changes indirectly by increasing the elimination of thyroid hormones (T4 and T3) through bile. In rats, 50 % of thyroxine is eliminated through bile. Inducers of hepatic microsomal enzymes, such as phenobarbitone sodium or polychlorinated biphenyls, result in increased thyroxine uptake by hepatocytes, glucuronic acid conjugation, and elimination through bile [23]. Hypolipidaemic agents also cause similar effects [24]. T4 glucuronidation is pivotal but T3 glucuronidation is also very significant. Other agents with similar effects include cimetidine and some calcium channel blockers. The mechanisms by which different agents act on the thyroid are varied and complex [25, 26].

Another class of agents inhibits enzymes required for peripheral conversion of T3 from thyroxine. The result is a decrease in circulating T3, which triggers TSH release and consequent follicular stimulation. FD&C Red, amiodarone, erythromycin, and some radiocontrast agents cause follicular proliferation in rats through this mechanism.

Thyroid function tests help in understanding the underlying mechanisms of thyroid toxicities. These tests include measurement of circulatory hormones (T4, T3,

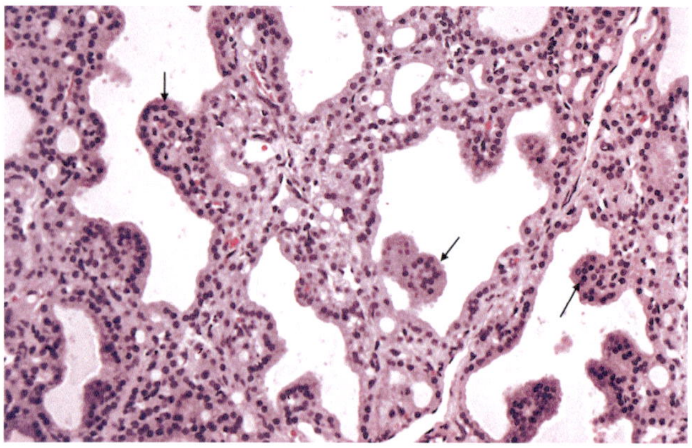

**FIGURE 8-40.** Follicular hyperplasia, thyroid, in a dog treated with a sulfonamide. Follicles reveal epithelial folding and hypertrophy (*arrows*). H&E (With kind permission from Springer Science+Business Media B.V [39]).

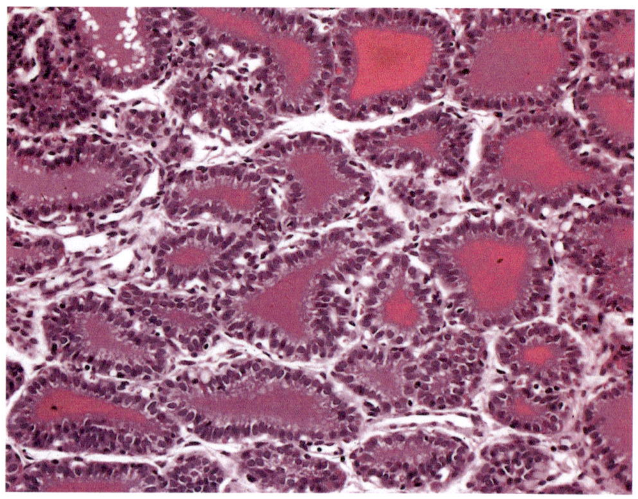

**FIGURE 8-41.** Follicular hyperplasia, thyroid, in a monkey treated with an industrial chemical. The epithelium is basophilic, with an increase in the number of tall cells. H&E.

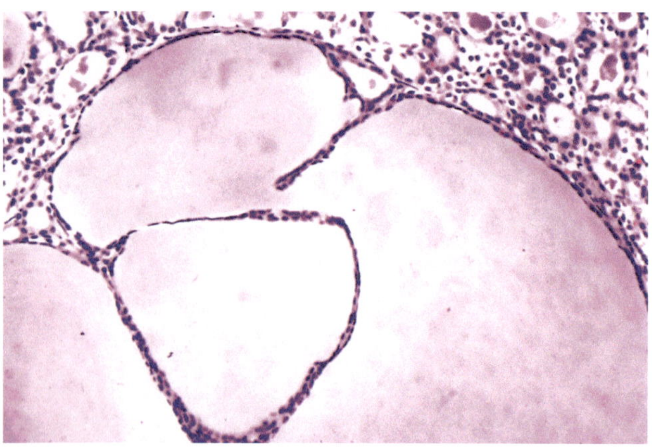

**FIGURE 8-42.** Cystic follicles, thyroid, in a rat. A focus of dilated follicles. H&E.

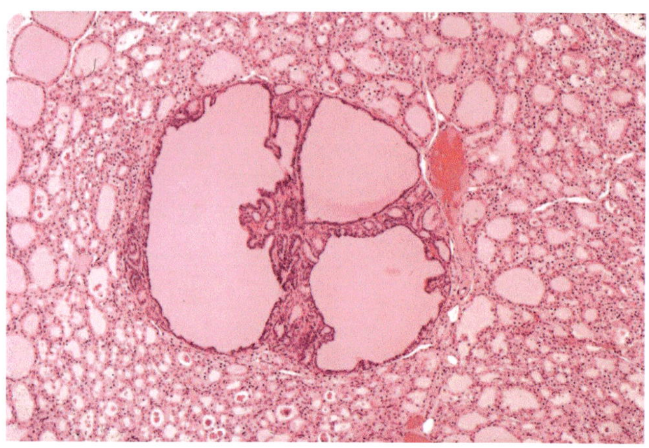

**FIGURE 8-43.** Cystic follicular hyperplasia in a rat. The cystic lesion consists of follicles of different sizes with basophilic epithelium. H&E.

rT3, and TSH), uptake of iodine by the thyroid, the perchlorate discharge test, clearance of $^{125}$I -T4, clearance of $^{125}$I- T3, biliary excretion of $^{125}$I -T4, and measurements of hepatic drug-metabolising enzymes. Irradiation and methylnitrosourea produce thyroid tumours by genotoxic mechanisms.

TSH-mediated stimulation frequently produces follicular tumours in the rat because of its species-specific exaggerated sensitivity (Figs. 8.44 and 8.45). These tumours are TSH dependent and regress on removal of trophic stimulation. Thyroid tumours produced in rats are not considered to be relevant to human safety because of the species-specific sensitivity of rat follicular epithelium. Many mechanisms that produce rat tumours do not operate in humans [27]. Furthermore, the threshold concept is applied for safe doses of nongenotoxic agents [27]. Epidemiologically, barbiturates and sulfonamides have been in human use for scores of years with no evidence of any thyroid effects. Some of the established species differences between rats and humans are summarised in Table 8.1.

Follicular atrophy is induced in monkeys treated with synthetic thyroid hormones (Fig. 8.46). Thyroid weight is reduced; microscopically, there is loss of follicles, follicular collapse, and atrophy of epithelium. Hypophysectomy induces follicular atrophy in rats (Fig. 8.47). Administration of a thyromimetic agent to dogs also resulted in follicular atrophy (Fig. 8.48). Gossypol is known to cause focal atrophy.

Pigmentation (brown to black) is seen in the follicular epithelium of laboratory animals treated with minocycline, vincamine alkaloids, or certain hair dyes or with

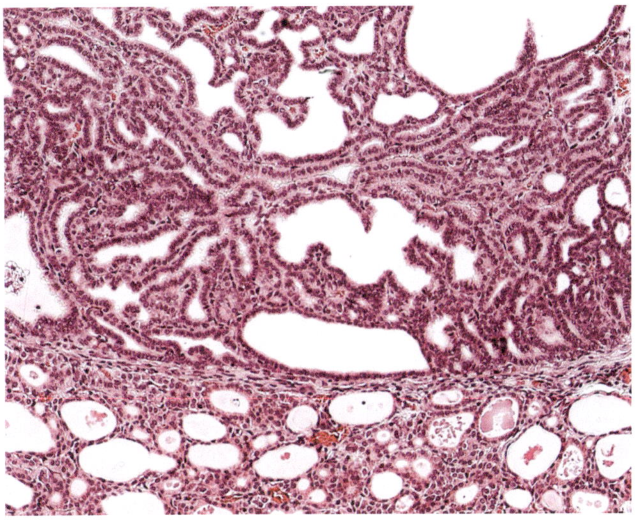

**Figure 8-44.** Follicular adenoma in a rat. Neoplastic follicles are basophilic and cause compression. H&E.

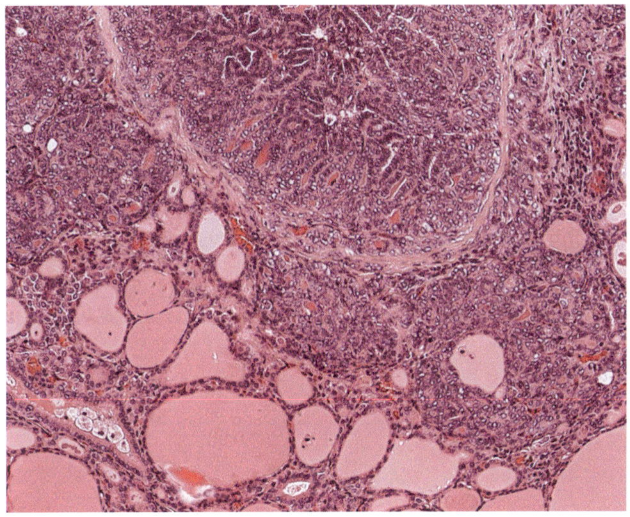

**Figure 8-45.** Follicular carcinoma in a rat. Neoplastic follicles appear in differing patterns, with evidence of local invasion. H&E.

**Table 8-1.** Species differences between rats and humans in thyroid hormones

| | Rat | Human |
|---|---|---|
| Biliary excretion of T4 (%) | 50 | 10–15 |
| TBG | Absent | ++ |
| Half-life of T4 (days) | >1 | 5–9 |
| Half-life of T3 (h) | 6 | 24 |
| TSH levels | Low | High |
| TRH response | Weak | Strong |

*TBG* thyroxine-binding globulin, *TRH* thyrotropin-releasing hormone, *TSH* thyroid-stimulating hormone

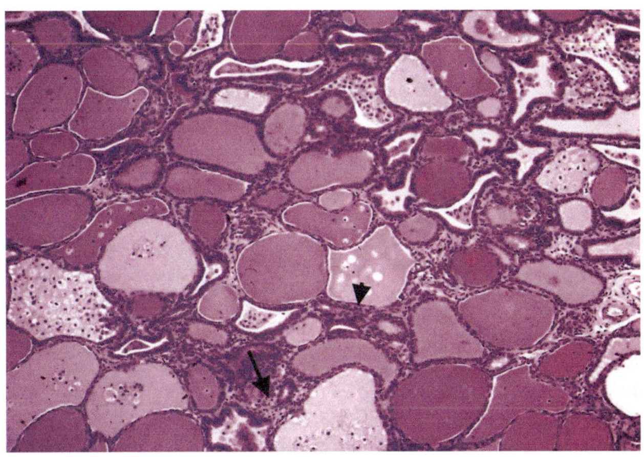

**Figure 8-46.** Follicular atrophy of the thyroid in a monkey treated with synthetic thyroid hormone. The follicular epithelium is flat, with focal collapse (*arrow*). H&E.

vitamin E deficiency (Fig. 8.49) [28]. In minocycline treatment, the pigment has similarities with melanin. Vincamine and minocycline produce accompanying follicular hypertrophy and hyperplasia in rodents. Pigments appear intracytoplasmically in follicular cells, and in severe cases the pigment is seen in the colloid and interstitial macrophages (Figs. 8.50 and 8.51). Clozapine produces brown pigmentation of follicular cells in rats but not in mice or dogs. Macroscopically, minocycline treatment makes the thyroid gland appear black.

Chronic thyroiditis is induced in mice, rats, and monkeys with trypan blue, methylcholanthrene, and 3, methyl-4-dimethylaminobenzene (Fig. 8.52). Frentizole causes thyroiditis in rats if treatment starts during immaturity. Certain synthetic estrogenic agents cause squamous metaplasia of follicles in dogs [29].

Follicular epithelial vacuolation is discernible in cases of phospholipidosis (Fig. 8.53). Epithelial vacuolation can also be seen spontaneously in rats.

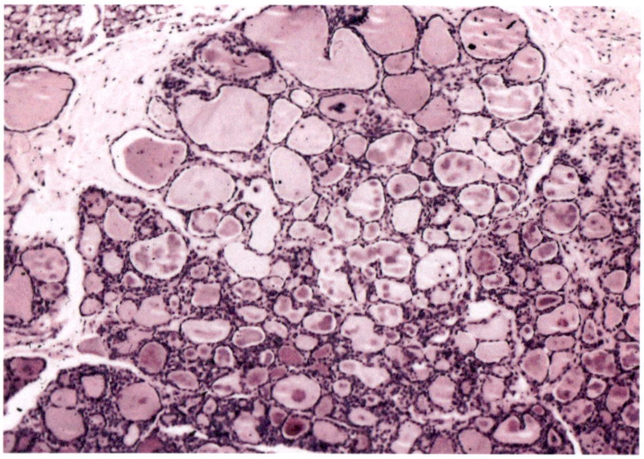

**Figure 8-47.** Follicular atrophy in a rat after hypophysectomy. Follicles lined by flat/thin cells, colloid distension. H&E.

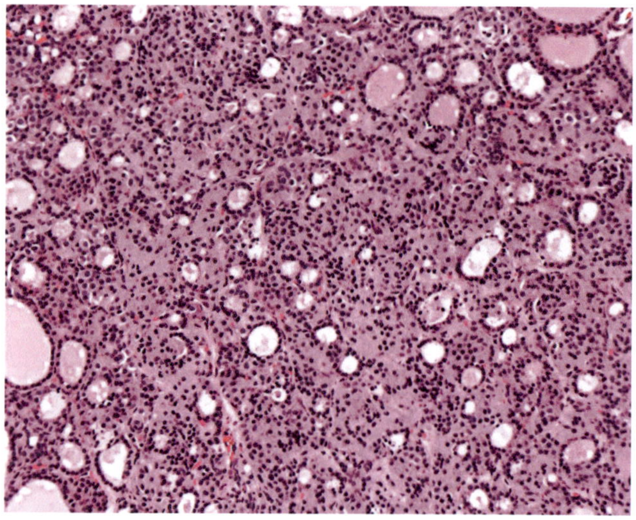

**Figure 8-48.** Follicular atrophy of the thyroid in a dog treated with a thyromimetic agent, showing collapse and loss of follicles. H&E.

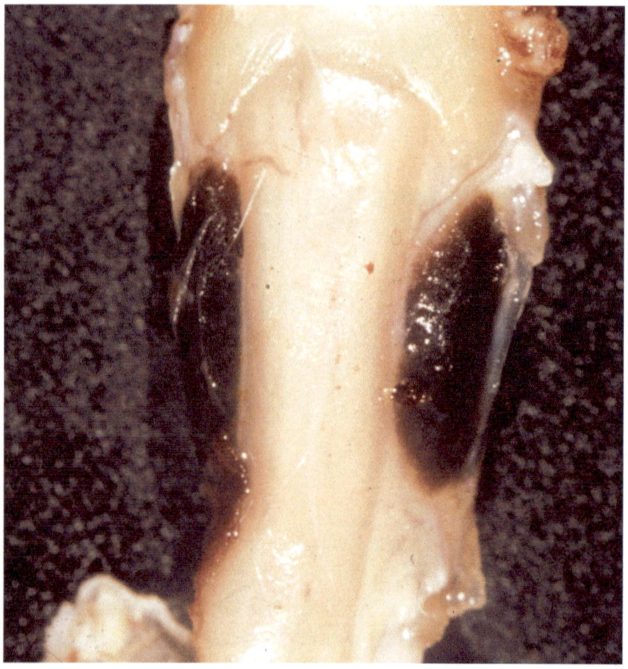

**Figure 8-49.** Dark thyroid in a rat treated with an antibiotic. The thyroid is enlarged and *dark brown* in colour.

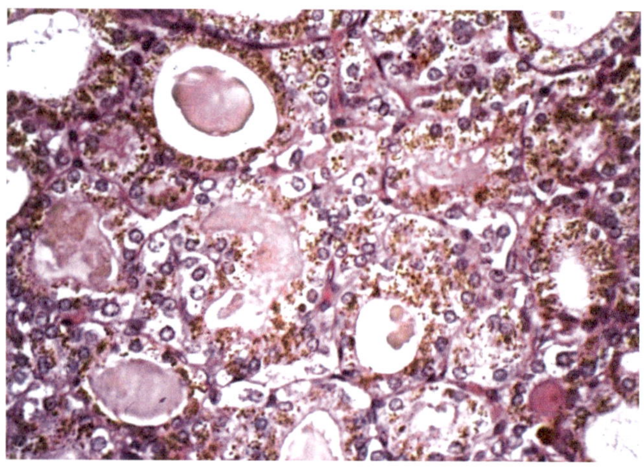

**Figure 8-50.** Pigmentation of the follicular cells of the thyroid in a rat treated with an antibiotic. Brown granular pigment is seen in follicular cells, colloid, and interstitium. H&E.

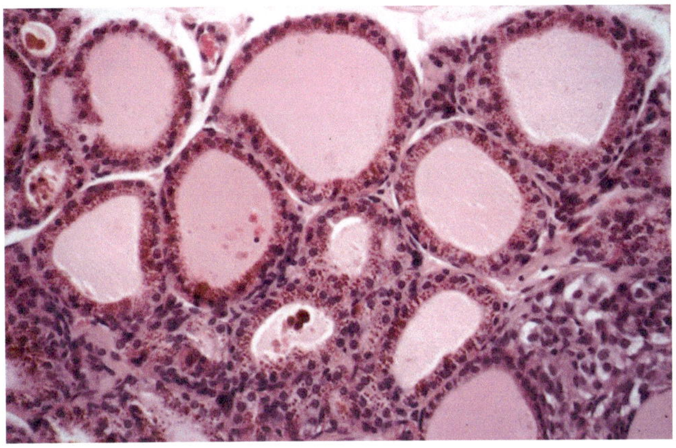

**Figure 8-51.** Pigmentation of follicular cells of the thyroid in a rat treated with a vincamine alkaloid. H&E (With kind permission from Springer Science + Business Media B.V [39]).

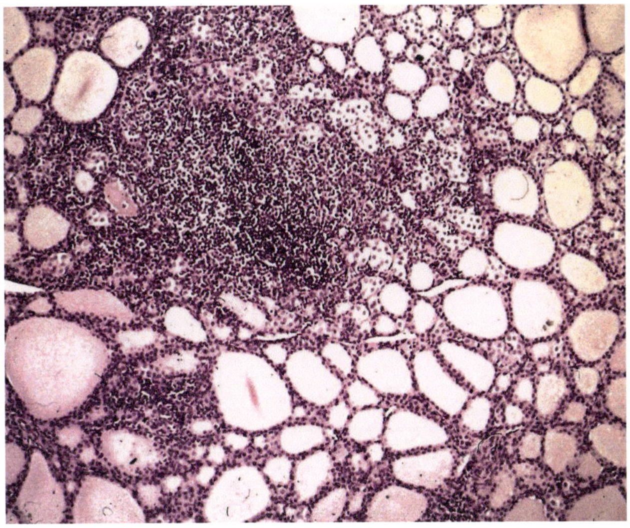

**Figure 8-52.** Lymphocytic thyroiditis in a rat, showing lymphocytic infiltration and aggregates and focal follicular cell hypertrophy. H&E.

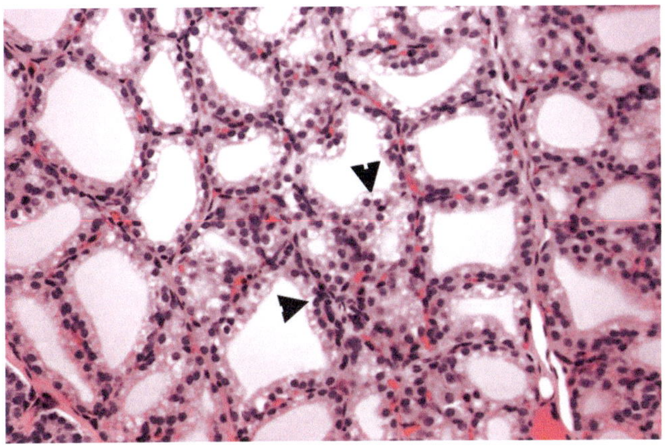

**Figure 8-53.** Follicular epithelial vacuolation (*arrow*) suggesting phospholipidosis in a rat. H&E.

C-cell hyperplasia is seen in rats as an age-related spontaneous change and may be focal or diffuse (Figs. 8.54–8.56). Immunohistochemical staining for calcitonin is useful to identify and quantify early proliferative changes of C cells in rodents. In young beagle dogs, C-cell aggregates are often present in the hilar region normally and should not be confused with hyperplasia (Fig. 8.57). C-cell tumours are common spontaneous age-related findings in rats but are rare in untreated mice (Figs. 8.58 and 8.59). High doses of vitamin D in the diet can cause hyperplasia of C cells. More recently, some antidiabetic agents such as glucagon-like peptide receptor agonists have produced hyperplasia and tumours of C cells in rats and mice (Figs. 8.60 and 8.61) [30, 31].

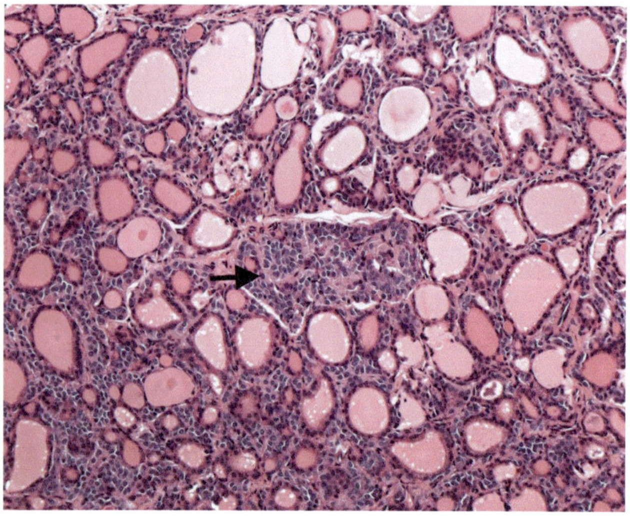

**Figure 8-54.** C-cell hyperplasia, focal (*arrow*), in a rat. H&E.

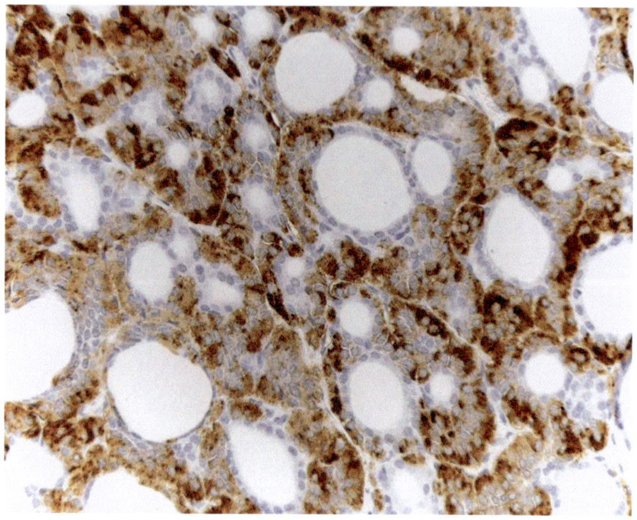

**Figure 8-55.** C-cell hyperplasia in a rat treated with a glucagon-like peptide (GLP) receptor agonist. Calcitonin, immunohistochemistry.

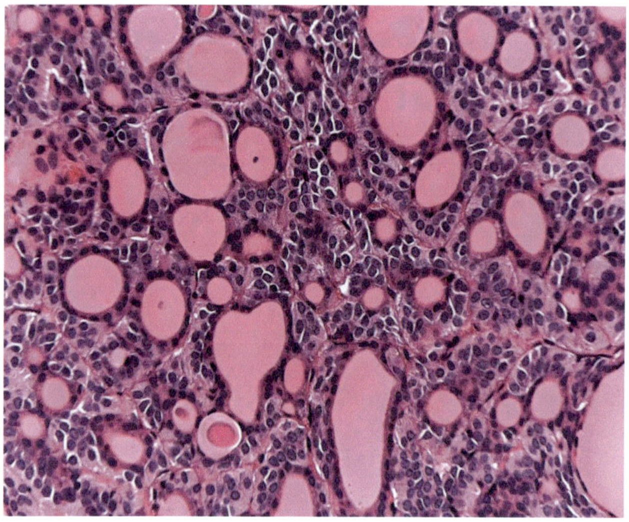

**Figure 8-56.** C-cell hyperplasia, diffuse, in a rat. H&E.

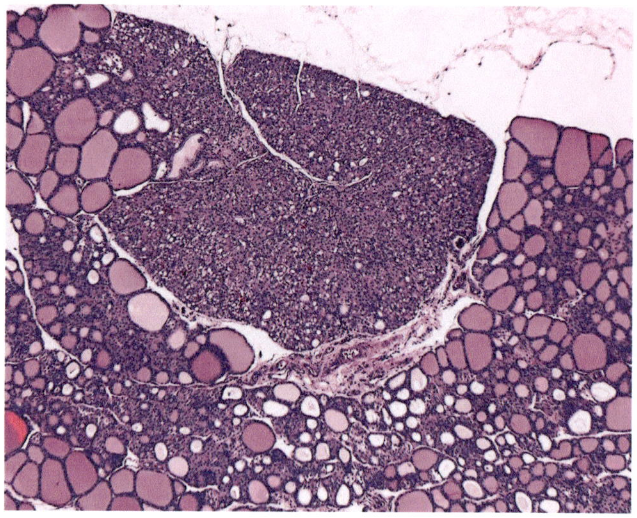

**Figure 8-57.** C-cell area, thyroid hilus, in a dog. H&E.

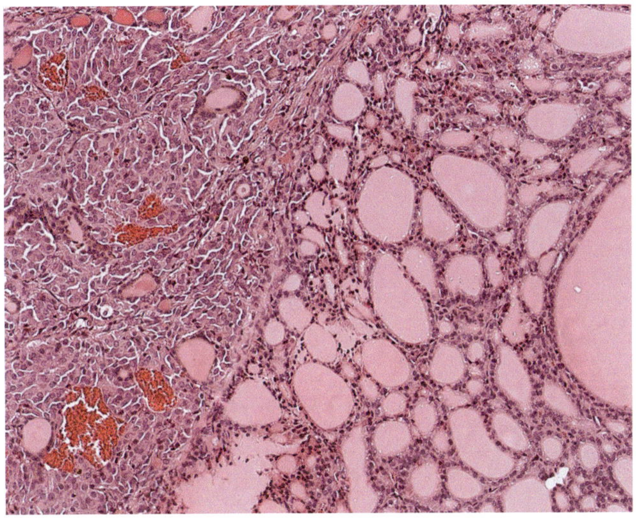

**FIGURE 8-58.** C-cell adenoma in a rat. H&E

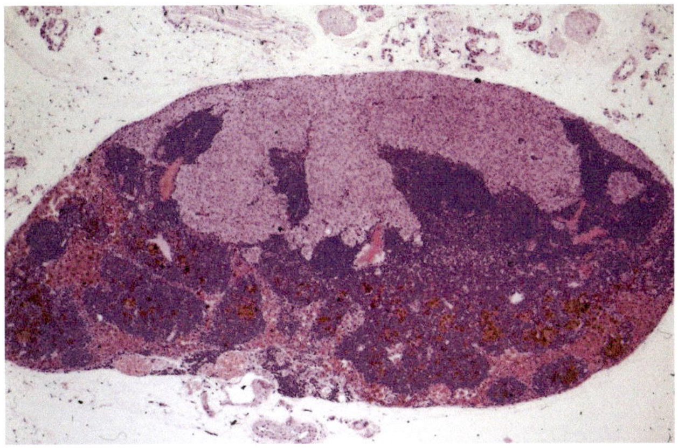

**FIGURE 8-59.** C-cell carcinoma, lymph node metastasis, in a rat. H&E

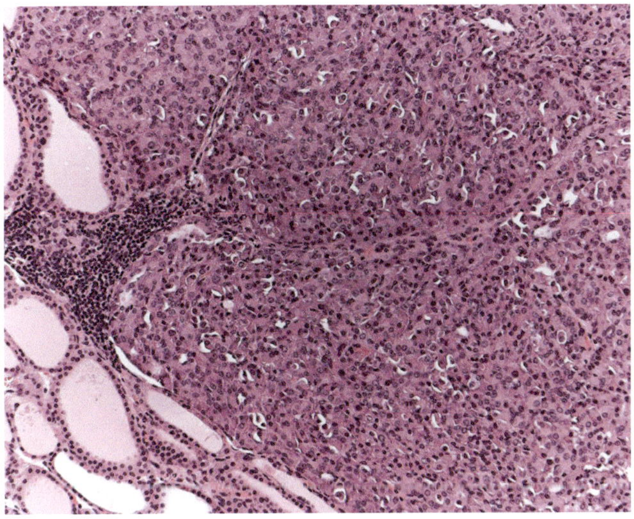

**FIGURE 8-60.** C-cell adenoma in a mouse treated with a GLP receptor agonist. H&E.

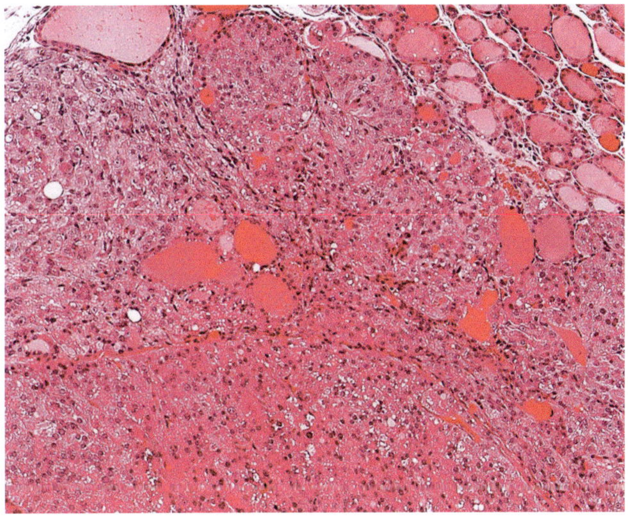

**FIGURE 8-61.** C-cell carcinoma in a mouse treated with a GLP receptor agonist. H&E.

## 8.4 Parathyroid Gland

Only a small number of changes are encountered in parathyroids during toxicity studies:

- Hyperplasia
- Atrophy/degeneration
- Parathyroiditis

Secondary parathyroid hyperplasia is seen in repeat-dose studies, with chronic nephrotoxicity as an endpoint (Figs. 8.62 and 8.63). Low calcium in the diet can result in hyperplasia of chief cells. Calcium homeostasis is linked with trophic/inhibitory effects on the chief cells. In rabbits, L-asparaginase results in apoptosis, degeneration, and loss of chief cells. Parathyroiditis is induced in dogs and rabbits exposed to ozone. The parathyroid shows lymphocytic infiltration, vasculitis, and haemorrhage. The change is suggested to be immune mediated. Hypercalcaemic conditions result in atrophy of chief cells. The pesticide rotenone increased the incidence of parathyroid adenomas during carcinogenicity studies in Fischer 344 rats.

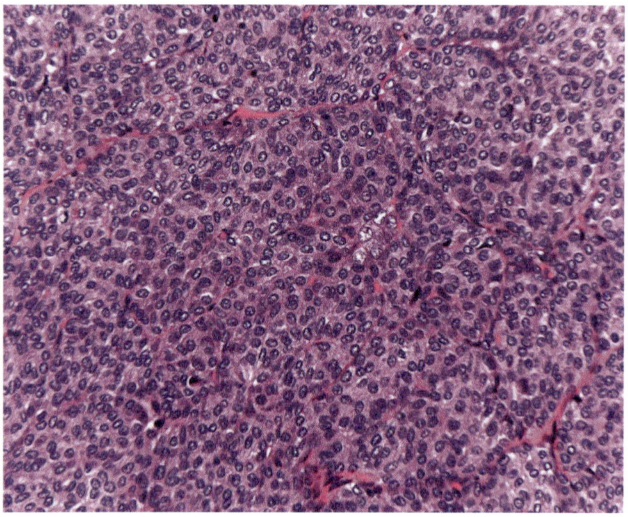

**FIGURE 8-62.** Diffuse hyperplasia of the parathyroid in a rat. H&E.

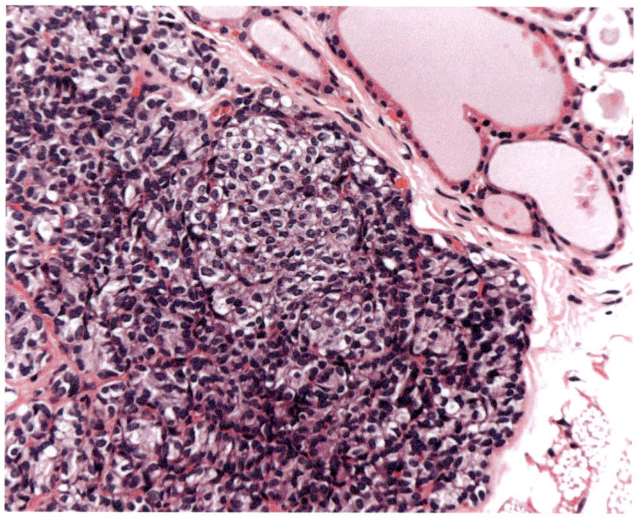

**FIGURE 8-63.** Focal hyperplasia of the parathyroid in a rat. H&E.

## 8.5 Pancreatic Islets

Pancreatic islets consist mainly of insulin-producing beta cells. Glucagon is produced by alpha cells located peripherally. A small number of delta cells are also located peripherally, producing somatostatin. Pancreatic polypeptide-containing cells are also encountered in small numbers. Toxicity studies have shown several types of changes in pancreatic islets:

- Vacuolation
- Necrosis
- Angiectasis
- Hyalinisation/fibrosis
- Hypertrophy/hyperplasia
- Metaplasia
- Tumours

Vacuolation of beta cells has been seen in rats given antihistamines like cyclizine and cyproheptadine [32]. The antibiotic gatifloxacin produces vacuolation in rats, dogs, and monkeys. Cyclosporine and similar immunosuppressive agents are also known to cause vacuolation and degranulation in rodents (Fig. 8.64). Benzothiadiazines and certain immunomodulators have caused increased eosinophilic granularity of beta cells (Fig. 8.65). Synthetic progestogens, megestrol acetate, or chlormadinone acetate given to dogs for long periods have induced diabetes mellitus and vacuolation of beta cells (Fig. 8.66) [7, 33].

Alloxan and streptozotocin are selective toxins for beta cells. Similar effects are seen with an antiprotozoan drug, pentamidine. These agents produce degranulation, vacuolation, and necrosis of the beta cells. The cytotoxic agent busulfan causes haemorrhage and fibrosis of islets. Oxine and dithizone, which bind with zinc, produce necrosis of beta cells, as does zinc deficiency. Angiectasis and loss of beta cells have been seen in monkeys treated with a novel immunomodulator (Figs. 8.67 and 8.68). Hyalinisation and fibrosis

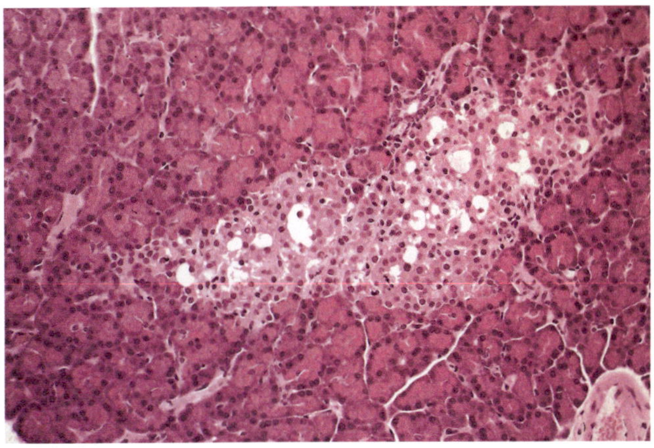

**Figure 8-64.** Vacuolated islet cells in a rat treated with an immunomodulator. H&E.

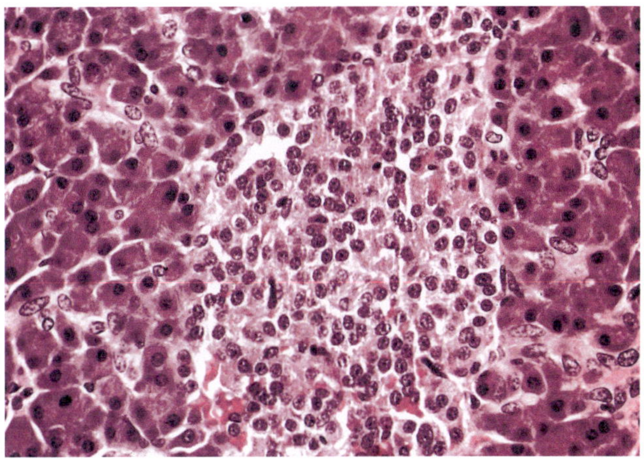

**Figure 8-65.** Eosinophilic granularity of the islet cell cytoplasm in a rat treated with an immunomodulator. H&E.

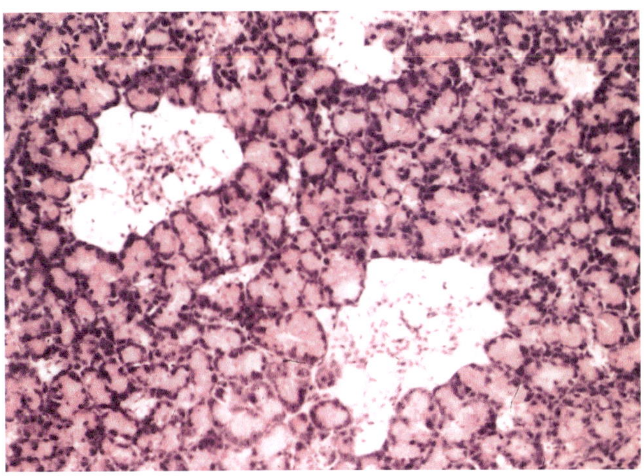

**Figure 8-66.** Vacuolated islet cells in a dog treated long term with a synthetic progestogen. H&E (With kind permission from Springer Science+Business Media B.V [39]).

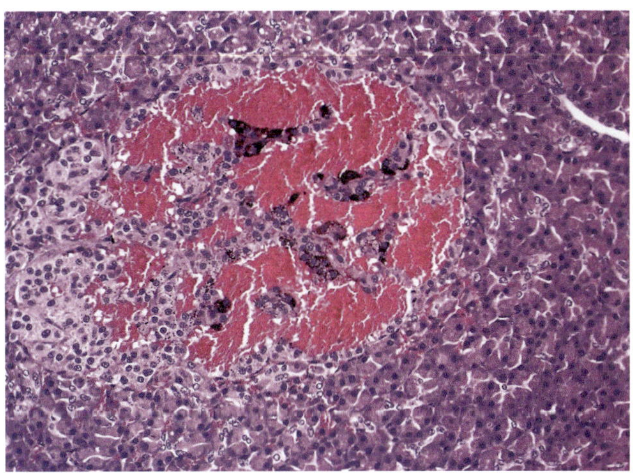

**Figure 8-67.** Angiectasis of pancreatic islets in a monkey treated with an immunomodulator. Note dilated vessels and pigmented macrophages. H&E.

are seen in islets of monkeys treated over long periods with synthetic progestogens (Figs. 8.69 and 8.70). Diazoacetate causes atrophy of beta cells. Growth hormone induces islet cell atrophy [34]. In such cases of islet cell atrophy, there is a reduction in the number of beta cells and a reduction in the number of islets. The cells may also display degenerative vacuolation (Fig. 8.71). Immunostaining for cellular hormones is valuable in this context.

Glucocorticoids cause hypertrophy of beta cells and hyperglycaemia (Fig. 8.72) [35]. Other trophic agents include growth hormone and glucagon. Hypertrophy may lead to hyperplasia. Hyperplasia in rodents appears as enlarged islets, an increase in the number of islets, or both (Figs. 8.73 and 8.74). Neuroleptics are known to induce hyperplasia in mice. It is interesting to note that continued stimulation of beta cells can lead to degeneration, vacuolation, atrophy, or loss of beta cells in treated animals.

Hepatocyte metaplasia adjacent to islets has been noted as an induced change with certain peroxisome proliferators (e.g. ciprofibrate) in rats [36]. Also in rats, two herbicides induced eosinophilic cells with a hepatoid appearance in the periphery of the islets during long-term exposure (Fig. 8.75). These cells did not stain positively for glycogen and did not have features of hepatocytes on electron microscopy. They possessed an abundance of mitochondria, suggesting that they were oncocytes. Islet cell degeneration and atrophy also can be induced by hormonal treatment.

Islet cell tumours can be induced by streptozotocin and alloxan. Many neuroleptic agents and heliotrine are known to increase the incidence of islet cell tumours in rodents (Figs. 8.76 and 8.77).

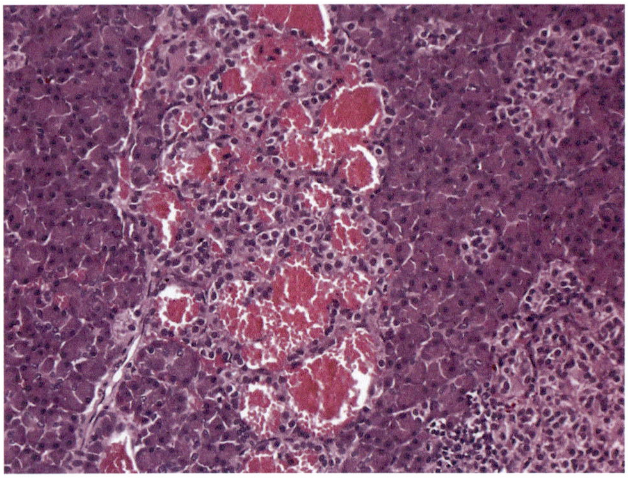

**Figure 8-68.** Angiectasis of pancreatic islets in a monkey. H&E.

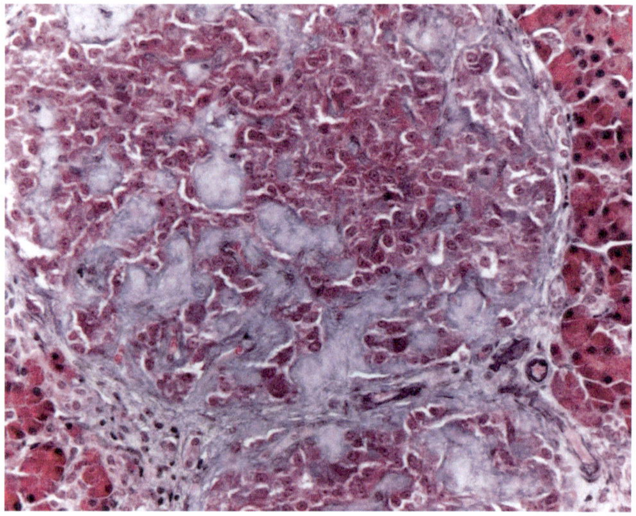

**Figure 8-69.** Hyalinisation of pancreatic islets in a monkey treated long term with a synthetic progestogen. Heidenhain's azan.

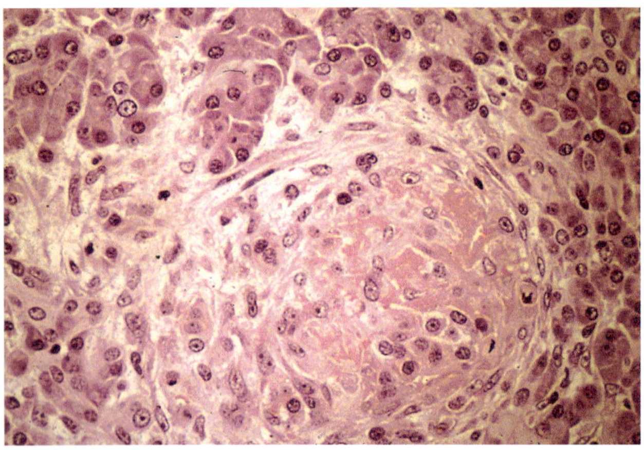

**Figure 8-70.** Fibrosis and loss of cells of pancreatic islets in a dog. H&E (With kind permission from Springer Science+Business Media B.V [39]).

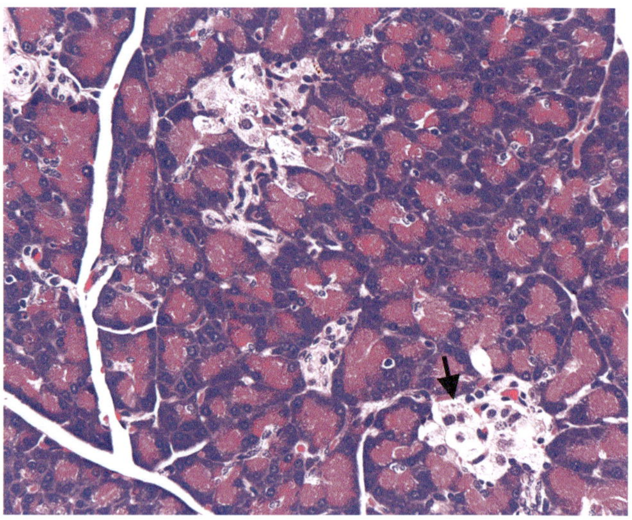

**Figure 8-71.** Islet cell atrophy and vacuolation (*arrow*) of the pancreas in a rat. H&E.

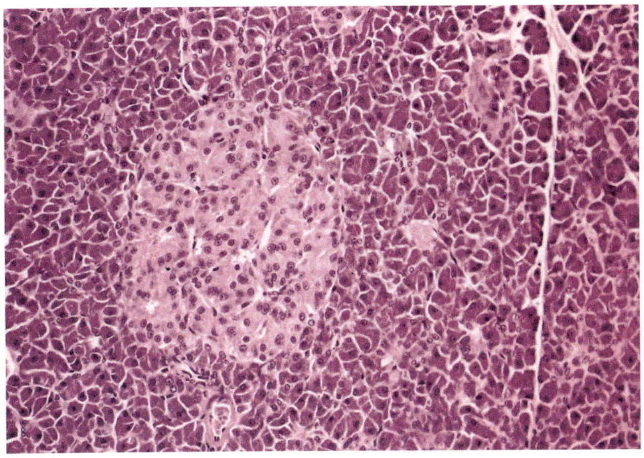

**Figure 8-72.** Hypertrophy of islet cells in a rat treated with a glucocorticoid. H&E.

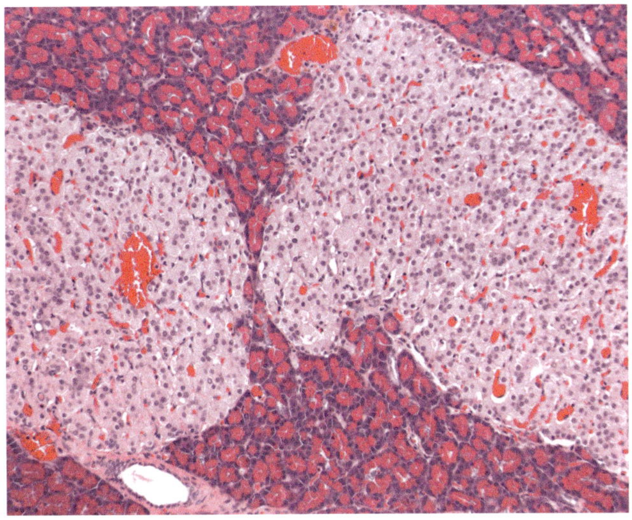

**Figure 8-73.** Islet cell hyperplasia in a rat treated with a hormonal agent. Note the increase in the size and number of islets. H&E.

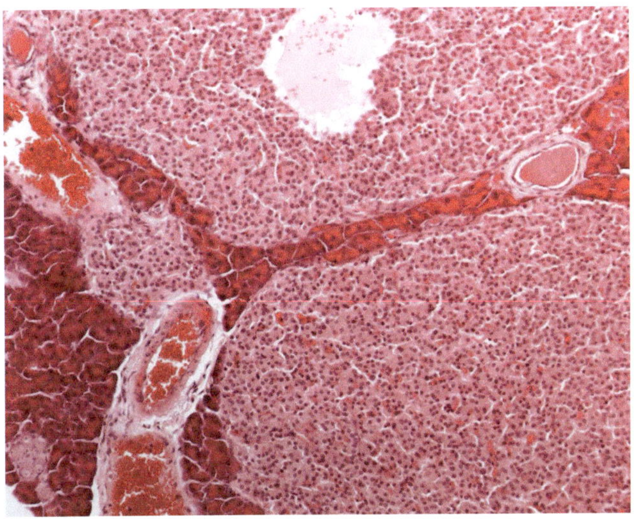

**Figure 8-74.** Islet cell hyperplasia in a mouse. The number and size of islets are increased. H&E.

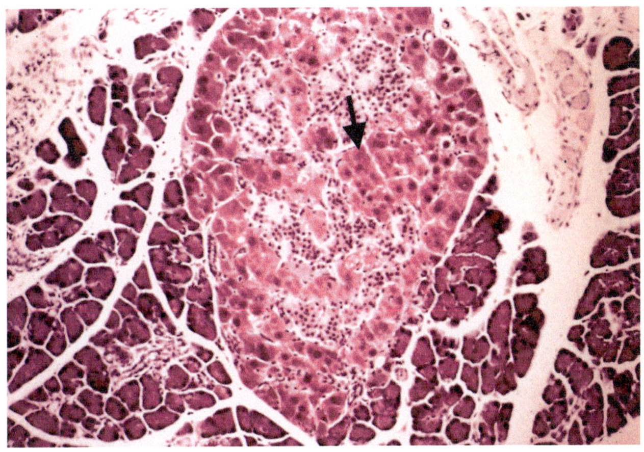

**Figure 8-75.** Hepatoid metaplasia (*arrow*) of the pancreatic islets in a rat. H&E.

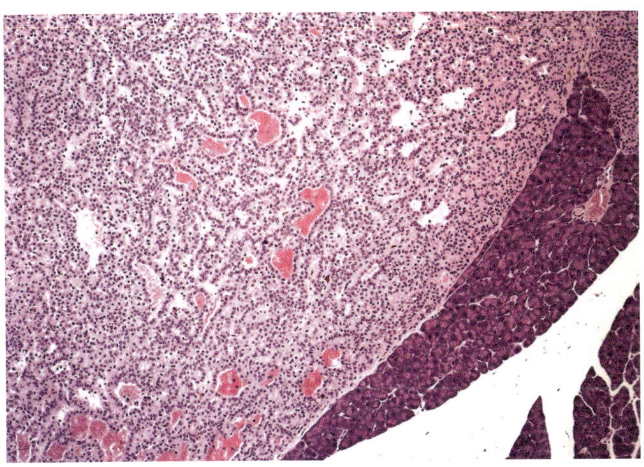

**Figure 8-76.** Islet cell adenoma in a rat treated with a neuroleptic agent. Neoplastic cells arranged as chords are causing compression. H&E.

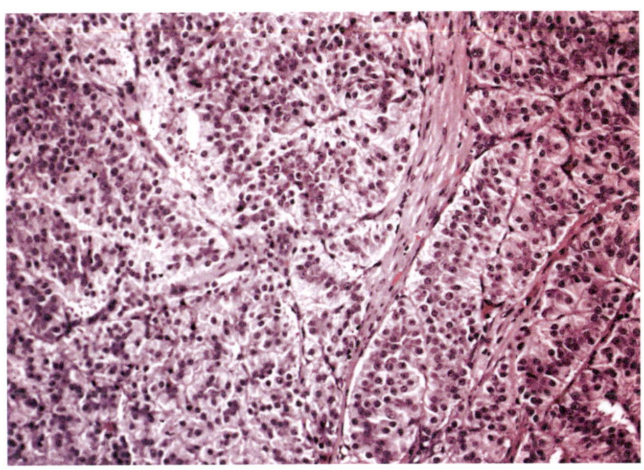

**Figure 8-77.** Islet cell carcinoma in a rat. Neoplastic cells are arranged in multicellular chords of differing patterns with evidence of local invasion. H&E.

## 8.6 Pituitary Gland

The pituitary gland seldom reveals toxic findings, except for hormonally mediated changes. Most changes reflect exaggerated pharmacological effects, which mirror alterations occurring during ageing, lactation, or stress. The cellular details of the anterior lobe are complex, and immunohistochemical techniques are essential to investigate changes. The cellular components of the anterior lobe include mammotrophs, somatotrophs, adrenocorticotrophs, thyrotrophs, and gonadotrophs. Most of the cell types have their own trophic and inhibitory mechanisms controlling their growth and hormonal output. Pituitary cells can be polyhormonal. Gonadotrophs can produce follicle-stimulating hormone (FSH), luteinising hormone (LH), or both. One cell can produce both growth hormone and prolactin. The cells also include undifferentiated cells (chromophobes) and interstitial stellate cells. Various types of changes may be encountered:

- Infarction/necrosis
- Vacuolation
- Apoptosis
- Hypertrophy/hyperplasia
- Tumours

Infarction has been reported in the pars anterior of the pituitary gland in rats treated with hexadimethrine. A similar necrotic lesion was seen in rats treated with an antiangiogenic agent (Figs. 8.78 and 8.79). The lesion reversed on withdrawal of the treatment. Diffuse vacuolation was seen in the anterior lobe in monkeys treated with an anticancer agent. Metals like selenium and lead are reported to be toxic to the pituitary gland. Most findings seen in pituitary glands are hormone mediated and usually affect one of the cell types in the pars anterior. Changes noted are degranulation, hypertrophy, hyperplasia, and/or vacuolation.

Thyroidectomy in rats and goitrogens result in hypertrophy or hyperplasia of thyrotrophs (Fig. 8.80) [37, 38]. Overstimulation results in vacuolation and degeneration, as seen in rats or dogs treated with certain goitrogens (Figs. 8.81 and 8.82). Pyridoxine deficiency causes degranulation of thyrotrophs. Administration of estrogens to rats induces prolactin cell hyperplasia (mammotrophs) [39]. Administration of a pituitary peptide resulted in hyperplasia of mammotrophs, and removal of the treatment caused increased apoptosis of prolactin cells (Fig. 8.83). Certain neuroleptic agents, when given to rodents, cause hyperplasia of prolactin cells; the result is mammary hyperplasia and later mammary tumours in these rodents. Neuroleptics exert their effects by inhibition of dopamine, which normally acts as an inhibitor of prolactin cells.

Treatment of dogs with progestogens and other contraceptive steroids causes hyperplasia of somatotrophs (Fig. 8.84) [6, 40]. Cyproterone acetate stimulates growth hormone cells in ovariectomised dogs [41]. The induction of mammary hyperplasia and mammary tumours in dogs treated long term with synthetic progestogens is mediated by growth hormone.

Gonadotrophs are increased following castration. Testicular atrophy induced by many agents (including anti-androgens such as flutamide) causes the presence of castration cells (enlarged and vacuolated gonadotrophs) (Fig. 8.85). Surgical adrenalectomy and treatment of experimental animals with antimycotic agents causing lipidosis of the adrenal cortex result in hypertrophy of adrenocorticotrophs.

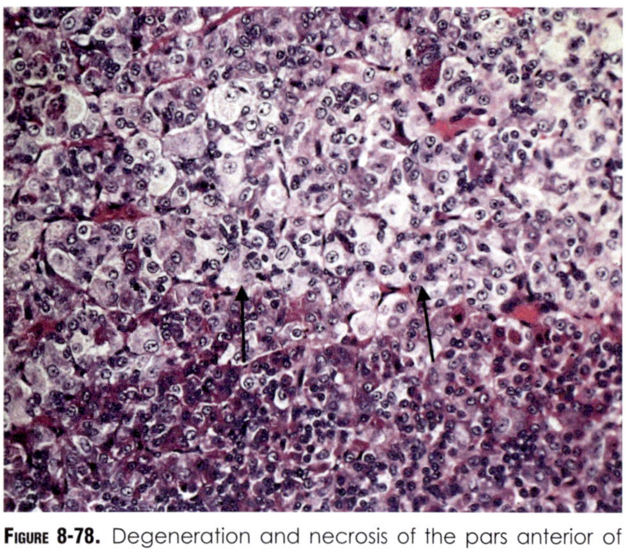

**FIGURE 8-78.** Degeneration and necrosis of the pars anterior of the pituitary gland (*arrows*) in a rat treated with an antiangiogenic agent. A zone of vacuolated and necrotic cells. H&E.

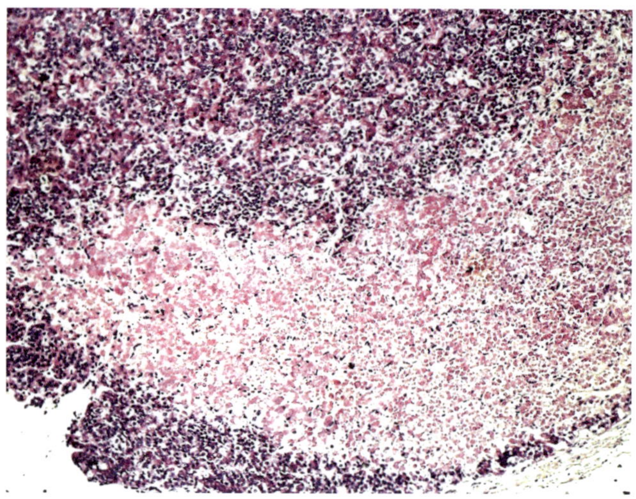

**FIGURE 8-79.** Necrosis of the pars anterior of the pituitary gland in a rat. The necrotic zone shows loss of cellular details. H&E.

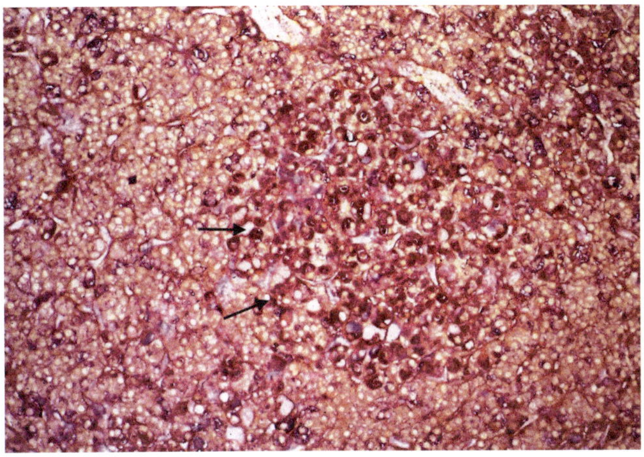

**Figure 8-80.** Focal hyperplasia of thyrotrophic cells (*arrows*) in the pituitary (PAS +ve) in a rat treated with a goitrogenic chemical. PAS/orange G.

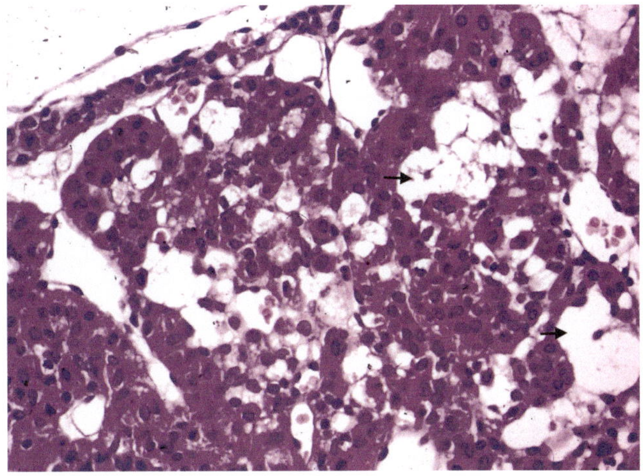

**Figure 8-81.** Vacuolated cells in the pars anterior (*arrows*), in a dog treated with a goitrogenic agent. Some cells are ballooned with pyknotic nuclei. H&E (With kind permission from Springer Science + Business Media B.V [39]).

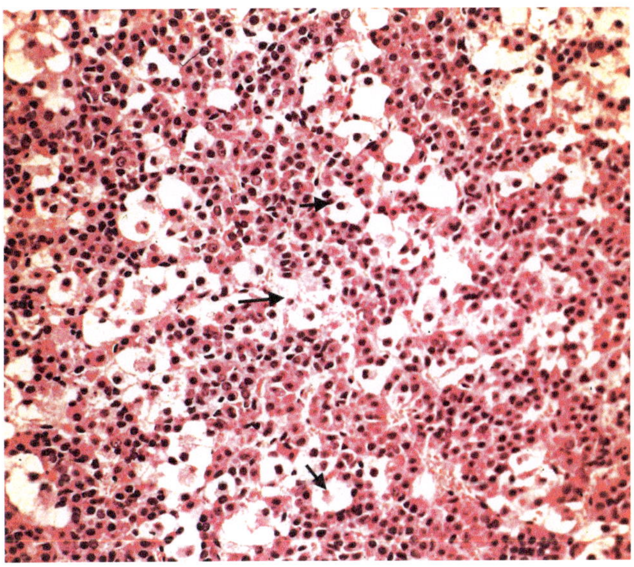

**Figure 8-82.** Vacuolated cells (*arrows*) in the pars anterior of a rat treated with a goitrogenic chemical. H&E

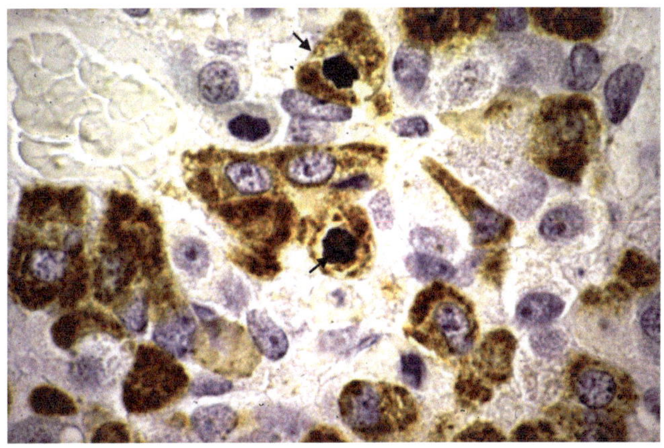

**Figure 8-83.** Apoptosis of prolactin-positive cells (*arrows*) in the pituitary in a dog treated with a hormonal agent. Immunohistochemistry

Pituitary tumours are common in aged rats. Their incidence can be increased by treatment with estrogens, luteinising hormone-releasing hormone (LHRH) analogues like goserelin and leuprolide, goitrogens, calcitonin, or radiation or by iodine deficiency [42]. Diets high in calories or protein increase the incidence of pituitary tumours in rodents [43]. Pituitary adenomas appear with different morphological patterns in the rat (Figs. 8.86–8.89). Restricted diets and tamoxifen (antiestrogen) reduce the incidence of pituitary tumours in rats. Pituitary adenomas are mostly hormone-dependent conditional neoplasms that regress if the trophic stimulation is withdrawn. Thus, they must be regarded separately from conventional neoplasms.

Melanocyte-stimulating cells of the pars intermedia are increased in hamsters treated with estrogens. Bromocriptine reduces the thickness of the pars intermedia in rats. Long-term treatment of mice with angiotensin-converting enzyme (ACE) inhibitors has produced deposition of amyloid-like material in the pars intermedia (Fig. 8.90).

The pars nervosa seldom exhibits any toxic lesions. A thyromimetic agent induced focal necrosis with cyst formation (infarct-like) in the pars nervosa of dogs (Figs. 8.91 and 8.92). In this instance, the affected animals showed polyuria and hyperplasia of the z. glomerulosa of the adrenal glands (personal observation).

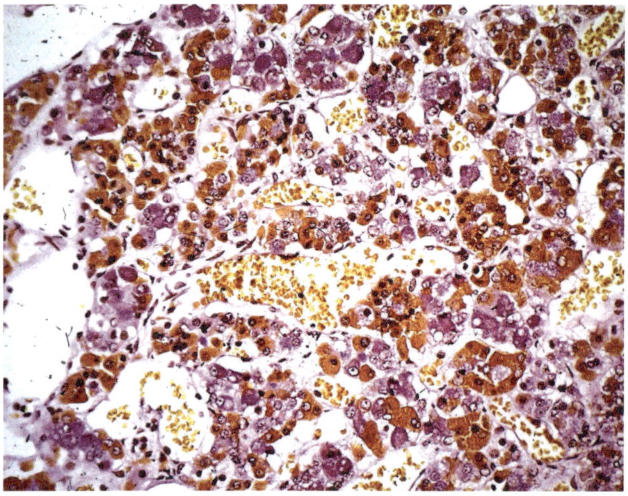

**Figure 8-84.** Increased somatotrophs (*golden yellow*) in the pars anterior of the pituitary in a dog treated with a synthetic progestogen. PAS/orange G.

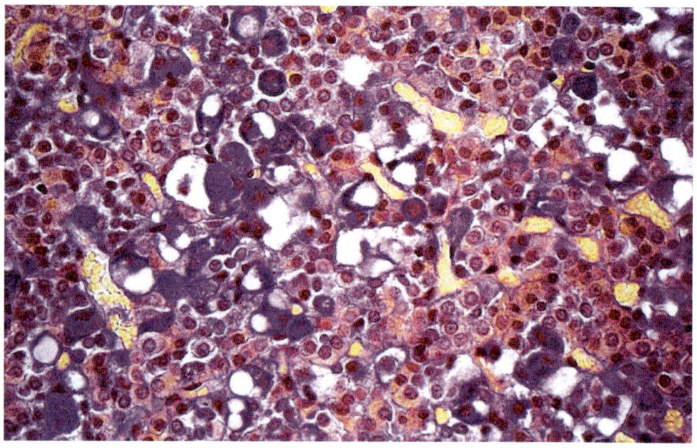

**Figure 8-85.** Castration cells (enlarged and vacuolated gonadotrophs) in the pars anterior of the pituitary in a rat treated with an anti-androgenic agent. PAS/orange G.

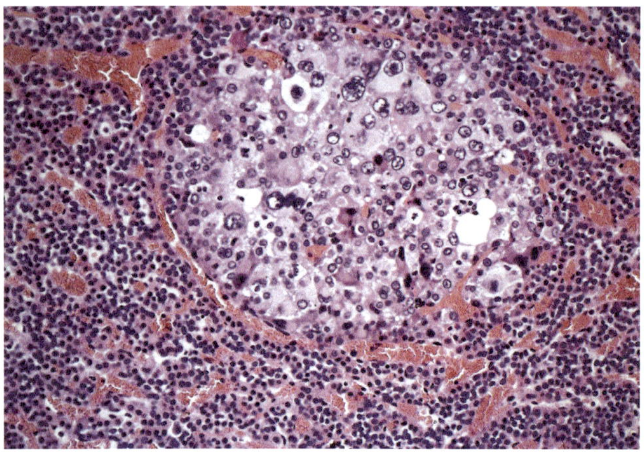

**Figure 8-86.** Pituitary adenoma in a rat. Pleomorphic neoplastic cells. H&E.

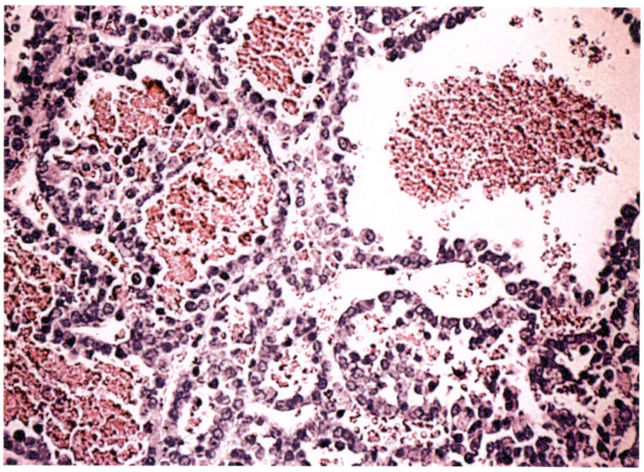

**Figure 8-87.** Pituitary adenoma in a rat. Pseudoglandular pattern. H&E.

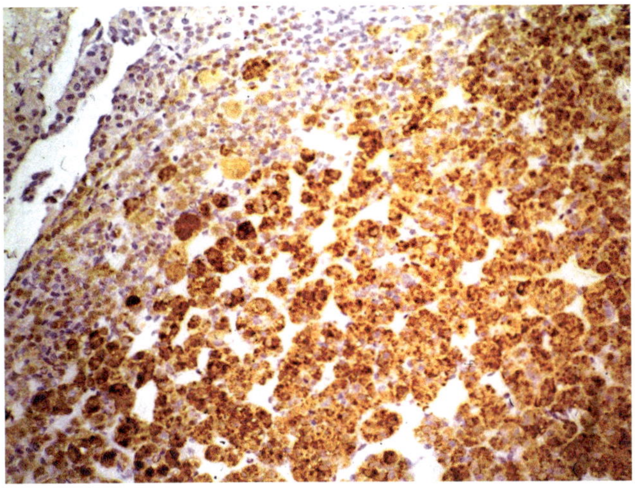

**FIGURE 8-88.** Pituitary adenoma with FSH-positive cells in a rat treated with an aromatase inhibitor. Immunocytochemistry.

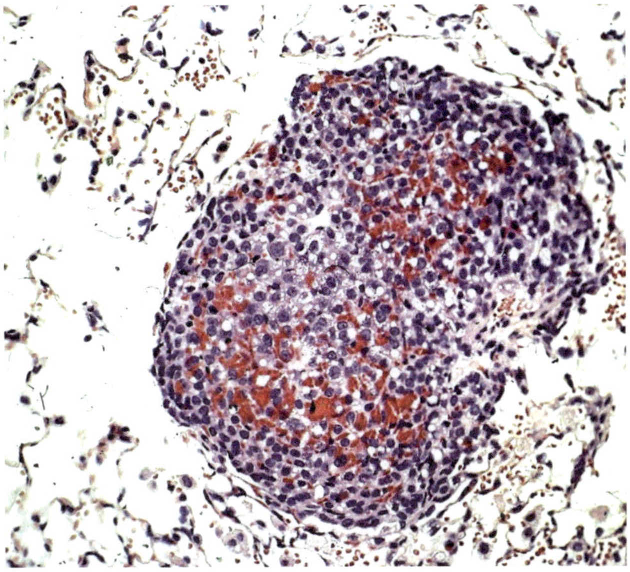

**FIGURE 8-89.** Pituitary carcinoma with metastasis into the lung of a rat. H&E.

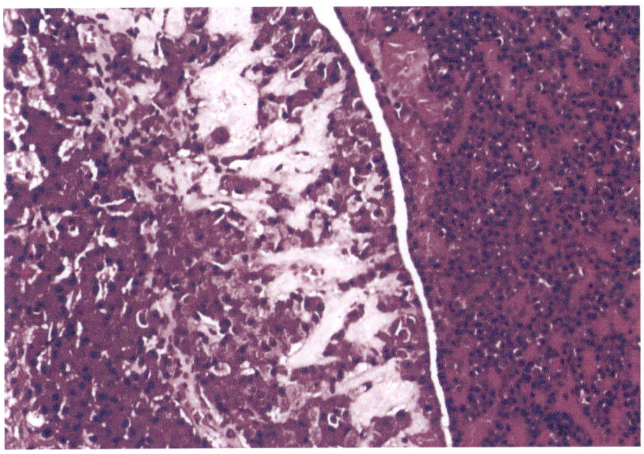

**FIGURE 8-90.** Amyloid deposition in the pars intermedia in a mouse treated long term with an angiotensin-converting enzyme (ACE) inhibitor. Note the areas of hyalinisation. H&E.

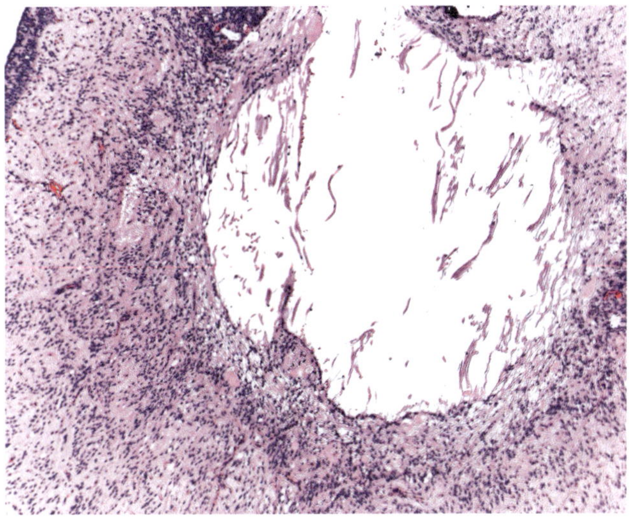

**FIGURE 8-91.** Liquefactive necrosis of the pars nervosa in a dog treated with a thyromimetic agent. A cystic area represents necrosis and loss of tissue. H&E.

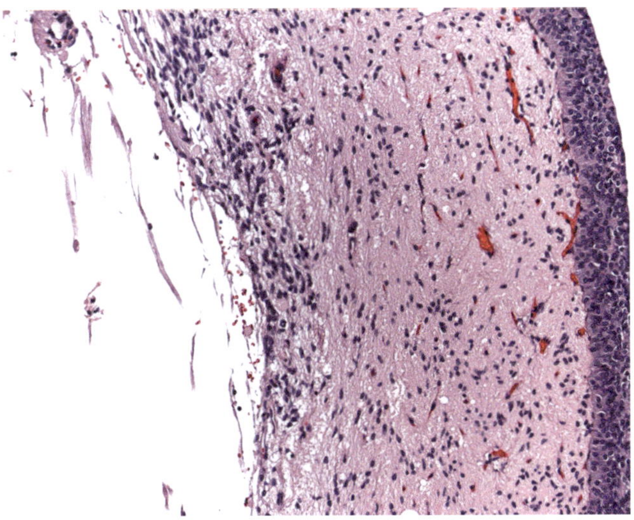

**FIGURE 8-92.** Necrosis of the pars nervosa in a dog. The cystic area with debris represents liquefactive necrosis. H&E.

## References


1. Colby HD, Eacho P. Chemical induced adrenal injury: role of metabolic activation. In: Thomas JA, Korach KS, McLachlan JA, editors. Endocrine toxicology. New York: Raven; 1985. p. 35.
2. Yarrington JT. Chemically induced adrenocortical lesions. In: Jones TC, Mohr U, Hunt RD, editors. Endocrine system. Berlin: Springer; 1983. p. 69.
3. Abbott EC, Monkhouse FE, Steiner JW, Laidlaw JC. Effect of a sulphated mucopolysaccharide (RO1-8307) on the zona glomerulosa of the rat adrenal gland. Endocrinology. 1966;78:651–4.
4. Mazzocchi G, Nussdorfer GG. Long-term effects of captopril on the morphology of normal rat adrenal zona glomerulosa. Exp Clin Endocrinol. 1984;84:148–52.
5. Kovacs K, Carroll R, Tapp E. The pathogenesis of hexadimethrine necrosis of the pituitary and adrenal. Arzneimittelforschung. 1966;16:516–9.
6. El Etreby MF, Graf KJ, Gunzel P, Neumann F. Evaluation of effects of sexual steroids on the hypothalamic-pituitary system of animals and man. Arch Toxicol Suppl. 1979;2:11–39.
7. Nelson LW, Kelly WA. Progestogen-related gross and microscopic changes in female beagles. Vet Pathol. 1976;13:143–56.
8. Szabo S, McComb DJ, Kovacs K, Huttner I. Adrenocortical haemorrhagic necrosis: the role of catecholamines and retrograde medullary-cell embolism. Arch Pathol Lab Med. 1981; 105:536–9.
9. Szabo S, Huttner I, Kovacs K, Horvath E, Szabo D, Homer HC. Pathogenesis of experimental adrenal haemorrhagic necrosis ('apoplexy'). Lab Invest. 1980;42:533–46.
10. Ribelin WE. The effects of drugs and chemicals upon the structure of adrenal gland. Fundam Appl Toxicol. 1984;4:105–19.
11. Tettenborn D. Toxicity of clotrimazole. Postgrad Med J. 1974;50 suppl 1:17–20.
12. Tachibana M, Noguchi Y, Monro AM. Toxicity of fluconazole in experimental animals. In: Fromtling RA, editor. Recent trends in the discovery, development and evaluation of antifungal agents. Barcelona: JR Prous; 1987. p. 93.
13. Gopinath C, Prentice DE, Lewis DJ. Endocrine system. In: Gopinath C, Prentice DE, Lewis DJ, editors. Atlas of experimental toxicological pathology. Lancaster: MTP Press; 1987. p. 104.
14. Zak F. Lipid hyperplasia, adrenal cortex, rat. In: Jones TC, Mohr U, Hunt RD, editors. Endocrine system. Berlin: Springer; 1983. p. 80.
15. Roe FJ, Bar A. Enzootic and epizootic adrenal medullary proliferative disease of rats: influence of dietary factors which affect calcium absorption. Hum Toxicol. 1985;4:27–30.
16. Boelsterli UA, Zbinden G. Early biochemical and morphological changes in the rat adrenal medulla induced by xylitol. Arch Toxicol. 1985;57:25–30.
17. Kurokawa Y, Hyashi Y, Maekawa A, et al. High incidence of pheochromocytomas after long-term administration of retinol acetate to F344/DuCrj rats. J Natl Cancer Inst. 1985;74:715–23.
18. Tischler AS, Riseberg JC. Different responses to mitogenic agents by adult rat and human chromaffin cells in vitro. Endocr Pathol. 1993;14:15–9.
19. Lumb GD, Rust JH. The pathologic response of the liver and thyroid of the rat to potassium prorenoate (SC-23992). Toxicol Pathol. 1985;13:315–24.
20. Heath JE, Littlefield NA. Morphological effects of subchronic oral sulfamethazine administration on Fischer 344 rats and B6C3F1 mice. Toxicol Pathol. 1984;12:3–9.
21. Collins WT, Capen CC, Kazsa L, et al. Effect of polychlorinated biphenyl (PCB) on the thyroid gland of rats. Am J Pathol. 1977;89:119–30.
22. Takayama S, Aihara K, Onodera T, Akimoto T. Antithyroid effects of propylthiouracil and sulfamonomethoxine in rats and monkeys. Toxicol Appl Pharmacol. 1986;82:191–9.
23. Hill RN, Erdreich LS, Paynter OE, Roberts PA, Rosenthal SL, Wilkinson CF. Thyroid follicular cell carcinogenesis. Fundam Appl Toxicol. 1989;12:629–97.
24. Price SC, Chescoe D, Grasso P, et al. Alterations in the thyroids of rats treated for long periods with di-(2-ethylhexyl) phthalate or with hypolipidaemic agents. Toxicol Lett. 1988;40:37–46.
25. Capen CC. Hormonal imbalances and mechanisms of chemical injury of thyroid gland. In: Jones TC, Capen CC, Mohr U, editors. Endocrine system. 2nd ed. Berlin: Springer; 1995. p. 217.
26. McClain RM. The significance of hepatic microsomal enzyme induction and altered thyroid function in rats. Implications for thyroid gland neoplasia. Toxicol Pathol. 1989;17:294–306.
27. Gopinath C. Comparative endocrine carcinogenesis. In: Harvey PW, Rush KC, Cockburn A, editors. Endocrine and hormonal toxicology. New York: Wiley; 1999. p. 155.
28. Benitz KF, Roberts GK, Yusa A. Morphological effects of minocycline in laboratory animals. Toxicol Appl Pharmacol. 1967;11: 150–70.
29. Zayed I, van Esch E, McConnell RF. Systemic and histopathological changes in beagle dogs after chronic daily oral administration of synthetic (ethenyl estradiol) or natural (estradiol) estrogens, with special reference to the kidney and thyroid. Toxicol Pathol. 1998;26:730–41.
30. Knudsen LB, Madsen LW, Andersen S, et al. Glucagon-like peptide-1 receptor agonists activate rodent thyroid-C-cells causing calcitonin release and C-cell proliferation. Endocrinology. 2010;15:1473–86.
31. Madsen LW, Knauf JA, Gottredsen C, et al. GLP-1 receptor agonists and thyroid C- cell effects in mice are mediated via GLP-1 receptor and not associated with RET activation. Endocrinology. 2012;153:1–10.
32. Greaves P. Endocrine pancreas. In: Histopathology of preclinical toxicity studies. 3rd ed. Amsterdam: Academic; 2007. p. 528.
33. Tucker M. Some effects of prolonged administration of progestogen to dogs. Proc Eur Soc Study Drug Toxicity. 1971;12: 228–38.
34. Campbell J, Pierluissi J, Kovacs K. Pancreatic islet ultrastructure, serum and pancreatic immunoreactive insulin in somatotrophic and metasomatotrophic diabetes in dogs. J Submicrosc Cytol. 1981;13:599–608.
35. Gopinath C, Prentice DE, Lewis DJ. Endocrine system. In: Gopinath C, Prentice DE, Lewis DJ, editors. Atlas of experimental toxicological pathology. Lancaster: MTP Press; 1987. p. 109.
36. Reddy JK, Rao MS, Qureshi SA, et al. Induction and origin of hepatocytes in rat pancreas. J Cell Biol. 1984;98:2577–81.
37. Tsuda H. Goitre, adenoma and carcinoma of thyroid gland induced by amitrol and ethylnitrosourea, rat. In: Jones TC, Mohr U, Hunt RD, editors. Endocrine system. Berlin: Springer; 1983. p. 204.
38. Farquahar MG. Lysosome function in regulating secretion: disposal of secretory granules in cells of the anterior pituitary gland. In: Dingle JT, Fell HB, editors. Lysosomes in biology and pathology. Amsterdam: North Holland; 1969. p. 462.

39. Gopinath C, Prentice DE, Lewis DJ. Endocrine system. In: Gopinath C, Prentice DE, Lewis DJ, editors. Atlas of experimental toxicological pathology. Lancaster: MTP Press; 1987. p. 113.

40. El Etreby MF. Practical application of immunocytochemistry of the pharmacology and toxicology of the endocrine system. Histochem J. 1981;13:821.

41. El Etreby MF, Fath El BaB MR. Effect of cyproterone acetate on cells of the pars distalis of the adenophysis in the beagle bitch. Cell Tissue Res. 1977;183:177–89.

42. Stefaneanu L, Kovacs K. Modern approaches to classification of pituitary tumours in human subjects and animals. In: Jones TC, Capen CC, Mohr U, editors. Endocrine system. 2nd ed. Berlin: Springer; 1995. p. 47.

43. Keenan KP, Soper KA, Smith PF, Ballam GC, Clark RL. Diet, overfeeding, and moderate dietary restriction in control Sprague–Dawley rats: I. Effects on spontaneous neoplasms. Toxicol Pathol. 1995;23:269–86.

# 9 The Lymphoid System

The organs included in this chapter include the thymus, lymph nodes, spleen, and bone marrow. The main responses seen in these organs are due to immunostimulation, immunosuppression, immunogenicity, or hypersensitivity. The changes in lymphoid organs are subject to many environmental factors. Changes in the thymus include apoptosis, atrophy, and a few proliferative responses. The lymph nodes and spleen display increases or decreases in the cellularity of their various compartments. Persistent stimulation sometimes can give rise to neoplasia. Bone marrow also undergoes increases or decreases in its cellularity in response to various agents, sometimes resulting in necrosis and fibrosis.

## 9.1 Introduction

The lymphoid system is highly disseminated, involving most of the organs and tissues of the body. For convenience, this chapter describes the pathology of the major lymphoid organs alone, including the primary lymphoid organs like the bone marrow and thymus and secondary organs such as the lymph nodes and spleen. The system also involves organs like the liver, brain, skin, and mucosa of the respiratory and gastrointestinal tracts, all of which are dealt with elsewhere.

The main cellular players of the system are bone marrow stem cells, macrophages (derived from bone marrow), T cells (from bone marrow or thymus), B cells and plasma cells (from bone marrow), and dendritic cells and natural killer (NK) cells (from the bone marrow). Macrophages have a role in antigen presentation, phagocytosis, and cytotoxicity. Various subsets of T cells are involved with tumour toxicity, immune regulation, memory, lymphokine production, hypersensitivity, and cytotoxicity. B cells and plasma cells have roles in the production of antibodies and lymphokines. Stem cells are sensitive to alkylating agents and folic acid analogues. Macrophages are sensitive to corticosteroids and are stimulated by particulate materials like silica and adjuvants. T cells are sensitive to alkylating agents, purine analogues, aromatic hydrocarbons, and certain antibiotics. Interleukin-2 and interferon gamma stimulate T cells. B cells are sensitive to hydrocarbons and are stimulated by interleukin-2.

Morphologically, these cells are organised in various compartments of the major lymphoid organs during health. In toxicity and other abnormal situations, the relative proportions of these cells in the various compartments of the lymphoid organs are subject to change, and their assessment is important in understanding the changes in lymphoid organs. Many immunohistochemical monoclonal antibody techniques are employed as markers for the various cell subtypes [1]. S-100, ED5, and KiM9R are useful for identifying dendritic cells. Similarly, CD3 is useful as a pan T-cell marker and CD45RA as a pan B-cell marker. These are important tools in enabling an assessment of increases or decreases in the cellularity of specific cell types within a lymphoid organ. The study of isolated cells by in vitro function studies provides useful information about the functional status of the cell. Although this type of study yields some useful information about the cell in question, in vitro tests tend to ignore whole-body status, particularly with regard to the huge reserve of the body. They also ignore interorgan and intercellular homeostatic influences. Thus it is important not to overemphasise in vitro test results in isolation, as they may not reflect the health

C. Gopinath, V. Mowat, *Atlas of Toxicological Pathology*,
DOI 10.1007/978-1-62703-998-7_9, © Springer Science+Business Media New York 2014

status of the whole individual. Generally speaking, histopathological examination provides much better and more balanced information on the health status of the individual. For specific groups of therapeutics such as immunomodulatory biologics, immunohistochemistry, and/or immunofluorescence, techniques may be added to the routine histopathology screening [2].

The literature contains several monographs on the structure and function of lymphoid tissues and organs of laboratory animals [3–7]. A basic understanding of the immune system's function is essential for the pathologist to be able to interpret changes and to predict when the immune system may be a target [8]. Assessment of juvenile immunotoxicity studies requires familiarity with immune system development and the functional and histologic differences between juveniles and adults [9]. Histopathological examinations of the thymus, spleen, and lymph nodes are important tools of investigation in regulatory immunotoxicity studies, with extensive literature describing histopathological changes in these organs and the use of enhanced screening protocols [10–23]. The position paper published by the Society of Toxicologic Pathology (STP) on best practices for pathology evaluation of the immune system and a monograph on histomorphologic evaluation of lymphoid organs also form excellent guides for practicing toxicologic pathologists [24, 25]. Guides to the nomenclature of neoplastic and nonneoplastic lesions also have been published by the STP [26, 27].

Generally, lymphoproliferative responses correlate with cell-mediated immunity. Plasma cell increases and germinal centre development are indicators of antibody-mediated reactions. Cell degeneration and depletion are evidence of immunosuppression or toxicity. Macrophage movement and prominence suggest antigen presentation or phagocytosis. Perivascular inflammatory cell infiltration indicates type IV hypersensitivity.

The lymphoid system is very vulnerable to influences by external factors, and the changes can often mimic those seen in toxicity studies. These factors include stress, steroids, nutrition, age, and antigen status. Experimental procedures, social ranking within the laboratory animal cage, and high-dose effects all induce stress, corticosteroid release, and consequent effects on lymphoid tissues. There are marked sex differences in the responses of lymphoid organs. Nutritional deficiencies have negative impacts on the appearance of lymphoid tissues. Age-related lymphoid depletion is well known. The antigen load of the environment also affects lymphoid organs; animals kept under germ-free conditions display inactive lymph nodes.

Generally speaking, responses of the lymphoid system manifest as immune stimulation, immune suppression, immunogenicity, or hypersensitivity. Immune responses may be innate or adaptive.

Immune stimulation causes the lymphoid organs to be enlarged and reactive, often with increased cellularity. The changes are not deleterious by themselves. Lymphokines, adjuvants, and lymphocytic mobilisers are examples of immunostimulants.

Immune suppression is a toxic response resulting in reduced resistance to infections. Many pesticides, metals, environmental agents, chemicals, and pharmaceuticals induce immunotoxicity, which generally manifests as degeneration and loss of lymphocytes in various tissues. The affected animals may develop bronchopneumonia, mycotic infection, increased dermal infections, papillomatosis, and/or viral encephalitis (Figs. 9.1–9.3). Agents such as cyclosporine (and others used in transplantation surgery), cyclophosphamide, purine analogues, folic acid analogues, certain antibiotics, and corticosteroids are known to induce immunosuppression in experimental animals and humans.

Hypersensitivity is another expression of immunotoxicity. Immunogenicity and hypersensitivity result from overstimulation of some aspects of immune function. There is an increase in immunoglobulins, C3, and deposition of immune complexes, leading to various pathologies. This condition can manifest as skin rashes, dermatitis, thrombocytopenia, haemorrhages, haemolytic anaemia, glomerulonephritis, vasculitis, or asthma (Fig. 9.4). Most agents used in toxicity studies are not immunogenic, but agents such as chlorpromazine, phenacetin, and amidopyrine can provoke drug-induced hypersensitivity. Immunogens are difficult to predict from animal studies, as these reactions can be species specific. Agents that are immunogenic in humans are not necessarily immunogenic or hypersensitivity inducing in animal studies, and vice versa.

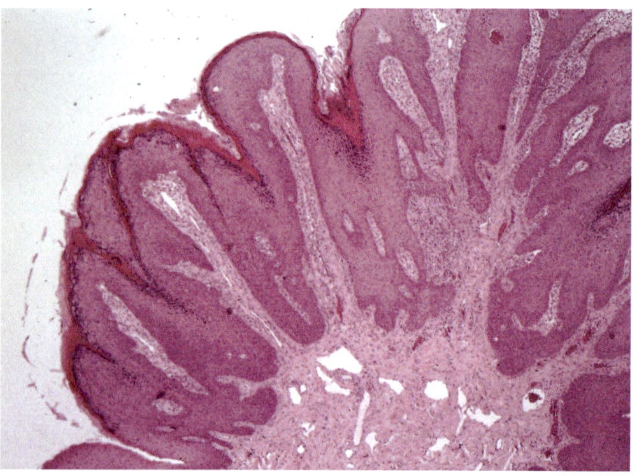

**FIGURE 9-1.** Squamous cell papilloma of the upper lip of a dog treated with high doses of a glucocorticoid. Haematoxylin and eosin (H&E).

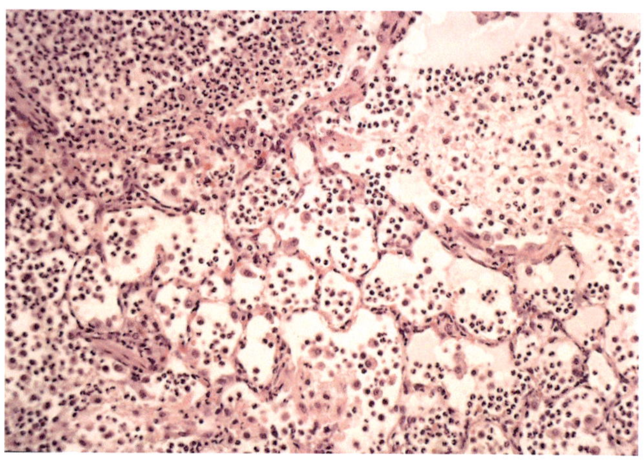

**FIGURE 9-2.** Bronchopneumonia in a dog treated with high doses of a glucocorticoid. H&E.

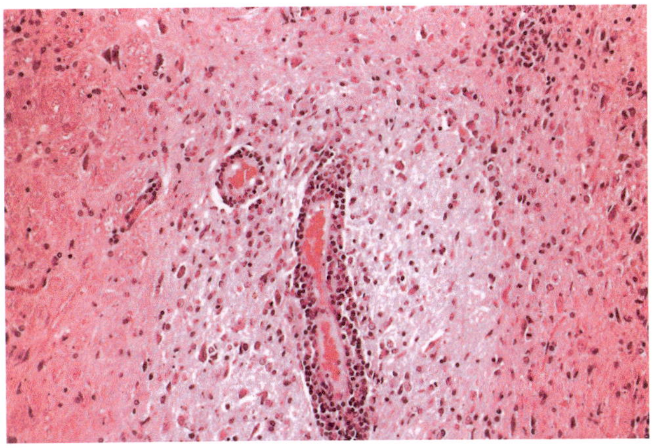

**Figure 9-3.** Encephalomyelitis in the cerebrum of a rat treated with an immunomodulator. Note focal gliosis and perivascular cuffing. H&E.

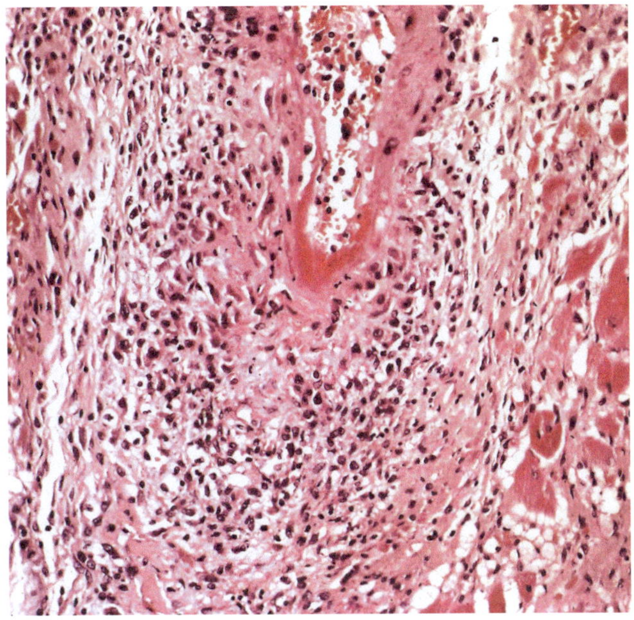

**Figure 9-4.** Vasculitis in a dog. Note inflammation and fibrinoid necrosis in the vascular wall. H&E.

## 9.2 Thymus

The most common finding in the thymus is atrophy, as this organ is highly vulnerable to nonspecific stress and age. The organ's weight is a sensitive tool for detection of alterations. A wide variety of industrial, environmental, and pharmaceutical agents induce thymic atrophy in laboratory animals. The thymus shows only a small number of induced changes:

- Thymic atrophy
- Apoptosis and loss of cells
- Lymphoid proliferation
- Germinal centre development
- Epithelial proliferation

Significant findings in the thymus have been described in detail [13]. Nonspecific stress caused by malnutrition, fighting, trauma, overcrowding, or disease produces thymic atrophy mediated by endogenous corticosteroids [28]. Glucocorticoids are thymolytic. Stress, cytotoxicity, and a decrease in growth hormone all reduce thymic size and cellularity. Organotin, cyclophosphamide, and other immunosuppressors are cytotoxic and cause increased apoptosis and loss of cortical lymphocytes. If minor, these effects appear as scattered apoptotic cells as tingible bodies within clear macrophages, giving a 'starry sky' appearance (Fig. 9.5). Severe effects first appear in large groups of cortical lymphocytes as hyperchromatosis, condensation (pyknosis), and nuclear breakdown, followed by marked loss of cells from the cortex (Fig. 9.6). In severe, long-standing cases of atrophy, the thymus appears as thin cords or strands and can disappear entirely (Figs. 9.7 and 9.8). Most induced thymic atrophy is reversible. The pathologist should be aware that the thymus also undergoes age-related involution, which presents a similar histologic appearance.

Certain potent immunomodulators can cause cortical loss of cells and a relative increase in medullary cellularity, causing the corticomedullary junction to become indistinct (Fig. 9.9). Some authors refer to this effect as 'medullary atrophy', but although certain cell types in the medulla are lost, concurrent mobilisation of B cells into the medulla occurs. Diethylstilboestrol causes thymic atrophy and epithelial proliferation [29, 30]. Age-related thymic involution features a loss of lymphoid cells and an apparent increase in epithelial components, which should not be confused with epithelial hyperplasia. Organotin and cyclophosphamide can cause thymic atrophy and fibrosis [30]. Medullary hyperplasia is an age-related incidental finding in mice (Fig. 9.10).

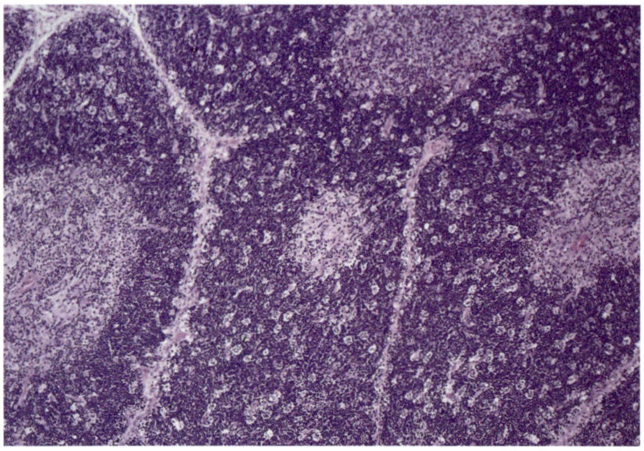

**FIGURE 9-5.** Lymphocyte apoptosis in the cortex of the thymus in a rat. Note the starry sky appearance. H&E (With kind permission from Springer Science + Business Media B.V [30]).

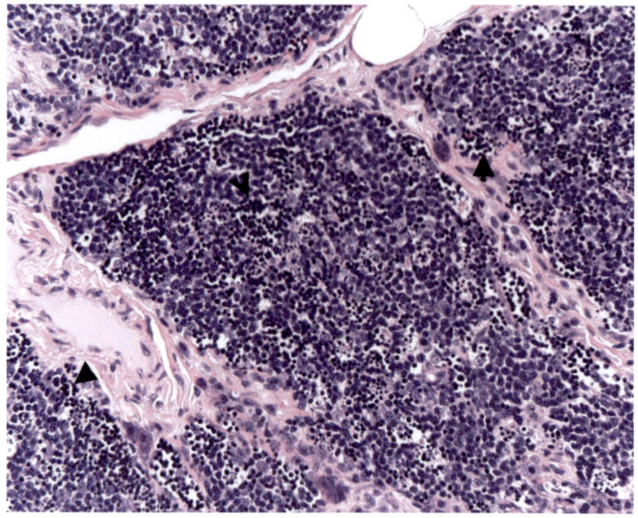

**FIGURE 9-6.** Severe apoptosis and loss of cells in the thymic cortex of a rat. Note aggregates of pyknotic lymphocytes (*arrows*) in the cortex. H&E.

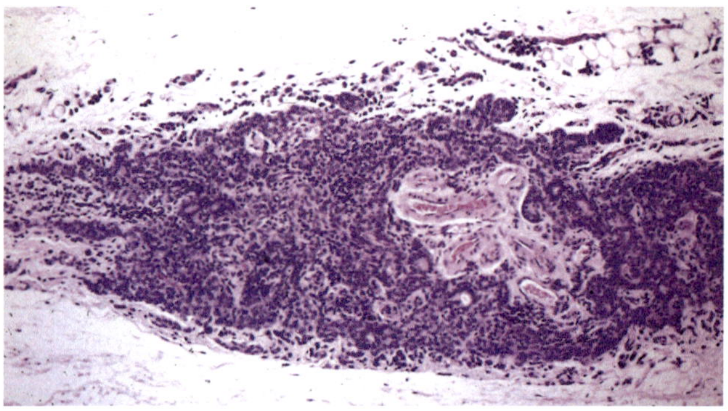

**FIGURE 9-7.** Atrophy of the thymus in a mouse treated with a corticosteroid. Note the loss of cortical lymphocytes and prominent epithelial structures in the medulla. H&E (With kind permission from Springer Science + Business Media B.V [30]).

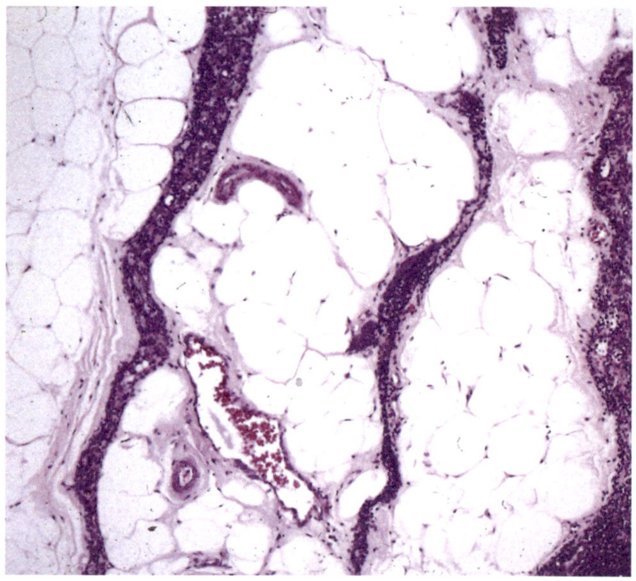

**FIGURE 9-8.** Atrophy of the thymus in a monkey treated with a corticosteroid. Note the loss of lymphocytes and cord-like appearance of the thymus. H&E (With kind permission from Springer Science + Business Media B.V [30]).

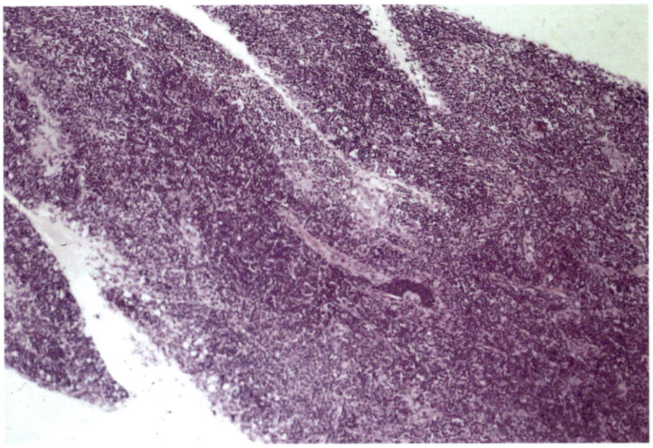

**Figure 9-9.** Indistinct cortex/medulla demarcation in a rat treated with an immunomodulator. Cellularity in the cortex is reduced, and there is some infiltration of lymphoid cells into the medulla. H&E.

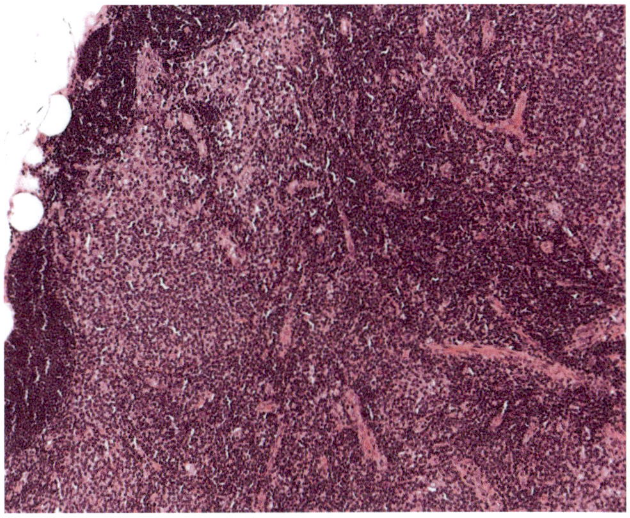

**Figure 9-10.** Medullary hyperplasia in the thymus of a 70-week-old mouse. Note the expansion of the medulla and the thin cortex. H&E.

## 9.3 Lymph Nodes

Antigenic stimulation and the administration of thyroxine produce lymphoid hyperplasia. Germinal centre development has been seen in monkeys treated with some immunostimulants in our laboratories. Antigenic stimulation also has similar effects. Inducible changes in lymph nodes include the following:

- Decreased cellularity in paracortex/follicles/germinal centres
- Increased cellularity in paracortex/follicles/germinal centres
- Cystic atrophy
- Haemorrhagic cystic degeneration
- Plasmacytosis
- Histiocytosis
- Mast cell increase

Specific areas in the lymph nodes can show increased or decreased cellularity [31]. Changes in the cellularity of the paracortex suggest a T-cell effect, whereas changes in the follicles, germinal centres, and plasma cells suggest a B-cell effect [11, 31]. Corticosteroids, cyclosporine, and cyclophosphamide all cause a decrease in cellularity (Fig. 9.11). Cyclophosphamide and triethyl tin decrease cellularity in B-cell areas. Some immunosuppressors decrease the cellularity of T-cell areas while simultaneously promoting B-cell areas and causing the development of germinal centres.

Cystic atrophy, characterised by marked loss of cells from the cortex and medulla and cystic dilatation of sinusoids, has been seen in the abdominal lymph nodes of rats treated with nonsteroidal anti-inflammatory agents for prolonged periods (Fig. 9.12). Haemorrhagic cystic degeneration of mesenteric lymph nodes was noted in rats treated with a novel pharmaceutical agent. The lesion was characterised by loss of cortical lymphocytes and markedly distended sinuses (cystic), which were often lined by one or more layers of erythrophagocytic cells (Fig. 9.13). The affected nodes were markedly enlarged and cystic.

Lymph nodes can show reactive stimulation with adjuvants, antigens, D-penicillamine, and diphenylhydantoin. Reactions can be localised, as seen in the popliteal lymph nodes following adjuvant/antigen load to the footpads of laboratory rodents. The nodes become enlarged and increased in weight, showing increased cellularity of the paracortex/cortex, prominent high endothelial venules, germinal centres, and plasmacytosis. Agents like diphenylhydantoin induce an increase in paracortical cellularity in mice. Interleukins stimulate lymph nodes in mice and monkeys (Fig. 9.14) [32, 33]. Antisense oligonucleotides induce hyperplasia of lymph nodes (hypercellularity) in laboratory animals [34]. Selective immunomodulators cause florid hyperplasia of germinal centres, which can be typical or atypical (Fig. 9.15) [35]. In atypical germinal centre hyperplasia, there is confluence of centres with loss of margins, giving a lymphomatous appearance. Muramyl dipeptide, an immunostimulant, causes hyperplasia of the paracortex and germinal centres and plasmacytosis in mice. Exogenous lymphokines stimulate germinal centres and induce plasmacytosis. Synthetic polysaccharides are lymphocyte mobilisers, which cause lymphocytosis of T or B cells in the circulation. Acute hypoxia preceding death or shock produces degeneration and necrosis of germinal centres. Germinal centres can be a site for antigen presentation (Fig. 9.16).

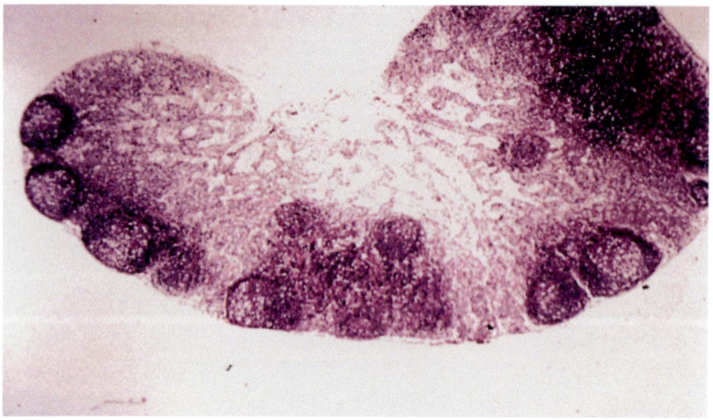

**Figure 9-11.** Decreased cellularity in the paracortex of a mesenteric lymph node of a rat treated with an immunosuppressive agent. H&E.

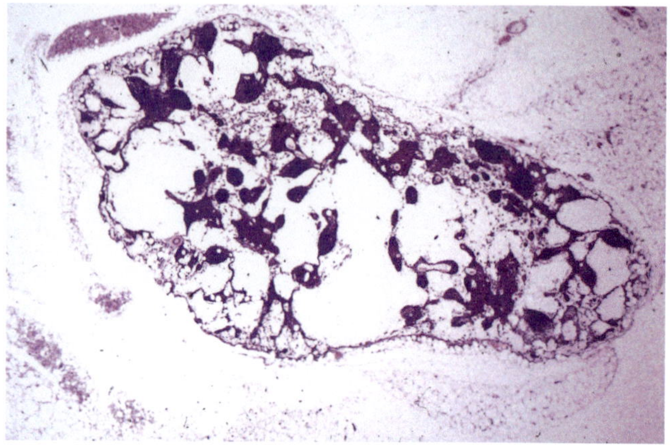

**Figure 9-12.** Cystic atrophy of a renal lymph node in a rat treated with a nonsteroidal anti-inflammatory agent. Note the marked depletion of cells and cystic dilatation of the sinuses. H&E (With kind permission from Springer Science + Business Media B.V [30]).

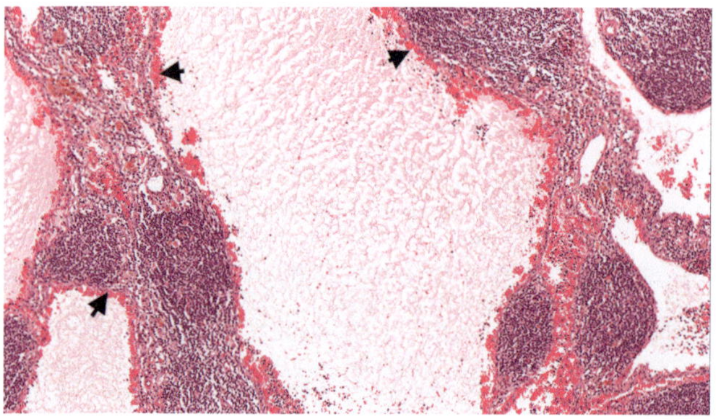

**Figure 9-13.** Cystic haemorrhagic degeneration of a mesenteric lymph node in a rat treated with a novel pharmaceutical agent. Note the cystic dilatation of the sinuses and cysts lined by erythrophagocytic cells (*arrows*). H&E.

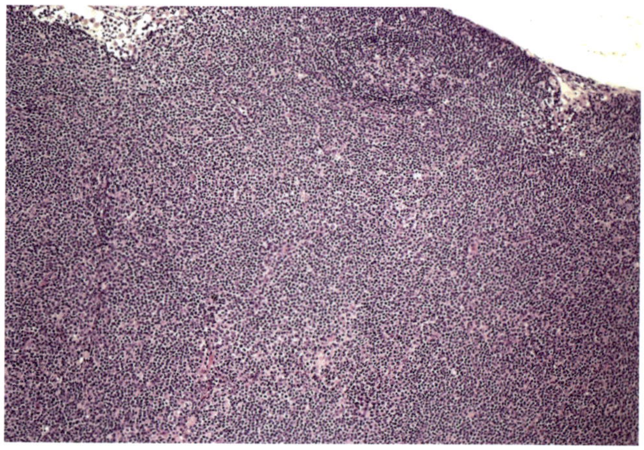

**Figure 9-14.** Increased cellularity in the paracortex of a mesenteric lymph node of a rat treated with an immunostimulant. H&E.

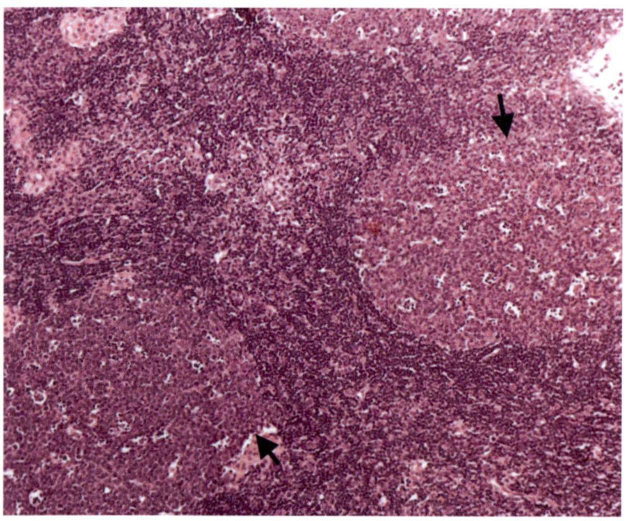

**Figure 9-15.** Increased cellularity in germinal centres of a mandibular lymph node of a rat treated with an immunostimulant. Germinal centres are prominent (*arrows*) and more numerous. H&E.

Lymph nodes can display histiocytosis, plasmacytosis, or mast cell increases (Figs. 9.17–9.19). Vacuolated histiocytes and vacuoles are seen in the sinuses of lymph nodes in rats treated subcutaneously with an oil-based compound (Fig. 9.20). Histiocytosis is seen in the bronchial and mediastinal lymph nodes of rodents that have inhaled dust, silicon, talcum, metal dusts, or quartz (Fig. 9.21). Histiocytes with distended cytoplasm are seen in subcapsular sinuses and medulla. Metallic dust or talcum administered intraperitoneally causes histiocytosis and granulomatous inflammation. Elmiron (pentosan polysulfate, a heparin-like agent) caused vacuolated histiocytes in lymph nodes [36]. Lymph nodes are affected by phospholipidosis and other lipidoses. Florid sinus histiocytosis/proliferation (staining positive with macrophage markers) can be induced in rodents by the injection of particulate materials such as latex particles and certain antigens (Fig. 9.22). Similar lesions are occasionally seen in untreated control rats and mice as a spontaneous change.

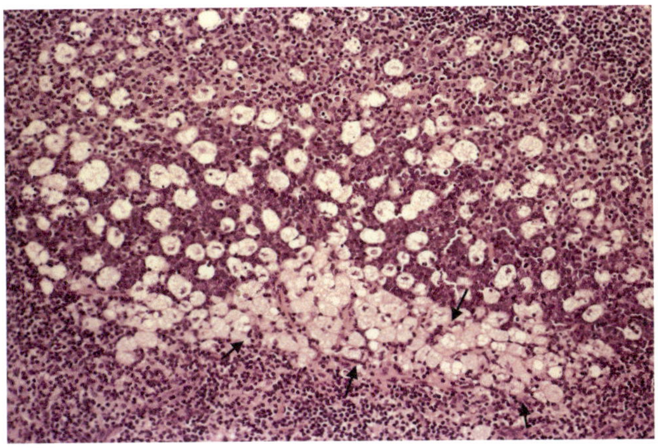

**Figure 9-16.** Accumulation of antigen-presenting cells (cells with clear cytoplasm) adjacent to and within a lymphoid follicle (*arrows*) of the popliteal lymph node of a rat. H&E.

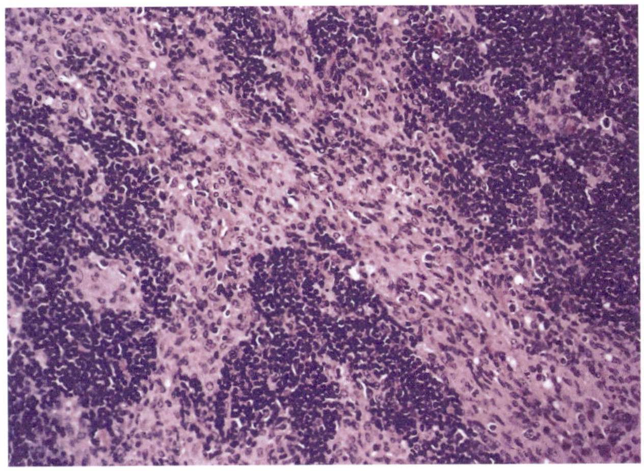

**Figure 9-17.** Histiocytosis in a popliteal lymph node of a rat. Note proliferating histiocytes in the sinuses, stained positive with macrophage markers. H&E.

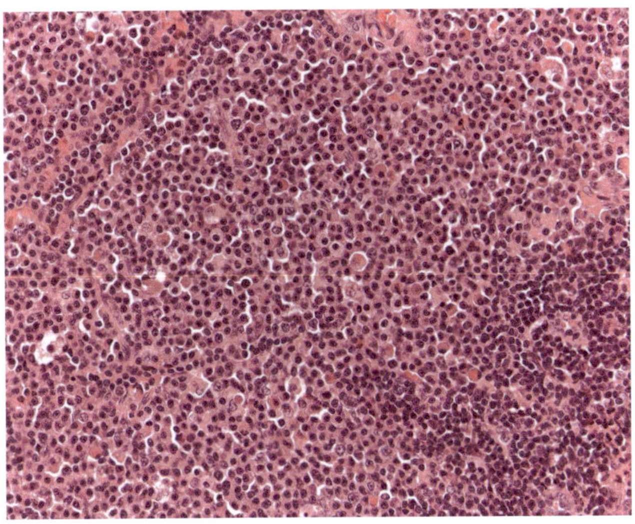

**Figure 9-18.** Plasmacytosis in a mandibular lymph node of a rat. Medullary chords are distended with plasma cells. H&E.

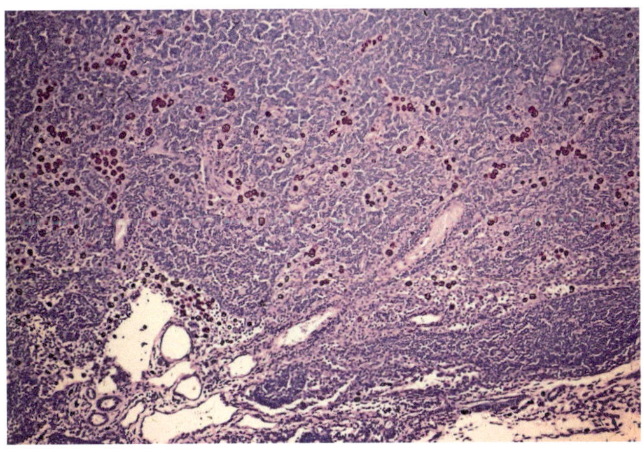

**Figure 9-19.** Mast cell infiltration of a mesenteric lymph node of a rat. Toluene blue (With kind permission from Springer Science + Business Media B.V [30]).

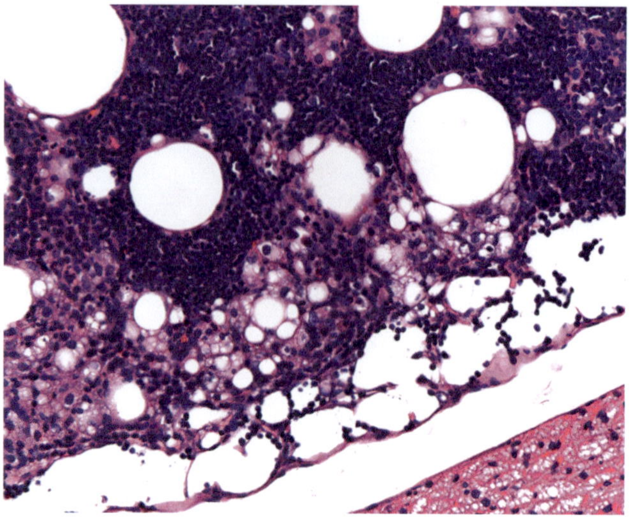

**Figure 9-20.** Vacuolated histiocytes and vacuoles in a lymph node of a rat given subcutaneous injection of an oil-containing compound. Vacuolated histiocytes are seen in the sinuses. H&E.

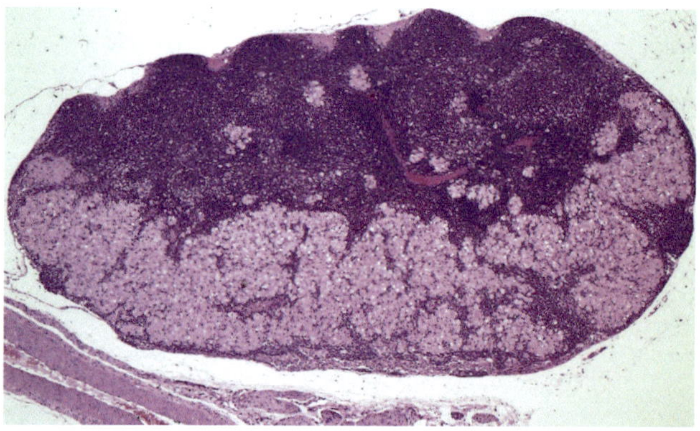

**Figure 9-21.** Histiocytosis in a mediastinal lymph node of a rat, from an inhalation study. Note the sinuses distended with histiocytes with eosinophilic/vacuolated cytoplasm. H&E (With kind permission from Springer Science + Business Media B.V [30]).

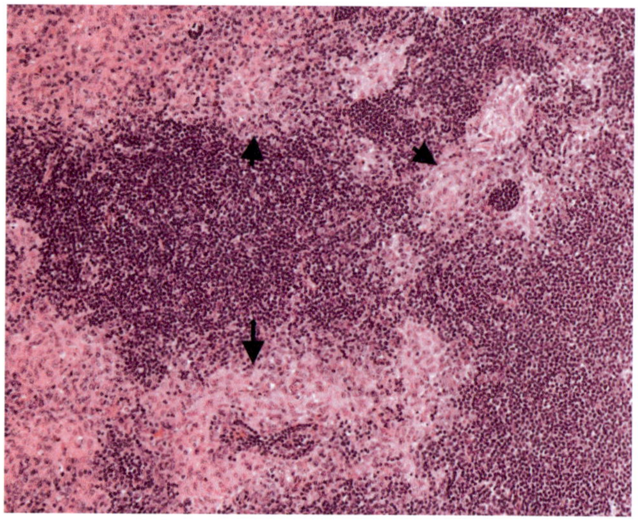

**Figure 9-22.** Histiocytosis in an axillary lymph node of a mouse from a subcutaneous injection study. Note proliferating histiocytes in sinuses (*arrows*). H&E.

Mast cell increases can be induced in the lymph nodes of rodents by agents like calcium channel blockers, cortisone, dextran, hydrazine sulphate, and monocrotaline [37].

Lymph nodes can be sites for pigment deposition involving ink, hair dyes, vegetable dyes, tobacco smoke, and other exogenous materials. Regional nodes can show erythrophagocytosis and/or haemosiderosis in areas of trauma or haemorrhage (Fig. 9.23) [30]. Lymph nodes also can be sites for extramedullary haemopoiesis (erythroid or myeloid) in rodents as a response to haematogenous stress. On rare occasions, as with the use of anticancer agents, lymph nodes can show necrosis (Fig. 9.24).

Changes in the cells of the high endothelial venules can be induced by antigens and estrogens in mice [38]. The affected endothelial cells become cuboidal and hyperplastic.

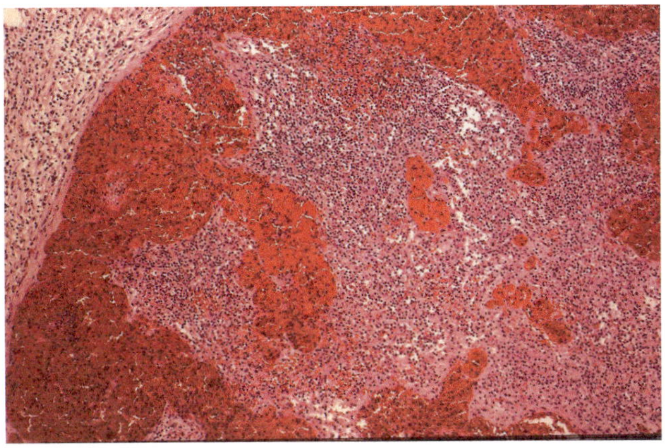

**Figure 9-23.** Erythrophagocytosis in an axillary lymph node of a rat. Note the presence of erythrocytes and macrophages containing erythrocytes in the sinuses. H&E.

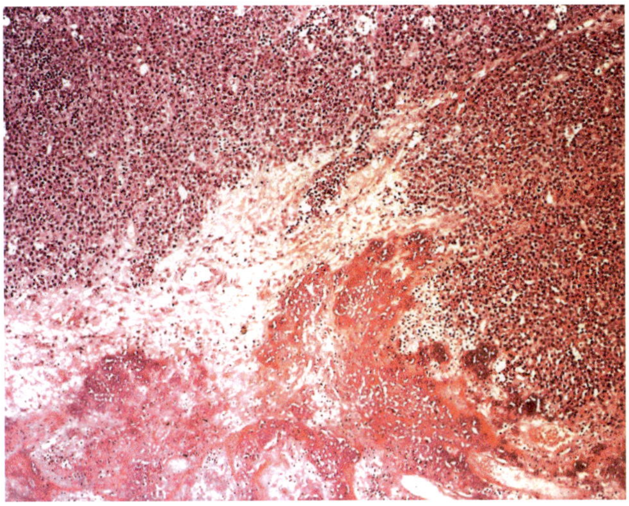

**Figure 9-24.** Necrosis and inflammation in an axillary lymph node of a dog treated with an anticancer drug. H&E.

## 9.4 Spleen

The types of spleens differ depending on species. They can be defensive, as in rodents, rabbits, nonhuman primates, and humans. They can be of the storage type, as seen in dogs, with thick capsules and muscular trabeculae (contractile). Spleens can also be of the intermediate type, as seen in pigs and ruminants.

A variety of inducible changes are commonly seen:

- Increased cellularity in T-cell areas or periarteriolar lymphoid sheath (PALS)
- Increased cellularity in B-cell areas or marginal zones
- Germinal centre (follicle) development
- Plasmacytosis
- Histiocytosis
- Decreased cellularity in T-cell or B-cell areas
- Necrosis/infarction
- Extramedullary haemopoiesis
- Haemosiderosis

In the spleen, the PALS is a T-cell area, follicles are mainly B-cell areas, and marginal zones have T cells, B cells (prominent), and macrophages (Figs. 9.25–9.27). There are interspecies differences in the morphology of the spleen, with reference to the relative prominence of the lymphoid compartments. The defensive spleens seen in rodents have better-developed PALS than those of the storage type, as seen in dogs, in which the PALS is less prominent. Primate spleens have distinct germinal centres and less-developed PALS.

Indomethacin and aspirin given to mice cause reduced cellularity of the PALS. This effect is prostaglandin mediated [39]. Corticosteroids, organotin, tilorone, and azathioprine produce decreased cellularity of T-cell areas (Fig. 9.28) [40]. Anticancer agents given to mice cause necrosis of the marginal zone with cell depletion (Fig. 9.29). Polychlorinated biphenyls, when given to monkeys, result in loss of the germinal centres. Immunosuppressors like cyclosporine cause reduction of T cells and B cells, producing lymphoid atrophy (Fig. 9.30).

Antigenic stimulation results in germinal centre development (Fig. 9.31). Several mitogens and adjuvants cause enlargement of the T-cell and B-cell areas in mice (Figs. 9.32 and 9.33). Macromolecular polymers, methylcellulose, and immunomodulators cause enlargement of the spleen due to red pulp expansion caused by histiocytosis (Fig. 9.34). Erythrophagocytosis, vacuolation, or foamy cells can all be seen on occasion. Marked histiocytosis of marginal zones with evidence of increased phagocytosis of other cell types has been noticed in animals exposed to certain novel biologically active agents (personal observation). Metallic tin causes plasmacytosis of red pulp. Hypersplenism is an autoimmune condition seen in dogs. Immune complex-mediated haemolytic anaemia develops in dogs treated with certain antibiotics, manifesting as increased immunoglobin and C3 levels and the development of immune complexes on erythrocytes. In autoimmune haemolytic anaemia, there is evidence of erythrocyte clumping in blood smear preparations, as well as the presence of fragmentation and the appearance of spherocytes.

A common reason for splenic enlargement in rodents is extramedullary haemopoiesis due to haematogenous stress, as a compensatory response, which can be erythroid or myeloid in character (Fig. 9.35). On rare occasions, increases in

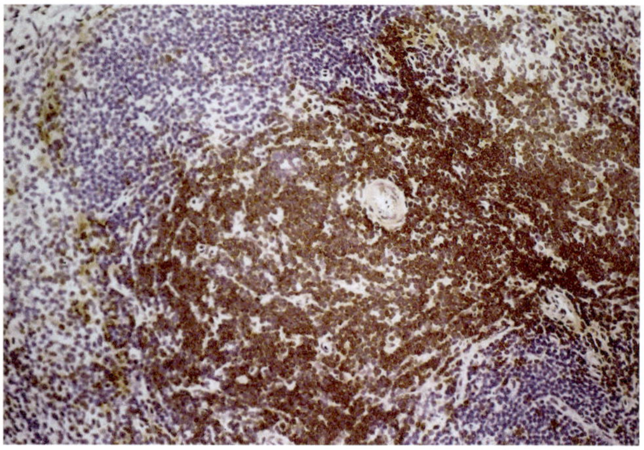

**Figure 9-25.** Spleen of a mouse, showing the PALS with T cells. CD3.

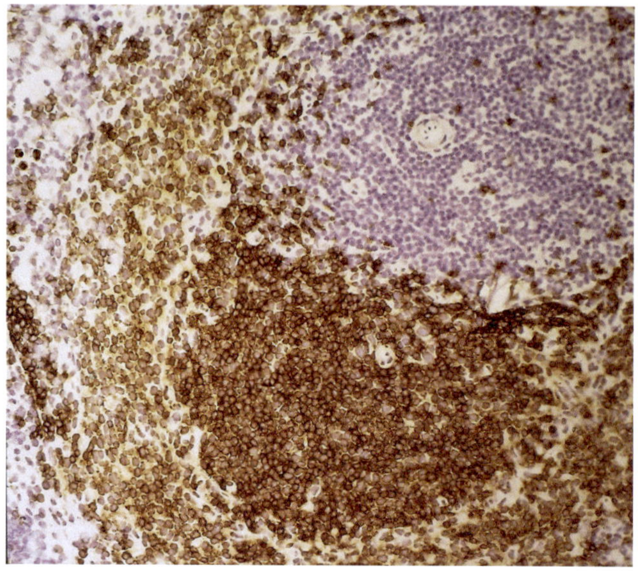

**Figure 9-26.** Spleen of a mouse, showing a germinal centre and marginal zone with B cells. CD45.

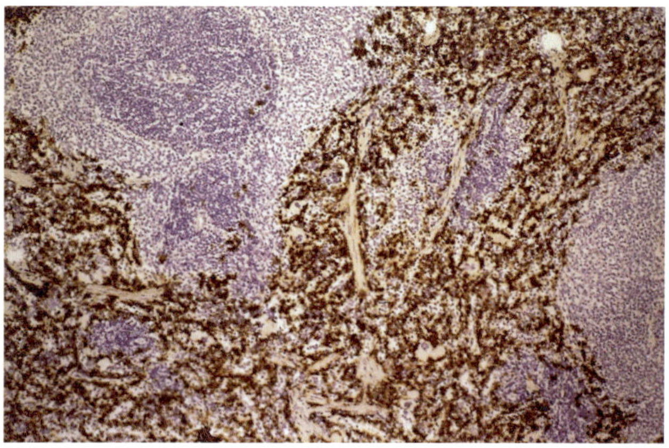

**Figure 9-27.** Spleen of a mouse, showing red pulp with macrophages. ED1.

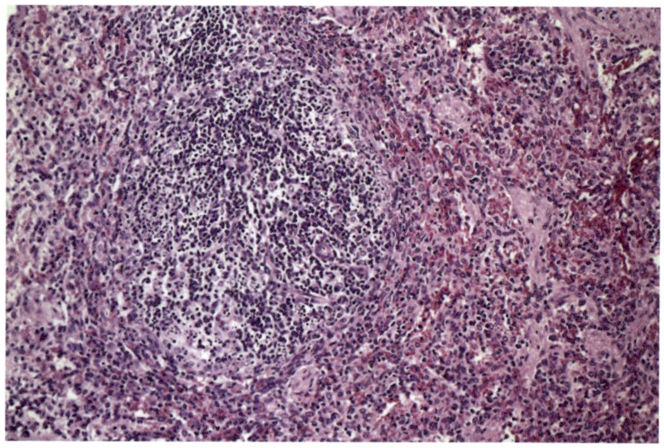

**Figure 9-28.** Loss of T cells in the PALS of a mouse treated with a cytotoxic agent. Note decreased cellularity and the presence of apoptotic cells (pyknotic). H&E.

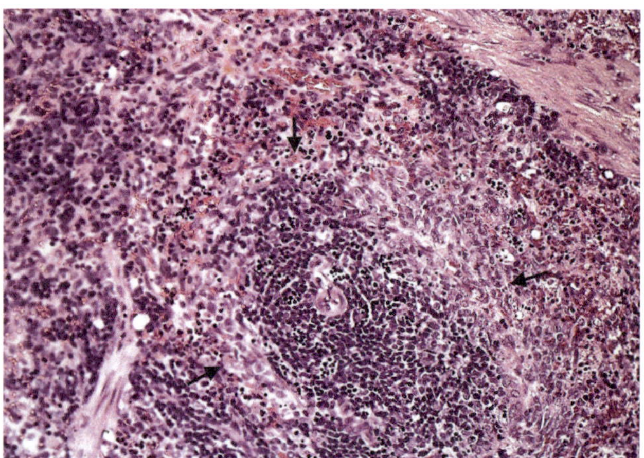

**Figure 9-29.** Loss of cells in the marginal zone (*arrows*) in a mouse treated with an anticancer drug. H&E.

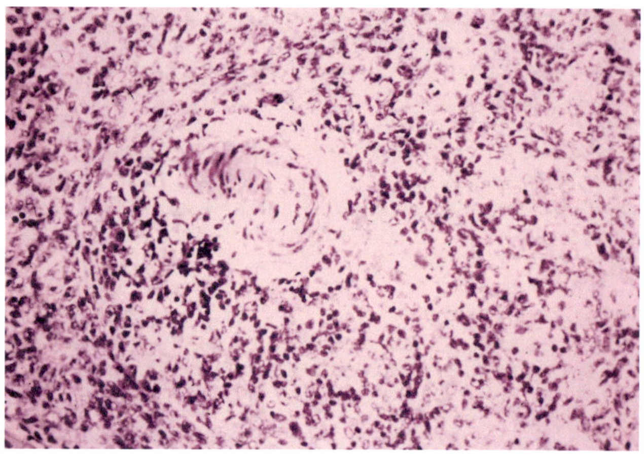

**Figure 9-30.** Atrophy of white pulp in a rat. Note marked loss of cells from the PALS and marginal zone. H&E.

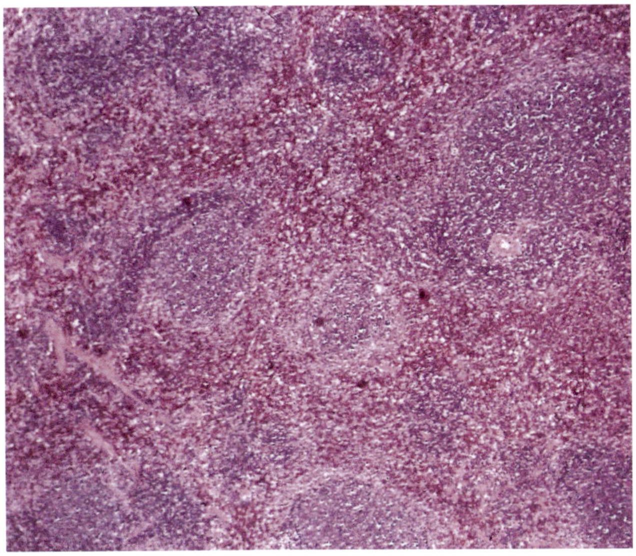

**Figure 9-31.** Increased cellularity and prominence of germinal centres in the spleen of a mouse. H&E.

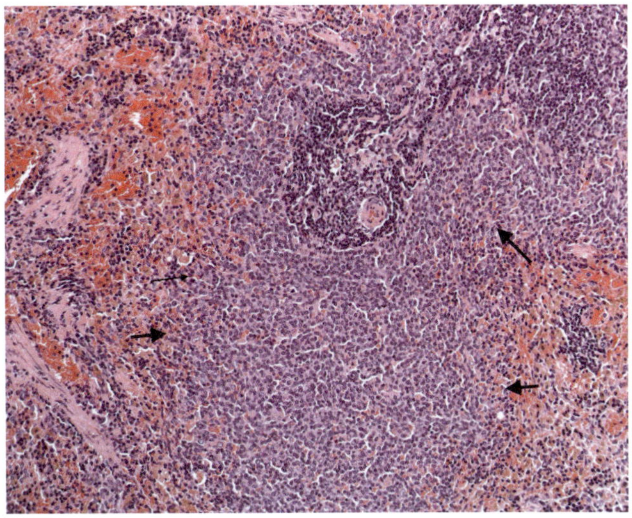

**Figure 9-32.** Increased cellularity and expansion of the marginal zone (*arrows*) in the spleen of a rat treated with an immunostimulant. H&E.

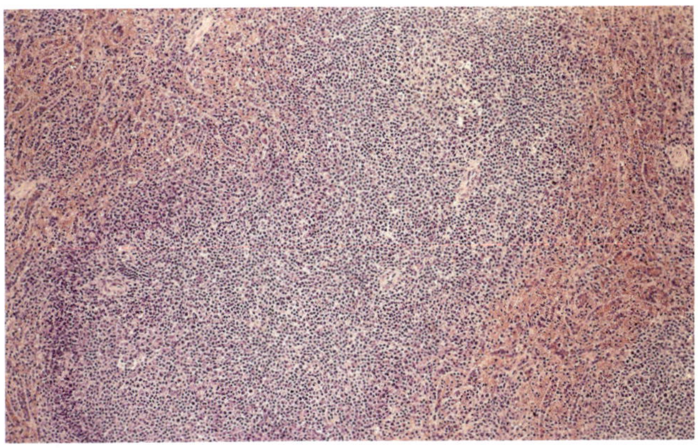

**Figure 9-33.** Increased cellularity of the PALS in the spleen of a monkey treated with a T-cell stimulant. H&E.

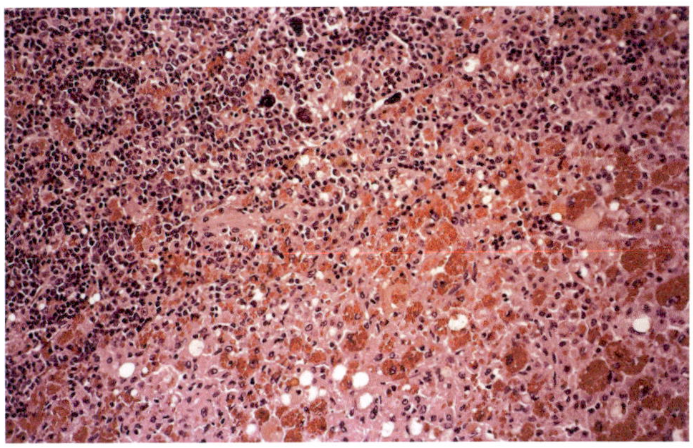

**Figure 9-34.** Histiocytosis in the spleen of a rat treated with a novel pharmaceutical agent. Note the presence of increased numbers of histiocytes in the red pulp. H&E.

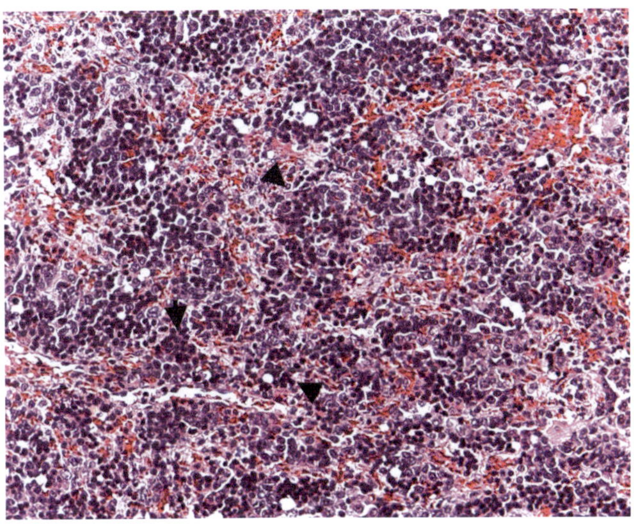

**Figure 9-35.** Extramedullary erythroid haemopoiesis (groups of darkly stained cells), in the spleen of a rat. Note the aggregates of erythroid cells (*arrowheads*) in the red pulp. H&E.

megakaryocytes in the red pulp are observed (Fig. 9.36). Extramedullary haemopoiesis of the spleen seldom occurs in dogs or primates. Certain biological agents (such as colony-stimulating factors) stimulate myeloid cells in the spleen (Fig. 9.37).

Aniline compounds induce necrosis and fibrosis in rats. In some instances, affected areas reveal adipose metaplasia (the presence of adipocyte clusters in fibrotic areas). Necrosis, inflammation, and infarction are produced by ethyl palmate and phenylephrine. Concanavalin A also produces necrosis. Necrosis of germinal centres is seen following shock or anoxia. In our laboratory, certain immunostimulants and thyromimetic drugs have induced capsular fibrosis and inflammation in rats (Fig. 9.38).

Long-term treatment of F344 rats with aniline compounds or dapsone produces necrosis, fibrosis, and tumours, including stromal cell sarcoma (Fig. 9.39) [41, 42]. Immunomodulators and azathioprine produce lymphoma in rodents after prolonged exposure. Vacuolation of splenic histiocytes in the red pulp is seen in rats treated with Elmiron [19].

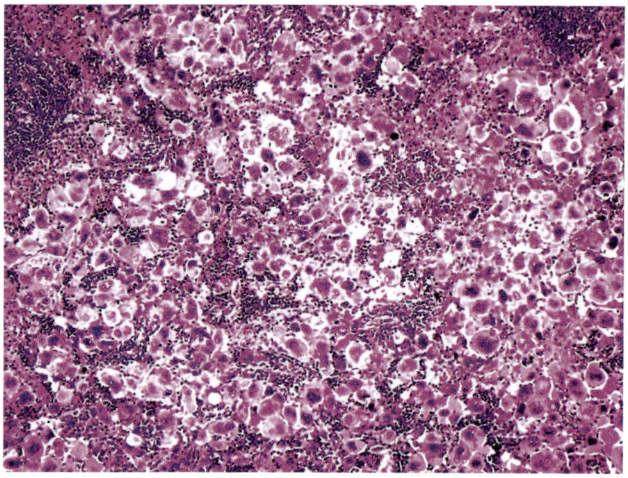

**FIGURE 9-36.** Megakaryocytosis in the spleen of a rat. Note increased numbers of megakaryocytes in the red pulp. H&E.

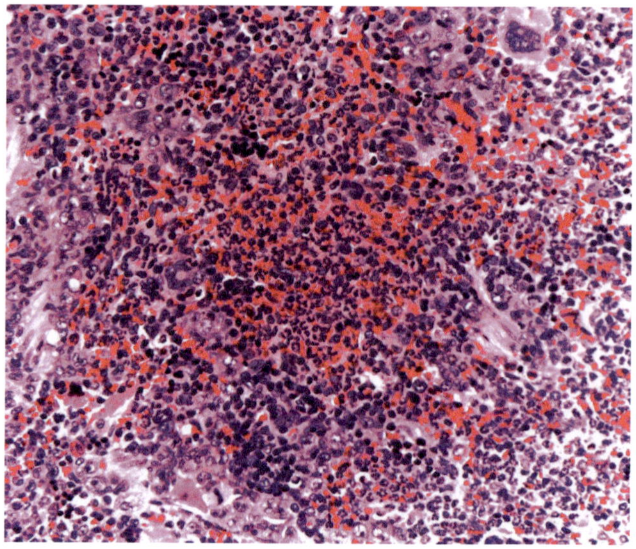

**FIGURE 9-37.** Increased numbers of polymorphonuclear cells in red pulp in the spleen of a rat treated with a colony-stimulating factor. H&E.

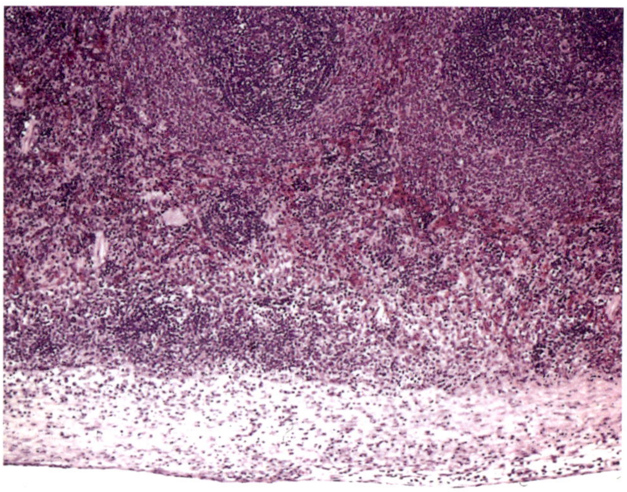

**FIGURE 9-38.** Capsular fibrosis and inflammation in the spleen of a rat treated with an industrial chemical. Note thickening of the capsule due to inflammation and fibroblastic proliferation. H&E.

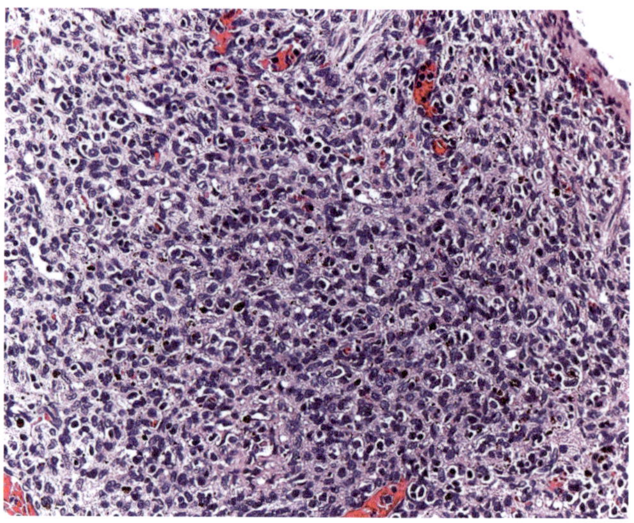

**FIGURE 9-39.** Stromal cell sarcoma in the spleen of a rat. The neoplastic cells are undifferentiated stromal cells. H&E.

## 9.5 Bone Marrow

Resin sections provide better cytologic detail than paraffin sections, and smears are better than paraffin sections for cytologic details. Estimation of the erythroid/myeloid ratio is useful for studying changes in the relative proportions of bone marrow cells. Several types of changes can be seen:

- Decreased cellularity/atrophy
- Necrosis
- Myelofibrosis
- Hyperplasia, erythroid/myeloid
- Megakaryocytosis
- Germinal centre development

In milder cases, decreased cellularity is seen as an increase in adipocytes, which replace marrow cells (Fig. 9.40). This also occurs as an age-related change. In cases of hypocellularity, megakaryocytes are usually spared (Figs. 9.41 and 9.42). Benzene causes bone marrow atrophy in mice. Cytosine arabinoside depletes erythroid cells in rats. Polychlorinated biphenyls reduce bone marrow cell populations in monkeys. Phenylbutazone, when given to dogs, causes bone marrow failure and aplastic anaemia [43]. Chromomycin in dogs depletes all bone marrow cells except megakaryocytes [44]. Cytotoxic anticancer agents and certain antibiotics are known to produce necrosis and haemorrhage (Fig. 9.43). Post-necrotic myelofibrosis is seen in dogs given estrogens, rabbits given saponins, and rodents given anticancer agents (Fig. 9.44) [45].

Increased cellularity is a common response to haematogenous stress and appears as erythroid or myeloid increases (Figs. 9.45 and 9.46). Germinal centre induction is seen with immunostimulants (Fig. 9.47).

Gold compounds produce immune-mediated thrombocytopenia and megakaryocytosis in dogs [46]. Hypersegmented megakaryocytes are seen in dogs treated with oxazolidinone [47]. An increase in mast cell numbers is noted in rats treated with β-aminopropionitrile

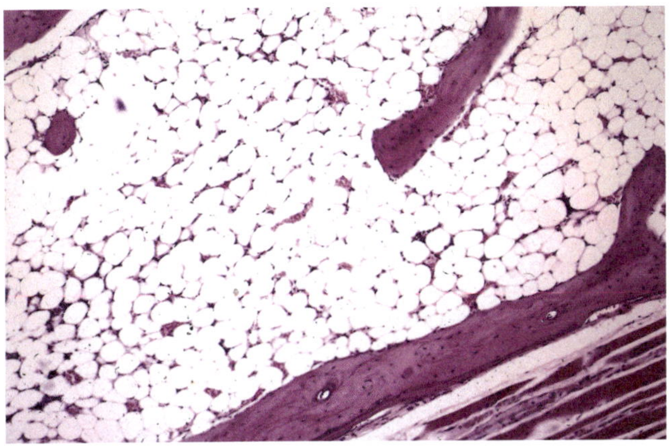

**Figure 9-40.** Reduced cellularity in bone marrow of a dog treated with a cytotoxic agent. Note the reduced cellularity of marrow cells and their replacement with adipocytes. H&E (With kind permission from Springer Science + Business Media B.V [30]).

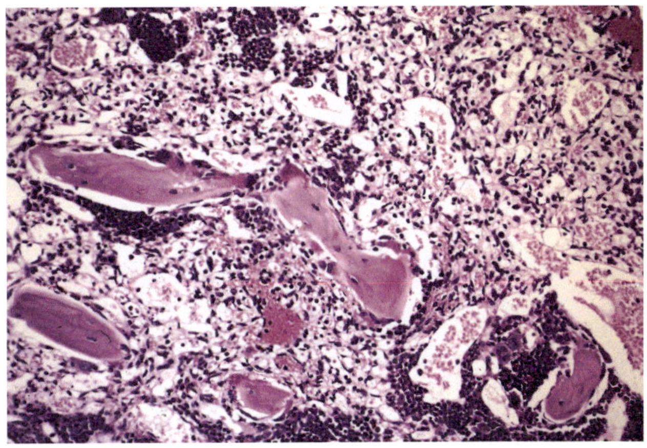

**Figure 9-41.** Reduced cellularity (especially of granulocytic series) of bone marrow from a dog treated with an anticancer agent. H&E (With kind permission from Springer Science + Business Media B.V [30]).

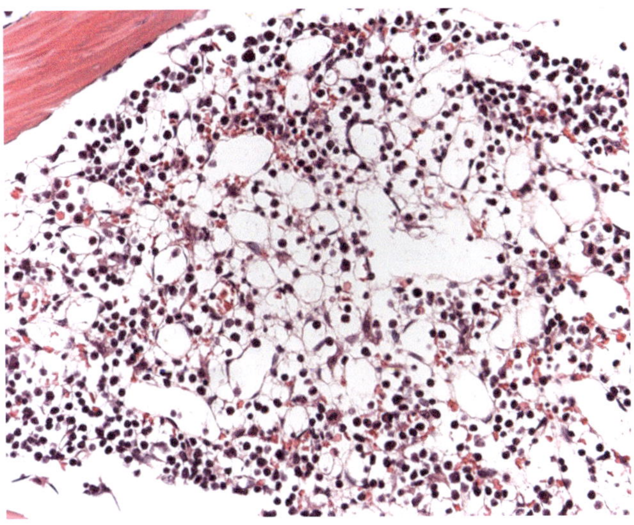

**Figure 9-42.** Reduced cellularity of bone marrow from a monkey treated with a cytotoxic agent. H&E.

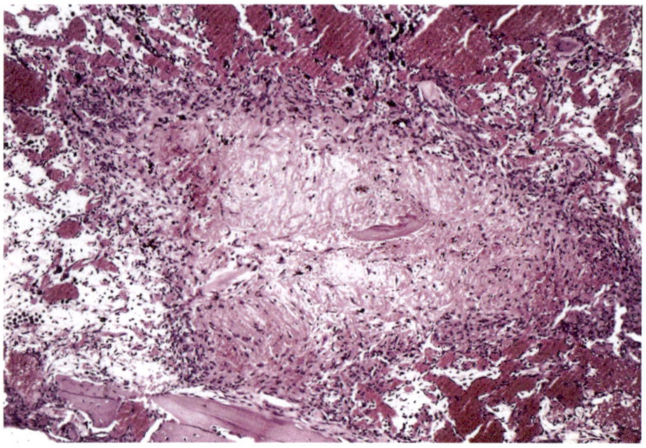

**Figure 9-43.** Necrosis, haemorrhage, and loss of cells in the bone marrow of a dog treated with an anticancer agent. H&E (With kind permission from Springer Science + Business Media B.V [30]).

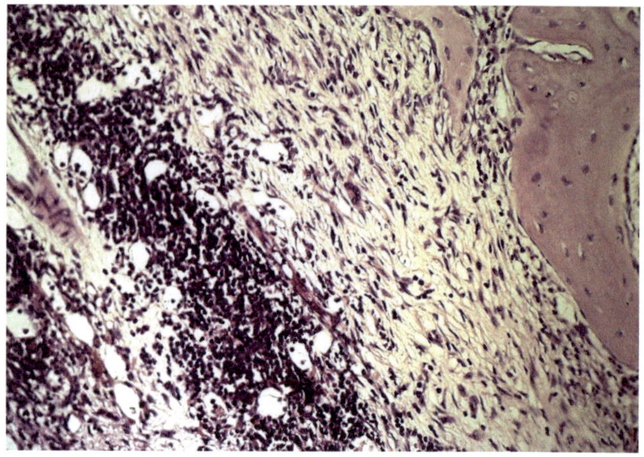

**Figure 9-44.** Myelofibrosis and loss of cellularity in the bone marrow of a dog treated with a cytotoxic agent. Note fibroblastic proliferation within the bone marrow. H&E.

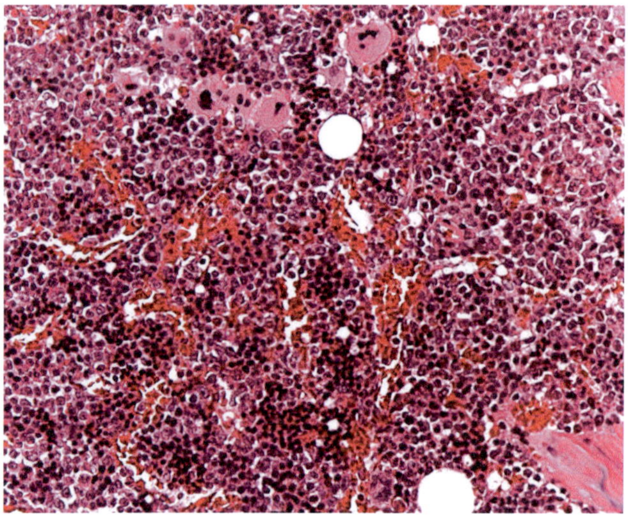

**Figure 9-45.** Increased erythroid cellularity in the bone marrow of a rat. H&E.

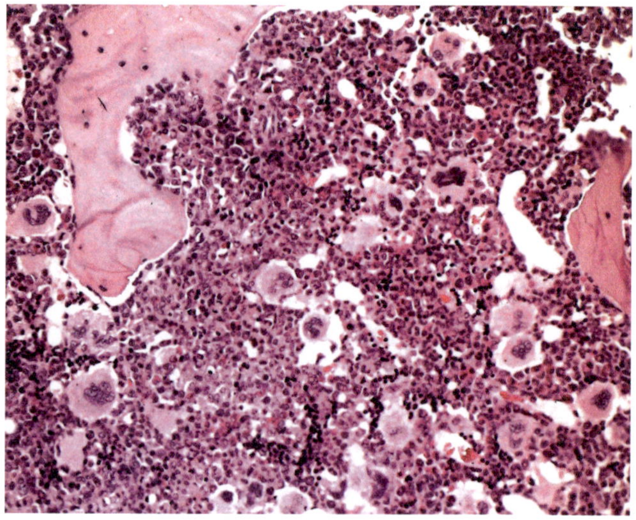

**Figure 9-46.** Increased granulocytic cellularity in the bone marrow of a rat. H&E.

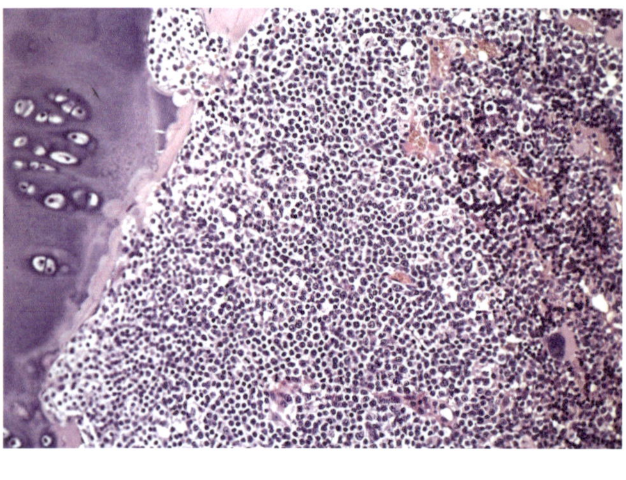

**Figure 9-47.** Lymphoid follicle in the bone marrow of a monkey treated with an immunomodulator. H&E.

and β-mercaptoethylamine [30, 48]. Histiocytosis was noted in rats treated long-term with a xenobiotic, as part of a systemic histiocytosis (Figs. 9.48 and 9.49). Similarly, cationic amphophilic drugs such as chloroquine and chlorphentermine, which cause systemic phospholipidosis, also can affect the bone marrow lymphocytes. Fibro-osseous lesions are a spontaneous age-related finding in the long bones of mice. Its incidence increases in mice receiving long-term treatment with sex steroids (Fig. 9.50).

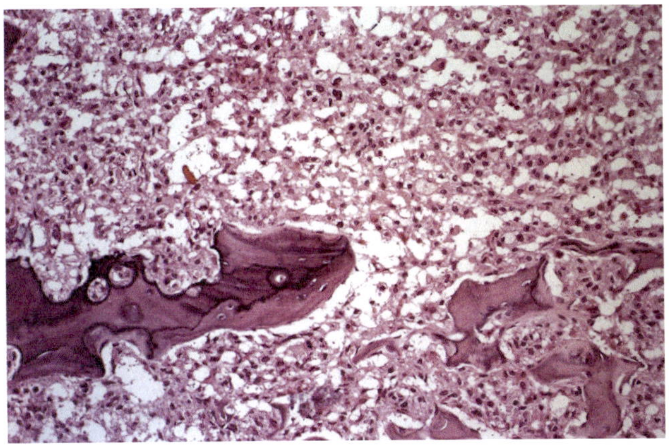

**Figure 9-48.** Histiocytosis in the bone marrow of a rat treated long term with a novel pharmaceutical agent. Note the replacement of marrow cells with histiocytes. H&E.

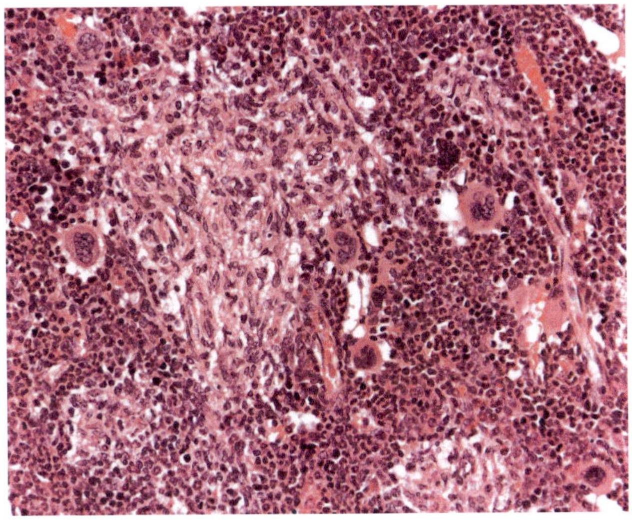

**Figure 9-49.** Multifocal histiocytosis in the bone marrow of a mouse from a subcutaneous injection study. H&E.

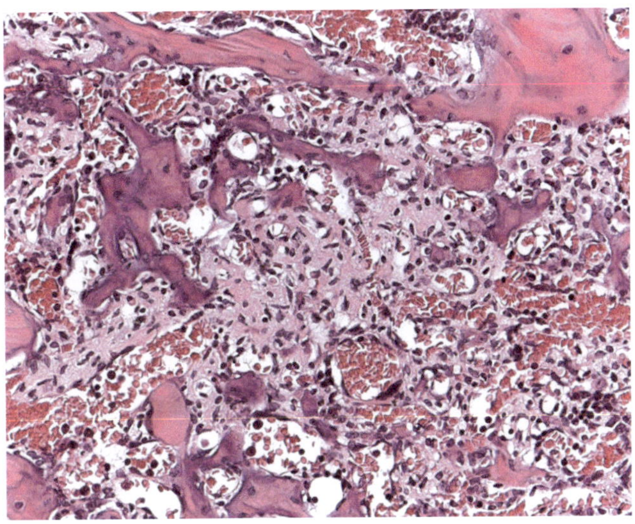

**Figure 9-50.** Fibro-osseous lesion in a 70-week-old mouse. Note the compact bone revealing extension of marrow spaces containing fibroblast proliferation and the presence of bony trabeculae. H&E.

## 9.6 Neoplasms

The lymphoid neoplasms encountered during routine rodent carcinogenicity bioassays are mostly spontaneous. In most situations in which an increased incidence of neoplasms is reported, their direct relationship to treatment is not clearly established. Lymphomas are common tumours in mice, with a greater incidence in females than in males. Their incidence is considerably lower among rats. In routine carcinogenicity studies, the various subtypes of lymphomas are grouped together for assessments. However, treatment-related lymphomas have become more frequent in humans and laboratory animals since the advent of newer immunomodulators, highlighting the need to establish the carcinogenic risk of these agents [49]. In safety studies, immunotyping has been found to be useful for the interpretation of lymphoreticular tumours [50–52]. The toxicologic pathologist often finds the diagnosis of lymphoid tumours somewhat problematic because of their widely variable morphology.

Generally, the lymphoid tumours of rodents are classified based on morphology. Excellent guidelines have been published by the STP and the International Agency for Research on Cancer (IARC) [24, 26]. For practical purposes, the following considerations may be helpful.

The tumours mainly composed of uniform sheets of lymphoblasts are referred to as lymphoblastic lymphoma (Fig. 9.51). The cells are basophilic with scanty cytoplasm and large open nuclei with finely dispersed chromatin. They frequently show a high mitotic index and several apoptotic cells (tingible bodies). Leukemic overspill is frequent. The cells may be of T-cell or B-cell origin (Fig. 9.52).

Lymphocytic lymphomas are rare and consist of sheets of small lymphocytes with compact nuclei and a relatively low mitotic index, but sheets of basophilic cells deface the architecture of the affected organ or tissue.

The lymphoid neoplasm most often encountered in mice (and to a lesser extent in rats) is the pleomorphic lymphoma, in which neoplastic lymphocytes with different morphologic features appear together (Fig. 9.53). In mice, these tumours usually are composed of follicular-centre cells of varying sizes, which are of B-cell origin. They have open nuclei (cleaved or non-cleaved), with polar location of the nucleoli. Cytoplasm can be faintly eosinophilic. Other cells of lymphoid lineage may be intermixed.

Immunoblastic lymphoma is a rare type of lymphoma consisting entirely of immunoblasts. The cells have large vesicular nuclei with prominent chromatin located peripherally and with a large central nucleolus. The cells have abundant amphophilic cytoplasm. Some plasmacytoid cells are also present. The cytoplasm stains strongly pyroninophilic (Fig. 9.54).

Plasma cell lymphoma is diagnosed when the tumour cell population is mostly of the plasma cell type. The cells display an eccentric nucleus with a 'clock face' chromatin arrangement. In such instances, the architecture of the affected lymph node is displaced by the neoplastic plasma cells.

Non-lymphoid tumours encountered include mast cell tumours, myeloid leukaemia, and histiocytic sarcomas (Fig. 9.55).

Fischer rat leukaemia, sometimes referred to as mononuclear cell leukaemia or large granular lymphocytic (LGL) leukaemia, occurs spontaneously among Fischer rats, with a strain-specific high incidence. The spleen and liver are enlarged and often reveal congestion of sinusoids. Isolated cases are encountered in other strains of rats.

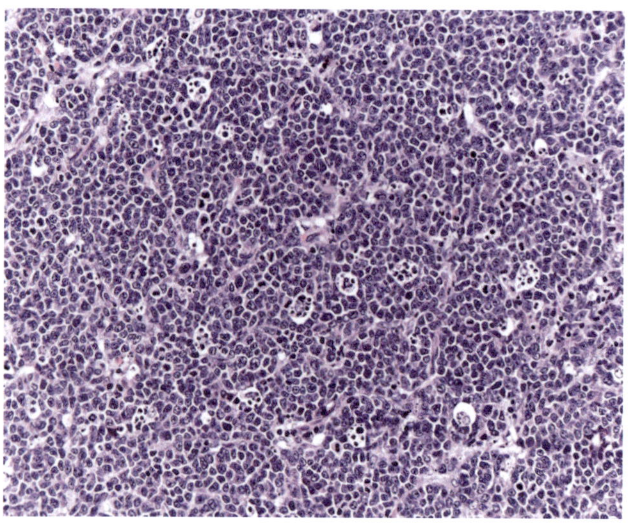

**Figure 9-51.** Lymphoblastic lymphoma in a mesenteric lymph node of a mouse. Note the uniform sheets of lymphoblasts and a few macrophages with apoptotic cells. Tumour cells have a large open nucleus, fine chromatin, and scanty, basophilic cytoplasm. H&E.

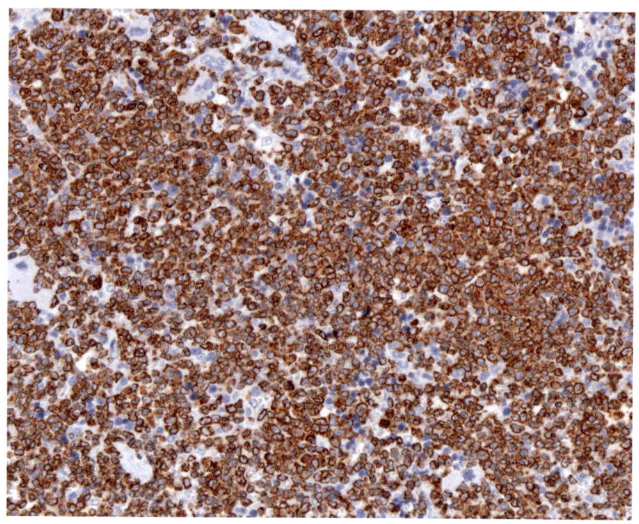

**Figure 9-52.** T-cell lymphoma (lymphoblastic) in a rat. CD3.

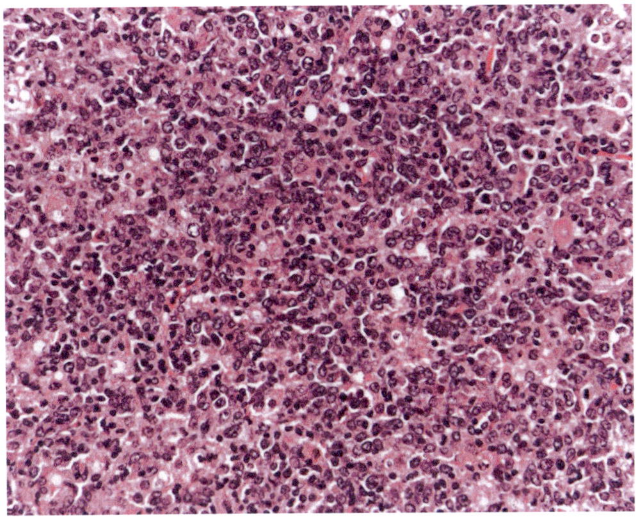

**Figure 9-53.** Pleomorphic lymphoma (mixed follicular-centre cells) in a mouse. Note the mixed lymphoid cells, mainly follicular-centre cells with open nuclei and faintly eosinophilic cytoplasm. H&E.

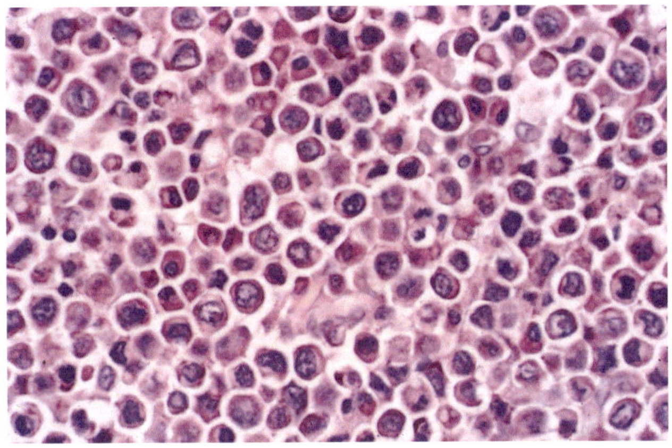

**Figure 9-54.** Immunoblastic lymphoma in a mouse. Note the large cells with open nuclei and prominent central nucleoli, peripheral chromatin, and pyroninophilic cytoplasm. Some plasmacytoid cells are also present. Methyl green-pyronin (MGP).

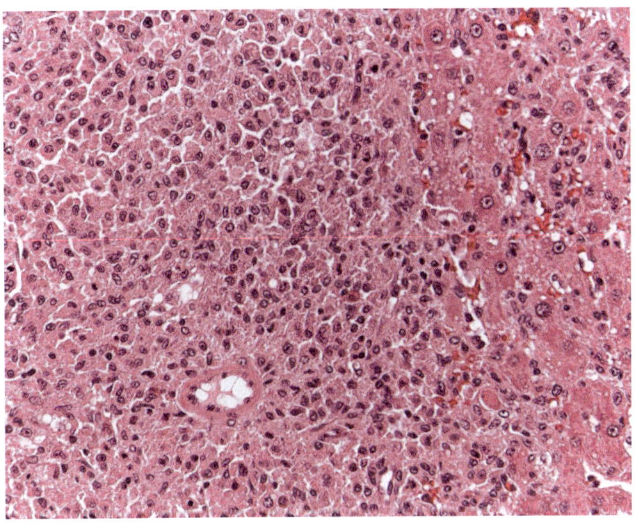

**Figure 9-55.** Histiocytic sarcoma in the liver of a rat. Note the monomorphic cells with eosinophilic cytoplasm, indistinct cell boundary, and compact nucleus. H&E.

## References


1. Ward JM, Erexson CR, Faucette LJ, Foley JF, Dijkstra C, Cattoretti G. Immunohistochemical markers for the rodent immune system. Toxicol Pathol. 2006;34:616–30.
2. Danilenko DM, Wang H. The yin and yang of immunomodulatory biologics: assessing the delicate balance between benefit and risk. Toxicol Pathol. 2012;40:272–87.
3. Cesta MF. Normal structure, function, and histology of the spleen. Toxicol Pathol. 2006;34:455–65.
4. Cesta MF. Normal structure, function, and histology of mucosa-associated lymphoid tissue. Toxicol Pathol. 2006;34:599–608.
5. Pearse G. Normal structure, function and histology of the thymus. Toxicol Pathol. 2006;34:504–14.
6. Travlos GS. Normal structure, function, and histology of the bone marrow. Toxicol Pathol. 2006;34:548–65.
7. Willard-Mack CL. Normal structure, function, and histology of lymph nodes. Toxicol Pathol. 2006;34:409–24.
8. Snyder PW. Immunology for the toxicologic pathologist. Toxicol Pathol. 2012;40:143–7.
9. Holsapple MP, O'Lone R. Juvenile immunotoxicology. Toxicol Pathol. 2012;40:248–54.
10. Elmore SA. Histopathology of the lymph nodes. Toxicol Pathol. 2006;34:425–54.
11. Elmore SA. Enhanced histopathology of the lymph nodes. Toxicol Pathol. 2006;34:634–47.

12. Elmore SA. Enhanced histopathology of the spleen. Toxicol Pathol. 2006;34:648–55.

13. Elmore SA. Enhanced histopathology of the thymus. Toxicol Pathol. 2006;34:656–65.

14. Elmore SA. Enhanced histopathology of the bone marrow. Toxicol Pathol. 2006;34:666–86.

15. Elmore SA. Enhanced histopathology of mucosa-associated lymphoid tissue. Toxicol Pathol. 2006;34:687–96.

16. Kuper CF. Histopathology of mucosa-associated lymphoid tissue. Toxicol Pathol. 2006;34:609–15.

17. Maronpot RR. Enhanced histopathology of lymphoid tissues. Toxicol Pathol. 2006;34:631–3.

18. Pearse G. Histopathology of the thymus. Toxicol Pathol. 2006;34:515–47.

19. Suttie AW. Histopathology of the spleen. Toxicol Pathol. 2006;34:466–503.

20. Travlos GS. Histopathology of bone marrow. Toxicol Pathol. 2006;34:566–98.

21. Elmore SA. Enhanced histopathology of the immune system: a review and update. Toxicol Pathol. 2012;40:148–56.

22. Elmore SA. Enhanced histopathology evaluation of lymphoid organs. Methods Mol Biol. 2010;598:323–39.

23. Kuper CF, Harleman JH, Richter-Reichelm HB, Vos JG. Histopathologic approaches to detect changes indicative of immunotoxicity. Toxicol Pathol. 2000;28:454–66.

24. Haley P, Perry R, Ennulat D, Frame S, Johnson C, Lapointe JM, et al. STP position paper: best practice guideline for the routine pathology evaluation of the immune system. Toxicol Pathol. 2005;33:404–7.

25. Maronpot RR. A monograph on histomorphologic evaluation of lymphoid organs. Toxicol Pathol. 2006;34:407–8.

26. Frith CH, Ward JM, Brown RH, Tyler RD, Chandra M, Stromberg PC. Proliferative lesions of the hematopoietic and lymphatic systems in rats. In: Guides for toxicologic pathology. Washington, DC: STP/ARP/AFIP; 1996.

27. Frith CH, Ward JM, Chandra M, Losco PE. Non-proliferative lesions of the hematopoietic system in rats. HL-1. In: Guides for toxicologic pathology. Washington, DC: STP/ARP/AFIP; 2000.

28. Trainin N. Thymic hormones and the immune response. Physiol Rev. 1974;4:272–315.

29. Lebish IJ, Hurvitz A, Lewis RM, Cramer DV, Krakowka S. Immunopathology of laboratory animals. Toxicol Pathol. 1986;14:129–34.

30. Gopinath C, Prentice DE, Lewis DJ. The lymphoid system. In: Gopinath C, Prentice DE, Lewis DJ, editors. Atlas of experimental toxicological pathology. Lancaster: MTP Press; 1987. p. 122–36.

31. Gopinath C. Pathology of toxic effects on the immune system. Inflamm Res. 1996;45 Suppl 2:S74–8.

32. Herzyk DJ, Bugelski PJ, Hart TK, Wier PJ. Preclinical safety of recombinant human interleukin-18. Toxicol Pathol. 2003;31:554–61.

33. Car BD, Eng VM, Lipman JM, Anderson TD. The toxicology of interleukin-12: a review. Toxicol Pathol. 1999;27:58–63.

34. Henry SP, Templin MV, Gillett N, Rojko J, Levin AA. Correlation of toxicity and pharmacokinetic properties of a phosphorothioate oligonucleotide designed to inhibit ICAM-1. Toxicol Pathol. 1999;27:95–100.

35. Pattengale PK, Taylor CR. Experimental models of lymphoproliferative disease. The mouse as a model for human non-Hodgkin's lymphomas and related leukemias. Am J Pathol. 1983;113:237–65.

36. Abdo KM, Johnson JD, Nyska A. Toxicity and carcinogenicity of Elmiron in F344/N rats and B6C3F1 mice following 2 years of gavage administration. Arch Toxicol. 2003;77:702–11.

37. Takeoka O, Angevine DM, Lalich JJ. Stimulation of mast cells in rats fed various chemicals. Am J Pathol. 1962;40:545–54.

38. Kittas C, Henry L. An electron microscopic study of the changes induced by oestrogens on the lymph-node post-capillary venules. J Pathol. 1979;129:21–9.

39. Koga Y, Taniguchi K, Kuba C, Nomoto K. Thymus-dependent increases in splenic T-cell population by indomethacin. Cell Immunol. 1983;75:43–51.

40. Levine S, Sowinski R, Albrecht WL. T-lymphocyte depletion induced in rats by analogs of tilorone hydrochloride. Toxicol Appl Pharmacol. 1977;40:137–45.

41. Goodman DG, Ward JM, Reichardt WD. Splenic fibrosis and sarcomas in F344 rats fed diets containing aniline hydrochloride, p-chloroaniline, azobenzene, o-toluidine hydrochloride, 4,4′-sulfonyldianiline, or D & C red No. 9. J Natl Cancer Inst. 1984;73:265–73.

42. Ward JM, Reznik G, Garner FM. Proliferative lesions of the spleen in male F344 rats fed diets containing P-chloroaniline. Vet Pathol. 1980;17:200–5.

43. Watson AD, Wilson JT, Turner DM, Culvenor JA. Phenylbutazone-induced blood dyscrasias suspected in three dogs. Vet Rec. 1980;107:239–41.

44. Fleischman RW, Schaeppi U, Heyman IA, Phelan RS, Rosenkrantz H, Ilievski V. Preclinical toxicologic evaluation of chromomycin A3 (NSC-58 514) in mice, dogs and monkeys. Toxicol Appl Pharmacol. 1974;27:259–70.

45. Hoshi H, Weiss L. Rabbit bone marrow after administration of saponin. An electron microscopic study. Lab Invest. 1978; 38:67–80.

46. Bloom JC, Blackmer SA, Bugelski PJ, Sowinski JM, Saunders LZ. Gold-induced immune thrombocytopenia in the dog. Vet Pathol. 1985;22:492–9.

47. Lund JE, Brown PK. Hypersegmented megakaryocytes and megakaryocytes with multiple separate nuclei in dogs treated with PNU-100592, an oxazolidinone antibiotic. Toxicol Pathol. 1997;25:339–43.

48. Takeoka O, Angevine DM, Lalich JJ. Proliferation of mast cells in the bone marrow of rats after feeding Beta-aminoproprionitrile and Beta-mercaptoethylamine. Am J Pathol. 1963;43:639–50.

49. Weaver JL. Establishing the carcinogenic risk of immunomodulatory drugs. Toxicol Pathol. 2012;40:267–71.

50. Frith CH, Ward JM, Chandra M. The morphology, immuno histochemistry, and incidence of hematopoietic neoplasms in mice and rats. Toxicol Pathol. 1993;21:206–18.

51. Ward JM, Uno H, Frith CH. Immunohistochemistry and morphology of reactive lesions in lymph nodes and spleen from rats and mice. Toxicol Pathol. 1993;21:199–205.

52. Rehg JE, Bush D, Ward JM. The utility of immunohistochemistry for the identification of hematopoietic and lymphoid cells in normal tissues and interpretation of proliferative and inflammatory lesions of mice and rats. Toxicol Pathol. 2012;40: 345–74.

# 10 The Nervous System

The importance of correct and adequate sampling of central nervous system in laboratory animals is stressed. Lesions pertaining to neurons such as necrosis, loss, and vacuolation are illustrated. Neuronal changes affecting the cerebrum and cerebellum are included. Distal and proximal axonopathies with examples are described with representative figures. Other changes discussed include demyelination, myelin oedema, and inflammatory lesions in different laboratory animals. Changes occurring in glial cells and choroid plexus are also described. A brief section on induced gliomas in rats is also included.

## 10.1 Introduction

In routine toxicity studies the sampling of tissues from the nervous system is very limited; this is a cause for concern among specialists because it includes only a small number of sections of brain (three to five), spinal cord (one to three), and one peripheral nerve. Reliance is mainly based on clinical signs. However, if there are signs of any involvement of the nervous system, then histopathological surveillance of the nervous system must be increased. A number of good publications with suggestions for routine or expanded sampling protocols for neurotoxicity studies exist [1–5]. On most occasions, the in-life data provide enough information to suggest possible target sites within the central nervous system (CNS) or peripheral nervous system (PNS).

Adequate fixation and preparation techniques are very important for tissues from the nervous system because they are uniquely susceptible to damage and preparation artefacts. Vascular perfusion of at least a proportion of animals provides better samples than routine immersion fixation. The routine haematoxylin and eosin staining provides surprisingly valuable data, although a large number of special staining techniques are essential for additional information on the nature of the lesion. These include silver impregnation methods, myelin staining, stains to differentiate live neurons from dead neurons, and many others [6–8]. Many neuropathologists prefer resin sections because they improve resolution. Electron microscopy is useful for subcellular details. Morphometry is used for quantification of certain types of injuries. Immunohistochemical stains such as glial fibrillary acidic protein (GFAP), neuron-specific enolase, and S-100 are also frequently used. Lesions of the CNS and PNS in rats and mice are well described [9].

The neurotoxic lesions commonly encountered are summarised as:

- Neuronopathies
- Axonopathies
- Myelinopathies
- Gliopathies
- Vascular changes
- Others

When studied, the role of the blood–brain barrier must be remembered to understand the significance of certain changes. It also explains susceptibilities of peripheral neurons as against the protected neurons of the central locations. Affinity of chemicals to specific receptor sites plays a crucial role in neurotoxicity.

C. Gopinath, V. Mowat, *Atlas of Toxicological Pathology*,
DOI 10.1007/978-1-62703-998-7_10, 

## 10.2 Neuronopathy

Neuronopathy describes changes pertaining to the neuronal body, these being the main target of the toxic agent. This, however, can lead to secondary changes, with dendritic and axonal injuries and even demyelination. The loss of neurons and nerve fibres in the CNS promotes local glial reaction. The damaged neurons become more eosinophilic with loss of Nissl granules and become shrunken and often reveal spaces when they are lost (Fig. 10.1). These must not be confused with artefactually produced dark neurons (Fig. 10.2) [10]. Neuronal necrosis usually produces nuclear changes and loss and most frequently causes local glial response. Loss of neurons, satellosis, and gliosis confirm neuronal damage (Figs. 10.3 and 10.4). Cytoplasmic vacuolation

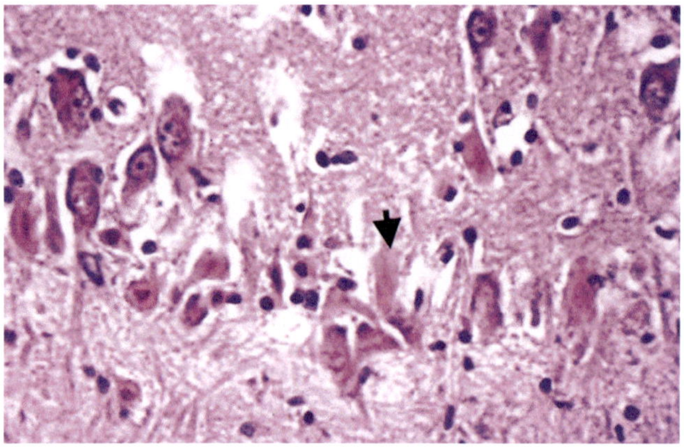

**Figure 10-1.** Neuronal necrosis and loss, hippocampus, in a dog treated with a novel pharmaceutical agent. Note loss of Nissl granules, increased cytoplasmic eosinophilia, and pyknotic nuclei (*arrow*). Haematoxylin and eosin (H&E).

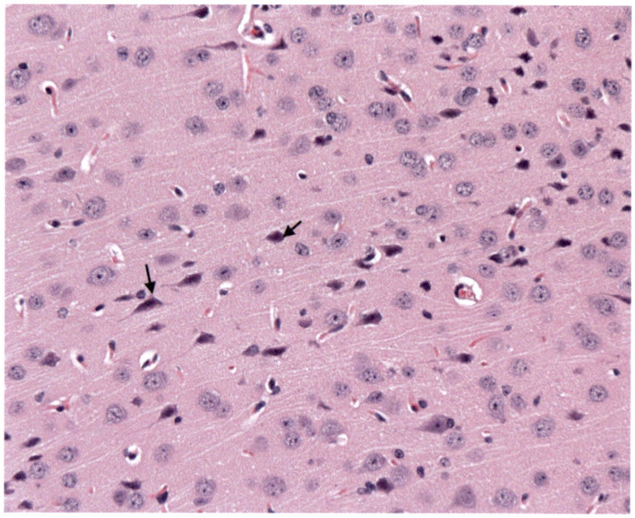

**Figure 10-2.** Dark neurons, cerebrum, in a mouse. This is a preparation artefact; neurons appear shrunken with loss of cellular details and dark (*arrows*). H&E.

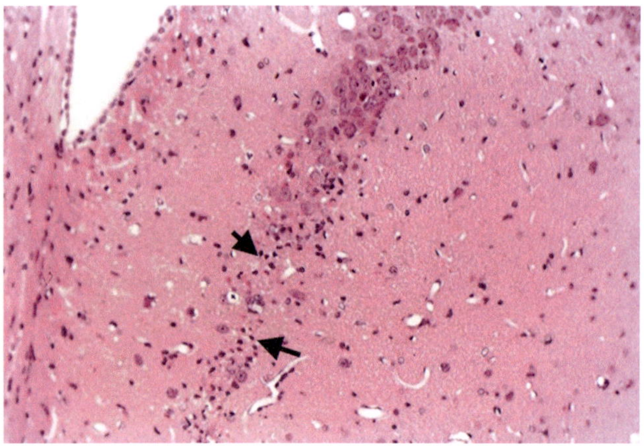

**Figure 10-3.** Neuronal loss and gliosis (*arrows*), hippocampus, in a hamster from an experimental ischaemic study. H&E.

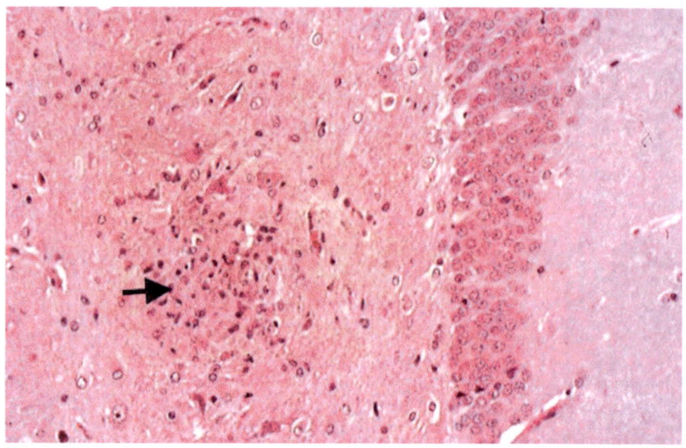

**Figure 10-4.** Neuronal loss and gliosis (*arrow*), hippocampus, in a rat treated with trimethyl tin. H&E.

is also a degenerative change seen in neurons (Fig. 10.5). Postsynaptic changes are also common in neuronopathies. Organic and inorganic mercury are toxic to neurons of humans and experimental animals [11, 12]. They can produce atrophy and loss of cells of the cerebellar granular layer (Fig. 10.6) [13, 14]. Peripheral neurons from dorsal root ganglia are affected in mercury poisoning. Tri- and tetramethyltin cause selective neuronal damage in experimental animals [13, 15, 16]. Inorganic lead causes neuronal necrosis and peripheral nerve fibre degeneration. High doses of pyridoxine to dogs result in neuronal degeneration in dorsal root and Gasserian ganglia. There is initial vacuolar degeneration followed by nerve fibre degeneration and demyelination. Nerve end damage also occurs in vitamin $B_6$ toxicity [17, 18].

Neurons are very susceptible to direct or indirect anoxia and hypoglycaemia. Excitatory neurotoxins cause neuronal damage and necrosis. Local neurotransmitters are released, become excitotoxic, and cause excessive stimulation of the receptors on the dendrosomal surfaces. Glutamate and kainic acid cause acute neuronal damage in experimental animals [19]. β-N-oxalylamino-L-alanine (BOAA) is another excitotoxic substance found in *Lathyrus sativus*, a toxic legume. This produces neuronal damage in monkeys with symptoms similar to lathyrism in humans. 1-Methyl-4-phenyl-1,2,3,6-tetrahydropyridine (MPTP) produces lesions in the neurons of the zona compacta of the substantia nigra in monkeys and humans [20]. This produces neuronal damage in the cerebral cortex, substantia nigra, and corpus striatum. MPTP is used as an agent to produce a Parkinson-like syndrome in monkeys as a model to study the efficacy of anti-Parkinson's drugs.

Anthracycline antibiotics like doxorubicin produce neuronal injuries in the dorsal root ganglia of rats, followed by Wallerian degeneration of sensory fibres. The CNS is spared owing to the blood–brain barrier. Suramin, an antitrypanosomicidal agent, and cisplatin cause damage to dorsal root ganglia [21]. Neuronal injury and vacuolation of the hippocampus major are reported in experimental animals due to several neurotoxins, including some pharmaceutical agents like hydroxyquinoline derivatives. Anticancer agents and certain antimalarial drugs like artemisinin produce damage of the brain stem in laboratory animals [22]. Phenytoin produces loss of Purkinje cells in experimental animals [23]. Taxol, a derivative from the yew tree, causes necrosis of cells in the granular layer of the cerebellum of treated mice (Fig. 10.7).

Phospholipidosis is induced in neurons of the cerebrum, cerebellum, spinal cord, and peripheral ganglia of experimental animals by agents like chloroquine and tamoxifen [24]. Crystalloid and lamellar bodies are observed in the nerve cell bodies by electron microscopy.

Neuronal pigmentation is noticed on rare occasions, without any signs of damage, owing to administration of certain neuroleptics [25] and coloured hair dyes (Fig. 10.8). A fragrant agent, acetyl-ethyl-tetramethyl tetralin (AETT), causes neurolipopigmentation, neuronal degeneration, and demyelination in rats [26, 27].

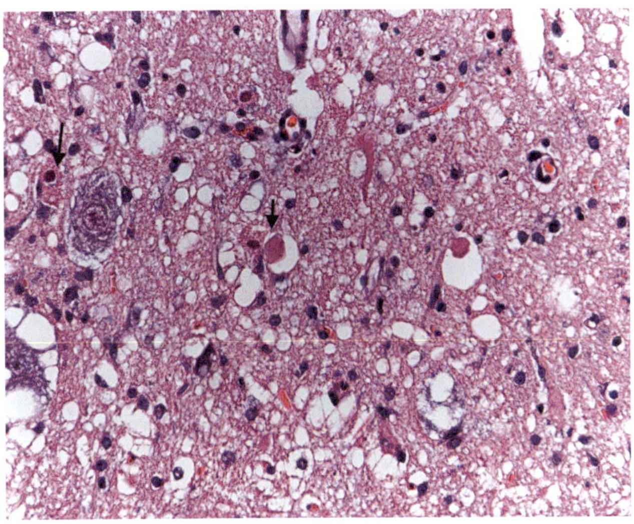

**Figure 10-5.** Neuronal vacuolation and necrosis, spinal cord, in a rat treated with an industrial chemical. Note the cytoplasmic vacuolation. Shrunken eosinophilic neurones without nuclei (*arrows*) are also seen. H&E.

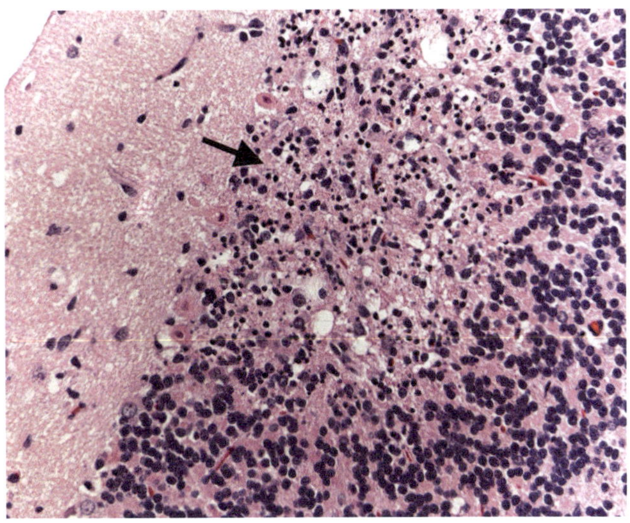

**Figure 10-6.** Necrosis, focal granular layer, cerebellum, in a rat treated with an industrial chemical. A distinct area with apoptotic/necrotic cells (*arrow*) in the granular layer and adjacent Purkinje cells show degeneration/necrosis. H&E.

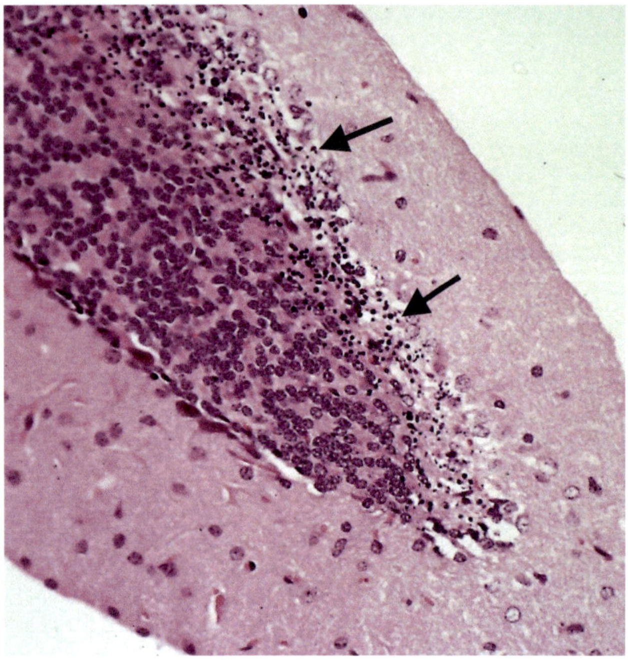

**Figure 10-7.** Necrosis, focal, granular layer, cerebellum, in a mouse treated with taxol. Area of cellular loss and necrosis (*arrows*) in the granular layer is present. H&E.

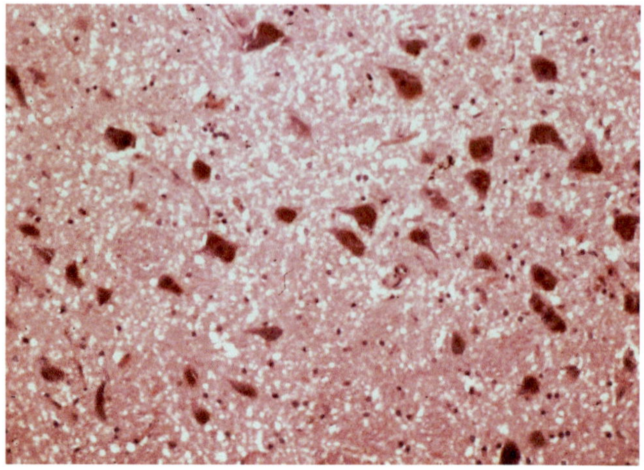

**Figure 10-8.** Pigmented neurones, cerebellum, in a monkey treated with a hair dye preparation. H&E.

## 10.3 Axonopathy

The length of axons and their distance from the cell body make them very vulnerable to injury. Axonal damage can result in secondary demyelination. Myelin spheroids and myelinophages are encountered in axonal degeneration (Fig. 10.9). Distal and proximal axonopathies exist; distal axonopathies are more frequent. Many pharmaceuticals (chloramphenicol, diphenylhydantoin, disulphuram, isoniazid, nitrofurantoin, and vincristine) and chemicals (acrylamide monomer, carbon disulphide, N-hexane methyl-N-butyl ketone, organophosphates, arsenic, polychlorinated benzenes, and thallium salts) cause axonal degeneration in experimental animals [28]. Distal axonopathies start multifocally in the distal segments of the long and large-diameter axons of the PNS and CNS. The clinical signs are delayed and degeneration precedes them. The stoppage of exposure can result in some recovery. The lesions reveal disruption, fragmentation, and distortion of axons (seen better with silver and other special stains) (Figs. 10.10 and 10.11). Variation of thickness and axonal balls is frequent. One-micron resin sections provide better resolution and results (Fig. 10.12).

Organophosphates are used as positive controls in delayed neurotoxicity assays in hens. Teasing of peripheral nerves for nerve fibre analysis is a useful but labour-intensive technique to demonstrate axonal degeneration (Fig. 10.13). Assessment of neurotoxic esterase in the brain and spinal cord is a useful adjunct in neurotoxicity studies. Specific sites such as the cervical cord and optic tract can be sensitive sites (Figs. 10.14–10.16). Distal axonopathy over a period can extend upwards, involving more proximal axons. A distal axonopathy, but mainly occurring in the CNS, is seen in beagle dogs treated with clioquinol. In this case cervical spinal cord dorsal, ventromedial, and lateral columns are affected, along with optic tracts, producing degeneration and secondary demyelination [29, 30].

Proximal axonopathies are rare and can be induced by β-iminodiproprionitrile (IDPN) in rodents. The compound causes impairment of axonal transport and results in proximal axonal swellings of the anterior horn and brain stem [31, 32]. The swellings appear as eosinophilic globoid bodies consisting of accumulations of neurofilaments (Fig. 10.17). This causes atrophy of distal axons and secondary demyelination and gliosis. Proximal axonopathy is noticed in allergic neuritis and experimental allergic encephalomyelitis.

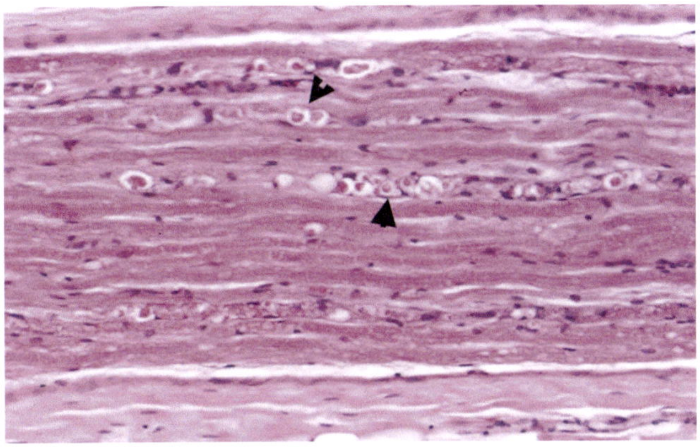

**Figure 10-9.** Axonal degeneration, sciatic nerve, in a rat treated with acrylamide. Affected nerve fibres show focal swelling, myelin breakdown, and digestion chambers with myelin spheroids (*arrowheads*). H&E.

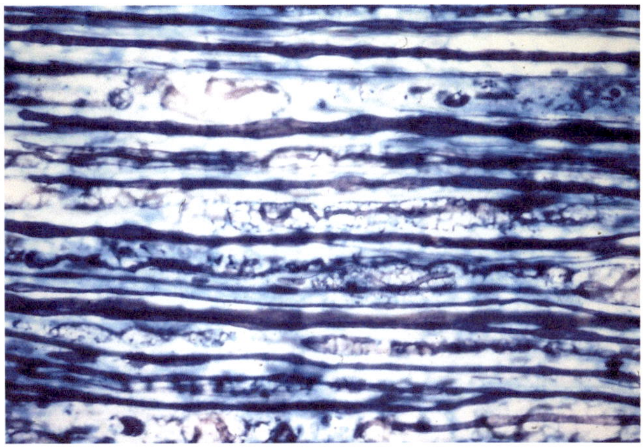

**Figure 10-10.** Axonal degeneration, tibial nerve, in a rat. Silver staining reveals axonal disruption, swellings, and distortion. Bodian with Luxol fast blue (LFB) (With kind permission from Springer Science + Business Media B.V [34]).

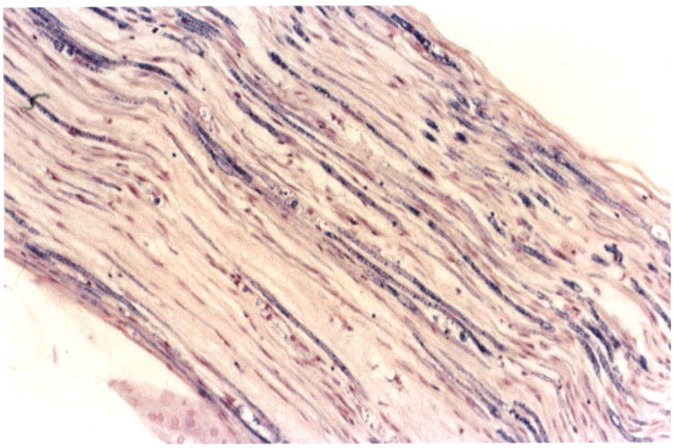

**Figure 10-11.** Axonal degeneration, tibial nerve, in a rat. Focal loss of myelin stain and axonal degeneration are shown. LFB.

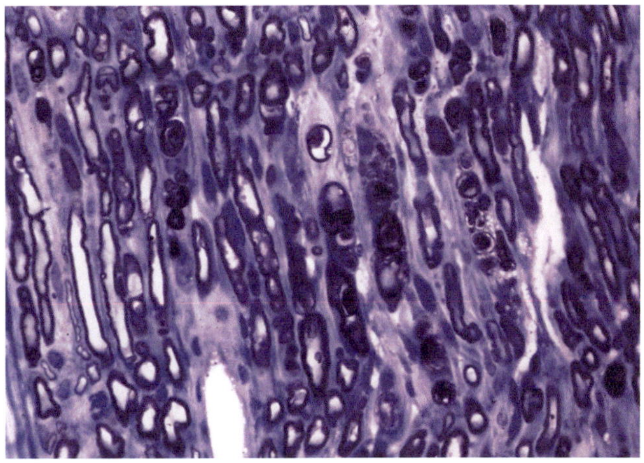

**Figure 10-12.** Axonal degeneration, tibial nerve, in a rat treated with acrylamide. Loss of myelin sheath, swelling, and myelin spheroids in the affected fibres are seen. Resin section, toluene blue.

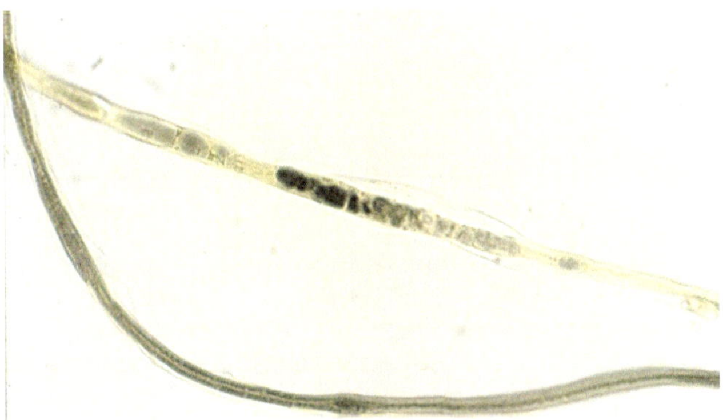

**Figure 10-13.** Axonal degeneration, tibial nerve, in a chick treated with tri-o-cresyl phosphate shows myelin fragmentation. Teased nerve fibre preparation.

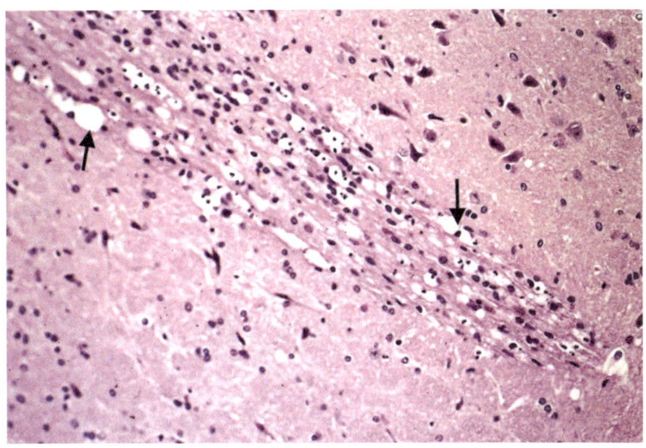

**Figure 10-14.** Axonal degeneration, optic tract, cerebrum in a rat treated with an industrial chemical. Note many swollen fibres (*arrows*). H&E.

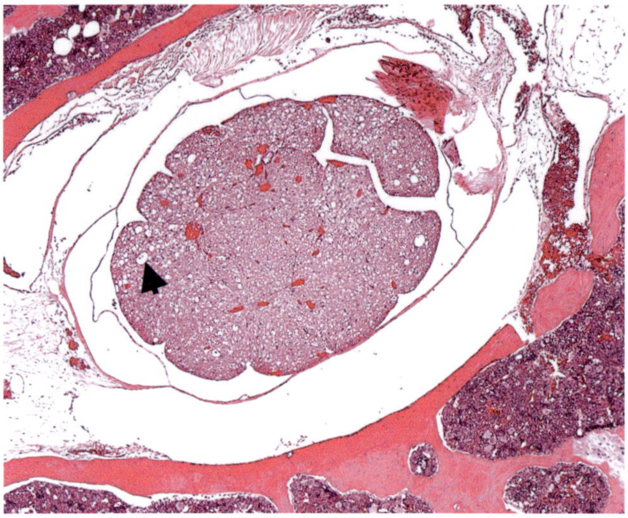

**Figure 10-15.** Axonal degeneration, dorsolateral column, spinal cord, in a mouse. Swollen fibres with larger diameters (*arrow*) represent degeneration. H&E.

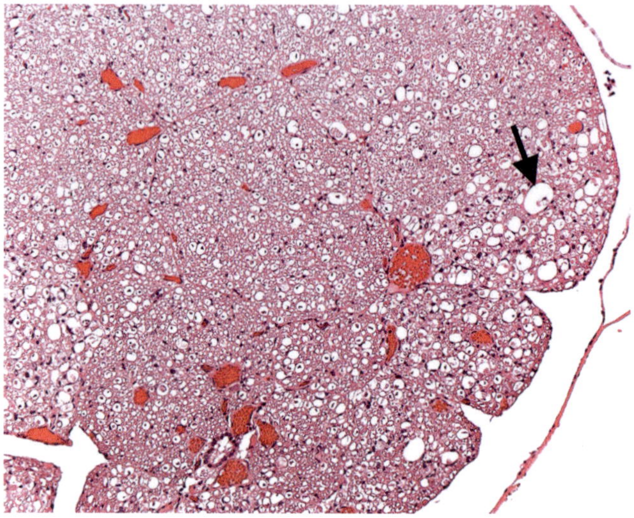

**Figure 10-16.** Axonal degeneration, multifocal, spinal cord, in a rat treated with an industrial chemical. Swollen fibres with larger diameter (*arrow*) represent degeneration. H&E.

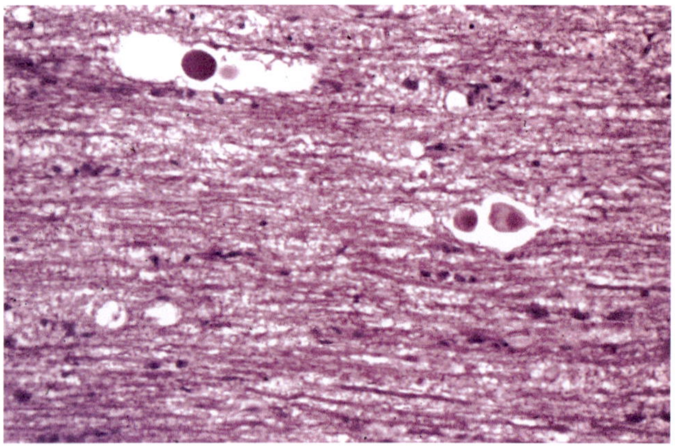

**Figure 10-17.** Eosinophilic bodies/swollen axons, spinal cord, longitudinal section, in a rat indicative of neurofilament accumulation. H&E. (With kind permission from Springer Science + Business Media B.V [34]).

## 10.4 Myelinopathy

Myelin damage can be due to direct action on myelin sheaths or on the cells producing myelin. Hexachlorophene and triethyl tin have a direct effect on the myelin sheath. Myelin damage occurs as splitting of lamellae, vacuolation, and oedema of myelin sheaths (Figs. 10.18 and 10.19). In our experience similar myelin oedema of the CNS has been observed in dogs and rodents treated with high doses of certain agrochemical agents (Fig. 10.20). Vigabatrin produces vacuolation of white matter in the cerebellum, pons, and optic tracts [33].

Myelin damage can be produced by agents such as buckthorn toxin and tellurium affecting Schwann cells or oligodendrocytes. Cuprizone produces injury to oligodendrocytes and causes spongiform myelinopathy in the CNS. Actinomycin D, ethidium dibromide, diphtheria toxin, and lead also produce similar demyelination in experimental animals [34]. The antifungal agent amphotericin produces demyelination and loss of oligodendrocytes in dogs [35]. Isoniazid produces vacuolation of white matter in dogs and rodents associated with damage to oligodendrocytes. Although myelin changes are visible in haematoxylin and eosin (H&E) preparations, myelin stains are used for confirmation. The presence of vacuolation in the CNS must carefully be separated from those produced by artefacts (Figs. 10.21 and 10.22) [10].

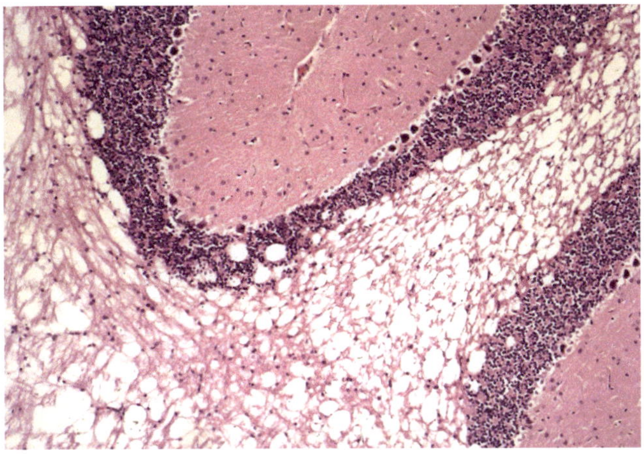

**Figure 10-18.** Myelin oedema, cerebellar white matter, in a rat treated with triethyl tin. An area of marked vacuolation (oval shaped) is seen in the white matter. H&E.

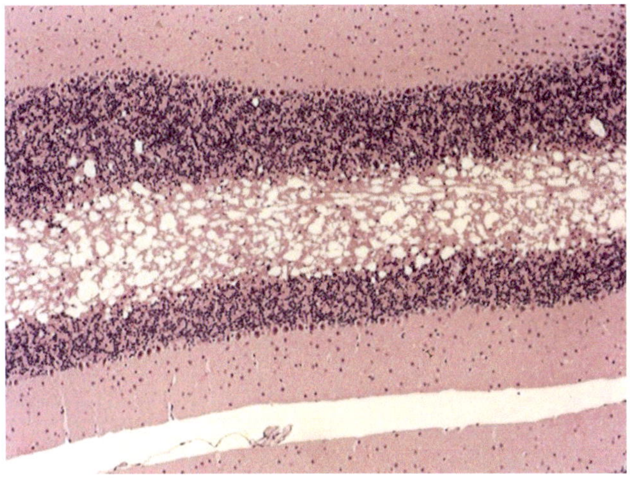

**Figure 10-19.** Myelin oedema, cerebellum, in a rat treated with triethyl tin. H&E.

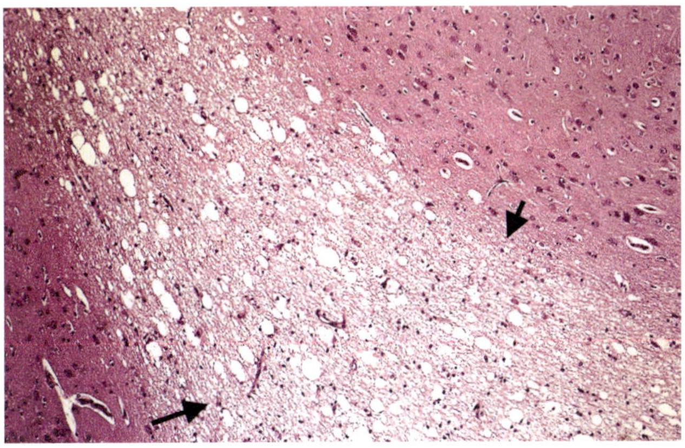

**Figure 10-20.** Myelin oedema, multifocal, cerebrum, in a dog treated with an agrochemical agent. Note vacuolation of white matter (*arrows*). H&E.

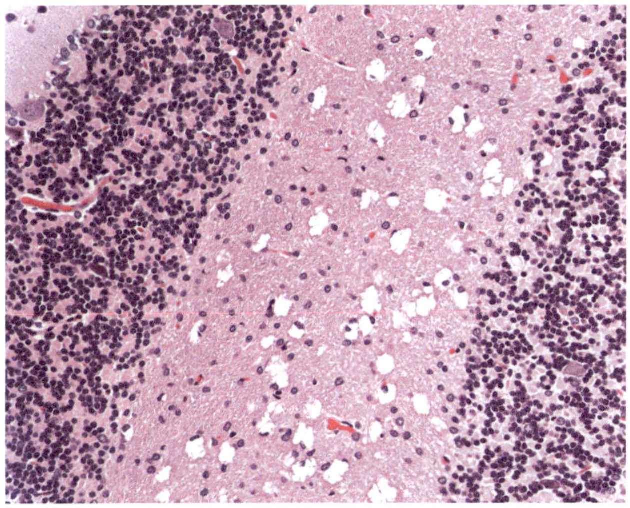

**Figure 10-21.** Artefactual vacuolation, cerebellar white matter in a rat. Note widespread clear vacuolation of white matter. H&E.

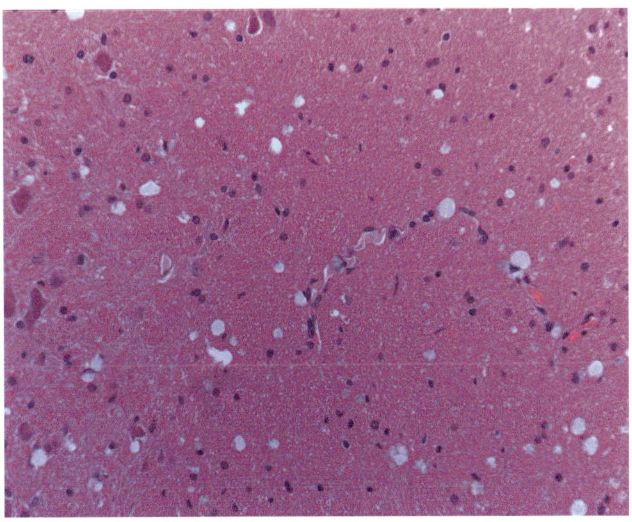

**Figure 10-22.** Mucocele, spinal cord, in a rat. Preparation artefact appears as basophilic vacuoles, widespread. H&E.

## 10.5 Gliopathies

Compounds such as tellurium and cuprizone can induce injuries to oligodendrocytes and produce demyelination and secondary axonopathy. Methionine sulphoximine (MSO) results in accumulation of glycogen in astrocytes. Astrocytic changes occur as multifocal vacuolation [36]. Agents producing astroglial changes include 6-chloro-6-deoxyglucose, 1-amino-3-chloro-2-propanol hydrochloride, certain male antifertility agents, monoamine oxidase inhibitors, and thiamine deficiency [37, 38]. The lesions appear as circumscribed foci of vacuolation in specific regions or nuclei of the brain stem and spinal cord (Figs. 10.23–10.25). Astrocyte changes may be accompanied by neuronal degeneration. GFAP is a useful marker for studying astrocytes (Fig. 10.26). Treatment of rhesus monkeys with a male fertility drug-induced focal vacuolation and encephalomalacia in the brain stem (Fig. 10.27) [34].

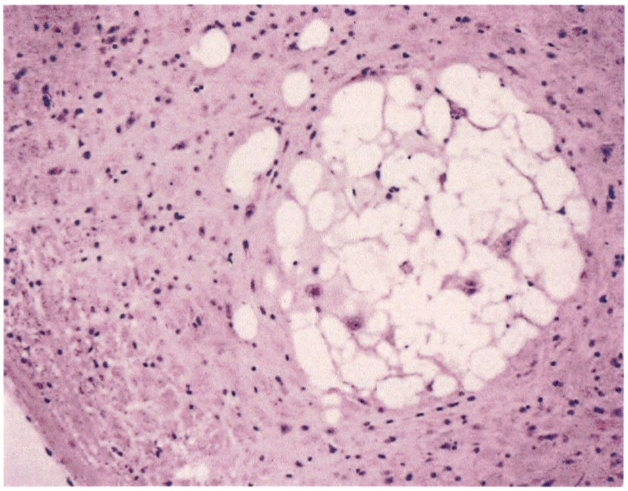

**Figure 10-23.** White matter vacuolation, cerebrum, in a mouse treated with a novel pharmaceutical agent. Note a distinct focus of vacuolation. H&E.

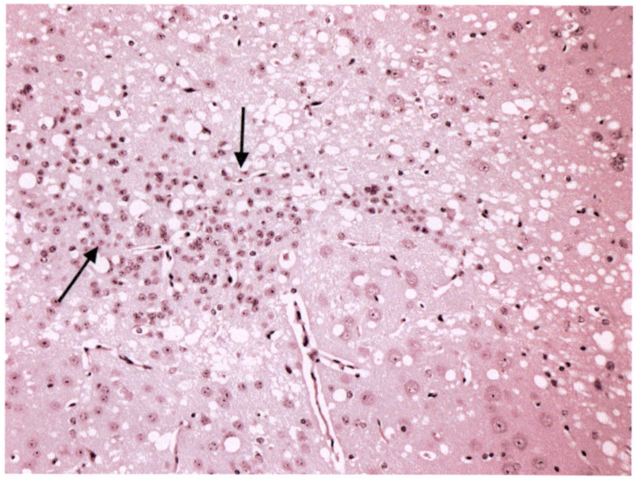

**Figure 10-24.** Vacuolation, gliosis (*arrows*), cerebral cortex, in a mouse treated with an antiviral agent. H&E.

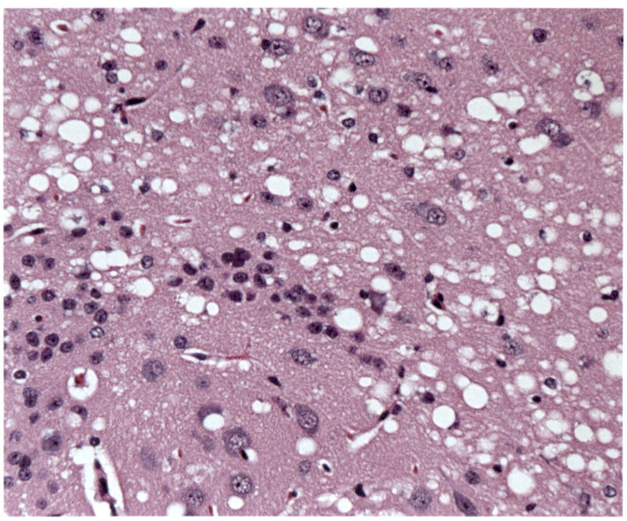

**Figure 10-25.** Vacuolation, gliosis, cerebral cortex, in a mouse. H&E.

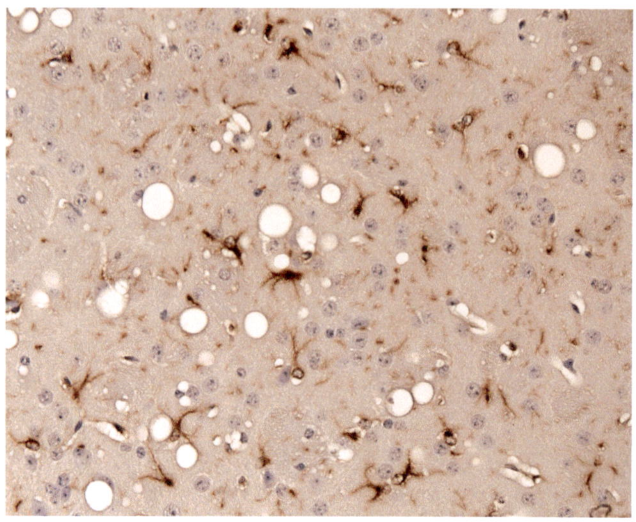

**Figure 10-26.** Vacuolation, reactive astrocytes, cerebral cortex, in a mouse. Glial fibrillary acidic protein (GFAP).

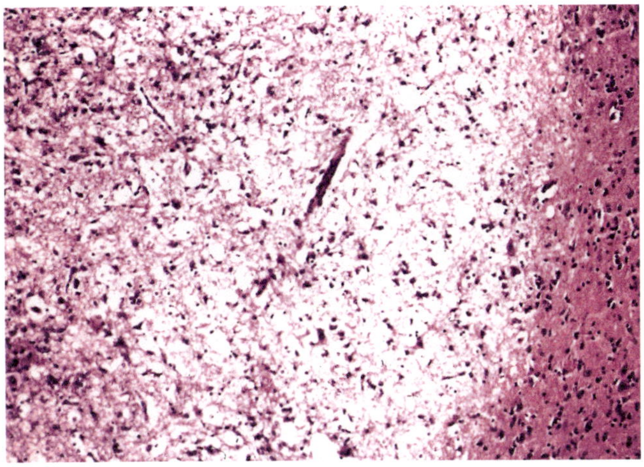

**Figure 10-27.** Vacuolation and loss of tissue, brain stem region, in a monkey treated with a male antifertility agent. Vacuolation, oedema, and loss of tissue in white matter, possibly affecting astrocytes. H&E (With kind permission from Springer Science + Business Media B.V [34]).

## 10.6 Other Changes

Experimental allergic encephalomyelitis (EAE), a model for autoimmune inflammatory disease, can be induced in guinea pigs or rats by injection of whole brain tissue or myelin basic proteins with complete Freund's adjuvant. This produces multifocal perivascular inflammation in the brain stem and spinal cord. In chronic or relapsing types, marked demyelination occurs.

A peripheral neuritis was seen in rodents treated with an immunomodulating agent (Fig. 10.28) [34]. Nonspecific vacuolar encephalopathy, noted occasionally in aged rodents, can be exacerbated by xenobiotic treatments (Figs. 10.29 and 10.30).

Cadmium and lead salts cause endothelial damage, and neonates appear more susceptible. Indium, terbium, thallium, mercury, and triethyl tin cause haemolytic encephalopathies. Lovastatin at high doses produces multifocal perivascular oedema in the brain of dogs with haemorrhage and damage to small vessels [39]. The optic nerve can often be subject to traumatic injury during retro-orbital bleeding procedures in rodents (Fig. 10.31). Multifocal foreign-body granulomata were seen in the brain of rats treated with an industrial chemical (Fig. 10.32), probably as a result of excessive concentration and precipitation.

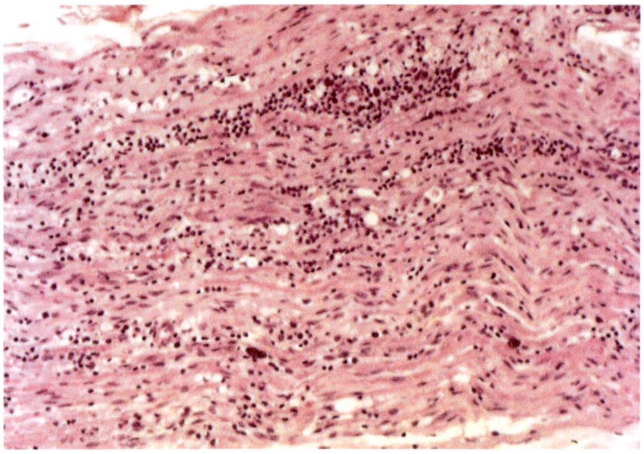

**Figure 10-28.** Neuritis, sciatic nerve, in a rat treated with an immunomodulator. Axonal degeneration and inflammatory cell infiltration (mainly lymphocytic) are present. H&E.

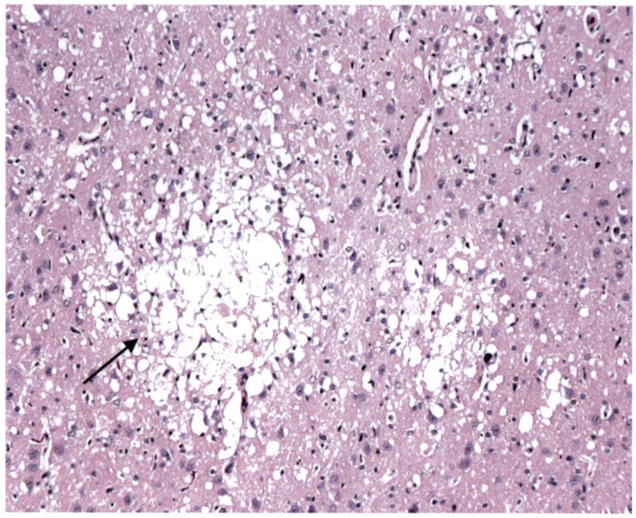

**Figure 10-29.** Vacuolar encephalopathy, cerebrum, in a rat from a chronic study. White matter shows multifocal vacuolation (*arrow*), sometimes at perivascular locations. H&E.

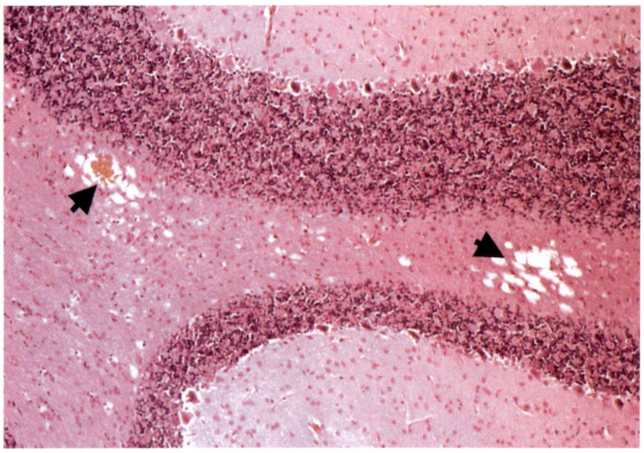

**Figure 10-30.** Vacuolar encephalopathy, cerebellum, in a rat from a chronic study. Cerebellar white matter with multifocal vacuolation (*arrows*) is present. H&E.

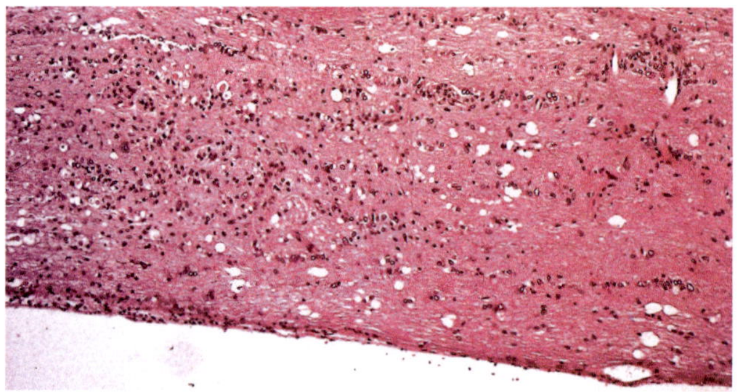

**Figure 10-31.** Traumatic injury, optic nerve, in a rat subjected to retro-orbital bleeding. Gliosis, degeneration, and necrosis are present. H&E.

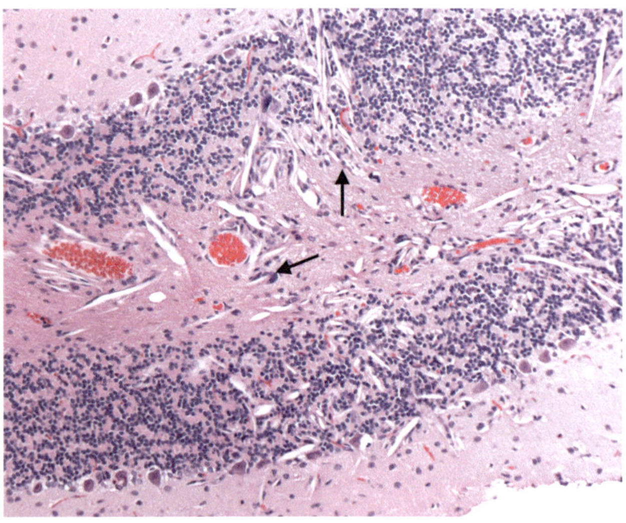

**Figure 10-32.** Foreign-body granuloma, multifocal, cerebellum, in a rat treated with an industrial chemical. Note deposition of clefts and granuloma (*arrows*) in white matter. H&E.

### 10.6.1 Choroid Plexus Vacuolation

Disobutamide given to monkeys results in marked vacuolation of cells of the choroid plexus, associated with increases in drug concentration. Clioquinol, triparanol, and chlorcyclizine also produce vacuolation of cells of the choroid plexus [40]. In these cases evidence of phospholipidosis was noted. The antitrypanosomal agent suramin and an immunomodulating agent produce vacuolation of cells of the choroid plexus. More recently a number of polyethylene glycol (PEG)-linked molecules, when given intravenously to monkeys, have resulted in varying degrees of vacuolation of cells of the choroid plexus (Fig. 10.33). In severe cases these vacuolar changes of the choroid plexus were associated with the presence of vacuolated macrophages in the lamina propria (Fig. 10.34). The change is attributed to PEG rather than to the active molecule in all cases.

### 10.6.2 CNS Tumours

Astrocytomas in rats are the only reported instance of treatment-related brain tumours in regulatory toxicity studies. Only a very small number of agents produce these, including acrylonitrile, ethylene oxide, and a few others. In most cases the increase in the incidence is small. In the rat, astrocytomas are the commonest spontaneous tumour of the brain (Figs. 10.35 and 10.36) [41]. Microscopically they appear as poorly circumscribed tumours with indistinct tumour borders, consisting of monomorphic cells with indistinct cell borders, eosinophilic cytoplasm, and ovoid nuclei. These rodent tumours behave somewhat differently than human or large animal astrocytomas because they seldom show any clear features of true astrocytomas, such as positivity for GFAP or other gliofibrillary properties of astrocytomas. Recent reports suggest that rat astrocytomas stain negatively with GFAP and have shown some features of microglial cells and some have shown staining features of histiocytic and lymphoid cells. So, at this juncture, they lack the specificity of true astrocytes, which suggests possible microglial or histiocytic origins [42].

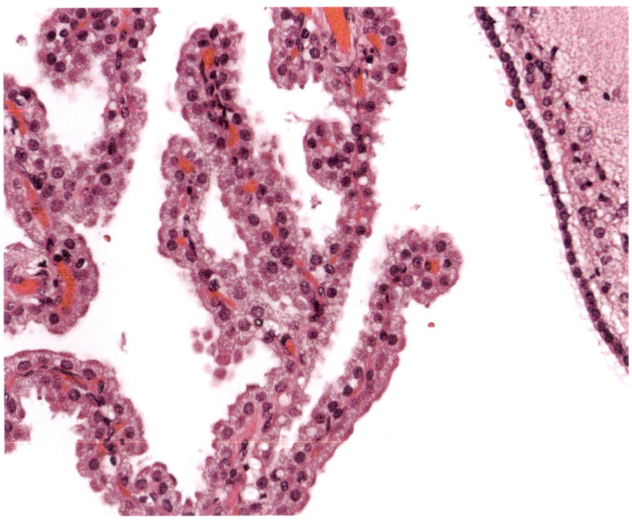

**Figure 10-33.** Vacuolation of choroid plexus, epithelium, in a monkey given a polyethylene-linked protein. Note intracytoplasmic vacuolation of the lining epithelium. H&E.

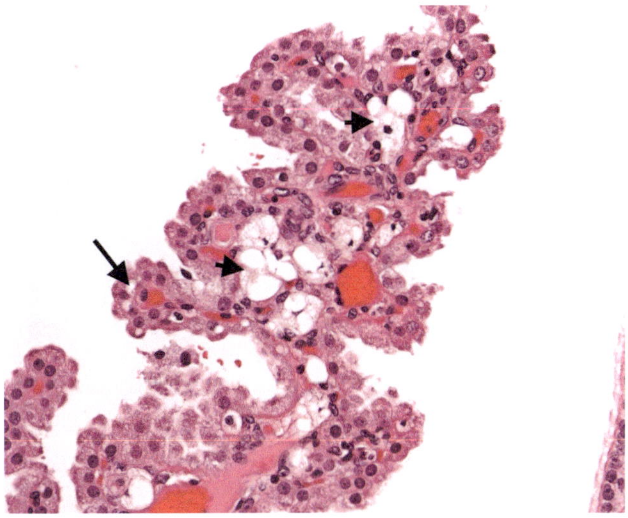

**Figure 10-34.** Vacuolation of choroid plexus, epithelium, in a monkey treated with a polyethylene glycol (PEG)-linked agent. Note intracytoplasmic vacuolation of the epithelium and also presence of vacuolated macrophages (*arrows*) in lamina propria. H&E.

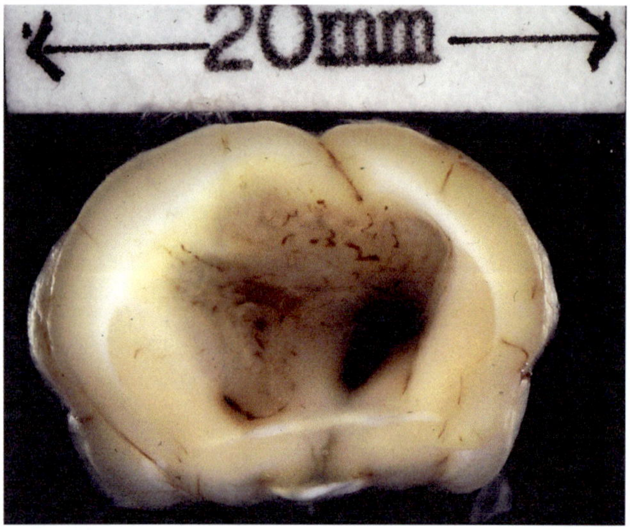


**FIGURE 10-35.** Glioma, cerebrum, in a rat. A gelatinous mass with dark brown discolouration is due to necrosis and haemorrhage.

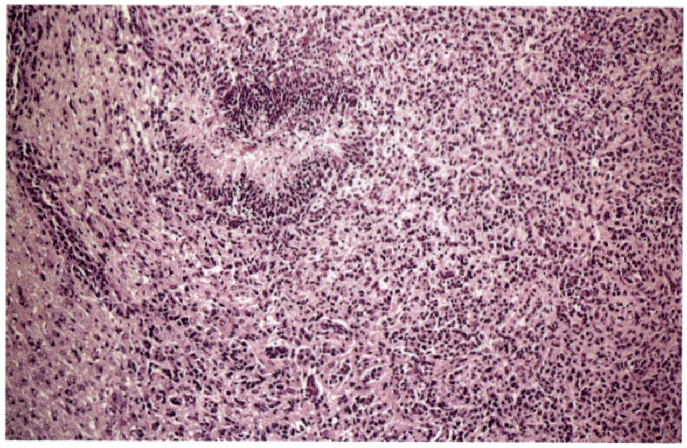

**FIGURE 10-36.** Glioma (astrocytoma), cerebrum in a rat. Monomorphic cells with slightly eosinophilic cytoplasm, indistinct cell borders and compact dark nuclei. The lesion has indistinct margins, areas of palisading necrosis. H&E.

## References


1. Garman RH. Evaluation of large-sized brains for neurotoxic endpoints. Toxicol Pathol. 2003;31(Suppl):32–43.
2. Jordan WH, Young JK, Hyten MJ, Hall DG. Preparation and analysis of the central nervous system. Toxicol Pathol. 2011;39:58–65.
3. Garman RH, Fix AS, Jortner BS, Jensen KF, Hardisty JF, Claudio L, et al. Methods to identify and characterize developmental neurotoxicity for human health risk assessment. II: neuropathology. Environ Health Perspect. 2001;109 Suppl 1:93–100.
4. Switzer III RC, Lowry-Franssen C, Benkovic SA. Recommended neuroanatomical sampling practices for comprehensive brain evaluation in nonclinical safety studies. Toxicol Pathol. 2011;39:73–84.
5. Jortner BS. Preparation and analysis of the peripheral nervous system. Toxicol Pathol. 2011;39:66–72.
6. Jortner BS. Mechanisms of toxic injury in the peripheral nervous system: neuropathologic considerations. Toxicol Pathol. 2000;28:54–69.
7. Switzer II RC. Application of silver degeneration stains for neurotoxicity testing. Toxicol Pathol. 2000;28:70–83.
8. Hale SL, Andrews-Jones L, Jordan WH, Jortner BS, Boyce RW, Boyce JT, et al. Modern pathology methods for neural investigations. Toxicol Pathol. 2011;39:52–7.
9. Kaufmann W, Bolon B, Bradley A, Butt M, Czasch S, Garman RH, et al. Proliferative and nonproliferative lesions of the rat and mouse central and peripheral nervous systems. Toxicol Pathol. 2012;40:87S–157.
10. Garman RH. Histology of the central nervous system. Toxicol Pathol. 2011;39:22–35.
11. Farina M, Rocha JB, Aschner M. Mechanisms of methylmercury-induced neurotoxicity: evidence from experimental studies. Life Sci. 2011;89:555–63.
12. Sakamoto M, Kakita A, de Oliveira RB, Sheng PH, Takahashi H. Dose-dependent effects of methylmercury administered during neonatal brain spurt in rats. Brain Res Dev Brain Res. 2004;152:171–6.
13. Chang LW. The neurotoxicology and pathology of organomercury, organolead, and organotin. J Toxicol Sci. 1990;15 Suppl 4:125–51.
14. Sorensen FW, Larsen JO, Eide R, Schionning JD. Neuron loss in cerebellar cortex of rats exposed to mercury vapor: a stereological study. Acta Neuropathol. 2000;100:95–100.
15. McCann MJ, O'Callaghan JP, Martin PM, Bertram T, Streit WJ. Differential activation of microglia and astrocytes following trimethyl tin-induced neurodegeneration. Neuroscience. 1996;72:273–81.
16. Barone Jr S. Developmental differences in neural damage following trimethyl-tin as demonstrated with GFAP immunohistochemistry. Ann N Y Acad Sci. 1993;679:306–16.
17. Chung JY, Choi JH, Hwang CY, Youn HY. Pyridoxine induced neuropathy by subcutaneous administration in dogs. J Vet Sci. 2008;9:127–31.
18. Krinke G, Schaumburg HH, Spencer PS, Suter J, Thomann P, Hess R. Pyridoxine megavitaminosis produces degeneration of peripheral sensory neurons (sensory neuronopathy) in the dog. Neurotoxicology. 1981;2:13–24.
19. Riljak V, Milotova M, Jandova K, Langmeier M, Maresova D, Pokorny J, et al. Repeated kainic acid administration and hippocampal neuronal degeneration. Prague Med Rep. 2005;106:75–8.
20. Lavoie B, Parent A, Bedard PJ. Effects of dopamine denervation on striatal peptide expression in parkinsonian monkeys. Can J Neurol Sci. 1991;18:373–5.
21. Peltier AC, Russell JW. Recent advances in drug-induced neuropathies. Curr Opin Neurol. 2002;15:633–8.
22. Genovese RF, Newman DB. Understanding artemisinin-induced brainstem neurotoxicity. Arch Toxicol. 2008;82:379–85.
23. Mimaki T, Deshmukh PP, Yamamura HI. Decreased benzodiazepine receptor density in rat cerebellum following neurotoxic doses of phenytoin. J Neurochem. 1980;35:1473–5.
24. Greaves P. Nervous system and special sense organs. In: Greaves P, editor. Histopathology of preclinical toxicity studies. Amsterdam: Elsevier; 2012. p. 799–866.

25. Dowson JH, Wilton-Cox W, James NT. Lipopigment in rat hippocampal and Purkinje neurones after chronic phenytoin administration. J Neurol Sci. 1992;107:105–10.
26. Akasaki Y, Takauchi S, Miyoshi K. Cerebellar degeneration induced by acetyl-ethyl-tetramethyl-tetralin (AETT). Acta Neuropathol. 1990;80:129–37.
27. Sterman AB, Spencer PS. The pathogenesis of primary internodal demyelination produced by acetyl ethyl tetramethyl tetralin: evidence for preserved Schwann cell somal function. J Neuropathol Exp Neurol. 1981;40:112–21.
28. Schaumburg HH, Spencer PS. Toxic models of certain disorders of nervous system—a teaching monograph. Neurotoxicology. 1979;1:209–20.
29. Krinke G, Schaumburg HH, Spencer PS, Thomann P, Hess R. Clioquinol and 2,5-hexanedione induce different types of distal axonopathy in the dog. Acta Neuropathol. 1979;47:213–21.
30. Thomas PK. Selective vulnerability of the centrifugal and centripetal axons of primary sensory neurons. Muscle Nerve. 1982;5:S117–21.
31. Llorens J, Crofton KM, O'Callaghan JP. Administration of 3,3′-iminodipropionitrile to the rat results in region-dependent damage to the central nervous system at levels above the brain stem. J Pharmacol Exp Ther. 1993;265:1492–8.
32. Schulze GE, Boysen BG. A neurotoxicity screening battery for use in safety evaluation: effects of acrylamide and 3′,3′-iminodipropionitrile. Fundam Appl Toxicol. 1991;16:602–15.
33. Powell HC, Myers RR, Lampert PW. Edema in neurotoxic injury. In: Shaumberg H, Spencer P, editors. Experimental and clinical neurotoxicology. Baltimore: Williams & Wilkins; 1980. p. 118–38.
34. Gopinath C, Prentice DE, Lewis DJ. The nervous system. In: Gopinath C, Prentice DE, Lewis DJ, editors. Atlas of experimental toxicologic pathology. Lancaster: MTP Press; 1987. p. 137–44.
35. Ellis WG, Bencken E, LeCouteur RA, Barbano JR, Wolfe BM, Jennings MB. Neurotoxicity of amphotericin B methyl ester in dogs. Toxicol Pathol. 1988;16:1–9.
36. Yamamoto T, Iwasaki Y, Sato Y, Yamamoto H, Konno H. Astrocytic pathology of methionine sulfoximine-induced encephalopathy. Acta Neuropathol (Berl). 1989;77:357–68.
37. Jacobs JM, Ford WC. The neurotoxicity and antifertility properties of 6-chloro-6-deoxyglucose in the mouse. Neurotoxicology. 1981;2:405–17.
38. Heywood R, Sortwell RJ, Prentice DE. The toxicity of 1-amino-3-chloro-2-propanol hydrochloride (CL88,236) in the rhesus monkey. Toxicology. 1978;9:219–25.
39. Berry PH, MacDonald JS, Alberts AW, Molon-Noblot S, Chen JS, Lo CY, et al. Brain and optic system pathology in hypocholesterolemic dogs treated with a competitive inhibitor of 3-hydroxy-3-methylglutaryl coenzyme A reductase. Am J Pathol. 1988;132:427–43.
40. Koizumi H, Watanabe M, Numata H, Sakai T, Morishita H. Species differences in vacuolation of the choroid plexus induced by the piperidine-ring drug disobutamide in the rat, dog, and monkey. Toxicol Appl Pharmacol. 1986;84:125–48.
41. Gopinath C. Spontaneous brain tumours in Sprague–Dawley rats. Food Chem Toxicol. 1986;24:113–20.
42. Nagatani M, Ando R, Yamakawa S, Saito T, Tamura K. Histological and immunohistochemical studies on spontaneous rat astrocytomas and malignant reticulosis. Toxicol Pathol. 2009;37:599–605.

# 11 The Musculoskeletal System and Skin

Induced lesions of the musculoskeletal system, skin, and adipose tissue have been identified with an increasing variety of test articles over the past two decades, including many biologics. The pathogenesis of these lesions is now being studied more intensively than in the past. In this chapter, mechanisms of toxicity are briefly discussed. Common induced lesions of these organ systems are described, with illustrations and examples of causative agents and their modes of action.

## 11.1 Muscle

Traditionally, the muscle was considered an unlikely target for primary toxicity in safety assessment studies. This was at least partially due to limited samples being routinely examined in toxicity studies. Myopathy due to dietary manipulation or secondary to other systemic changes was well documented, but, of recent years, direct adverse effects in man and laboratory species have been recognised with increasing frequency. This trend has led to more emphasis being placed on sampling protocols, which are now designed to include more samples and techniques if myotoxicity is expected.

Routine skeletal muscle samples in laboratory species are generally taken from the proximal hind limb. Muscle artefacts are easily produced by faulty handling and fixation techniques, and procedures that reduce artefact should be consistently applied [1]. If the route of administration or implantation is intramuscular, sampling and trimming procedures should be designed to optimise coverage of the target areas for consistency.

Muscles fibres are broadly divided into type I (slow-twitch) and type II (fast-twitch) based on physiological characteristics and composition. Type II muscles are further divided into A, B, and C on the basis of myosin ATPase activity and pH sensitivity. Different muscles are comprised of different proportions of these fibre types, depending on their function. The soleus in most species is comprised mostly of type I fibres. Histochemical stains for myosin, ATPase, NADH-TR, electron microscopy, and immunocytochemical staining for myosin isoforms are used to differentiate myofibre types. Muscle susceptibility to toxicants often depends on their metabolic type and function.

Plasma creatine kinase is the most sensitive and specific marker of muscle damage; three isoenzymes can be measured in the blood. Serum glutamic-pyruvic transaminase (SGPT), serum glutamic oxaloacetic transaminase (SGOT), aldolase, and lactic dehydrogenase can also be measured but are less specific.

Muscle cells are very long and multinucleated, generally extending from tendon to tendon. Nuclei are located beneath the sarcolemma, and satellite cells, which are instrumental in regeneration, are located between the sarcolemma and external lamina. The muscle responds differently to a wide range of physiological conditions and insults [1], although it generally shows a limited range of histopathological responses to injury or impairment of function in safety assessment. Commonly seen induced changes in the muscle are as follows:

- Myofibre degeneration/necrosis
- Vacuolation/fatty degeneration
- Atrophy

C. Gopinath, V. Mowat, *Atlas of Toxicological Pathology*,
DOI 10.1007/978-1-62703-998-7_11, © Springer Science+Business Media New York 2014

- Hypertrophy
- Regeneration

Pathologic changes in the muscle are broadly mediated by three general mechanisms: (1) direct effects on muscle fibres, (2) indirectly through altered function of peripheral nerves, and (3) indirectly by disturbance of neuromuscular transmission. Immunologically mediated changes and ischaemia are also occasionally seen as mechanisms of indirect toxicity. In addition, intramuscular injections and implants can result in localised damage, inflammatory reaction, and tumour development.

Isolated degenerate muscle fibres, often accompanied by inflammatory cell infiltrate, are seen as a background finding in most laboratory species. The incidence of these lesions can be exacerbated by various compound classes.

Early degenerative changes in the muscle include loss of cross-striations, eosinophilia, vacuolation, and pallor (Figs. 11.1 and 11.2). Special stains such as phosphotungstic acid haematoxylin (PTAH) can be used for detection of early degenerative changes, such as loss of cross-striation, which may not be obvious with haematoxylin and eosin (H&E) stains. Variable degrees of inflammatory cell infiltrate appear as the lesions progress, and fibres shrink due to loss of sarcoplasm, becoming paler (Fig. 11.3). Although some neutrophils may be present in acute necrosis, inflammatory cells are usually macrophagic. Industrial chemicals can form clefts and crystals between the muscle fibres, causing myofibre degeneration and eliciting a histiocytic reaction with foreign-body giant cell formation (Fig. 11.4).

Barring damage to the sarcolemmal membrane or satellite cells, regeneration usually occurs. Myoblasts with central chains of nuclei and basophilic cytoplasm appear, and these are often seen alongside degenerating fibres. As regenerating fibres mature,

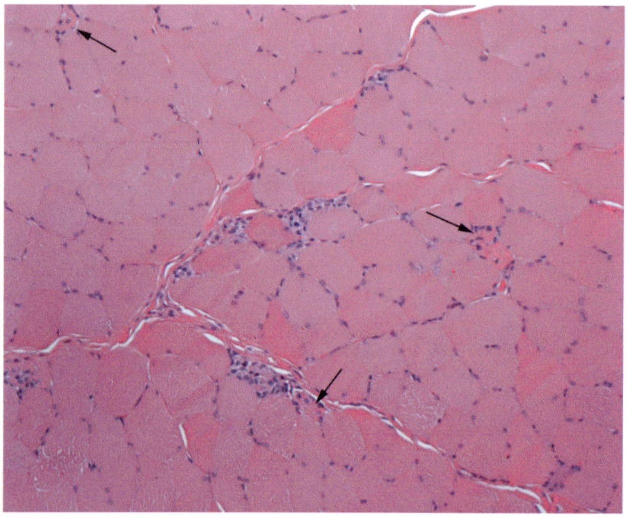

**Figure 11-1.** Myofibre degeneration in a cynomolgus monkey given a kinase inhibitor. Early degenerative changes are characterised by eosinophilia and condensation of the sarcoplasm, with a few inflammatory cells (*arrows*). More chronic degenerating fibres are pale and shrunken with loss of cytoplasm and more inflammatory cells. H&E.

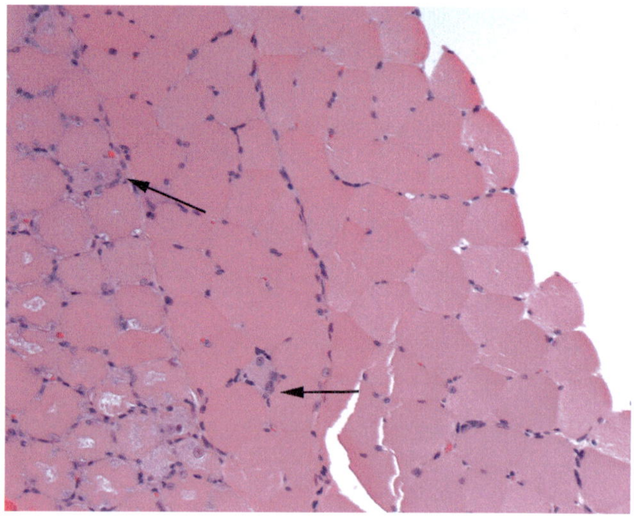

**Figure 11-2.** Myofibre degeneration in a cynomolgus monkey given a kinase inhibitor Degenerating myofibres appear pale with vacuolated, lacy cytoplasm, and increased numbers of nuclei (*arrows*), which is sometimes moving towards the fibre's centre. H&E.

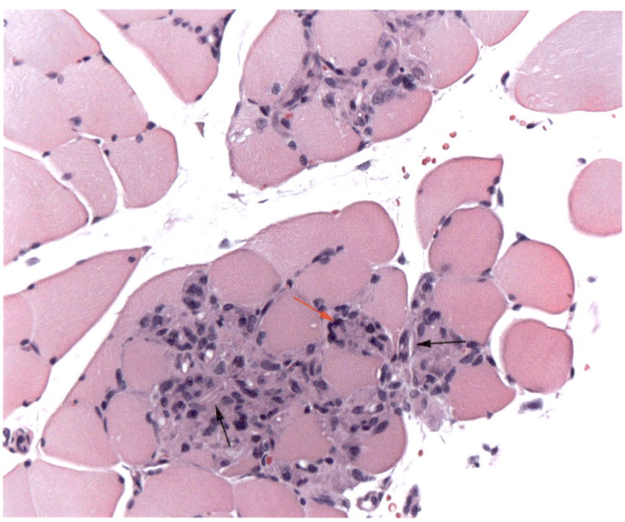

**Figure 11-3.** Foreign-body reaction in the muscle of a rat given an industrial chemical orally. The test article is present as crystals and clefts (*black arrows*) that have elicited a foreign-body giant cell response (*red arrow*). Similar lesions were seen in several other organs. H&E.

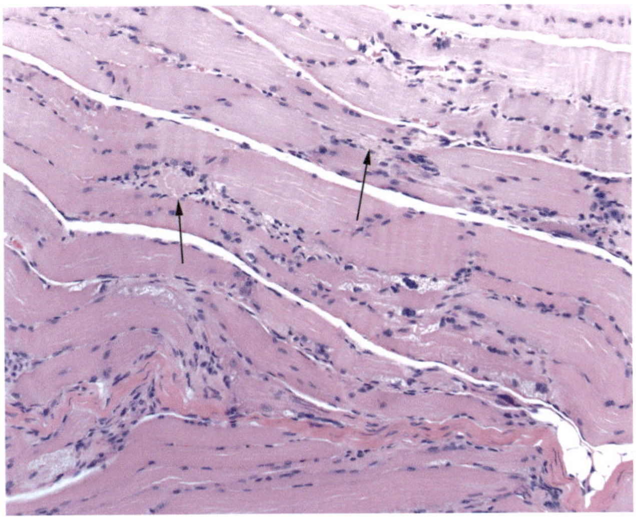

**Figure 11-4.** Myopathy in the muscles of a rat given a phospholipidotic. Several fibres show early degenerative changes, with eosinophilic debris and infiltration by macrophages and lymphocytes (*arrows*). Loss of sarcoplasm in some fibres has left a lacy appearance. H&E.

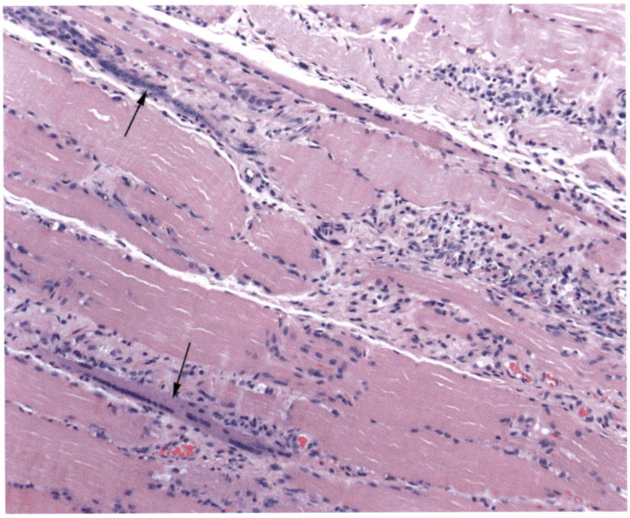

**Figure 11-5.** Chronic myopathy in the muscles of a rat given a phospholipidotic. Several fibres are degenerating, with eosinophilic debris and mixed inflammatory cell infiltration. Several myotubes (*arrows*) with basophilic cytoplasm and central columns of nuclei are also present, indicating regeneration. H&E.

eosinophilia is restored and central nuclei migrate peripherally. In rodent muscles nuclei remain centrally located postregeneration for a long period. With continuous dosing with myotoxic compounds, a combination of degenerating and regenerating myofibres is usually seen (Fig. 11.5). If the sarcolemma or satellite cells are damaged, or the vasculature affected, fibrosis may follow.

Morphologically, degenerative changes in the muscle can be broadly divided into hyaline degeneration and granular degeneration. In the hyaline type, sections of affected fibres appear swollen and eosinophilic, with loss of cross-striations. The sarcoplasm undergoes coagulative or hyaline necrosis, forming eosinophilic fragments or discs that remain within the intact lamina of the muscle cell.

In granular degeneration, the damaged sarcoplasm appears granular due to the presence of mineralised mitochondria. In both types, recruitment of inflammatory cells (usually macrophages with some lymphocytes) can appear as the lesions progress.

Vitamin E and selenium deficiency induce muscular dystrophy in many laboratory species. The rabbit is particularly susceptible to vitamin E deficiency, and pale mineralised streaks may be seen at necropsy. Histologically, hyaline degeneration of myofibres with clumping of the sarcoplasm is seen, often with mineralisation and sometimes macrophage infiltration. Muscle atrophy with fatty replacement is seen in rats injected subcutaneously with 6-mercaptopurine, but mice and hamsters are unaffected [2–4].

Direct effects on the muscle fibres are probably the commonest mechanism of toxicity in safety studies. These include alteration of the cell membrane, cell organelles or cytoskeleton, altered protein synthesis, and changes in intracellular calcium concentration. Compounds may preferentially target one particular type of muscle fibre or affect several fibre types, depending on mode of action.

Many classes of hypolipidaemics are associated with myopathies. Statins cause muscle fibre degeneration, with type II fibres, particularly type IIB, being more sensitive than type I. The mechanism of action is thought to be directly due to HMG-CoA reductase inhibition, with ultrastructural changes being seen in the mitochondria first. Histologically, vacuolation and myelinoid vesicular bodies are seen in the sarcolemma initially, progressing to necrosis [5, 6]. Peroxisome proliferator associated receptor (PPAR)$\alpha$-agonists cause myofibre degeneration with accompanying regeneration, probably due to oxidative injury resulting from increased $\beta$-oxidation [7]. Fibrates cause myopathy of type I and II fibres in rats, with type I fibres showing greater susceptibility and the soleus muscle thus being targeted [8–10]. This effect is possibly due to cell membrane alteration resulting from altered cholesterol biosynthesis, which can lead to changes in cell electrolyte content. Hypokalaemia results from a decrease in cell membrane excitability.

Colchicine and vincristine produce myopathy in rats by microtubule disruption, leading to development of spheromembranous bodies containing lipid and debris within the fibres [11, 12]. Plasmocid causes degeneration of the myofilaments. Loss of cross-striations is seen with emetine [13]. Adriamycin causes lipid droplets in skeletal muscle at low exposure levels, but higher exposures result in interstitial oedema, sarcoplasmic vacuolation due to dilation of sarcoplasmic reticulum, and mitochondrial degeneration [14]. Monensin toxicity is thought to be due to calcium overloading. Mitogen-activated protein (MAP) kinase inhibitors have been associated with myofibre degeneration in primates (personal observation).

Malignant hyperthermia is seen in pigs and humans with a genetic predisposition and is known by a variety of names including lactic acidosis or porcine stress syndrome in pigs. This syndrome often occurs during anaesthesia or transport in animal species. Stress results in excessive leakage of Ca2+ from the sarcoplasmic reticulum, leading to glycolysis and elevated lactic acid, resulting in overheating. Macroscopically, widespread pale exudative myopathy may be apparent. In pigs, oedematous, hypercontracted, and fragmented muscle fibres are seen histologically [15].

Fatty degeneration appears histologically as micro- or macrovacuolation of the myofibres. This change can develop as a sequel to atrophy, with adipocytes replacing atrophic fibres, or as primary vacuolation. Cationic amphophilic compounds (CADs), which induce generalised phospholipidosis, produce myopathy due to accumulation of drug-lipid complexes that delay enzymatic breakdown within lysosomes. Vacuolation and extensive replacement of muscle fibres by adipocytes are seen histologically (Figs. 11.6 and 11.7). On electron microscopy, the characteristic lamellar bodies are seen (Fig. 11.8). Chloroquine, when given to rats, causes vacuolar myopathy in type I fibres and also neurogenic-type atrophy in type II fibres [16]. Degeneration of muscle fibres independent of vacuolation is also seen with CADs [17].

Atrophy can be caused by malnutrition, denervation, disuse, direct effects, and vascular compromise. Atrophy appears histologically as a reduction in the size of the muscle fibres, and, if mild, may only be detectable when compared carefully with controls. It is more easily recognised on transverse muscle sections than

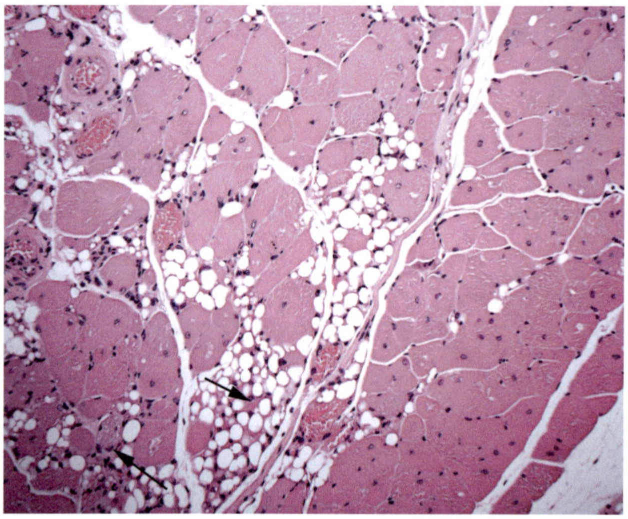

**Figure 11-6.** Fatty vacuolation in the skeletal muscle of a mouse given a phospholipidotic compound. Patchy lipid vacuoles are evident in the myofibres and interstitium. Mild interstitial inflammatory cell infiltration is present, and a few myofibres show degenerative changes (*arrows*). H&E.

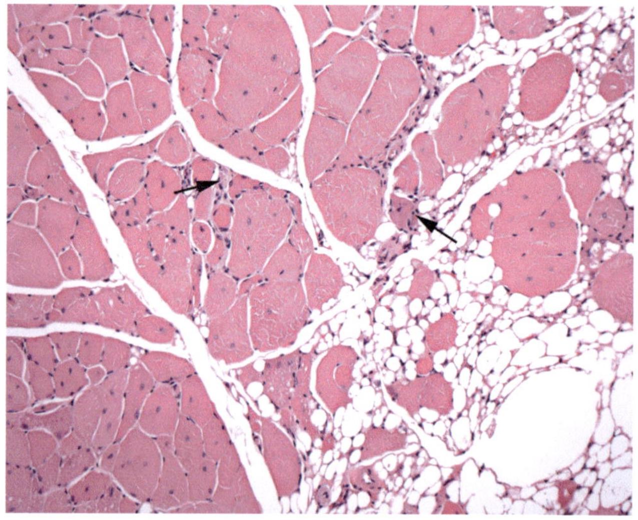

**Figure 11-7.** Fatty vacuolation in the skeletal muscle of a mouse given a phospholipidotic compound. The muscle has been partially replaced by lipid vacuoles of varying sizes. The diameter of the remaining muscle fibres is variable, with some degenerating fibres (*arrows*). H&E.

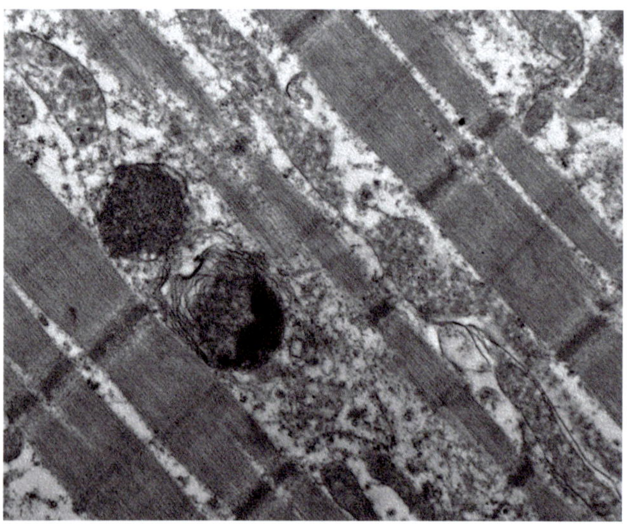

**Figure 11-8.** Lamellar bodies in the muscle of a dog given a phospholipidotic. Two lamellar bodies, with the characteristic whorling pattern, are present between myofibres. Transmission electron microscopy.

longitudinal ones. If marked, the change is often reported at necropsy due to the reduced muscle mass, which gives a thin appearance. If secondary to malnutrition, type II fibres are predominantly involved. Small groups of myofibres are affected and appear shrunken with angular margins due to pressure from unaffected fibres nearby. Induced muscle atrophy associated with corticosteroids has been widely recorded in both man and a variety of laboratory species, and generally appears as a diffuse reduction in fibre diameter (Fig. 11.9a, b). Reduced protein synthesis is considered to be the likely mechanism, with steroids that are fluorinated in the nine position most likely to be myotoxic (*e.g.* triamcinolone, dexamethasone) [13]. Dexamethasone-induced atrophy of the extensor digitorum muscles of the rat is mainly due to changes in fast glycolytic fibres [18].

Denervation atrophy is secondary to impairment to peripheral nerve function. In older rodents, muscle atrophy of the hind limbs, secondary to radiculoneuropathy and consequent sciatic nerve degeneration, is a common background finding (Fig. 11.10a, b). Peripheral neuropathy caused by 2,5-hexanedione administration results in muscle atrophy in dogs [19]. Thiamine deficiency causes peripheral neuropathy and muscle fibre atrophy in rats which is exacerbated by alcohol [20]. With denervation-mediated muscle atrophy, fibres appear thinner and shorter than normal. In muscle fibres allowed to recover from atrophy, fibre type may change depending on re-enervation.

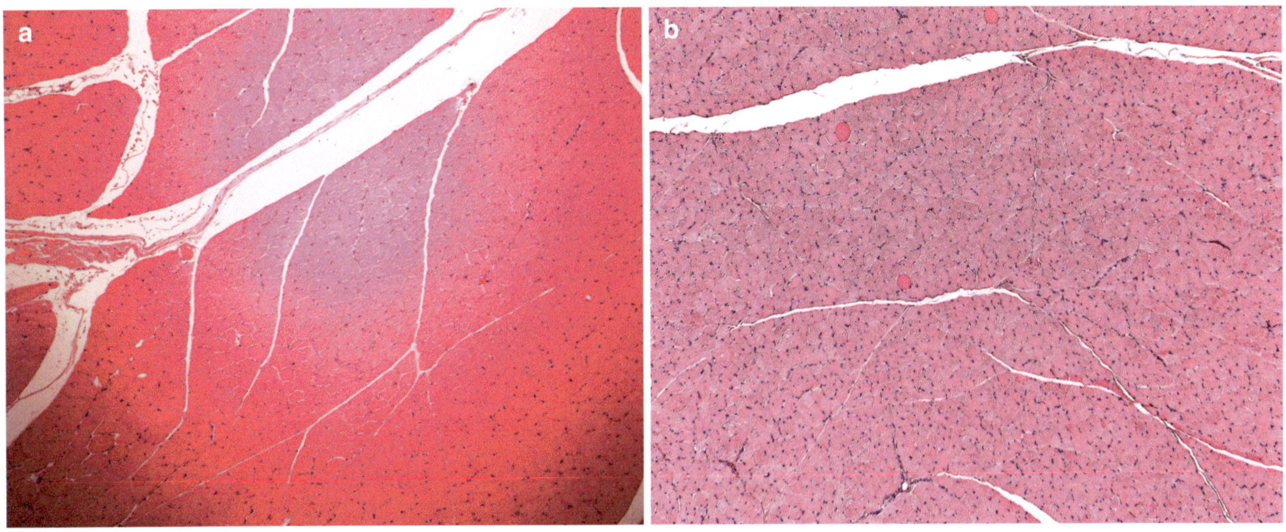


**Figure 11-9.** (**a**) Skeletal muscle from a normal control dog. H&E. (**b**) Atrophy of the skeletal muscle in a dog given a corticosteroid. Muscle fibres are much smaller in diameter than those of the control. Macroscopically, the muscle appeared pale and atrophic. H&E.

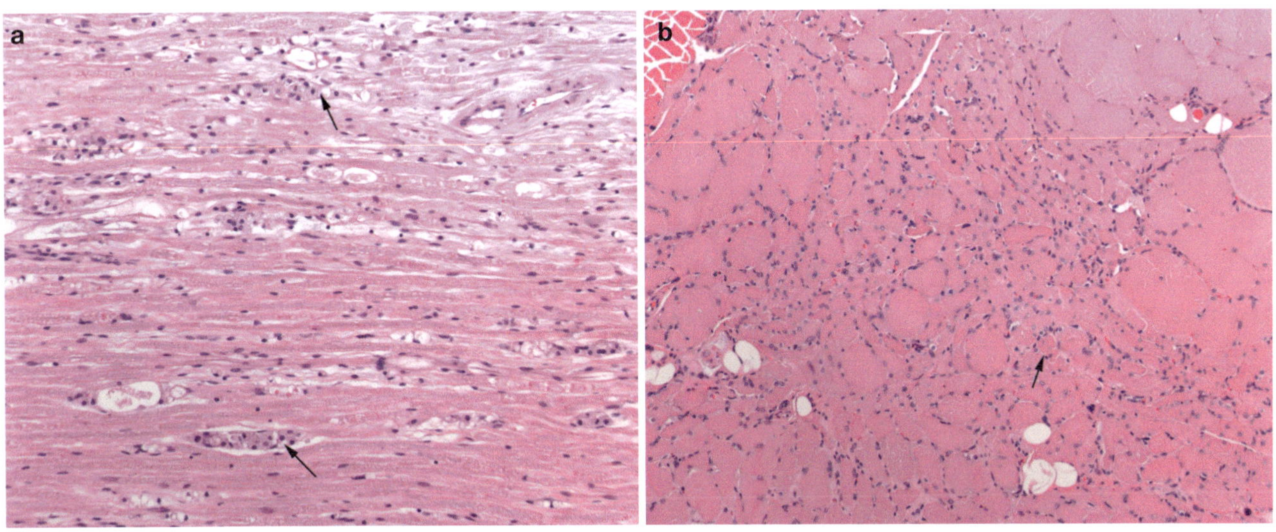


**Figure 11-10.** (**a**) Peripheral neuropathy of the sciatic nerve, rat. Several nerve fibres are degenerating, with digestion chambers present, some containing eosinophilic material and some containing phagocytic cells (*arrows*). H&E. (**b**) Hind-limb muscle from the same animal. Patchy focal atrophy is evident, with several myofibres showing reduced diameter. A few degenerative fibres are present (*arrow*). H&E.

Many xenobiotics and pharmaceuticals exert their effects at the neuromuscular junction. With anticholinesterase inhibitors, myopathy is often localised to the regions near the motor endplates. Pyridostigmine bromide produces postsynaptic areas of affected myofibres with myofilament dissolution, mitochondrial inclusions and vacuolisation in the extraocular muscles of rats, secondary to accumulation of excessive amounts of acetylcholine [21]. Recognition of motor endplates, or neuromuscular junctions, requires special techniques including histochemistry, electron microscopy (EM), intravital dyes, and metallic impregnation techniques. In humans, heroin addiction also causes myopathy, probably due to motor nerve excitation.

Hypertrophy of the skeletal muscle is induced by growth hormone in dogs and primates, mediated by somatomedins or insulin-like growth factors rather than as a direct effect. Hypertrophy is due to increased protein synthesis, leading to an increase in numbers of myonuclei, fibre length, and diameter. Administration of $T_4$ to rats causes an increase in numbers of satellite cell nuclei and also in the numbers of satellite cells per muscle fibre [22]. Increased workload also results in physiological hypertrophy. Histologically, muscle fibres are increased in size, presumably due to increased amounts of inter-myofibrillar material and numbers of myofibrils [23]. Increased capillarisation of the skeletal muscle develops in rats treated with dipyridamole, due to proliferation of capillary walls, and is possibly due to vasodilation [24].

Indirect effects on the muscle can be immunologically mediated, as is seen with procainamide and D-penicillamine, both of which induce an inflammatory myopathy [25]. Vasoactive amines, such as serotonin, induce a form of myopathy which is believed to involve ischaemia [26, 27].

Localised muscle changes are often seen with intramuscular injections in safety studies. Myopathy can be associated with vehicles as well as test substances and should be clearly differentiated (Fig. 11.11). Inflammatory infiltrates are usually lymphohistiocytic and often track down between muscle fibres and bundles. Adjuvants, such as aluminium hydroxide, and vaccines can induce a persistent granulomatous inflammation, with degenerating macrophages releasing the agent, which is then taken up again by macrophages (Fig. 11.12). Granulomas and fibrosis may also occur with vaccines and adjuvants, which cause necrosis and sarcolemmal damage.

Implantation of solid materials can elicit a foreign-body reaction with macrophages, giant cells, and fibrotic reaction, which can progress to fibrosarcomas. Rhabdomyosarcomas have been induced in rats by implanting and/or injecting a variety of materials [28, 29].

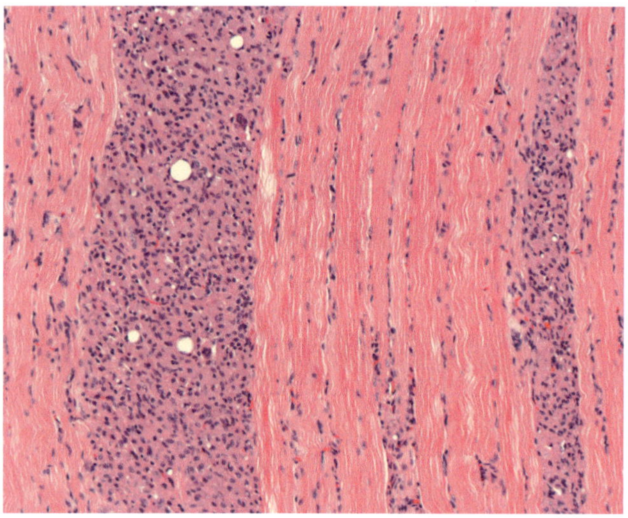

**Figure 11-11.** Muscle from a minipig injected intramuscularly with a saline vehicle. Marked interstitial macrophage infiltration with tracking between muscle bundles is seen. The reaction is possibly due to a contaminant in the vehicle. H&E.

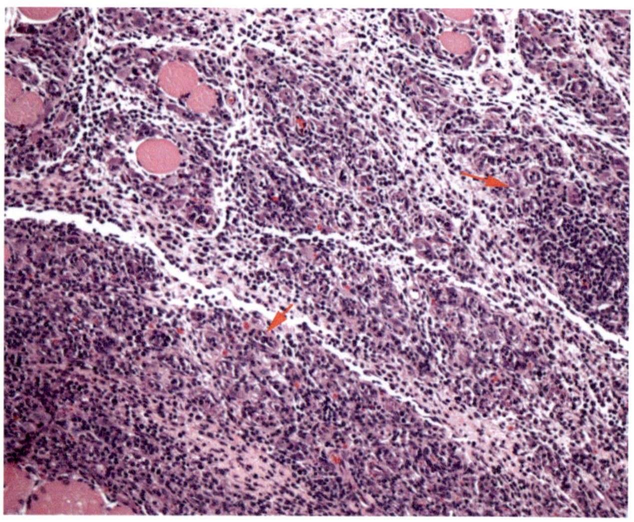

**Figure 11-12.** Muscle from a rat injected intramuscularly with a vaccine. The site shows chronic inflammation with localised loss of muscle fibres and prominent neovascularisation (*arrows*). Inflammatory cells are mostly macrophages and lymphocytes. H&E.

## 11.2 Bones

In routine safety assessment studies, a joint should be included so that articular cartilage, synovium, and growth plates can be examined. Routine sections of decalcified bone are adequate for general assessments of toxicity. Specialised investigations usually involve histomorphometry and may require more rigorous processing and sectioning protocols, such as fluorochrome labelling and plastic sections [30].

Bone remodelling is an ongoing process throughout life and is regulated by a wide range of physiological and mechanical factors. Bone matrix is produced by osteoblasts and bone resorption is effected by osteoclasts, with the two processes being closely intertwined. A wide range of hormones and cytokines influence bone formation and resorption, often acting on both osteoblasts and osteoclasts. Lesions of the cartilage/bone and joints are uncommon as induced changes in non rodents. A few spontaneous and induced changes are seen in old rodents. Direct toxicity is somewhat rare, with most changes being secondary. Direct mechanisms include mitotic inhibition by anticancerals like cyclophosphamide and accumulation of elements like fluoride and lead, which cause hypomineralisation and increase resorption and remodelling, resulting in thinning. Alterations in hormonal controls, mineral balances, and blood supply are some of the mechanisms commonly involved in secondary toxicity. Most toxicologic changes represent increases or decreases of a particular component. Induced changes of the skeletal system are listed below.

- Cartilage—increase/decrease
- Cartilage—erosion/degeneration
- Osteosclerosis
- Osteoid—increase/decrease
- Fibrous osteodystrophy
- Bone atrophy/necrosis
- Tumours—osteosarcomas

Increased or reduced thickness of the articular cartilage and/or growth plate is associated with a range of pharmaceuticals and is often secondary to hormonal perturbations. Growth plate changes are most easily recognised in rodents, where they stay open throughout life. The growth plate consists of proliferative, hypertrophic, and mineralisation zones from the epiphysis towards the diaphysis. Increased thickness of the articular cartilage and/or growth plate has been recorded with several compound classes including growth hormone, insulin, vascular endothelial growth factor inhibitors, metalloproteinase inhibitors, and tyrosine kinase inhibitors in several laboratory species, including primates (Fig. 11.13a, b) [31, 32]. In many cases, thickening of the growth plate is due to an increase in the zone of

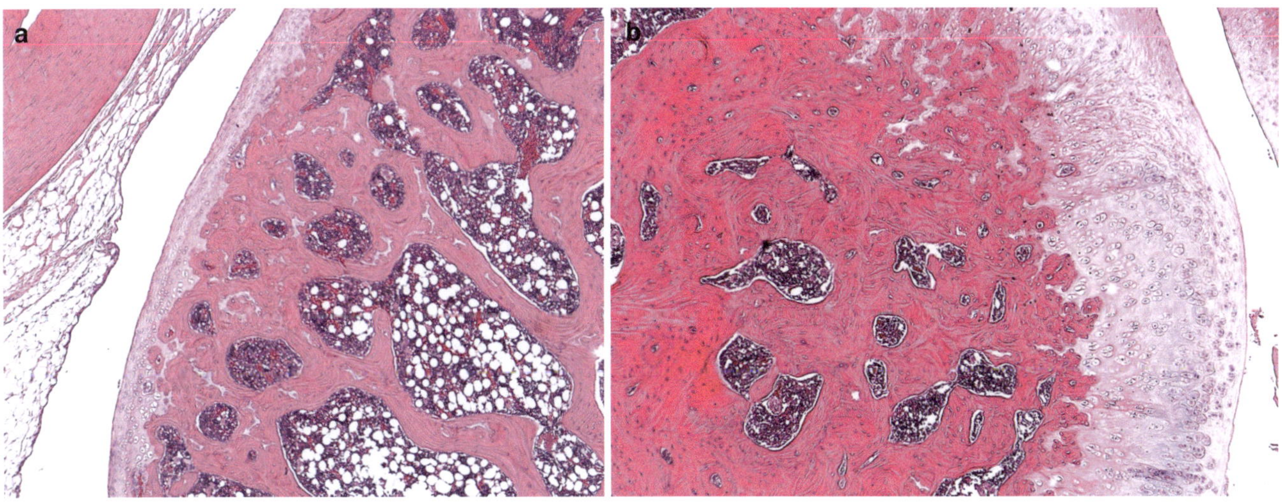


**Figure 11-13.** (**a**) Normal articular cartilage, distal femur of a rat. Cartilage comprises four to five layers of cells distributed in tangential, transitional, radial, and calcified layers. H&E. (**b**) Thickening of the articular cartilage of the distal femur in a rat given a growth hormone. The cartilage is thicker than normal, with expansion of the transition and radial zones and chondrocyte clustering. H&E.

hypertrophic chondrocytes (Figs. 11.14a, b and 11.15a, b) [33]. Chondroid hyperplasia has also been recorded in rats receiving growth hormones (Fig. 11.16). ALK5 inhibitors induce physeal dysplasia, including expansion of the hypertrophic and proliferative zones, chondroid hypertrophy and hyperplasia, and hyperostosis (Fig. 11.17) [34].

Physiological thinning and closure of the growth plate occur spontaneously with maturity in nonrodent species, with intersex differences. This process can be accelerated or retarded by several classes of compounds. Retention of the growth plate in dogs has been seen with glucocorticoid agonists (personal observation). Quinolones and warfarin cause premature closure of the growth plate in rats, with warfarin causing excessive mineralisation as well [35]. Vitamin A toxicity is associated with growth plate closure in man and several animal species including rats.

In safety assessment studies, thinning of the growth plate is seen in many laboratory species, including minipigs, given glucocorticoids and glucocorticoid agonists (Figs. 11.18 and 11.19). Histologically, this generally appears as thinning of the hypertrophic zone and zone of calcification. Age influences the pattern of changes seen, with younger animals generally being more susceptible. Semicarbazide hydrochloride, a metabolite of nitrofurazone, caused severe disarrangement and deformation of articular cartilage in young rats, whereas adult rats showed relatively mild osteochondral lesions [36]. HhAntag, a hedgehog pathway inhibitor, causes

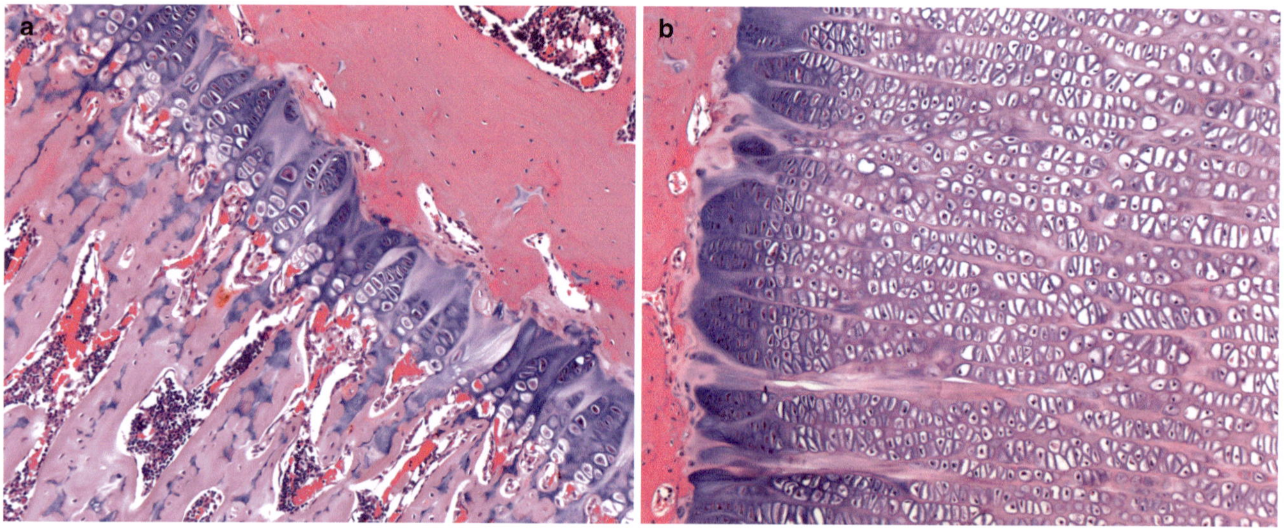

**Figure 11-14.** (**a**) Femoro-tibial joint, control rat with normal tibial growth plate. H&E. (**b**) Femoro-tibial joint, rat treated with a biologically active compound. Marked widening of the tibial growth plate is present, largely due to expansion of the hypertrophic zone. Growth factor inhibitors and tyrosine kinase inhibitors are often associated with this change. H&E.

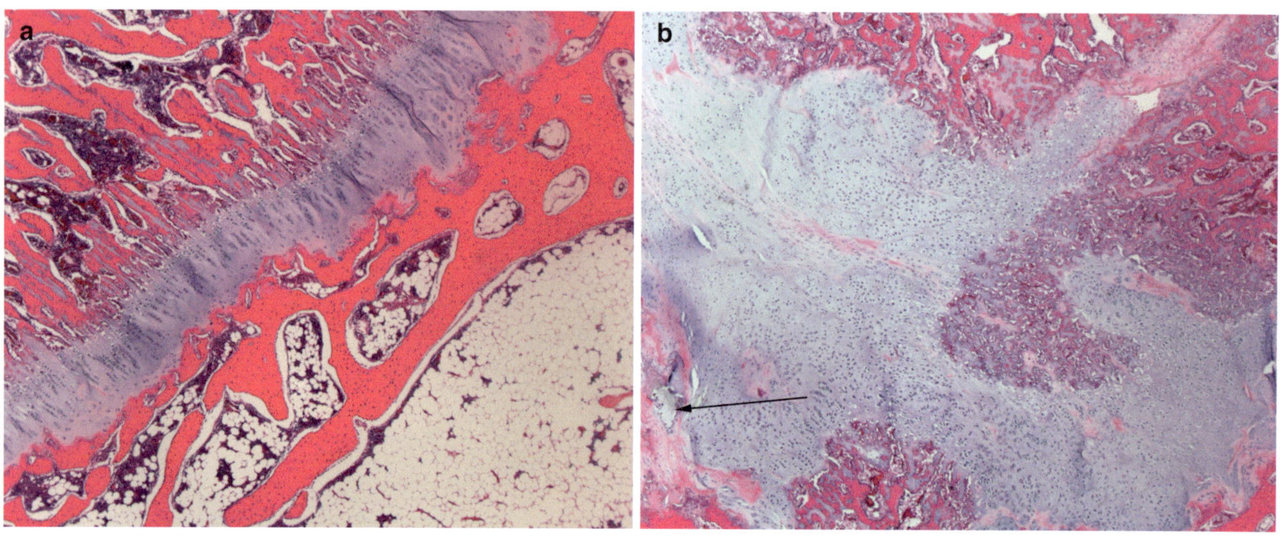

**Figure 11-15.** (**a**) Normal growth plate, distal femur, in a cynomolgus monkey. H&E. (**b**) Hypertrophic growth plate with disruption, distal femur, in a cynomolgus monkey given a biologic. Disorganisation and localised hypertrophy of the growth plate are seen, with focal cartilage necrosis (*arrow*). The growth plate extends focally into the epiphysis and metaphysis, areas of cartilage being surrounded by osteogenic zones. H&E.

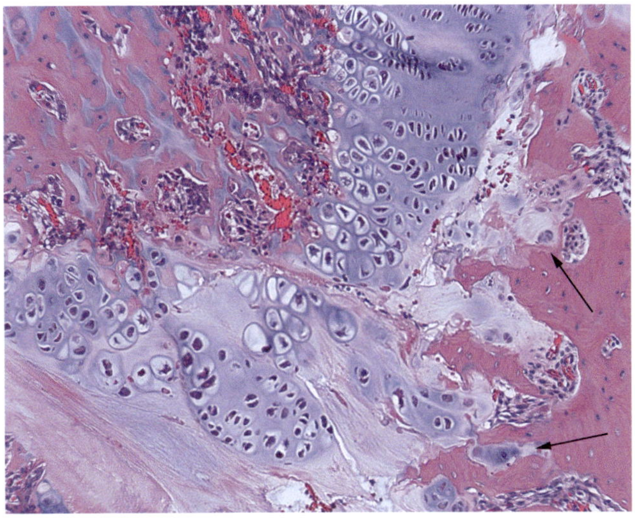

**Figure 11-16.** Chondroid hyperplasia in the femoral growth plate of a rat. The growth plate shows loss of architecture, with islands of chondrocytes in the epiphyseal bone above the growth plate (*arrows*). Growth hormones and ALK5 inhibitors can produce these changes. H&E.

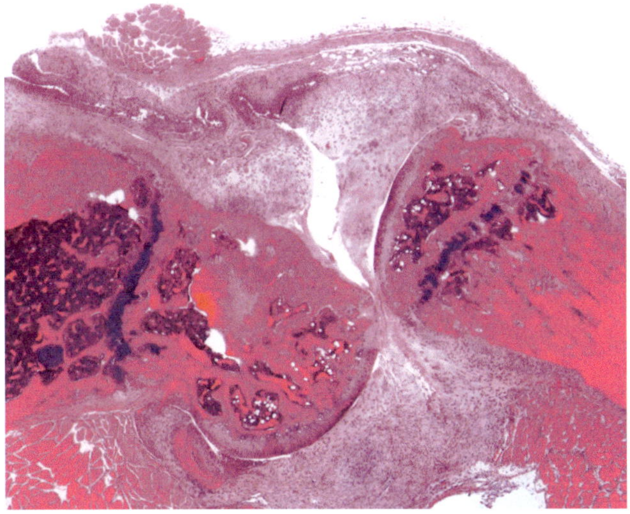

**Figure 11-17.** Chondroid hyperplasia in the femoro-tibial joint of a mouse. Marked cartilaginous proliferation is present within the joint, involving the synovial membranes, tendon insertions, and capsule. The articular cartilage is mildly thickened. H&E.

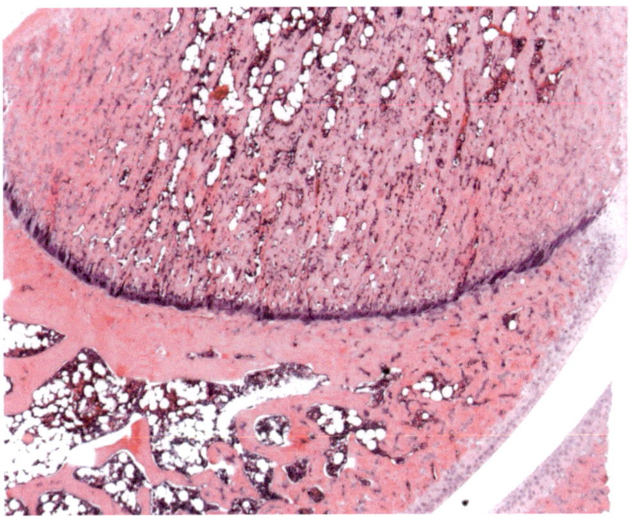

**Figure 11-18.** Thinning of the femoral growth plate in a rat treated with a steroid. Marked thinning of the distal femoral growth plate is evident. H&E.

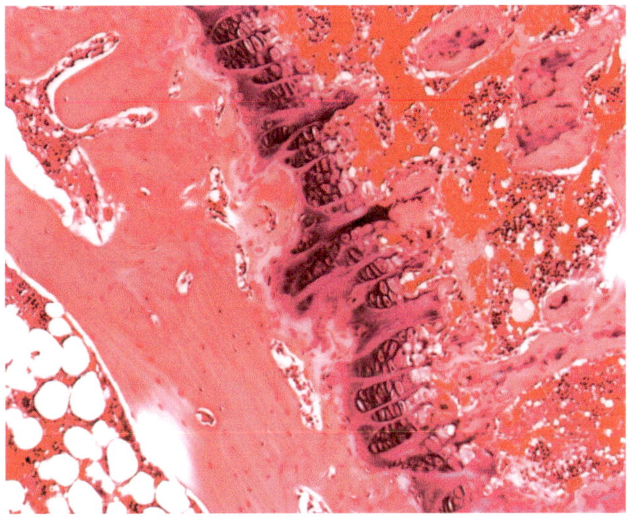

**Figure 11-19.** Thinning of the growth plate of the tibia of a rat treated with a steroid. The zone of proliferation appears normal, but the zones of hypertrophy and mineralisation are largely absent. H&E.

premature differentiation of chondrocytes, thinning of cortical bone, and fusion of the growth plate in young mice [37].

Thyromimetics can be associated with articular cartilage erosion and degeneration (personal observation). Degeneration, erosion, and necrosis of the articular cartilage are induced in several species with quinolone derivatives (*e.g.* nalidixic acid) (Figs. 11.20 and 11.21). In juvenile dogs, quinolones cause vesicles on the articular surfaces, which are grossly visible. Histologically, cavities and fissures within the articular cartilage are seen, with disorganisation of the normal architecture (Fig. 11.22) [38]. Similar changes are induced by compounds of this class in juvenile rats [39]. Inhibition of proteoglycan synthesis is thought to be partially responsible for these changes.

Chondromucinous degeneration, particularly seen in the sternal cartilage, is a common spontaneous finding in older rodents. Its incidence can be reduced by caloric restriction [40]. T-2, a mycotoxin, causes chondrocyte degeneration and necrosis of the articular cartilage in rats [41]. Thinning of the growth plate and necrosis of cartilage and bone are seen with 2-butoxyethanol, due to ischaemia associated with microthrombi [42]. Radiation osteopathy is partially mediated by vascular injury.

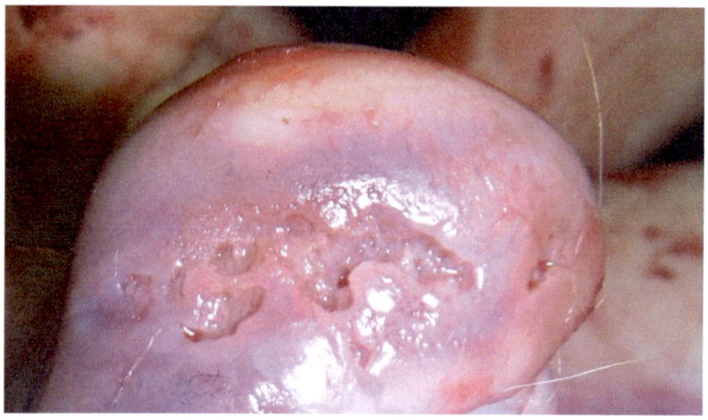

**Figure 11-20.** Erosion of the head of the femur in a juvenile dog, seen at necropsy. Coalescing deep erosions of the articular cartilage are present. Such changes are typically seen with quinolone derivatives.

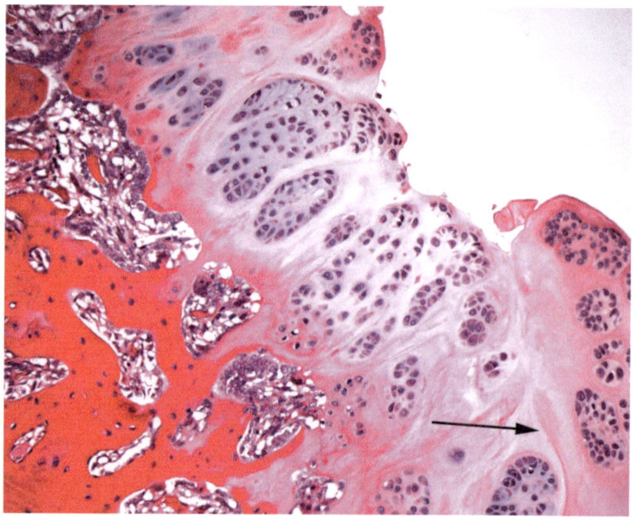

**Figure 11-21.** Erosion of the articular cartilage in a rabbit, with chondrocyte hyperplasia and clustering around and below the erosion. Early fissure formation is also present (*arrow*). H&E.

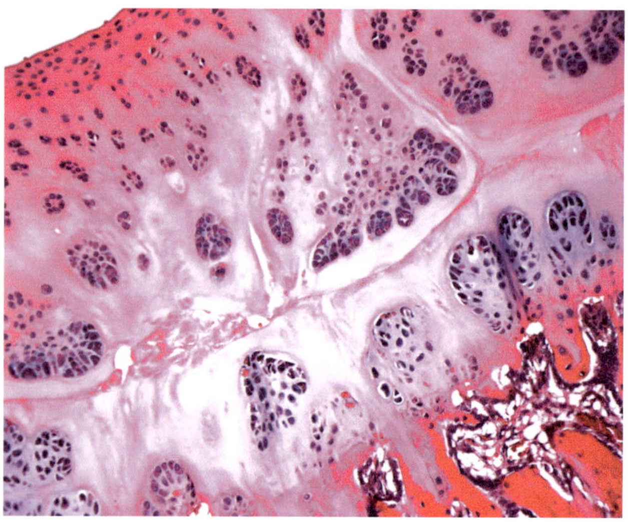

**Figure 11-22.** Early degenerative changes in the articular cartilage in a rabbit. Fissure formation is evident, with chondrocyte clustering and hyperplasia. H&E.

Bone thinning is seen with a variety of compound such as corticosteroids, anticonvulsants, bisphosphonates, antidiabetic compounds, vascular endothelial growth factors (VEGFs), and thyromimetics, among others. Anticonvulsants such as phenytoin affect membrane cation transport, impairing calcium absorption. 2-Hydroxypropyl-β-cyclodextrin caused thinning of bones in a long-term rodent study, possibly through increased osteoclastic resorption [43]. The thickness of the cortical bone is reduced, predisposing to pathologic fractures in rabbits and rodents (Fig. 11.23).

A wide variety of mechanisms including high dietary phosphorus, kidney disease, and agents that impair calcium absorption or vitamin D synthesis lead to hyperparathyroidism and increased bone resorption, causing fibrous osteodystrophy. Histologically, loss of osteoid with replacement by fibroblasts and collagen is seen in the bones (Fig. 11.24). Fibro-osseous lesions are a spontaneous lesion in aging mice (Fig. 11.25). Their incidence can be exacerbated by oestrogen administration [44].

Widening of the zones of mineralisation or ossification due to impaired calcification occurs with several compound classes that affect mineralisation or bone formation. Histologically, expansion of the zone of mineralisation is evident, with increased osteoid and formation surfaces (Fig. 11.26a–c). Accumulation of fluoride,

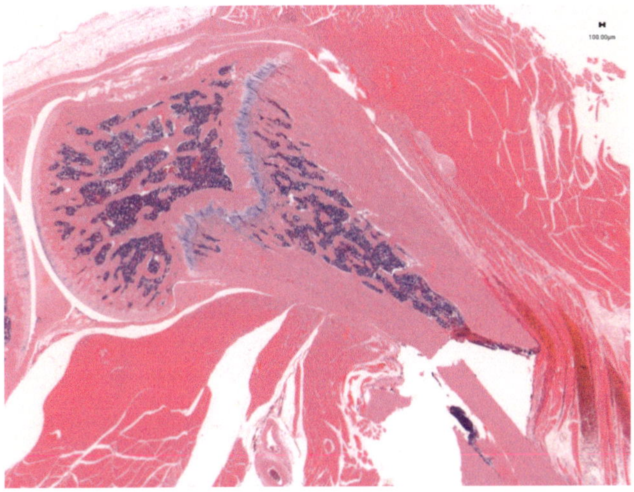

**Figure 11-23.** Pathologic fracture of the femur in a rabbit which received a biologically active compound. The femur has a midshaft fracture, with haemorrhage in the adjacent muscle. The bone appears normal otherwise. H&E.

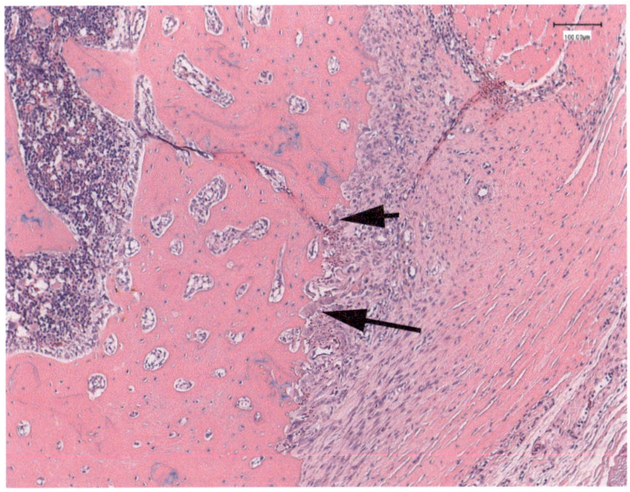

**Figure 11-24.** Increased remodelling activity in a rabbit humerus. Several osteoclasts (*arrow*) are present at the bone margin, which appears irregular with indentations. H&E.

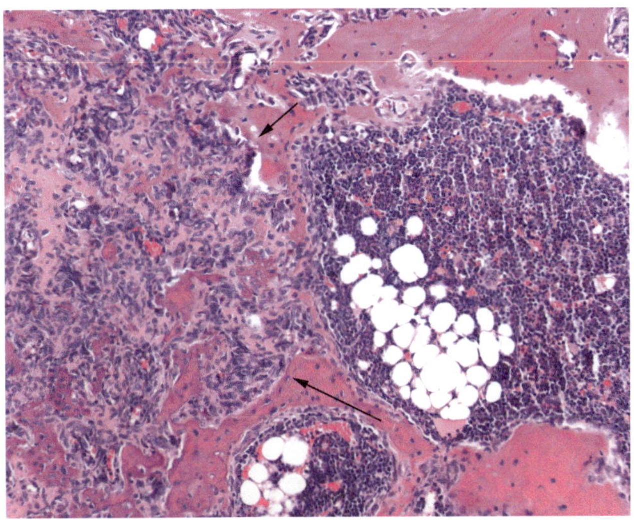

**Figure 11-25.** Fibro-osseous lesion in the sternum of a female mouse (*arrows*). There is focal loss of bone with fibrosis and increased remodelling. These lesions occur spontaneously, particularly in females, but can be increased by oestrogen administration.

tetracyclines and metals such as aluminium interferes with matrix mineralisation, resulting in osteoporosis. Because control of bone remodelling is complex, agents that cause thinning can also initially cause reduced bone resorption and osteosclerosis through inhibition of osteoclast activity. Bisphosphonates, calcitonin, and lead can lead to osteosclerosis by this mechanism. Increased bone growth due to higher cell proliferation occurs with growth hormone and androgens. Increased bone formation, both periosteal and endosteal, is caused by hormone classes such as oestrogens, vitamin D analogues, and prostaglandins. In long-term studies in rodents with vitamin D analogues, the marrow cavities of affected bones may be completely obliterated due to extensive endosteal hyperostosis (Figs. 11.27 and 11.28), resulting in a compensatory increase in splenic extramedullary haemopoiesis. Altered blood flow, causing increases or decreases in oxygen tension, leads to increased bone resorption and new bone formation respectively. This is probably the mechanism for subperiosteal new bone formation induced by prostaglandin $E_2$ and is also seen with pulmonary tumours in dogs.

In most species, osteosarcomas are the commonest spontaneous and induced tumour of the bone. Agents associated with osteosarcoma induction in rodents are numerous and include irradiation, intraosseous injection of viruses or genotoxic carcinogens, and implantation of foreign materials. Systemically administered oestrogens are associated with osteoma and osteosarcoma development, probably due to their promoting effect on bone proliferation. Teriparatide, a parathormone fragment, induces formation of osteomas, osteoblastomas, and osteosarcomas [45, 46].

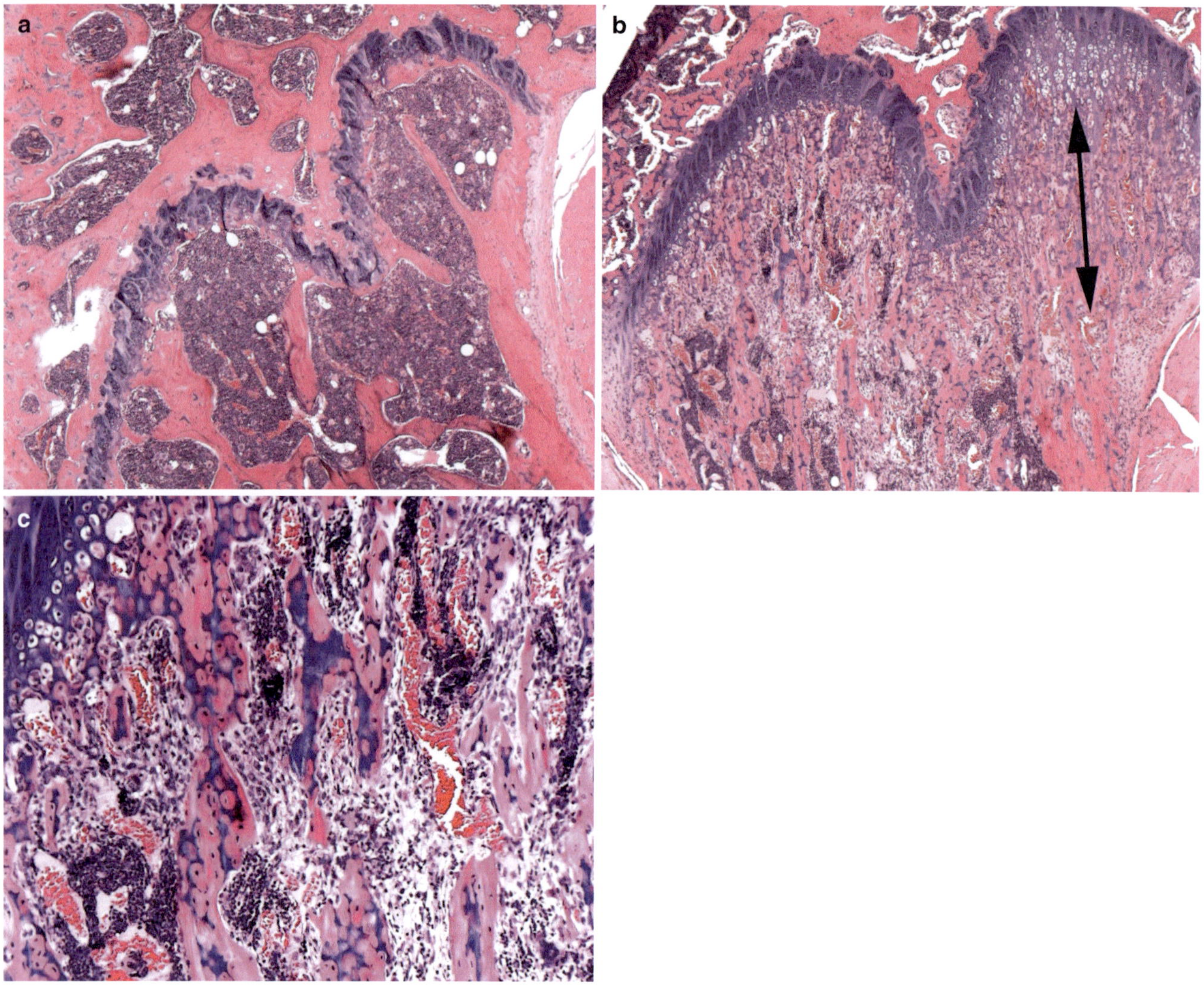


**FIGURE 11-26.** (**a**) Control mouse showing normal epiphyseal architecture of distal femur. (**b**) Treated mouse showing osteosclerosis, with expanded zones of hypertrophy, mineralisation, and osteogenesis, and increased trabeculae in the metaphysis. (**c**) High power of 11.26b. Islets of mineralised cartilage persist within the trabeculae due to delayed mineralisation and osteogenesis. Trabeculae are more numerous than normal, with fibrous replacement of the marrow. Fluoride, metals, and growth factor inhibitors are often associated with these lesions. H&E.

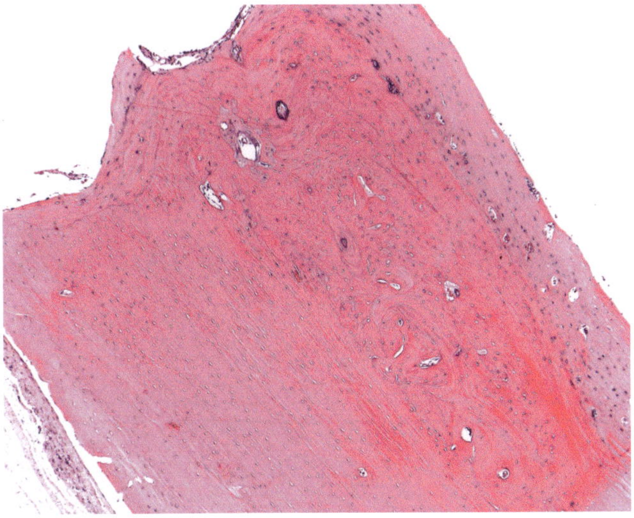

**Figure 11-27.** Hyperostosis of the cranium of a rat given a vitamin D analogue. The cranium is markedly thickened due to diffuse new bone formation on the surface. H&E.

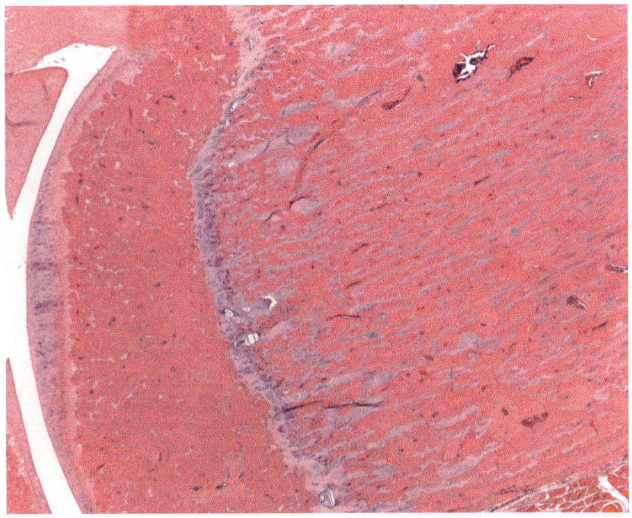

**Figure 11-28.** Endosteal hyperostosis of the distal femur, in a rat. Both epiphyseal and diaphyseal cavities are completely filled by compact bone. The rat received a vitamin D analogue. H&E.

## 11.3 Joints

Intra-articular injections of numerous test articles, including polysaccharides and peptides, cause inflammation, but induced changes in the joints are rare with systemically administered compounds. Toxicologically induced changes in the joints are listed below:

- Synovial epithelial vacuolation
- Synovial hyperplasia
- Synovial inflammation/arthritis
- Tendons—thickening/inflammation

When administered systemically, antibodies bound to polyethylene glycol (PEG) have been known to accumulate in the synovial membrane in dogs and primates. Histologically, vacuolation of the epithelial cells is seen, sometimes with foamy macrophage infiltration, but generally with no inflammatory response. Synovial hyperplasia with lymphocytic infiltration has been seen with a muramyl peptide in our laboratory (Fig. 11.29) [18]. Synovial hyperplasia and degeneration with subsynovial fibrodysplasia have been recorded with a metalloproteinase inhibitor in dogs (Fig. 11.30) [47]. Similar changes have been recorded in rats with this class of compound [32].

Spontaneous arthritis, particularly of the hind legs, is a common background finding in old rats, often accompanying pododermatitis. Incidence of this finding can be altered by hormonal treatment, with androgens increasing its incidence and oestrogens reducing it. A number of animal models of arthritis have been developed to study the human condition and to assess the efficacy of therapeutic compounds. Injections of various adjuvants into the footpad induce arthritis. 6-Sulphanil-aminoindazole induces arthritis in rats when given orally [48]. Histologically, fibrin deposition and neutrophilic infiltrate are seen in acute arthritis (Fig. 11.31). In longer-standing cases, synovial hyperplasia, periarticular fibrosis, and chronic inflammation develop. Induced arthritis may also be immune mediated. Immune-mediated arthritis can occur due to deposition of antigen in the joint, eliciting a delayed hypersensitivity response. Antigen–antibody complex deposition in the joint, triggering an inflammatory reaction, is the mechanism of induction with trimethoprim and sulfadiazine. Lysosomal membrane destabilisers, enzymes, and contrast agents can induce synovial membrane inflammation and hypertrophy. Deposition of urate crystals in the joint occurs with compounds such as salicylates, ethambutol, and some diuretics, resulting in arthritis. Tendon degeneration occurs with quinolone antibiotics, which causes mononuclear cell infiltration and oedema initially, followed by necrosis of the cells and matrix [39, 49, 50]. Metalloproteinase inhibitors cause fibrodysplasia of the tendons, characterised by collagen replacement with active fibroblasts and irregularly placed collagen bundles in dogs, with similar effects in other species including man (Fig. 11.32) [47].

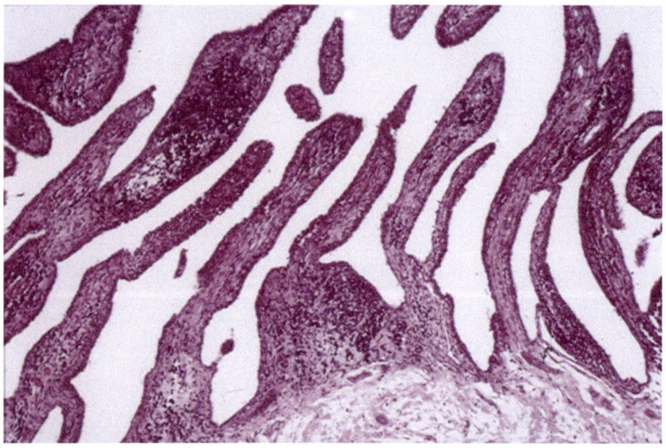

**Figure 11-29.** Synovial hyperplasia with extensive villus formation in the joint of a dog given a novel immunostimulant drug. An associated lymphocytic infiltration is also present. H&E (With kind permission from Springer Science+Business Media B.V [18]).

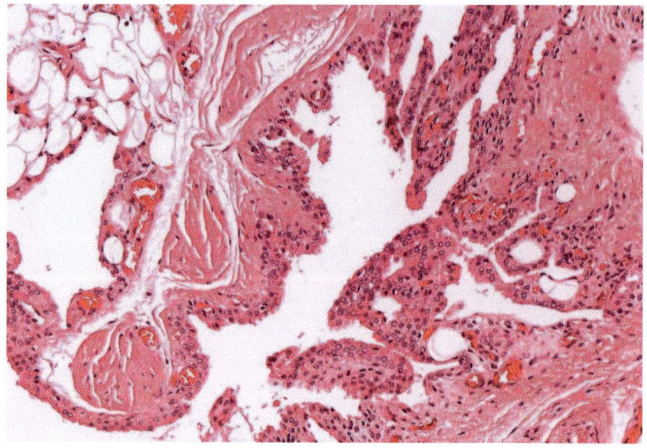

**Figure 11-30.** Synovial hyperplasia in a monkey. The synovial membrane is forming fronds and papillary projections. H&E.

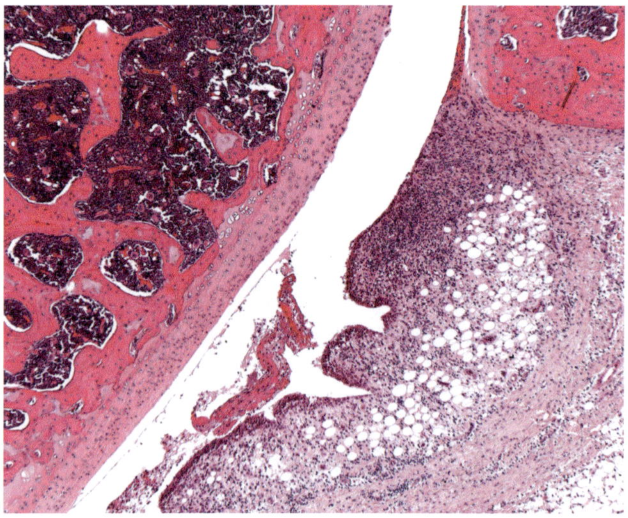

**Figure 11-31.** Arthritis in the femoro-tibial joint of a rat. Fibrinous exudate is present within the joint cavity, and the synovial capsule is infiltrated by inflammatory cells. Septic emboli from other organs can result in arthritis. H&E.

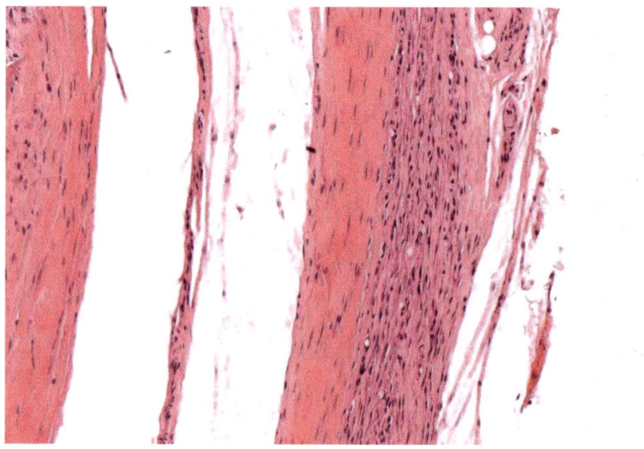

**Figure 11-32.** Thickening of the tendon sheath with fibroblasts and collagen in a monkey. These lesions can be induced by metalloproteinase inhibitors. H&E.

## 11.4 Skin and Adipose Tissue

### 11.4.1 Skin

The skin is usually an effective barrier against insult, despite its large surface area and its exposure to a wide variety of toxic agents. In safety assessment studies, lesions of the skin are most frequently seen with an administration route that involves the skin. These include topical applications and intradermal, subcutaneous, and intramuscular injections. A certain level of procedural changes is to be expected with these routes of application and should be clearly differentiated from any treatment-related changes. In addition, changes due to the vehicle are common, such as with oil-based vehicles and adjuvants, and should be clearly identified as disparate from any effect of the test article.

Testing of skin irritancy potential is routinely done for topically applied pharmaceuticals and chemicals that are likely to contact human skin, although relevance of animal models for man is much debated. The species most commonly employed for these studies are rabbits, mice, and pigs. The pig is considered to be the most similar to man in terms of skin structure. Scoring of clinical signs such as reddening, thickening, and oedema is routinely done in vivo. A semiquantitative scoring system is used for grading macroscopic and microscopic findings. Models commonly used for detection of chloracnegens include the rabbit pinnae, skin of the hairless mouse, and facial skin of the rhesus monkey. Wound healing models are also used for assessment of different types of wounds under different conditions, such as in diabetic models. Recently developed models include transgenic mice and rats for investigating molecular pathways [51, 52]. Guinea pigs are generally used as sensitisation models.

To accurately assess effects in local application or injection studies, the site of treatment should be clearly identified to ensure correct sampling at necropsy. The histology protocol should be designed to ensure that sections are consistently taken from the centre of the treated site, with more than one section being examined where necessary.

Broadly, the skin is comprised of epidermis, dermis, and adnexal structures. Effects on the skin can be due to irritation or to toxicity, which can be direct or indirect, and may involve one or more of the components of the skin. Cutaneous toxicity can be caused by test materials administered locally or systemically and can be due to the test article itself or a metabolite. The skin has a high capacity for metabolism, so cutaneous pathology can be caused by toxic metabolites generated either locally or systemically. More rarely, cutaneous toxicity develops through immune-mediated processes or phototoxicity. Secondary effects can also occur, such as ulceration due to altered folate metabolism with antibiotics or viral papilloma development with immunosuppressants.

The skin has a wide range of responses to insult, usually including one or more of the following processes: inflammation, degeneration, and hyperplasia. Commonly seen histologic changes in dermal studies are hyperkeratosis, oedema, congestion, inflammation, erosion, ulceration, and necrosis. Proliferative changes that may be seen are fibrosis, epidermal hyperplasia, and adnexal hyperplasia. Epidermal and adnexal hyperplasia may be regenerative, secondary to inflammatory or degenerative processes, or a primary response to a test article causing increased epithelial cell replication such as epidermal growth factor.

Changes associated with systemically and dermally administered compounds include the following:

- Hyperkeratosis
- Disturbances of pigmentation
- Inflammation/ulceration/vesicles and degenerative changes, epidermal/adnexal
- Chloracne
- Hyperplasia—epidermal/adnexal
- Atrophy—epidermal/adnexal
- Toxic epidermal necrolysis
- Xanthomas
- Papillomas, keratoacanthomas, squamous cell carcinomas, basal cell tumours

Subcutaneous tissue:

- Increased collagen/fibrosis
- Inflammation
- Fibrosarcomas
- Lipomas/liposarcomas
- Haemangiomas/haemangiosarcomas

Hyperkeratosis, appearing as increased thickness of the cornified layer, can be induced as an independent finding or as part of a spectrum of changes. Hyperkeratosis represents a protective response of the skin to minimal irritation and is often seen in topical application studies in untreated areas of shaved skin. Parakeratosis, where the cornified layer contains nuclei, is seen in increased epithelial turnover. It is induced by zinc deficiency in pigs.

Epidermal pigmentation can result from accumulation of an exogenous substance, either on its own or as a complex with an endogenous substance, or due to increased synthesis and accumulation of an endogenous pigment. Greyish colouration of the skin is seen with silver in man and rodents. Orange discolouration of the fur occurs in rats given β-carotene. Sodium xylenesulfonate, a constituent of several household products including shampoos, causes brown skin discolouration in rats [53]. Bile pigments produce yellow discolouration of the skin in animals suffering from jaundice. Several compound classes, including hormones and hydantoin derivatives, stimulate melanogenesis, resulting in hyperpigmentation (Fig. 11.33a, b). Size and distribution of

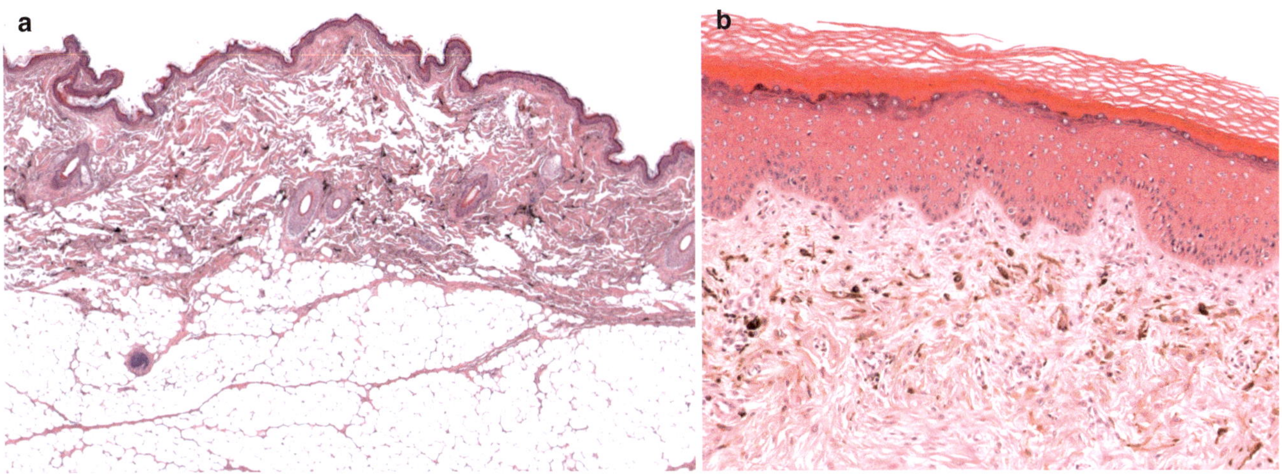


**Figure 11-33.** (**a**) Hyperpigmentation in a cynomolgus monkey, noted in vivo. Large pigmented aggregates are present in the dermis. (**b**) Hyperpigmentation in a cynomolgus monkey, noted in vivo. Numerous melanocytes are seen in the dermis, some with large melanosomes. H&E.

melanosomes in the melanocyte, and the level of tyrosinase activity, influence the degree of pigmentation [54]. Immunostaining for tyrosinase activity is used to identify melanocytes.

Hypopigmentation of normally pigmented skin has been recorded in the dog with a platelet aggregate inhibitor PD89454, with ultrastructural findings suggesting an interference in melanosome formation and/or melanisation [55]. Cabergoline, a dopaminergic agonist, is associated with skin discolouration in dogs, possibly due to inhibition of melanocyte-stimulating hormone [56]. Grey discolouration of the fur has been recorded in hamsters given oxidosqualene cyclase inhibitors [57]. Depigmenting agents such as retinoic acid and melanocytotoxic agents like cysteaminylphenol are associated with depigmentation in man.

A variety of different compound classes induce inflammatory and degenerative changes in the epidermis and/or adnexal structures. These changes include inflammation, erosion, ulceration, vesicles, and scab formation. Direct irritation occurs with acidic or alkaline agents applied topically.

Folliculitis and dermal inflammation are induced by a wide variety of compound classes. Biological agents associated with these changes include erbB receptor inhibitors, tyrosine kinase inhibitors, and cytokines such as IL-2 (Fig. 11.34) [58]. Lymphohistiocytic inflammation of the dermis, often centred on the follicles, is seen histologically. If the follicles are specifically affected, folliculitis often progresses to degeneration and subsequent atrophy.

Degeneration and necrosis of the external ear margins in some species and the tail tip in rodents are seen with test materials that cause vasoconstriction, such as ergot-containing compounds (Fig. 11.35). Bleomycin causes alopecia, ulceration of the footpads, and loss of nails in dogs, probably by an antimitotic effect [59]. Acyclovir and nucleoside analogues have similar effects [60, 61].

Compounds like 2,3,7,8-tetrachlorobenzo-p-dioxin (TCDD) and other polyhalogenated aromatic hydrocarbons induce chloracne in laboratory animal models, seen as large keratin cysts. These cysts develop from the hair follicles and sebaceous glands whose ducts undergo squamous metaplasia, resulting in blockage and atrophy with keratin accumulation (Figs. 11.36 and 11.37) [18].

Hyperplasia of various adnexal structures is seen with some test materials. Sebaceous gland hyperplasia is associated with administration of androgens and androgen promoters such as citral and L-arginine [62]. Emollients such as oleic acid diethanolamine cause dermal inflammation with epidermal and sebaceous gland hyperplasia in rodents [63].

Immune-mediated skin toxicity occurs in man with many antibiotics including sulphonamides and ampicillin. Sulphonamide hypersensitivity is also seen in dogs [64]. In susceptible individuals, sulphonamides are bioactivated to a nitroso metabolite that binds with a protein to form adducts, and possibly elicits an antibody-mediated immune response [64].

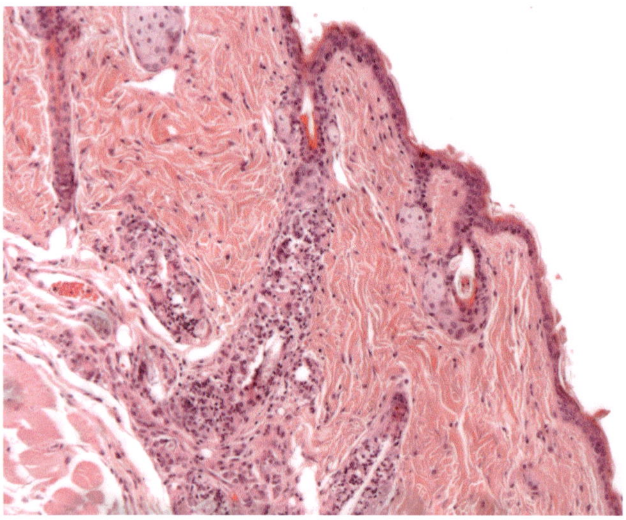

**Figure 11-34.** Folliculitis in the skin of a rat. Inflammatory cells are predominantly macrophages and lymphocytes, infiltrating degenerating hair follicles and adnexal structures. Many biologics including growth factor inhibitors induce similar changes. H&E.

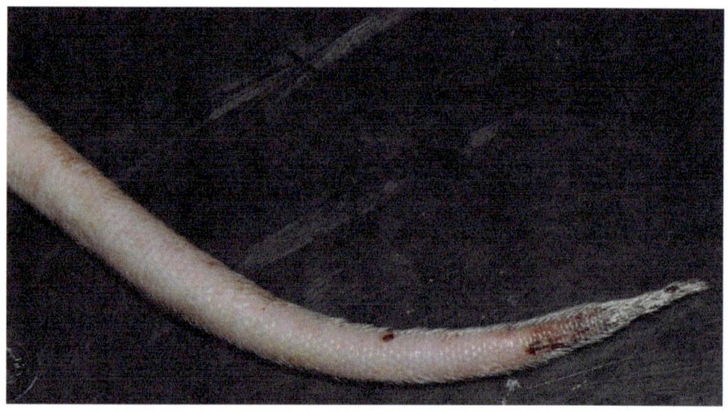

**Figure 11-35.** Necrosis of the tail tip in a rat, which appears dark and shrunken. Test articles causing vasoconstriction can induce these changes in the tail and ear tips of laboratory species. H&E.

In humans, phototoxicity occurs with a number of pharmaceuticals, including tetracyclines, sulphonamides, and chlorpromazine. It is difficult to predict from safety studies. In rats and cattle, quinoxaline derivates are associated with photoallergic reactions.

A wide range of compound classes, including anticancerals, thallium, selenium, and halogenated hydrocarbons, target the hair follicles resulting in alopecia. Anticancerals such as doxorubicin, vincristine, and cyclophosphamide affect the anagen phase due to their antimitotic activity. Propranolol, mercury, thallium, and anticoagulants, among many other agents, prolong the telogen phase. Corticosteroid administration results in thinning of the epidermis, arrest of hair follicle growth, and atrophy of adnexal structures (Fig. 11.38). The mechanism is not clear but corticosteroids have been shown to lower the epithelial mitotic rate and fibroblast growth rate. Areas subject to rubbing, such as around the nose in steroid inhalation studies in rodents, are common sites of alopecia (personal observation). Sex hormones and bromocriptine also cause alopecia in rodents.

Bleomycin causes sebaceous gland atrophy in rats, along with thickening and hyperpigmentation of the skin [65] (Fig. 11.39). In hamsters the flank organ, which consists of large sebaceous glands, is androgen-dependent and partially atrophies after castration.

Xanthomas in the skin have been induced in monkeys and rabbits given high-cholesterol diets [66]. These appear as accumulations of foamy macrophages with

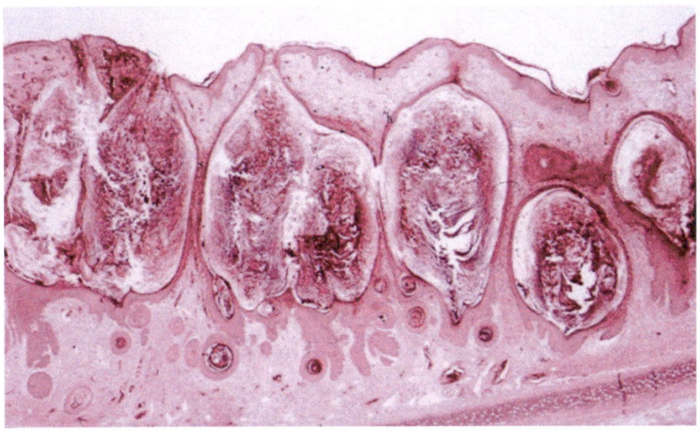

**Figure 11-36.** Chloracne in a rabbit pinna induced by a potent chloracnegen. The pilosebaceous follicles are grossly distended with keratin debris. The lining epithelium shows acanthosis and hyperkeratosis. Note the absence of sebaceous glands. H&E (With kind permission from Springer Science+Business Media B.V [18]).

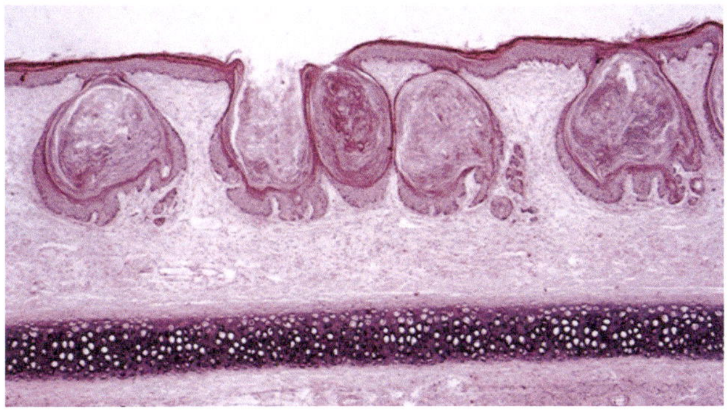

**Figure 11-37.** The same condition as in Fig. 11.36 but with a lower dose of the chloracnegen. The follicles are slightly dilated with acanthosis and hyperkeratosis of the lining epithelium. H&E (With kind permission from Springer Science+Business Media B.V [18]).

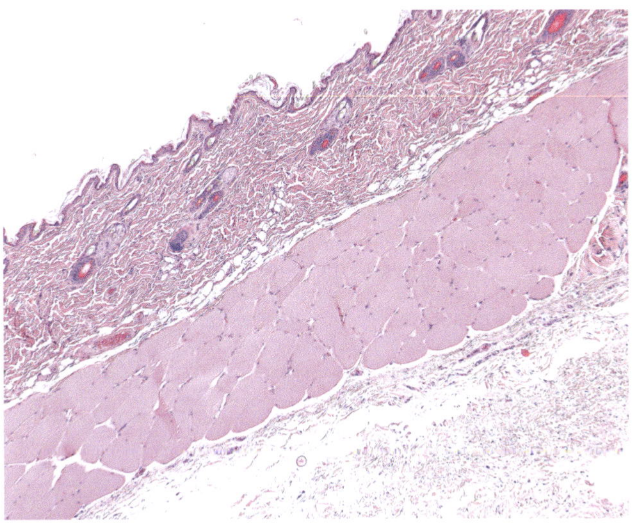

**Figure 11-38.** Increased telogen hair follicles in the skin of a rat treated with a steroid. Many compound classes, including steroids, induce this change. H&E.

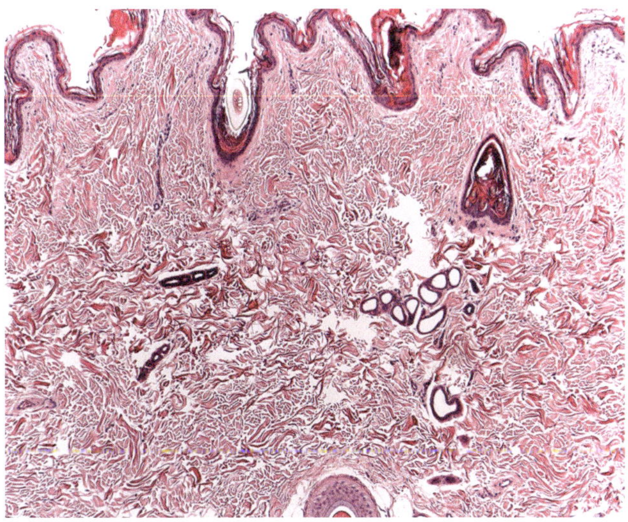

**Figure 11-39.** Sebaceous gland atrophy in the skin of a dog. Hair follicles and sweat glands are seen, but sebaceous glands are not evident. H&E.

cholesterol clefts in the dermis, sometimes associated with mild lymphocytic infiltration (Fig. 11.40).

Toxic epidermal necrolysis is associated with many pharmaceuticals including penicillin and phenytoin in man. Diffuse severe epidermal necrosis, with clefts and blisters at the dermoepidermal junction, is seen histologically. Similar lesions have been seen in dogs treated with sulphonamides, penicillin, and anthelminthics such as thiabendazole [67].

Epidermal hyperplasia can be secondary to irritant or degenerative changes in the skin or primary due to a direct effect of the test article. Proliferation can also be secondary to effects on other systems; for example, hormonal perturbations. Oxidosqualene cyclase inhibitors induce squamous hyperplasia and dermal inflammation in hamsters and dogs, with folliculitis leading to follicular atrophy in dogs [57, 68]. Epidermal growth factor and growth hormones are associated with primary epithelial hyperplasia or acanthosis. Histologically, this appears as thickening of the epidermis with increased layers of cells and increased numbers of spinous cells. Growth hormones also increase dermal collagen.

A wide range of genotoxic compounds, including dioxins and polycyclic hydrocarbons, cause epithelial hyperplasia and skin tumours. These tumours include papillomas, squamous cell carcinomas, and other epithelial tumours (Figs. 11.41 and 11.42). Both one-stage and two-stage models of carcinogenesis are used for detection of

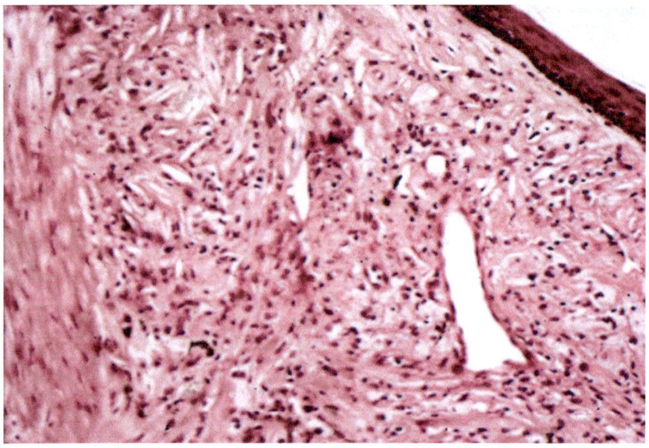

**Figure 11-40.** Xanthoma in the skin of a monkey that received a high-cholesterol diet. Cholesterol clefts and foamy macrophages in the dermis, as seen here, are characteristic of this lesion. H&E (With kind permission from Springer Science+Business Media B.V [18]).

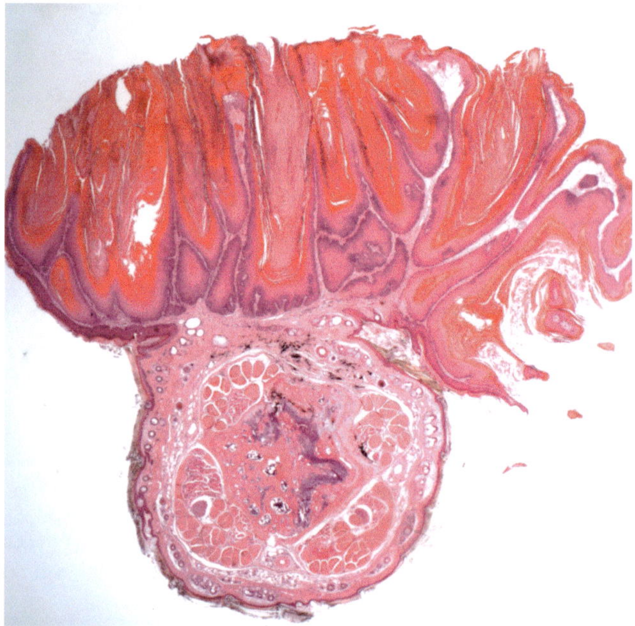

**Figure 11-41.** Papilloma on the tail of a transgenic mouse given methylnitrosourea. Branching stromal projections covered by hyperplastic squamous epithelium are characteristic of this tumour type. Marked keratosis is also evident. H&E.

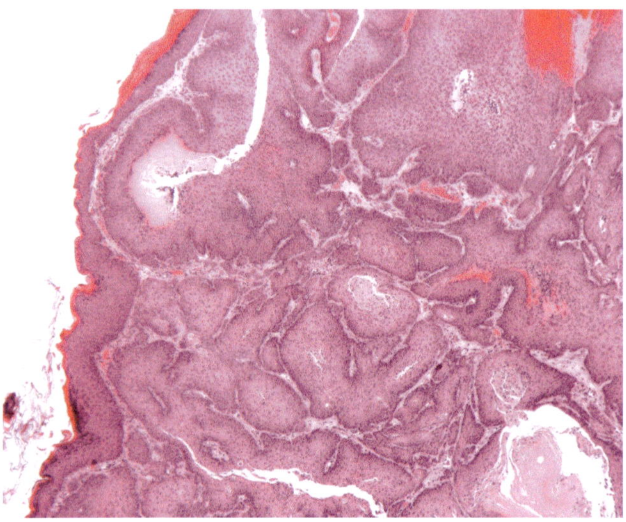

**Figure 11-42.** Squamous cell carcinoma in the skin of a transgenic mouse given methylnitrosourea. Nests and sheets of well-differentiated squamous epithelium have invaded the dermis. H&E.

dermal carcinogenic agents. Carcinogenesis bioassays for contact dermal carcinogens are preferentially performed on mice, although other rodent species are sometimes used [69].

Dermal and subcutaneous injections are often associated with nonprocedural changes. Subcutaneous injections of proteins often induce some degree of acute or granulomatous inflammation and/or granulomas in the subcutis. Growth hormone injected subcutaneously produces a localised increase in dermal collagen, unaccompanied by inflammation (Fig. 11.43). Subcutaneous injection with oil-based vehicles results in lipogranulomas in the subcutis, sometimes with necrosis and abscess formation of the subcutaneous fascia (Figs. 11.44 and 11.45a, b). Rats treated by this route can also develop lipogranulomas in the lung (personal observation) and the peritoneal cavity by an incompletely understood mechanism [70].

Inflammation and proliferation of the subcutaneous connective tissue occur in man and animals given metalloproteinase inhibitors. These agents cause fibrodysplasia of the subcutaneous tissue, characterised by myofibroblastic cell proliferation around blood vessels, in dogs [47]. Bleomycin is associated with an increase in dermal collagen in rats [65]. Multifocal granulomas in several organs including the subcutaneous tissue have been induced in dogs with a thromboxane receptor antagonist [71].

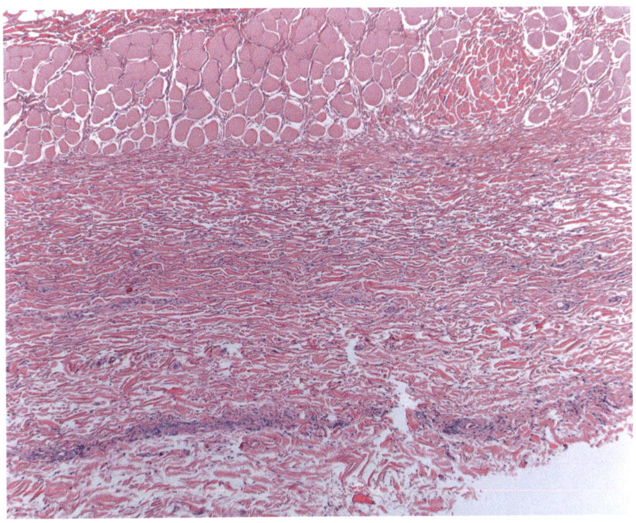

**Figure 11-43.** Increased dermal collagen in the skin of a rat given a growth promoter locally. Many compound classes can cause this change, either by a direct proliferative effect or secondary to inflammation. H&E.

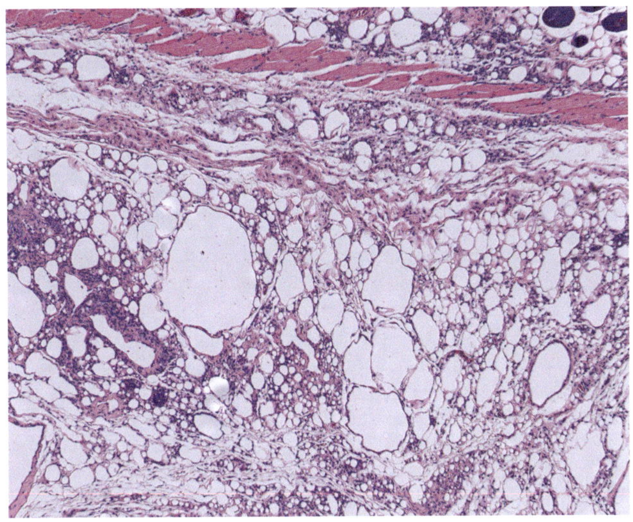

**Figure 11-44.** Subcutaneous lipogranuloma following injection of an oil-based vehicle in a rat. Numerous variably sized lipid vacuoles are seen in the dermis and subcutis, with subcutaneous macrophage infiltration. H&E.

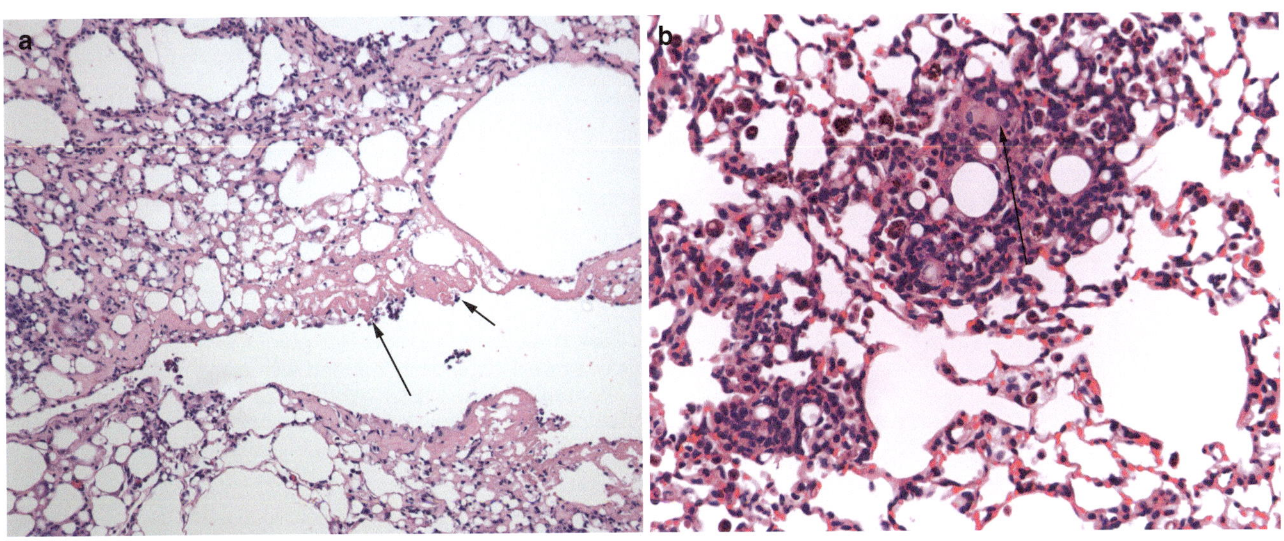


**Figure 11-45.** (**a**) Subcutaneous injection of an oil-based vehicle in a rat. The subcutaneous tissue shows early degenerative changes, appearing homogenous and eosinophilic with lack of cellular detail (*arrows*). H&E. (**b**) Lipogranuloma in the lung of a rat injected subcutaneously with an oil-based vehicle. Variably sized lipid vacuoles are surrounded by macrophages and dark brown pigmented macrophages, with a foreign-body giant cell evident (*arrow*). H&E.

Peroxisome proliferator associated receptor agonists (PPARs) are associated with the development of several types of tumours. Stimulation of adipogenesis, with subsequent release of cytokines and growth factors that stimulate mesenchymal and endothelial proliferation, is considered to be the mechanism of induction for these tumours [72]. Development of angiomatous hyperplasia, haemangiomas, and haemangiosarcomas in the skin/subcutis of mice has been recorded with PPARα and γ-agonists. One of these, troglitazone, has been shown to increase the survival of mouse, but not human, endothelial cells in vitro [73]. Pregabalin, a γ-hydroxybutyric acid (GABA) inhibitor, also induces haemangiosarcomas in mice, possibly via growth factors that stimulate endothelial cell proliferation [74]. The susceptibility of mice to the induction of these tumours is possibly due to their background level of endothelial proliferation, which is higher than that of humans and rats [75]. Subcutaneous fibrosarcomas in rodents are also associated with PPAR-γ and dual α-/γ-agonists [76].

Subcutaneous implants of various types, including plastics, are known to cause subcutaneous mesenchymal tumours in a range of species including man [77]. Tumour development may depend on the physical characteristics of the implant. Tumours associated with microchips have been recorded in dogs and some strains of rodents, including the B6C3F1 mouse and F344 rat (Fig. 11.46) [78, 79]. Undifferentiated pleomorphic sarcomas and fibrosarcomas are the tumour types most commonly diagnosed in association with microchips and implants. Injection of a range of carcinogenic chemicals such as polycyclic hydrocarbons, and noncarcinogenic substances such as macromolecular dextrans and vaccines, also induces mesenchymal tumours.

## 11.4.2 Adipose Tissue

Induced changes in adipose tissue comprise the following:

- Increased adipose tissue
- Decreased adipose tissue
- Transformation of brown to white adipose tissue
- Transformation of white to brown adipose tissue
- Inflammation/necrosis
- Lipomas/liposarcomas

In safety assessment studies, the commonest changes in the adipose tissue are increases or decreases in quantity. These can be either due to primary toxicity or, more often, secondary to systemic effects.

Increases in body fat can be related to dietary manipulation. Sympathomimetic agents, cold, and hypoxia stimulate the brown fat, resulting in hyperplasia due to increased demand for energy [80]. Troglitazone increases brown fat, accompanied by a reduction in white fat.

Nonspecific reductions in adipose tissue are often seen with reduced food intake, which can be associated with a range of agents including antidiabetic and antiobesity treatments such as GLP-1 peptide agonists. Hypocholesterolemics, through their effects on lipid metabolism, result in a reduction in body fat. Recombinant human leptin produces atrophy of brown and white fat in C57BL/6 mice.

Administration of PPAR-γ and dual α-/γ-agonists is often associated with changes in adipose tissue. Transformation of brown fat to white, caused by this compound class, is seen histologically as macrovesicular vacuolation of brown adipocytes (Fig. 11.47a, b). Growth hormones can cause a similar transformation. Transformation of white fat to brown, seen histologically as microvesiculation of adipocytes, giving it the appearance of brown

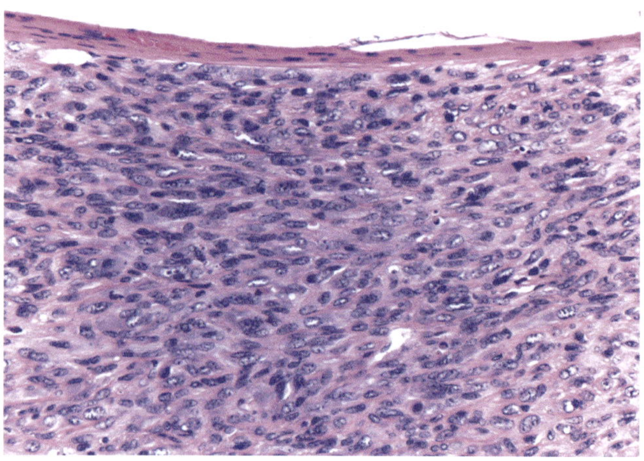

**Figure 11-46.** Subcutaneous fibrosarcoma in a rat. The tumour developed around an implant, with a thin fibrous tissue capsule between the implant and the tumour. Tumour cells resemble fibroblasts, with large oval- or spindle-shaped nuclei, eosinophilic cytoplasm, and indistinct cell membranes. H&E.

fat, is also associated with PPAR-γ and dual α-/γ-agonists (Fig. 11.48a, b). Inflammation of brown fat sometimes occurs as an induced change with β3 agonists and PPARs.

Focal fat necrosis in rodents occurs as a spontaneous finding in the abdominal adipose tissue usually due to strangulation of focal areas of adipose tissue. Grossly these appear as yellow nodules of necrotic adipocytes in the abdominal fat or, less frequently, in the epididymal fat pad. Fat necrosis can be induced in several species including rats by feeding a vitamin E-deficient diet.

Lipomas, liposarcomas, and angiolipomas—the latter comprising both proliferating adipocytes and vascular endothelial cells—have been induced by PPAR-γ and dual α-/γ-agonists in rodents, the postulated mechanism being a direct stimulatory effect on white adipocytes and mesenchymal cells [76]. Diagnostic criteria and recommended nomenclature for these soft tissue tumours have been published [72]. An increase in hibernomas has been recorded with phentolamine, an α-adrenergic, and is thought to represent an exaggerated pharmacological response [81]. Mesenchymal tumours, predominantly fibrosarcomas, are also induced by PPAR-γ and dual α-/γ-agonists [76, 82]. The mechanism of induction for these tumours is thought to be proliferation of mesenchymal cells in the adipose tissue, concomitant with inflammation and fibrosis [83] (Fig. 11.49).

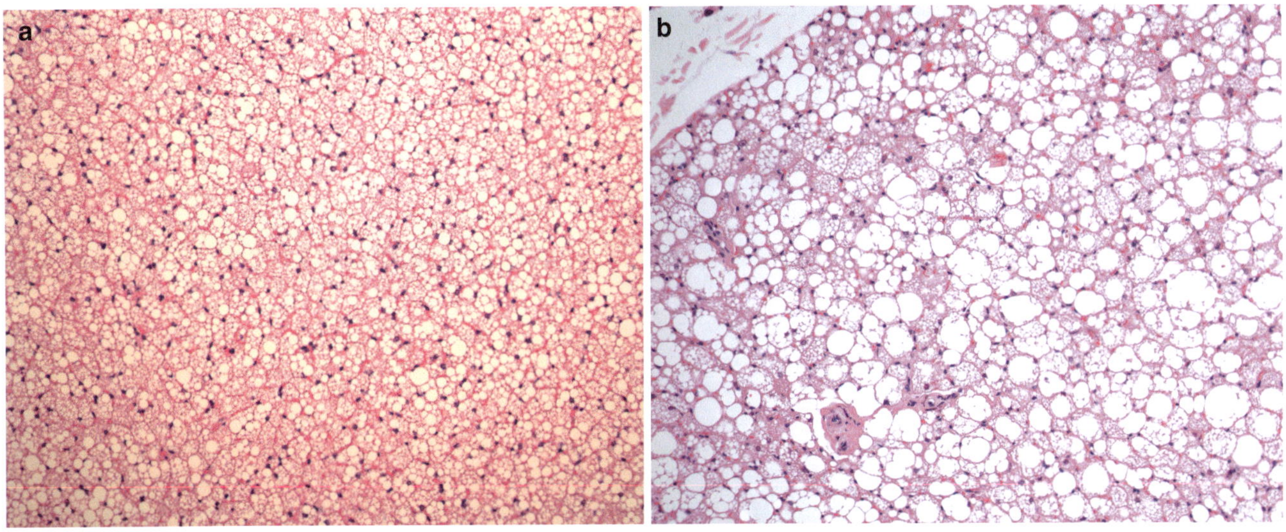

**Figure 11-47.** (**a**) Normal interscapular brown adipose tissue from a rat. (**b**) Brown adipose tissue transformation in a rat. Macro- and microvesicular vacuolation of the adipocytes are present. This change can be adaptive or due to a direct effect on adipocyte receptors. PPARs are often associated with this change. H&E.

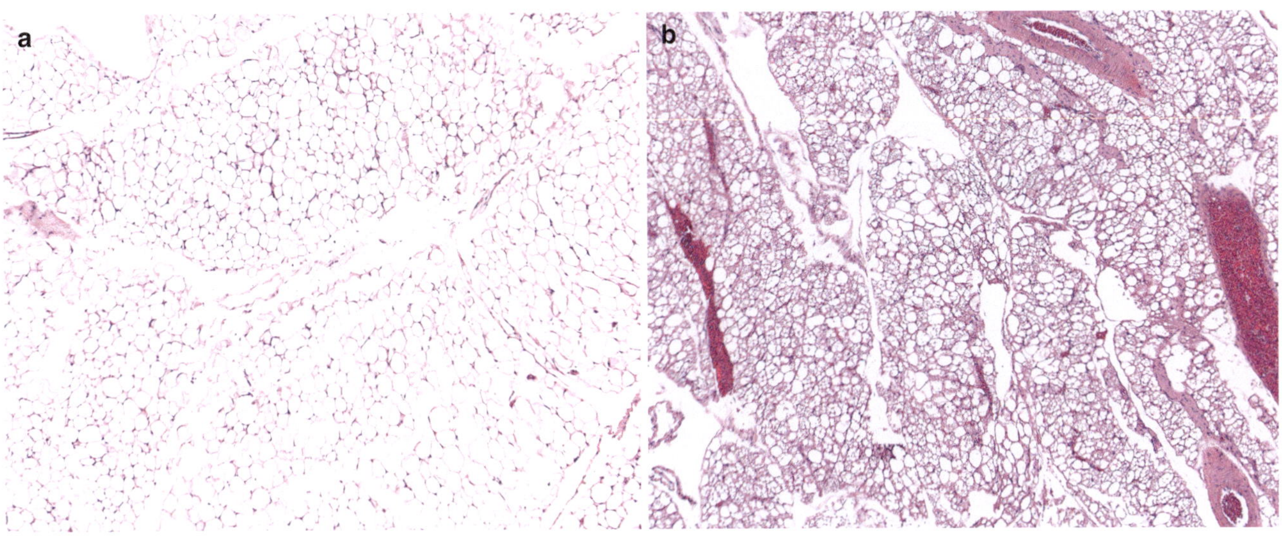

**Figure 11-48.** (**a**) Normal mesenteric white adipose tissue in a rat. H&E. (**b**) White adipose tissue transformation in a rat. Micro- and macrovesicular vacuolation of the adipocytes are present, giving the appearance of brown fat. B-agonists can be associated with this change. H&E.

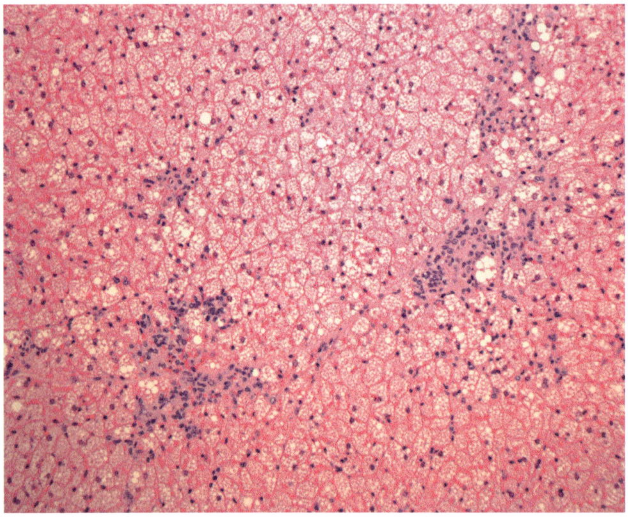

**Figure 11-49.** Eosinophilia and inflammation of brown adipose tissue in a rat. The tissue appears more eosinophilic than normal with focal vacuolation and inflammation. Inflammatory cells are predominantly lymphocytic.

## References


1. Valentine BA, Hermanson JW. Pathology methods in nonclinical neurotoxicity studies: evaluation of muscle. In: Bolon B, Butt MT, editors. Fundamental neuropathology for pathologists and toxicologists. Hoboken: John Wiley and Sons; 2011. p. 239–52.
2. Alleva FR, Haberman BH, Slaughter LJ, Balazs T. Muscular degeneration in rats after postnatal treatment with 6-mercaptopurine. Drug Chem Toxicol. 1981;4:133–46.
3. Alleva FR, Slaughter LJ, Abraham AA, Balazs T. Further studies on 6-mercaptopurine-induced muscle atrophy in rats, mice, and hamsters treated as neonates. Pediatr Pharmacol (New York). 1984;4:39–48.
4. Alleva FR, Slaughter LJ, Abraham AA, Balazs T. Toxicological studies with 6-mercaptopurine in neonates. Toxicol Ind Health. 1986;2:11–23.
5. Westwood FR, Bigley A, Randall K, Marsden AM, Scott RC. Statin-induced muscle necrosis in the rat: distribution, development, and fibre selectivity. Toxicol Pathol. 2005;33:246–57.
6. Westwood FR, Scott RC, Marsden AM, Bigley A, Randall K. Rosuvastatin: characterization of induced myopathy in the rat. Toxicol Pathol. 2008;36:345–52.
7. Pettersen JC, Pruimboom-Brees I, Francone OL, Amacher DE, Boldt SE, Kerlin RL, et al. The PPAR alpha agonists fenofibrate and CP-778875 cause increased beta oxidation, leading to oxidative injury in skeletal and cardiac muscle in the rat. Toxicol Pathol. 2012;40:435–47.
8. Teravainen H, Larsen A, Hillbom M. Clofibrate-induced myopathy in the rat. Acta Neuropathol. 1997;39:135–8.
9. Okada M, Inoue Y, Ube M, Sano F, Ikeda I, Sugimoto J, et al. Skeletal muscle susceptibility to clofibrate induction of lesions in rats. Toxicol Pathol. 2007;35:517–20.
10. Okada M, Sano F, Ikeda I, Sugimoto J, Takagi S, Sakai H, et al. Fenofibrate-induced muscular toxicity is associated with a metabolic shift limited to type-1 muscles in rats. Toxicol Pathol. 2009;37:517–20.
11. Clarke JT, Karpati G, Carpenter S, Wolfe LS. The effect of vincristine on skeletal muscle in the rat. A correlative histochemical, ultrastructural and chemical study. J Neuropathol Exp Neurol. 1972;31:247–66.
12. Karpati G, Carpenter S, Clarke JT, Wolfe LS. Experimental vincristine myopathy—a histochemical, ultrastructural and biochemical study. J Neuropathol Exp Neurol. 1971;30:137.
13. Haschek WM, Rousseaux CG, Wallig MA. Cardiovascular and skeletal muscle systems; section III. In: Fundamentals of toxicologic pathology. London: Elsevier; 2010. p. 365–76.
14. Doroshow JH, Tallent C, Schechter JE. Ultrastructural features of adriamycin-induced skeletal and cardiac muscle toxicity. Am J Pathol. 1985;118:288–97.
15. Sims LD, Glastonbury JRW. Skeletal muscle. In: Pathology of the pig. Bendigo: Pig Research and Development Corporation; 1996. p. 284.
16. Velasco W, Finol HJ, Marquez A. Toxic and neurogenic factors in chloroquine myopathy fibre selectivity. J Submicrosc Cytol Pathol. 1995;27:451–7.
17. Greaves P. Musculoskeletal system. In: Histopathology of preclinical safety studies. Philadelphia: Elsevier; 2012. p. 157–206.
18. Gopinath C, Prentice DE, Lewis DJ. The musculoskeletal system and skin. In: Atlas of experimental toxicological pathology. Lancaster/Boston: MTP Press; 1987. p. 156–66.
19. Krinke G, Schaumburg HH, Spencer PS, Thomann P, Hess R. Clioquinol and 2,5-hexanedione induce different types of distal axonopathy in the dog. Acta Neuropathol. 1979;47:213–21.
20. Juntunen J, Teravainen H, Eriksson K, Larsen A, Hillbom M. Peripheral neuropathy and myopathy. An experimental study of rats on alcohol and variable dietary thiamine. Virchows Arch A Pathol Anat Histol. 1979;383:241–52.
21. Schuschereba ST, Bowman PD, Vargas JA, Johnson TW, Woo FJ, McKinney L. Myopathic alterations in extraocular muscle of rats subchronically fed pyridostigmine bromide. Toxicol Pathol. 1990;18:387–95.
22. Beermann DH, Liboff M, Wilson DB, Hood LF. Effects of exogenous thyroxine and growth hormone on satellite cell and myonuclei populations in rapidly growing rat skeletal muscle. Growth. 1983;47:426–36.
23. Montgomery CA. Muscle diseases. In: Benirschke K, Garner FM, Jones TC, editors. Pathology of laboratory animals. New York: Springer; 2013. p. 821–87.

24. Adolfsson J. Time dependence of dipyridamole-induced increase in skeletal muscle capillarization. Arzneimittelforschung. 1986;36:1768–9.
25. Grasedyck K. D-penicillamine—side effects, pathogenesis and decreasing the risks. Z Rheumatol. 1998;47 Suppl 1:17–9.
26. Laskowski MB, Dettbarn WD. The pharmacology of experimental myopathies. Annu Rev Pharmacol Toxicol. 1977;17:387–409.
27. Mastaglia FL. Adverse effects of drugs on muscle. Drugs. 1982; 24:304–21.
28. Kirkpatrick CJ, Alves A, Kohler H, Kriegsmann J, Bittinger F, Otto M, et al. Biomaterial-induced sarcoma: a novel model to study preneoplastic change. Am J Pathol. 2000;156: 1455–67.
29. Maenza RM, Pradhan AM, Sunderman Jr FW. Rapid induction of sarcomas in rats by combination of nickel sulfide and 3,4-benzpyrene. Cancer Res. 1971;31:2067–71.
30. Haschek WM, Rousseaux CG, Wallig MA. Bones and joints. San Diego: Elsevier; 2010. p. 411–50.
31. Patyna S, Arrigoni C, Terron A, Kim TW, Heward JK, Vonderfecht SL, et al. Nonclinical safety evaluation of sunitinib: a potent inhibitor of VEGF, PDGF, KIT, FLT3, and RET receptors. Toxicol Pathol. 2008;36:905–16.
32. Renkiewicz R, Qiu L, Lesch C, Sun X, Devalaraja R, Cody T, et al. Broad-spectrum matrix metalloproteinase inhibitor marimastat-induced musculoskeletal side effects in rats. Arthritis Rheum. 2003;48:1742–9.
33. Hall AP, Westwood FR, Wadsworth PF. Review of the effects of anti-angiogenic compounds on the epiphyseal growth plate. Toxicol Pathol. 2006;34:131–47.
34. Frazier K, Thomas R, Scicchitano M, Mirabile R, Boyce R, Zimmerman D, et al. Inhibition of ALK5 signaling induces physeal dysplasia in rats. Toxicol Pathol. 2007;35:284–95.
35. Price PA, Williamson MK, Haba T, Dell RB, Jee WS. Excessive mineralization with growth plate closure in rats on chronic warfarin treatment. Proc Natl Acad Sci U S A. 1982;79: 7734–8.
36. Takahashi M, Yoshida M, Inoue K, Morikawa T, Nishikawa A. Age-related susceptibility to induction of osteochondral and vascular lesions by semicarbazide hydrochloride in rats. Toxicol Pathol. 2010;38:598–605.
37. Brechbiel JL, Ng JM, Curran T. PTHrP treatment fails to rescue bone defects caused by Hedgehog pathway inhibition in young mice. Toxicol Pathol. 2011;39:478–85.
38. Yabe K, Satoh H, Ishii Y, Jindo T, Sugawara T, Furuhama K, et al. Early pathophysiologic feature of arthropathy in juvenile dogs induced by ofloxacin, a quinolone antimicrobial agent. Vet Pathol Online. 2004;41:673–81.
39. Kashida Y, Kato M. Toxic effects of quinolone antibacterial agents on the musculoskeletal system in juvenile rats. Toxicol Pathol. 1997;25:635–43.
40. Kawahara T, Shimokawa I, Tomita M, Hirano T, Shindo H. Effects of caloric restriction on development of the proximal growth plate and metaphysis of the caput femoris in spontaneously hypertensive rats: microscopic and computer-assisted image analyses. Microsc Res Tech. 2002;59:306–12.
41. Wang LH, Fu Y, Shi YX, Wang WG. T-2 toxin induces degenerative articular changes in rodents: link to Kaschin-Beck disease. Toxicol Pathol. 2011;39:502–7.
42. Lewis DN, Nyska A, Johnson K, Malarkey DE, Ward S, Streicker M, et al. 2-Butoxyethanol female-rat model of hemolysis and disseminated thrombosis: X-ray characterization of osteonecrosis and growth-plate suppression. Toxicol Pathol. 2005;33:272–82.
43. Kantner I, Erben RG. Long-term parenteral administration of 2-hydroxypropyl-beta-cyclodextrin causes bone loss. Toxicol Pathol. 2012;40:742–50.
44. Highman B, Roth SI, Greenman DL. Osseous changes and osteosarcomas in mice continuously fed diets containing diethylstilbestrol or 17 beta-estradiol. J Natl Cancer Inst. 1981;67:653–62.
45. Vahle JL, Long GG, Sandusky G, Westmore M, Ma YL, Sato M. Bone neoplasms in F344 rats given teriparatide [rhPTH(1–34)] are dependent on duration of treatment and dose. Toxicol Pathol. 2004;32:426–38.
46. Jolette J, Wilker CE, Smith SY, Doyle N, Hardisty JF, Metcalfe AJ, et al. Defining a noncarcinogenic dose of recombinant human parathyroid hormone 1–84 in a 2-year study in Fischer 344 rats. Toxicol Pathol. 2006;34:929–40.
47. Westwood R, Scott RC, Somers RL, Coulson M, Maciewicz RA. Characterization of fibrodysplasia in the dog following inhibition of metalloproteinases. Toxicol Pathol. 2009;37:860–72.
48. Alspaugh MA, Van Hoosier GLJ. Naturally-occurring and experimentally-induced arthritides in rodents: a review of the literature. Lab Anim Sci. 1973;23:722–42.
49. Kashida Y, Kato M. Characterization of fluoroquinolone-induced Achilles tendon toxicity in rats: comparison of toxicities of 10 fluoroquinolones and effects of anti-inflammatory compounds. Antimicrob Agents Chemother. 1997;41:2389–93.
50. Kato M, Takada S, Kashida Y, Nomura M. Histological examination on Achilles tendon lesions induced by quinolone antibacterial agents in juvenile rats. Toxicol Pathol. 1995;23:385–92.
51. Tkalcevic VI, Cuzic S, Brajsa K, Mildner B, Bokulic A, Situm K, et al. Enhancement by PL 14736 of granulation and collagen organization in healing wounds and the potential role of egr-1 expression 2. Eur J Pharmacol. 2007;570:212–21.
52. Tkalcevic VI, Cuzic S, Parnham MJ, Pasalic I, Brajsa K. Differential evaluation of excisional non-occluded wound healing in db/db mice 1. Toxicol Pathol. 2009;37:183–92.
53. National Toxicology Program. NTP toxicology and carcinogenesis studies of technical grade sodium xylenesulfonate (CAS No. 1300-72-7) in F344/N rats and B6C3F1 mice (dermal studies). Natl Toxicol Program Tech Rep Ser. 1998;464:1–272.
54. Wojcinski ZW, Andrews-Jones L, Aibo DI, Dunstan R. Skin. In: Sahota PS, Popp JA, Hardisty JF, Gopinath C, editors. Toxicologic pathology. Boca Raton: CRC Press; 2013. p. 831–93.
55. Walsh KM, Gough AW. Hypopigmentation in dogs treated with an inhibitor of platelet aggregation. Toxicol Pathol. 1989;17:549–53.
56. Gobello C, Castex G, Broglia G, Corrada Y. Coat colour changes associated with cabergoline administration in bitches. J Small Anim Pract. 2003;44:352–4.
57. Funk J, Landes C. Histopathologic findings after treatment with different oxidosqualene cyclase (OSC) inhibitors in hamsters and dogs. Exp Toxicol Pathol. 2005;57:29–38.
58. Brown AP, Dunstan RW, Courtney CL, Criswell KA, Graziano MJ. Cutaneous lesions in the rat following administration of an irreversible inhibitor of erbB receptors, including the epidermal growth factor receptor. Toxicol Pathol. 2008;36:410–9.
59. Ito K, Handa J, Mori M, Ezura H, Kumagai M, Suzuki A, et al. Toxicity test of bleomycin oil suspension. Chronic toxicity in beagle dogs (author's translation). Jpn J Antibiot. 1980;33: 29–72.
60. Szczech GM, Tucker Jr WE. Nail loss and footpad erosions in beagle dogs given BW 134U, a nucleoside analog. Toxicol Pathol. 1985;13:181–4.
61. Tucker Jr WE, Krasny HC, de Miranda P, Goldenthal EI, Elion GB, Hajian G, et al. Preclinical toxicology studies with acyclovir:

carcinogenicity bioassays and chronic toxicity tests. Fundam Appl Toxicol. 1983;3:579–86.

62. Yin YR, Bai L, Wang F. Mechanism of L-arginine-induced sebaceous gland hyperplasia in rats. Di Yi Jun Yi Da Xue Xue Bao. 2005;25:766–8.

63. National Toxicology Program. Toxicology and carcinogenesis studies of oleic acid diethanolamine condensate. Natl Toxicol Program Tech Rep Ser. 1999;481:1–198.

64. Lavergne SN, Danhof RS, Volkman EM, Trepanier LA. Association of drug-serum protein adducts and anti-drug antibodies in dogs with sulphonamide hypersensitivity: a naturally occurring model of idiosyncratic drug toxicity 1. Clin Exp Allergy. 2006;36:907–15.

65. Mountz JD, Downs Minor MD, Turner R, Thomas MB, Richards F, Pisko E. Bleomycin-induced cutaneous toxicity in the rat: analysis of histopathology and ultrastructure compared with progressive systemic sclerosis (scleroderma). Br J Dermatol. 1983;108:679–86.

66. Armstrong ML, Mathur SN, Sando GN, Megan MB. Lipid metabolism in xanthomatous skin of hypercholesterolemic rabbits. Am J Pathol. 1986;125:339–48.

67. Scott DW, Wolfe MJ, Smith CA, Lewis RM. The comparative pathology of non-viral bullous skin diseases in domestic animals. Vet Pathol. 1980;17:257–81.

68. Pyrah IT, Kalinowski A, Jackson D, Davies W, Davis S, Aldridge A, et al. Toxicologic lesions associated with two related inhibitors of oxidosqualene cyclase in the dog and mouse. Toxicol Pathol. 2001;29:174–9.

69. Lynch D, Svoboda J, Putta S, Hofland HE, Chern WH, Hansen LA. Mouse skin models for carcinogenic hazard identification: utilities and challenges. Toxicol Pathol. 2007;35:853–64.

70. Ramot Y, Ben-Eliahu S, Kagan L, Ezov N, Nyska A. Subcutaneous and intraperitoneal lipogranulomas following subcutaneous injection of olive oil in Sprague–Dawley rats. Toxicol Pathol. 2009;37:882–6.

71. Westwood FR, Duffy PA, Malpass DA, Jones HB, Topham JC. Disturbance of macrophage and monocyte function in the dog by a thromboxane receptor antagonist: ICI 185,282. Toxicol Pathol. 1995;23:373–84.

72. Hardisty JF, Elwell MR, Ernst H, Greaves P, Kolenda-Roberts H, Malarkey DE, Mann PC, Tellier PA. Histopathology of hemangiosarcomas in mice and hamsters and liposarcomas/fibrosarcomas in rats associated with PPAR agonists. Toxicol Pathol. 2007;35:928–41.

73. Kakiuchi-Kiyota S, Vetro JA, Suzuki S, Varney ML, Han HY, Nascimento M, et al. Effects of the PPAR gamma agonist troglitazone on endothelial cells in vivo and in vitro: differences between human and mouse. Toxicol Appl Pharmacol. 2009;237:83–90.

74. Lyrica. INN-Pregabalin; 2012. http://www.ema.europa.eu/docs/en_GB/document_library/EPAR_-_Scientific_Discussion/human/000546/WC500046600.pdf.

75. Ohnishi T, Arnold LL, Clark NM, Wisecarver JL, Cohen SM. Comparison of endothelial cell proliferation in normal liver and adipose tissue in B6C3F1 mice, F344 rats, and humans. Toxicol Pathol. 2007;35:904–9.

76. Pruimboom-Brees IM, Francone O, Pettersen JC, Kerlin RL, Will Y, Amacher DE, Boucher GG, Morton D. The development of subcutaneous sarcomas in rodents exposed to peroxisome proliferators agonists: hypothetical mechanisms of action and de-risking attitude. Toxicol Pathol. 2012;40:810–8.

77. Morgan RW, Elcock M. Artificial implants and soft tissue sarcomas. J Clin Epidemiol. 1995;48:545–9.

78. Le CS, Perron-Lepage MF, Burnett R. Subcutaneous microchip-associated tumours in B6C3F1 mice: a retrospective study to attempt to determine their histogenesis. Exp Toxicol Pathol. 2006;57:255–65.

79. Tillmann T, Kamino K, Dasenbrock C, Ernst H, Kohler M, Morawietz G, et al. Subcutaneous soft tissue tumours at the site of implanted microchips in mice. Exp Toxicol Pathol. 1997;49:197–200.

80. Nagase I, Sasaki N, Tsukazaki K, Yoshida T, Morimatsu M, Saito M. Hyperplasia of brown adipose tissue after chronic stimulation of beta 3-adrenergic receptor in rats. Jpn J Vet Res. 1994;42:137–45.

81. Poulet FM, Berardi MR, Halliwell W, Hartman B, Auletta C, Bolte H. Development of hibernomas in rats dosed with phentolamine mesylate during the 24-month carcinogenicity study. Toxicol Pathol. 2004;32:558–66.

82. Long GG, Reynolds VL, Dochterman LW, Ryan TE. Neoplastic and non-neoplastic changes in F-344 rats treated with Naveglitazar, a gamma-dominant PPAR alpha/gamma agonist. Toxicol Pathol. 2009;37:741–53.

83. Glinghammar B, Berg AL, Bjurstrom S, Stockling K, Blomgren B, Westerberg R, et al. Proliferative and molecular effects of the dual PPAR alpha/gamma agonist tesaglitazar in rat adipose tissues: relevance for induction of fibrosarcoma. Toxicol Pathol. 2011;39:325–36.

# 12 The Eye and Ear

## 12.1 The Eye

The eye is a complex organ with unique anatomical, functional, and physiological features that render it susceptible to a range of highly specific pathologic changes. In addition, increased longevity in recent decades, particularly in developed countries, has raised the prevalence of age-related diseases such as macular degeneration and glaucoma, increasing the demand for effective treatments for these conditions. Because visual impairment has serious implications for quality of life and independent function, as well as high-cost implications for governments in countries with centrally funded healthcare services, specially targeted new drugs and therapies have been developed.

The eye's many unique barriers to drug delivery have also led to the development of novel technologies for ocular drug administration [1]. Ocular bioavailability after topical ocular administration is less than 5 %, and currently, only diseases of the anterior segment can be treated by this route [1]. Other modes of administration are necessary to administer therapeutics to the posterior segment of the eye.

Among the eye's specialised features are its immunoprivileged status due to innate immunoregulatory mechanisms; the avascular nature of the cornea and lens the retina, which contains photosensitive pigments; and the ciliary bodies, which produce aqueous humour and maintain the blood–aqueous barrier [2]. The features forming the blood–ocular barrier include ciliary and retinal pigmented epithelial layers with their interepithelial tight junction complexes, nonfenestrated capillaries, and efflux pumps. Another unusual feature is the high concentration of zinc in ocular tissues, especially the retina and choroid, when compared with other organs [3].

Knowledge of the eye's unique features is essential for understanding and interpreting induced ocular pathologic changes in laboratory animal species and evaluating their implications for human safety. Any potential toxicologic effects must be identified and cautiously interpreted in safety studies. Familiarity with the different anatomical and physiological characteristics of each laboratory species is also necessary for appropriate study design and species selection and to ensure accurate examination and interpretation of ocular histopathology [2, 4]. Toxic and spontaneous changes can be influenced by the species, strain, and age of the animal [5].

Rodent strains commonly used in safety testing are albino and lack ocular pigmentation. This may make them inappropriate models for testing compounds that bind to melanin to induce ocular toxicity. The tapetum lucidum, which reflects light, is found in the choroid of dogs, but not in other common laboratory species or in humans. Humans and nonhuman primates possess a macula densa and fovea in the retina, which may be a potential target for xenobiotics; routine eye sections from primates should include this area. Primates are frequently used in ocular studies, as their ocular anatomy and physiology most closely resemble those of humans.

Protocols for assessing ocular toxicity require careful selection of examination techniques and appropriate timing of these examinations [6]. Recent developments in visualising, imaging, and electrophysiological technologies have increased the potential for in-life observations [7, 8]. These techniques include fluorescein angiography, electroretinography, confocal scanning laser ophthalmoscopy, and spectral domain optical

C. Gopinath, V. Mowat, *Atlas of Toxicological Pathology*,
DOI 10.1007/978-1-62703-998-7_12, © Springer Science+Business Media New York 2014

coherence tomography, some of which are already being used in safety assessment studies [2].

Careful sampling at necropsy, fixation in appropriate media such as Davidson's fluid [9], and the use of standardised trimming procedures are all required to produce high-quality histologic sections of the eye containing all ocular structures [5, 10]. Potentially, treatment-related changes seen ophthalmoscopically should also be captured in the eye sections and examined microscopically. Depending on the species, periocular structures to be examined can include harderian glands, lacrimal glands, meibomian glands, and nictitating glands.

Induced changes in the eye are infrequent when compared with other organs or tissues. Changes can be induced by topical or systemic administration of a xenobiotic. With systemic administration, the drug can act on the eye directly or through a metabolite. Lesions in the eye also can be secondary to toxicologically induced changes in the meibomian or lacrimal glands, which keep the eye lubricated, so these should also be evaluated microscopically.

The Draize test, which is a regulatory requirement for a variety of pharmaceuticals and chemicals, is a safety assessment test performed on the eye to assess irritant potential. This procedure is performed on rabbits because of their higher sensitivity to ocular irritants. The Draize test involves topical application of the xenobiotic to the eye, using a standardised terminology and grading scheme to assess the significance of clinical and macroscopic findings. Because the Draize test involves a level of overdosing to ensure irritancy is not missed, various modifications or alternatives to the Draize method are increasingly being used instead [11, 12].

In addition to conventional routes of treatment such as systemic administration and topical application, specialised techniques such as intraocular implants and injection by subconjunctival, retrobulbar, peribulbar, and intravitreal routes are used to ensure more targeted delivery of drugs to specific regions of the eye. However, many of these techniques are associated with procedural changes, which must be clearly differentiated from test article-related changes in safety assessment studies. A wide variety of therapies, including oligonucleotides, nanoparticles, microparticles, and stem cells, are being developed for intraocular use by these routes. Intraocular injections are also traditionally used to administer steroids and immunosuppressants (e.g. cyclosporine) to treat macular degeneration.

Permeability enhancers such as surfactants and preservatives are used to enhance corneal penetration. Highly lipophilic compounds penetrate the cornea better. Regulatory requirements for these drugs depend on indication-specific factors including route of administration, systemic exposure, and other variables [13].

### 12.1.1 Cornea

The cornea is an avascular structure that consists of an epithelial layer overlying an acellular, collagenous Bowman's membrane (in primates only) and a thick, transparent stroma. The epithelial layer is composed (externally to internally) of squamous, wing, and basal epithelial cells, the latter overlying a basement membrane. The stroma contains specialised keratocytes and is bordered internally by Descemet's membrane.

The clarity of the cornea, essential for transmitting light, depends on its relative dehydration, maintained by the pumping of fluid into the anterior chamber across a pressure gradient created by the corneal endothelial cells. Thus, even a slight increase in fluid results in translucency. The cornea's lack of vascularisation, the arrangement of collagenous and noncollagenous components, and the function of the stromal keratocytes are also important in maintaining its transparency.

Several types of induced changes can occur in the cornea:

- Mineralisation
- Vacuolation
- Lipidosis
- Keratitis (inflammation, oedema, erosion, ulceration, fibrosis, neovascularisation)
- Epithelial hyperplasia, cutaneous metaplasia
- Atrophy
- Papillomas, squamous cell carcinoma

Mineralisation may occur as a spontaneous finding in older rodents and can sometimes be a sequel to inflammatory changes, owing to calcium depositing in damaged tissues. Corneal mineralisation also occurs as a primary change in conditions resulting in hypercalcaemia and can be induced by treatment with vitamin D analogues. Histologically, multifocal mineral deposits can be seen in the epithelial basement membrane and subepithelial corneal stroma (Fig. 12.1). These mineral deposits may evoke a mild inflammatory response in the adjacent stroma.

Amphophilic cationic drugs such as chlorphentermine and iprindole cause vacuolation of the corneal epithelial cells. Electron microscopy of these vacuoles shows the multilamellar bodies characteristic of phospholipidosis. Vacuolation of the basal corneal epithelial cells has been recorded in our laboratory in cynomolgus monkeys treated with a novel antineoplastic agent (Fig. 12.2). Electron microscopy of the cornea revealed large, empty cytoplasmic vacuoles [14].

Corneal lipidosis appears as cholesterol clefts, with or without foamy macrophages, in the corneal stroma in the dog, guinea pig, and rabbit. This can be spontaneous or induced by feeding high-fat diets [15].

Keratitis can be primary or secondary. Primary keratitis is often due to irritant drugs or chemicals making direct contact with the cornea. Accidental exposure to a wide variety of industrial chemicals, including solvents, detergents, and gases, can cause corneal irritation in humans and animals. In addition, xenobiotics administered systemically (or their metabolites) may be excreted via the lacrimal fluid and exert local irritant effects.

Administration of narcotic analgesics or prolonged anaesthesia, particularly if the eyes are open, results in corneal dryness secondary to impaired tear production and blinking. If the function of the lacrimal or meibomian glands is affected, secondary keratitis frequently develops as a result of reduced tear production. Reductions in aqueous tear production can be monitored by in-life Schirmer's tear test.

Systemically administered compounds also can result in nonirritant corneal changes after absorption, directly or through metabolites. Regardless of mechanism, the pathology is similar and often manifests in life as corneal opacity if severe or chronic. Histologically, if the irritation is mild, keratitis with minimal to slight neutrophilic infiltration is seen, and the conjunctiva frequently is also involved (Fig. 12.3). If treatment is of a longer duration or the irritation is more severe, inflammation is pronounced, with diffuse, marked neutrophilic infiltration and corneal hyperplasia.

Keratinisation, corneal erosion, and ulceration also can result, with neutrophilic debris and scabs overlying the cornea (Fig. 12.4). Prolonged inflammation, fibrosis, and neovascularisation cause marked hyperplasia of the corneal epithelium and stromal proliferation, manifesting clinically as opacity (Fig. 12.5). Epithelial hyperplasia of the cornea, involving one or more of the corneal cell types, can progress to cutaneous metaplasia and keratinisation with prolonged irritation.

Malonaldehyde, a metabolic product of prostaglandin synthesis, causes corneal inflammation in rats and mice [16]. Topical administration of an EP4 prostaglandin E2 receptor agonist caused irritation and corneal neovascularisation, with inflammatory mediators and a direct effect on vascular endothelial cells being postulated as mechanisms of pathogenesis for the neovascularisation [17]. Ultraviolet irradiation causes opacity in mice, seen histologically as loss of keratocytes, corneal stromal thinning, keratitis, and fibrosis [18].

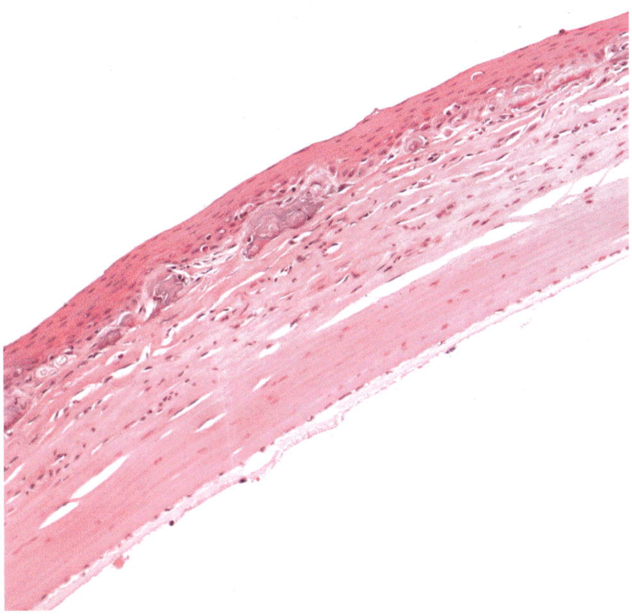

**Figure 12-1.** Multifocal corneal mineralisation and keratitis in a rat given a vitamin D analogue. The cornea displays multifocal mineral deposits in the basement membrane and mild neutrophilic inflammation of the underlying stroma. Haematoxylin and eosin (H&E).

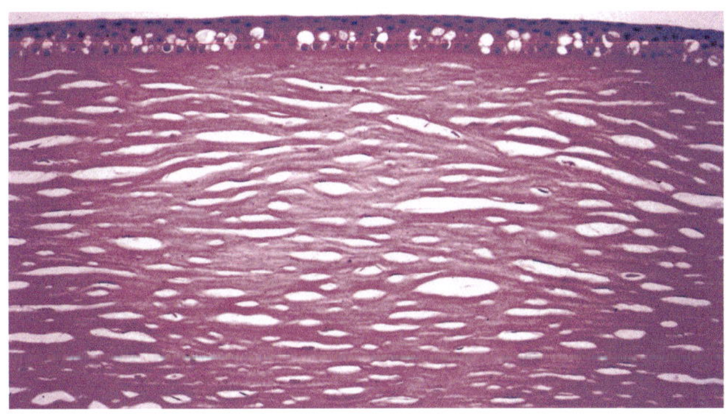

**Figure 12-2.** Vacuolation in the corneal epithelium of a monkey treated with an antineoplastic agent. The vacuoles are confined to the basal cells. H&E (With kind permission from Springer Science+Business Media B.V [14]).

Certain nutritional deficiencies, including deficiencies of lysine, tryptophan, vitamin A, and zinc, are associated with neovascularisation with no apparent inflammatory process, although inflammation may have occurred at an early stage [12, 19].

The corneal epithelium has a high concentration of acetylcholine, which helps to maintain the flow of aqueous humour. A number of organophosphorus pesticides (e.g. dichlorvos) induce keratitis and conjunctivitis through their cholinesterase-inhibiting effect. This results in a build-up of acetylcholine, resulting in corneal oedema and inflammation. Epidermal growth factor receptor (EGFR) inhibitors can cause oedema, erosion, inflammation, and ulceration of the cornea in dogs.

Cadmium causes severe corneal oedema in pregnant rats. Ultrastructurally, prominent swelling of mitochondria with cadmium–oxine complexes and vacuoles in the corneal endothelium is seen. These imply disturbance of pump and barrier function due to primary toxic effects on mitochondria [20].

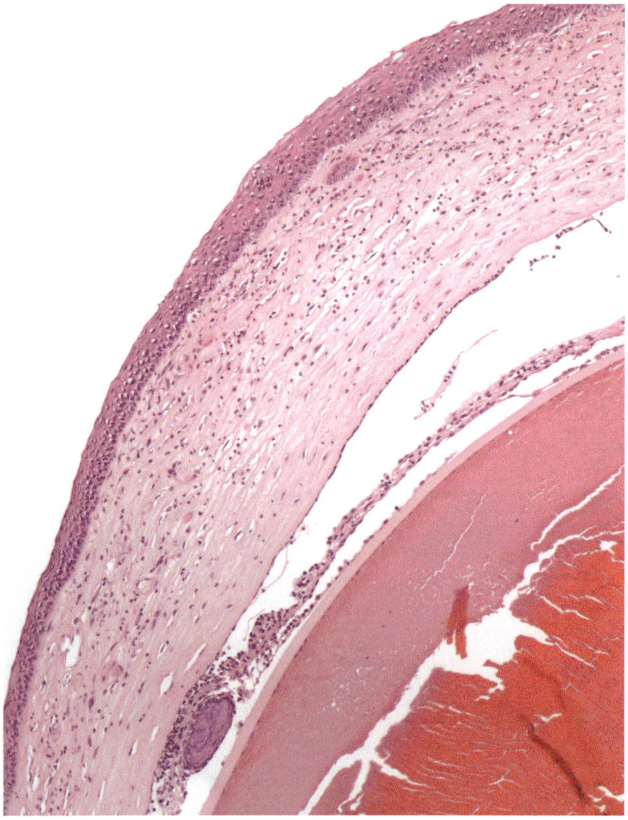

**Figure 12-3.** Keratitis and dystrophic mineralisation, from a mouse on a short-term study. The corneal epithelium is hyperplastic, with loss of architecture. The corneal stroma shows neovascularisation and neutrophilic infiltration, with focal mineral deposition in the iris. H&E.

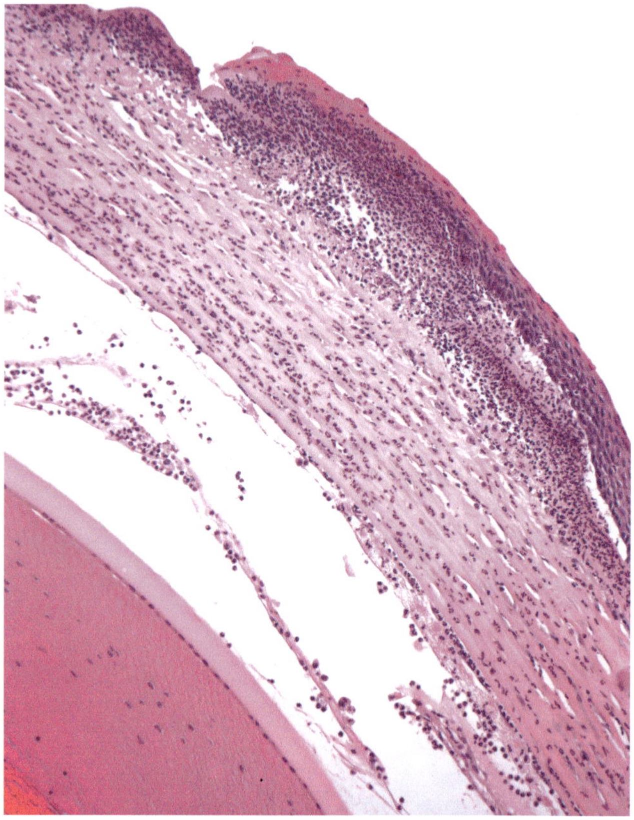

**Figure 12-4.** Focal corneal ulceration from a mouse on a long-term study. Marked inflammation is present, with epithelial ulceration and necrosis. The corneal epithelium is sloughing, with marked suppurative exudate, stromal inflammation, and pyaemia.

Hyperplasia of the corneal epithelium is generally secondary to inflammatory changes or irritation, but it also may be a primary effect of a xenobiotic. Recombinant human epidermal growth factor (rhEGF) causes diffuse corneal hyperplasia in cynomolgus monkeys [21].

Epidermal growth factor inhibitors and vascular endothelial growth factor inhibitors interfere with corneal epithelial replication, resulting in corneal atrophy in several laboratory species (Fig. 12.6). Histologically, the cornea appears thinner, with fewer layers of cells than in control animals. In some, only two or three layers of flattened cells remain, with complete loss of polygonal and basal cell layers. Mild neutrophilic infiltration is sometimes associated with epithelial atrophy. Corneal atrophy and ulceration in the dog have been induced by novel hypolipidaemic agents that inhibit oxidosqualene cyclase, possibly through inhibition of corneal epithelial division [22]. Similar changes have been recorded with triparanol, another hypocholesterolaemic drug [23].

In short-term studies, 4-hydroxyphenylpyruvate dioxygenase (4-HPPD) inhibitors, such as topramezone, cause slight corneal irritation owing to increased tyrosine levels, with keratitis and corneal opacity developing in rats and beagles [24]. In carcinogenicity studies, ocular papillomas and squamous cell carcinomas of the cornea have been recorded in rats; these appear to be a species-specific phenomenon [personal observation].

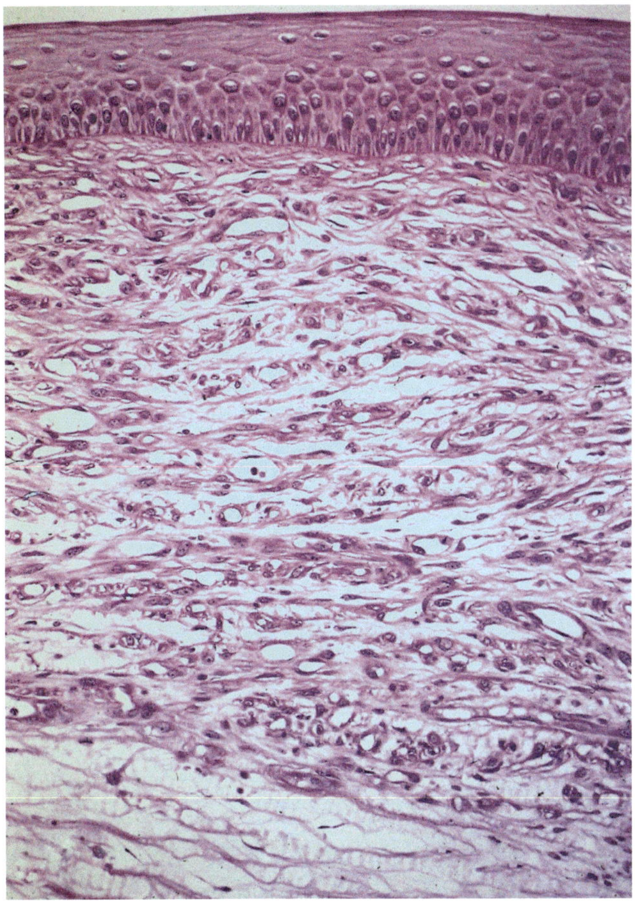

**Figure 12-5.** Vascularisation of the cornea of a dog treated with a novel antispasmodic compound. The lesion developed following keratoconjunctivitis sicca and is characterised by neovascularisation and fibroblasts in the stroma. Little inflammatory cell involvement is present, and the overlying epithelium appears normal. H&E (With kind permission from Springer Science+Business Media B.V [14]).

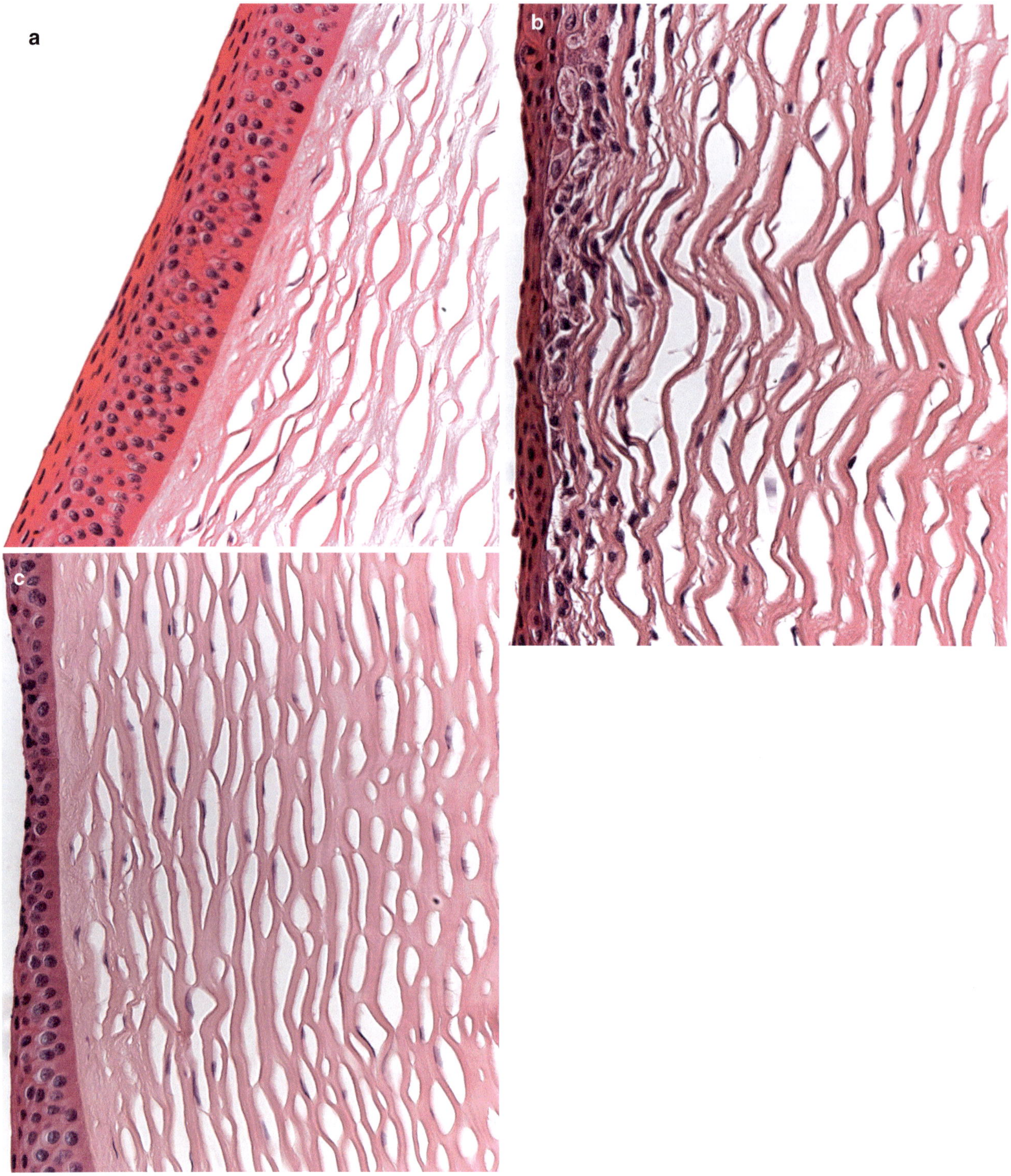


**Figure 12-6.** (**a**) Normal corneal epithelium from a control dog, comprising five to seven layers of squamous, wing, and basal cells. H&E. (**b**) The corneal epithelium is focally atrophic and consists of two to three layers of squamous cells, with loss of other cell layers. Corneal atrophy can be induced by vascular endothelial growth factor (vEGF) inhibitors and EGF-receptor (EGFR) inhibitors, among other drugs. H&E. (**c**) Focal corneal epithelial atrophy is present, with partial loss of cells from all layers. Normal corneal epithelium is evident ventral to the atrophic area. H&E.

### 12.1.2 Retina

The retina is highly complex in structure and function and consists of ten layers of specialised cells that function closely with each other. The main layers (from the interior towards the choroid) are nerve fibres, ganglion, inner plexiform, inner nuclear, outer plexiform, and outer nuclear layers, with the latter overlying the photoreceptor layer. The photoreceptor cells have a very high-energy demand. The retinal pigmented epithelium (RPE), which lies between the photoreceptor layer and the choroid, is essential for retinal function. Together with the tight junctions between the retinal vascular endothelial cells, the RPE forms the blood–retinal barrier.

Although retinal components are easily identified on routine paraffin-embedded haematoxylin and eosin (H&E) sections, plastic-embedded, semi-thin sections are used if finer detail of cell morphology is required.

Several types of retinal changes can be induced:

- Degeneration or atrophy
- Pigment deposition
- Phospholipidosis
- Retinoblastomas or teratomas
- Papilloedema

Retinal degeneration or atrophy is associated with a wide variety of environmental and physiological factors and varies greatly with species, age, and strain [25]. Albino animals' eyes are highly sensitive to light and develop progressive retinal degeneration under continued exposure to fluorescent light, as is seen in mice on the top cage racks in safety studies. Rhesus and cynomolgus monkeys also can show light-related retinal lesions even though pigmented eyes are less susceptible. Retinal degeneration also can be secondary to injury in another area or structure of the eye (e.g. in glaucoma, in which intraocular pressure results in damage to the retina and subsequent atrophy) or to panophthalmitis caused by a variety of agents, in which several or all of the ocular structures are involved.

Retinal changes are caused by a wide range of pharmaceuticals and chemicals, as well as nutritional deficiencies and metabolic disorders. Retinopathy can be classified according to the nature of the causative agent (e.g. nutritional, age related, induced), but sometimes, more than one factor may be involved; for instance, light may potentiate toxic retinopathy.

Oculotoxic compounds can be broadly divided into those primarily affecting the photoreceptors or ganglion cells and those affecting the RPE [26]. Atrophy of the tapetum lucidum in dogs is considered species specific and is generally accepted as being without relevance for humans if it is confined to this area. Ethambutol, diethyl dithiocarbamate, and several compounds with metal-chelating properties target this area (possibly because of the high zinc concentration of the tapetum), resulting in disruption of rods within the tapetal cells. Degeneration and partial or complete loss of cells are apparent histologically; all layers may be affected (Figs. 12.7 and 12.8).

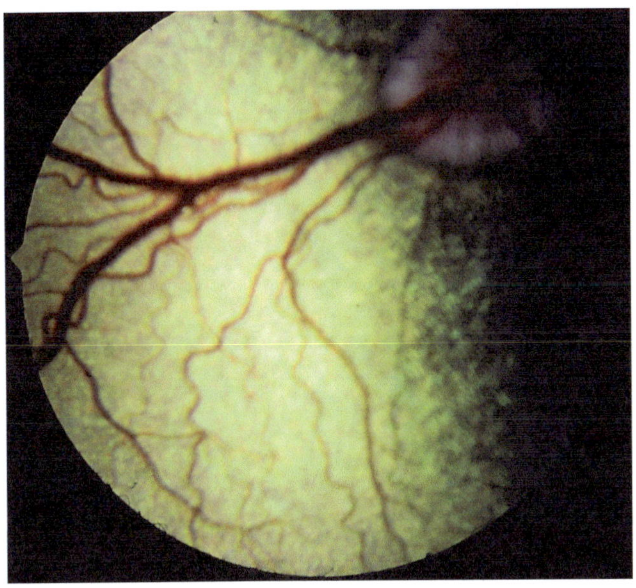

**Figure 12-7.** Degeneration of the retina of a dog seen at ophthalmoscopy. Diffuse degeneration of the tapetum lucidum is present, giving a granular appearance.

Different compounds target different layers of the retina via various mechanisms. Ethambutol causes vacuolation of retinal ganglion cells in vivo and in vitro in rats, possibly by mitochondrial perturbation or by lysosomal activation [27, 28]. Doxorubicin causes axonal swelling and necrosis by inhibition of slow transport. Glutamate causes swelling and necrosis of the ganglion cells in rodents [29].

Diets deficient in vitamin K and agents that reduce vitamin K-dependent clotting factors result in intraocular haemorrhage (and sometimes secondary retinal detachment) in rats [14]. Hydroxypyridinethionine causes localised haemorrhage and retinal detachment in the tapetum in dogs.

The outer nuclear and photoreceptor layers of the retina are generally considered the layers most susceptible to toxicity. GABA inhibitors used as antiepileptic drugs (e.g. vigabatrin) cause disorganisation of the outer nuclear layer in rats and visual disturbances in humans [30, 31]. Fluoroquinolones cause retinal damage and blindness in cats; enrofloxacin at high doses produces attenuation and loss of retinal blood vessels at ophthalmoscopy, with retinal pigment deposition and retinal degeneration involving the outer nuclear and photoreceptor layers histologically [32, 33].

In both spontaneous and induced retinal degeneration, the outer layer is most commonly affected; sometimes, the outer layer is completely lost while the inner layer remains intact (Figs. 12.9–12.11). Rarely, just the inner nuclear layer is targeted. Vacuolation of the inner nuclear layer has been seen in our laboratory in monkeys treated with a novel antineoplastic compound (Fig. 12.12). Both the outer and inner layers are sometimes affected, with reduction of retinal thickness; the remaining cells of the outer and inner layers form a single band of cells (Fig. 12.13). *N*-ethyl-*N*-nitrosourea (ENU) causes retinal degeneration in mice after a single intraperitoneal injection, with the outer nuclear and photoreceptor layers showing cell loss [34]. Cationic amphophilic agents such as chloroquines produce phospholipidosis of the retina. In rats with phospholipidosis, the characteristic lamellar bodies may be seen in the RPE, neural cells, and Muller cells on semi-thin, toluidine blue-stained sections.

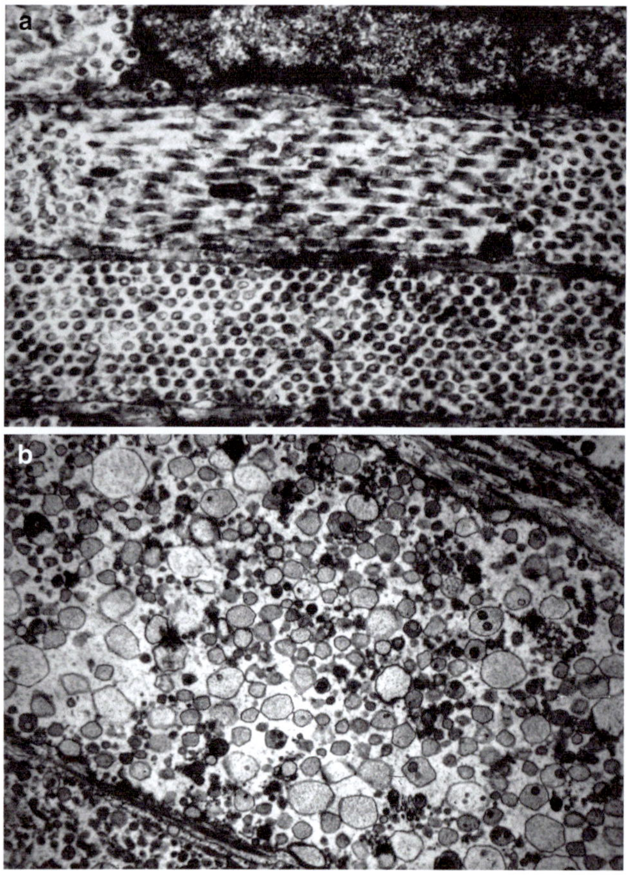

**Figure 12-8.** (**a**) Normal tapetum lucidum from the eye of a dog. Note the orderly arrangement of cells in layers. The tapetal cells are packed with electron-dense rods. Transmission electron micrograph. (**b**) Marked degeneration of the tapetum lucidum of a dog treated with a compound with chelating properties. The cells are swollen and architecture has been lost. Rods are decreased in number and swollen. Transmission electron micrograph (**a** With kind permission from Springer Science+Business Media B.V [14]).

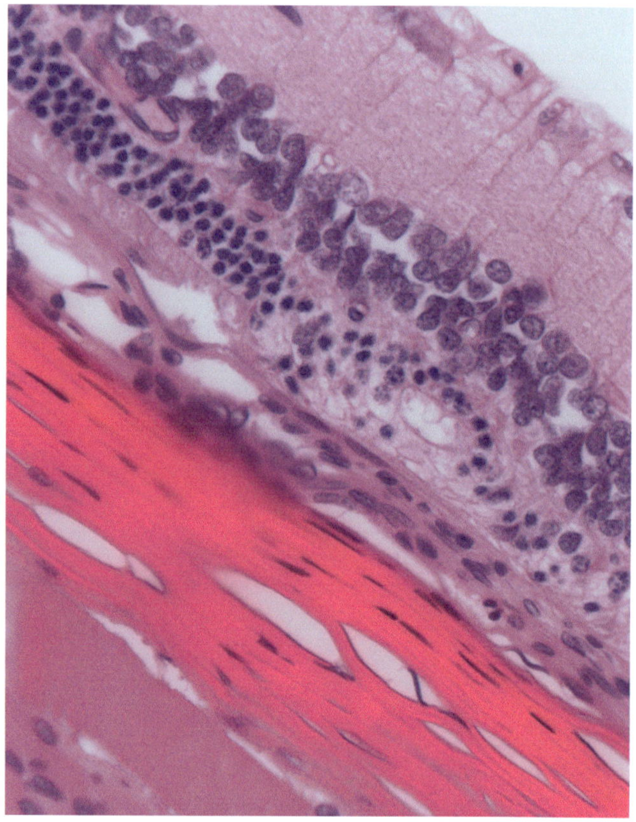

**Figure 12-9.** Retinal degeneration in a rat treated with a chemical with chelating properties. The outer nuclear layer is focally disorganised with cell loss, and several apoptotic cells are present.

The melanin content of the RPE in pigmented species protects against retinal atrophy but also makes the RPE a potential target for melanin-binding compounds. Changes in the RPE are believed to reflect the phagocytic activity of these cells secondary to degenerative changes in other retinal layers, so lipofuscin contents of these cells can increase with age and spontaneous or induced degeneration. A range of compounds including lead, naphthalene, and oxalates are thought to affect the retina primarily through the RPE [35].

Compounds affecting the RPE after systemic administration can cause increased pigment, intracytoplasmic accumulation, hypertrophy, hyperplasia, and degeneration of retinal pigmented cells. Hyperplasia and metaplasia of the RPE cells, as well as formation of subretinal membranes and colloid bodies, can also occur secondary to toxic cell injury (Fig. 12.14) [35]. Toxicity can result in fibroplasia, macrophage accumulation, and haemorrhage in the subretinal space (Fig. 12.15).

Vacuolation of the RPE has been recorded in rabbits with 6-aminonicotinamide, in association with ciliary and iridal epithelial cell swelling. These lesions appear to be due to nicotinamide deficiency, as administration of nicotinamide prevented development of ocular lesions [36]. Cyclin-dependent kinase inhibitors induce retinal atrophy in various species, causing damage to the outer retinal layers, with aggregates of pigmented cells in the RPE in monkeys [37, 38].

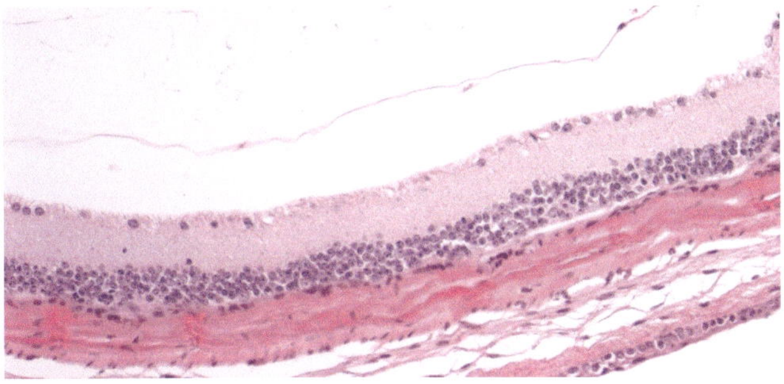

**Figure 12-10.** Retinal atrophy in a mouse on a long-term study. The inner nuclear layer is largely intact, with loss of the outer nuclear, outer plexiform, and rods and cones layers. This change can be spontaneous or induced, with the outer nuclear layer being much more commonly affected. H&E.

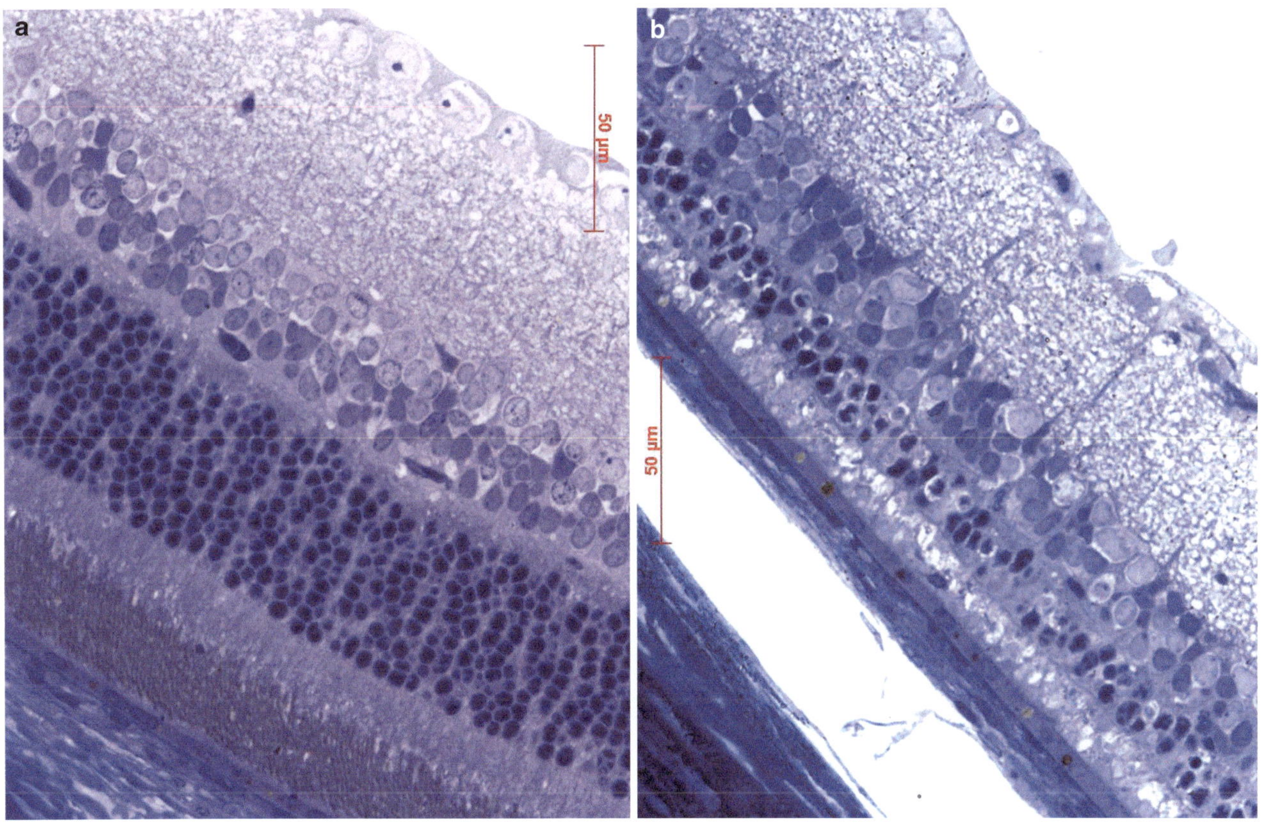


**Figure 12-11.** (**a**) Normal populations of retinal cells in all layers of a specimen from a control rat. Resin section, toluidine blue. (**b**) In a treated rat, moderate loss of cells from the outer nuclear layer is evident, with the presence of swollen, apoptotic, and degenerative cells. The outer plexiform layer and rods and cones are largely absent. Semi-thin section, toluidine blue.

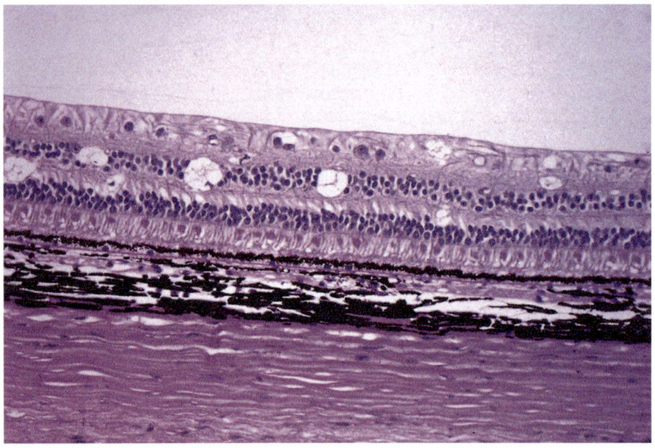

**Figure 12-12.** Vacuolar degeneration in the retina, primarily affecting the inner nuclear layer, in a specimen from a monkey treated with an antineoplastic compound. H&E (With kind permission from Springer Science+Business Media B.V [14]).

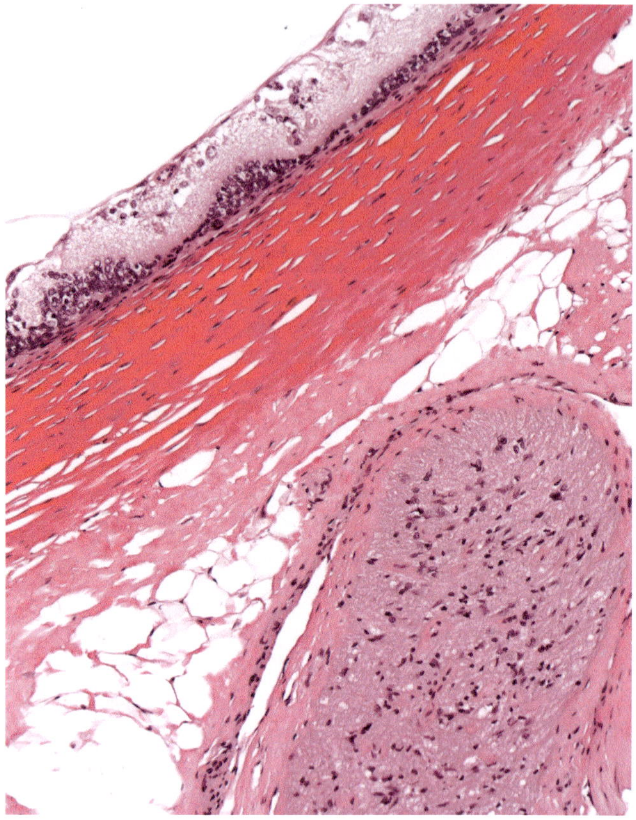

**Figure 12-13.** Severe retinal degeneration in a rat on a 13-week study. All layers of the retina are affected, with the remaining cells of the inner and outer nuclear layers forming a single, uneven band. H&E.

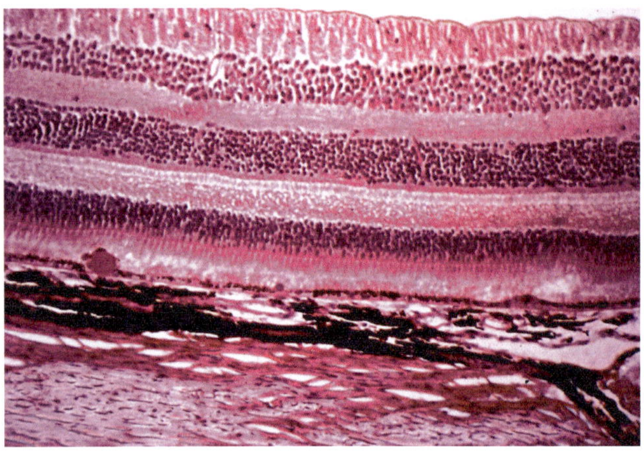

**Figure 12-14.** Swelling of retinal pigmented epithelial (RPE) cells from a nonhuman primate. Note the body lying on Bruch's membrane (drusen). H&E.

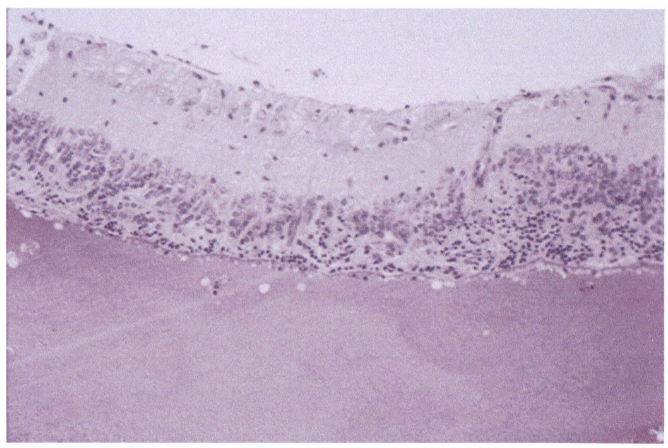

**Figure 12-15.** Subretinal haemorrhage in a rat given a diet deficient in vitamin K. The retina is detached, with atrophy of the outer nuclear and photoreceptor layers. H&E (With kind permission from Springer Science+Business Media B.V [14]).

Triparanol affects the Muller cells and RPE. The varying affinities of drugs for particular polar lipids may explain differences in target cell populations [12].

The development of ocular tumours, including teratomas and retinoblastomas, has resulted from intraocular injection of viruses, stem cells, and a variety of chemicals, including nickel subsulphide and nitrosoureas (Figs. 12.16 and 12.17).

Oedema of the optic disc is an uncommon finding in safety assessment studies (Fig. 12.18). In spontaneous occurrences, it is generally associated with intracranial pressure. It has been described in monkeys given trimethyltin acetate and in dogs given salicylanilide [14, 39]. In dogs, guinea pigs, and monkeys, β, β′ iminodipropionitrile given systemically causes optic disc swelling due to massive accumulation of neurofilaments [40]. In humans, this lesion is associated with ethylene glycol, lead, and nalidixic acid, among other agents. Because of differences in metabolic pathways, methanol causes papilloedema in primates but not in other species [14].

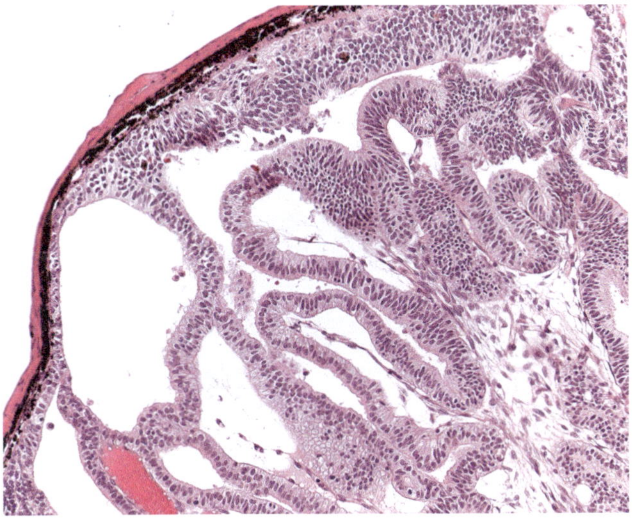

**Figure 12-16.** A retinoblastoma in a rat. The retina is disorganised and hyperplastic, forming multilayered folds and projections. The cells are columnar, with oval to spindloid nuclei. Mild pleomorphism and anisokaryosis are present. Such tumours can be induced by intraocular injection of many agents, including nitrosourea, viruses, and stem cells. H&E.

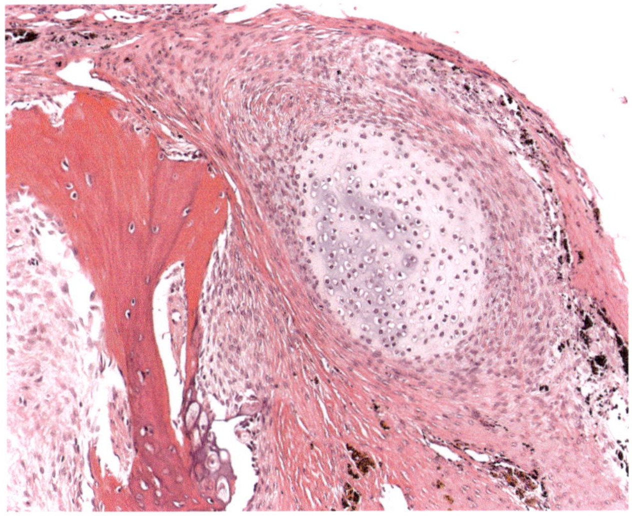

**Figure 12-17.** Teratoma in the eye of a rat; a large, heterogenous mass replaces the normal structures. Areas resembling cartilage, bone, and nervous tissue are present within the tumour, with multifocal pigment. As with the tumour shown in Fig. 12.16, tumours of this sort can be associated with intraocular injection of a variety of agents. H&E.

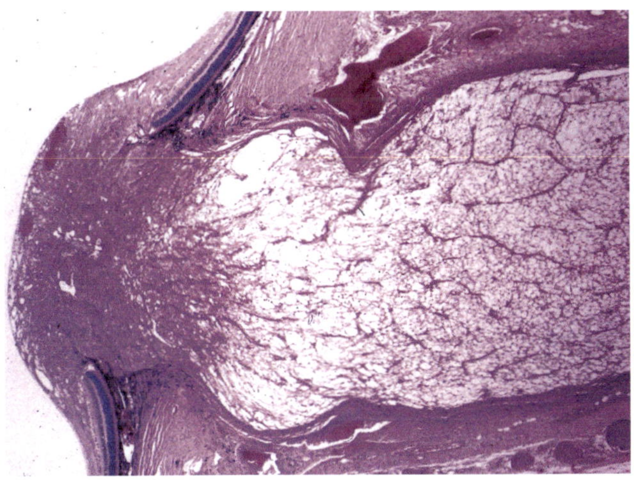

**Figure 12-18.** Papilloedema, which developed in the eye of a dog following systemic administration of a novel agrochemical. The swollen optic disc projects into the posterior chamber, with severe swelling, oedema, and vacuolation of the optic nerve. H&E (With kind permission from Springer Science+Business Media B.V [14]).

## 12.1.3 Uveal Tract

The uveal tract comprises the choroid, iris, and ciliary body. It provides most of the blood supply for the intraocular structures, and the ciliary body produces the aqueous humour. Obstruction to drainage of this fluid into the canal of Schlemm in the corneo-iridal angle leads to raised intraocular pressure and glaucoma.

Several induced changes can affect this tract:

- Uveitis
- Accumulations or vacuolation in the ciliary body
- Pigmentation of the iris
- Glaucoma

In laboratory animals, induced inflammation of the iris is rare. Lymphocytic infiltration in the iris and ciliary body is seen as a spontaneous finding in cynomolgus monkeys. Inflammation seen in rodents is generally secondary to inflammatory processes in the anterior chamber. Lymphoplasmacytic infiltrates in the ciliary body and iris have been induced by an EP4 prostaglandin E2 receptor agonist applied topically in dogs [17]. An antiviral agent induced uveitis, with lymphoplasmacytic infiltration in the ciliary body, in baboons in our laboratory (Fig. 12.19). In humans, drug-induced uveitis is associated with sulphonamides, rifabutin, and cidovir, an antiviral agent, among other therapies. Iritis, congestion, and haemorrhage, along with hydropic change, have been induced in rabbits with 6-aminonicotinamide [36]. Vacuolation and swelling of the ciliary body, predominantly affecting the pigmented cells, have been recorded in monkeys in our laboratory treated with a novel anticancer agent (Figs. 12.20 and 12.21) [14].

Prostaglandins, notably latanoprost, are associated with increased pigmentation of the iris in humans and cynomolgus monkeys, resulting in marked darkening of the iris and sometimes pigmented epithelial cysts [41–43]. This pigmentation results from an increase in melanin synthesis; transmission electron microscopy has shown extracellular pigment in the stroma and intracellular pigment in fibroblasts, melanocytes, and trabecular endothelial cells [43].

Long-term administration of silver or exposure to silver results in silver granule deposits in the eyes of several species, including humans and rats. In rats, silver accumulates in the ciliary bodies and Bruch's membrane [44].

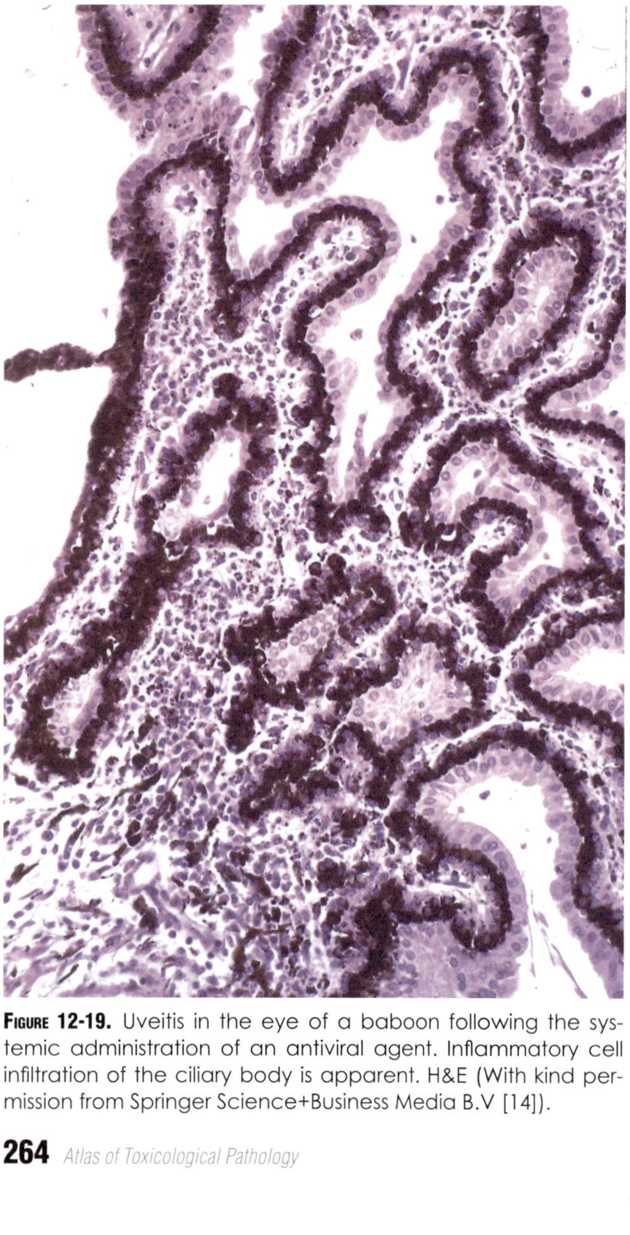

**Figure 12-19.** Uveitis in the eye of a baboon following the systemic administration of an antiviral agent. Inflammatory cell infiltration of the ciliary body is apparent. H&E (With kind permission from Springer Science+Business Media B.V [14]).

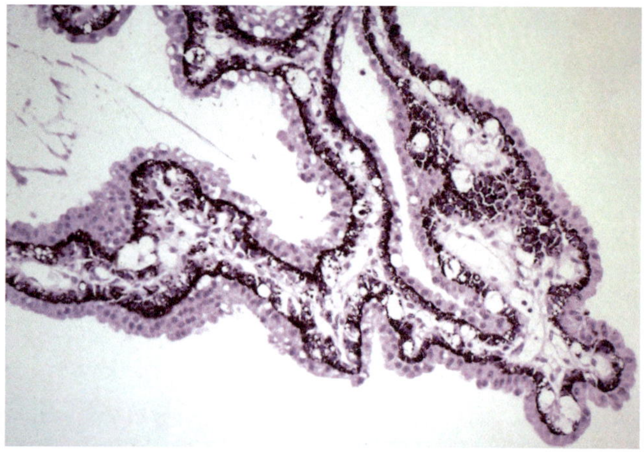

**Figure 12-20.** Minimal vacuolation of the ciliary body from a monkey treated with a novel anticancer agent. The vacuolation is largely confined to the pigmented cells. H&E (With kind permission from Springer Science+Business Media B.V [14]).

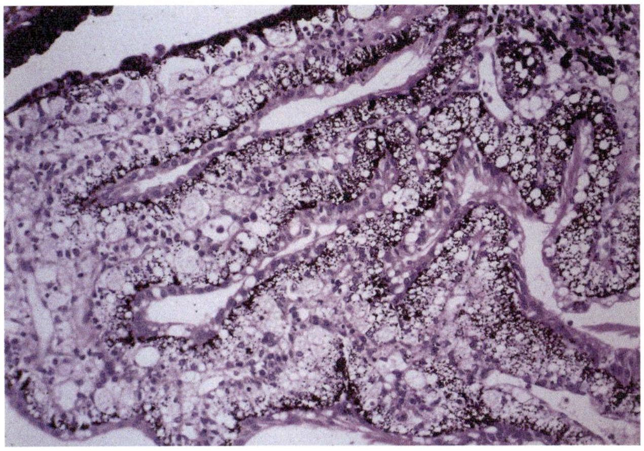

**Figure 12-21.** Pronounced vacuolation and swelling of the ciliary body of a monkey. The animal received a higher dose of the same test compound as the monkey shown in Fig. 12.20. H&E (With kind permission from Springer Science+Business Media B.V [14]).

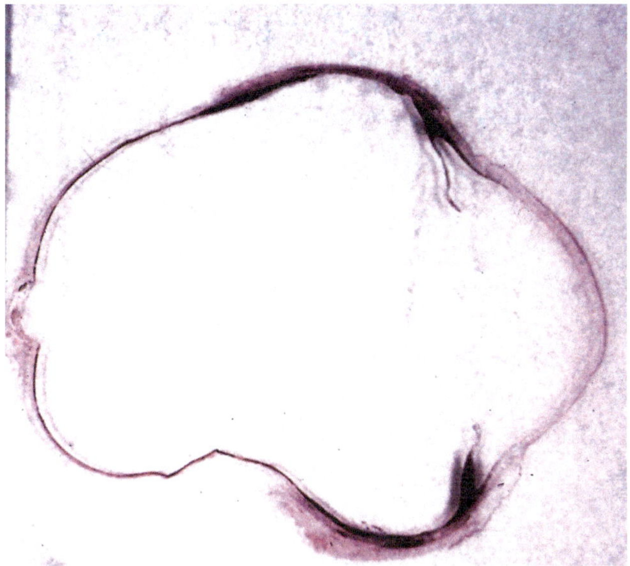

**Figure 12-22.** Glaucoma in the eye of a dog. The eye bulb is noticeably misshapen, with protrusion of the cornea and bulging of the posterior chamber behind the iris.

Compounds that impair filtration and cause fluid accumulation can lead to glaucoma (Fig. 12.22). Topically applied dexamethasone induces glaucoma in rats. Topical anticholinergic or sympathomimetic dilating drops, tricyclic antidepressants, monoamine oxidase inhibitors, antihistamines, antiparkinsonian drugs, and antipsychotic medications all have the potential to induce glaucoma in humans, affecting susceptible individuals.

## 12.1.4 Lens

The lens has a simple structure and is composed predominantly of fibres. Swelling, vacuolation, and degeneration of these fibres may be followed by rupture and liquefaction of the lens fibres, with formation of Morgagnian globules (Figs. 12.23–12.25). If changes are severe, distortion and collapse of the lens may occur, with subsequent calcification. Most degenerative lenticular changes are associated with cataract formation, which is seen in life as opacity. The avascular nature of the lens and the impermeability of the capsule generally prevent an inflammatory reaction, but capsule rupture can lead to inflammation and fibrosis.

Certain compounds induce disorganisation, pigmentation, hypertrophy, and hyperplasia of the lenticular epithelium, sometimes secondary to inflammatory changes in other ocular structures (Figs. 12.26 and 12.27). Administration of 4-diethylaminoethoxy-α-ethylbenyhydrol causes lenticular epithelial proliferative changes in rats that progress to cataracts, subsequent to keratitis and iridocyclitis [45].

A wide variety of drugs and xenobiotics, including metals, sugars, hypolipidaemic agents, and morphine-like compounds, acting by various mechanisms, have been linked with cataract development in humans and laboratory animals. High doses of sugars such as xylose and glucose result in cataracts owing to the formation of sugar alcohols and osmotic stress on the lens fibres. Agents such as streptozocin, used to induce diabetes in experimental models, cause secondary cataracts as increases in blood glucose, and consequently aldose reductase, lead to sorbitol formation in the lens. The formation of naphthalene-induced cataracts in rats, used as a model for age-related cataracts in humans, is reduced by aldose reductase inhibitors, which probably inhibit the conversion of naphthalene dihydrodiol to 1,2-dihydroxynaphthalene [46, 47]. *N*-methyl-*N*-nitrosourea (MNU) is cataractogenic in rats [48], with accompanying reductions in levels of several α amino acids and glutathione in the lens [49].

Long-term administration of steroids is known to cause cataract formation in humans. Rats are less susceptible, but topical or systemic administration of prednisolone accompanied by a single dose of irradiation induces cataracts in Brown Norway rats, with lens fibre degeneration and Y-suture dissociation [50, 51].

A number of hypolipidaemic agents induce cataracts in laboratory species and humans. Impaired cholesterol synthesis, perturbation of lens membrane function, or both have been implicated [52]. Hydroxymethylglutaryl (HMG)-CoA reductase inhibitors such as lovastatin induce cataracts in dogs [53, 54]. Triparanol causes cataracts in rats and humans due to inhibition of cholesterol synthesis and accumulation of lipid, leading to swelling and disruption [23]. In rats, these cataracts are characterised histologically by hydropic change, lens fibre degeneration, epithelial proliferation, and microvesicular lipid accumulation [55]. Oxidosqualene cyclase inhibitors cause cataracts in mice, dogs, and hamsters, with early lesions manifesting as swelling and degeneration of the lens fibres [22, 52, 56]. Phospholipidotics such as chloroquine and iprindole produce cataracts through the formation of intralysosomal drug–lipid complexes.

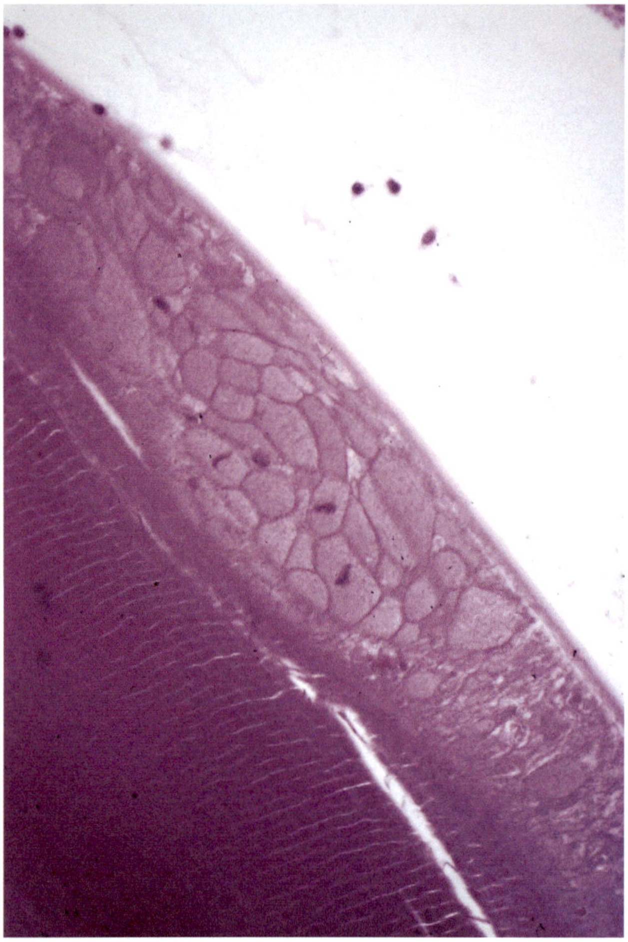

**Figure 12-23.** Lens from a rat treated with a herbicide. Focally, subcapsular fibres are moderately swollen and normal architecture is lost. H&E.

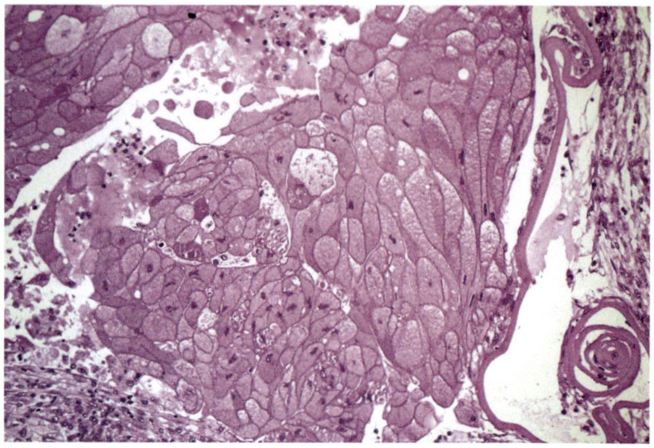

**Figure 12-24.** Severe swelling, rupture, and degeneration of the lenticular fibres from the eye of a rat treated systemically with a novel herbicide. H&E (With kind permission from Springer Science+Business Media B.V [14]).

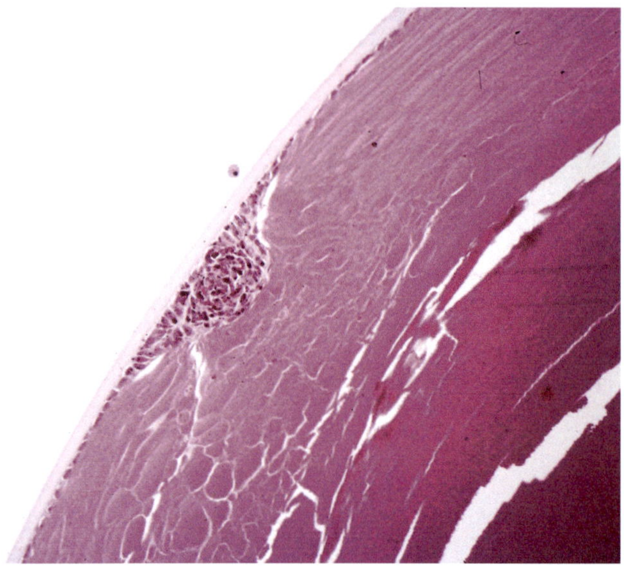

**Figure 12-25.** Focal lenticular epithelial hypertrophy and hyperplasia in a rat. The lenticular epithelial cells are hypertrophic and pigmented, with minimal hyperplasia and disorganisation of epithelial architecture. H&E.

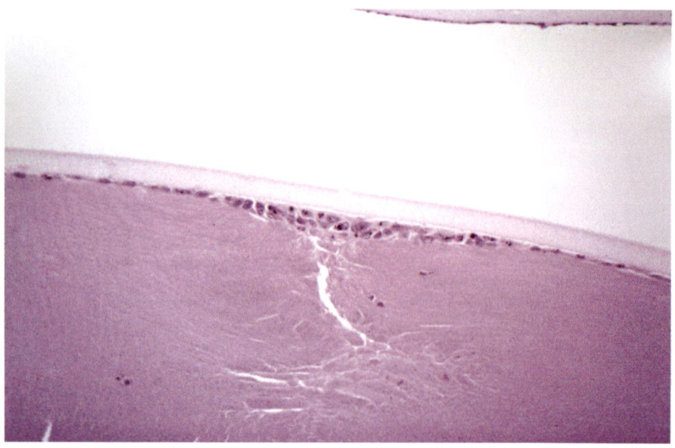

**Figure 12-26.** Lenticular epithelial hyperplasia in a rat. The lenticular epithelium shows focal subcapsular proliferation of epithelial cells. Some of the hyperplastic cells contain large pigment granules. H&E.

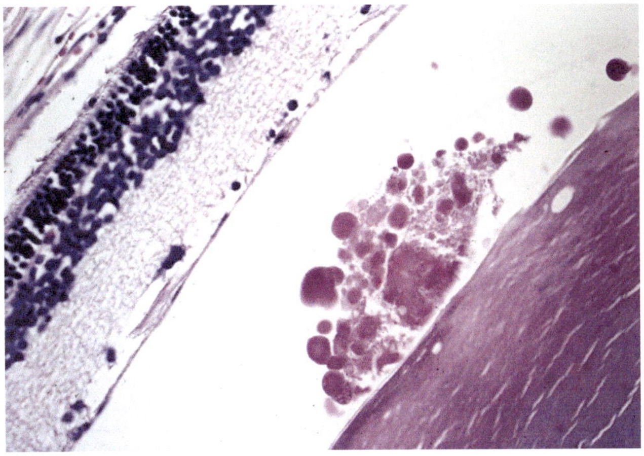

**Figure 12-27.** Hyaline bodies lying between the retina and lens in a rodent. H&E.

## 12.1.5 Harderian Glands

Harderian glands are specific to certain species, including the rat, mouse, and hamster. Sexual dimorphism is evident, with the porphyrin content being higher in females. This content can be manipulated in both sexes by hormone administration and by castration in males. Hyperprolactinaemia, associated with dopamine antagonists, increases the porphyrin content in mice. In rats, β-adrenergics and atropine sulphate increase porphyrin content through inhibitory effects on secretion [57]. Local irritation and cholinergics increase Harderian gland secretion, resulting in characteristic chromodacryorrhoea.

Inflammation, degeneration, and acinar atrophy occur as background findings in older animals (Fig. 12.28). These are also associated with orbital bleeding and in the past have been associated with the sialodacryoadenitis virus. Dacryoadenitis has been recorded with phosphodiesterase inhibitors [58]. Anticholinesterase agents can induce harderian gland atrophy, manifesting histologically as decreased cytoplasmic vacuolation, dilated lumina, and increased single-cell necrosis [14]. Recombinant human EGF causes acinar hypertrophy and hyperplasia, with anisokaryosis and areas of brown pigmentation in rats [59].

Hyperplasia and neoplasia can be induced in rodents by irradiation and by a wide range of agents. Genotoxic carcinogens administered by various routes, such as 1,3-butadiene, ethylene oxide, and *N-ethyl-N*-nitrosourea (ENU) followed by urethane, produce tumours of the Harderian gland (Fig. 12.29) [60, 61]. Activation of the H-*ras* gene has been implicated in spontaneous and induced tumours [62]. These tumours are considered to be of little relevance to humans, as the gland is rodent-specific.

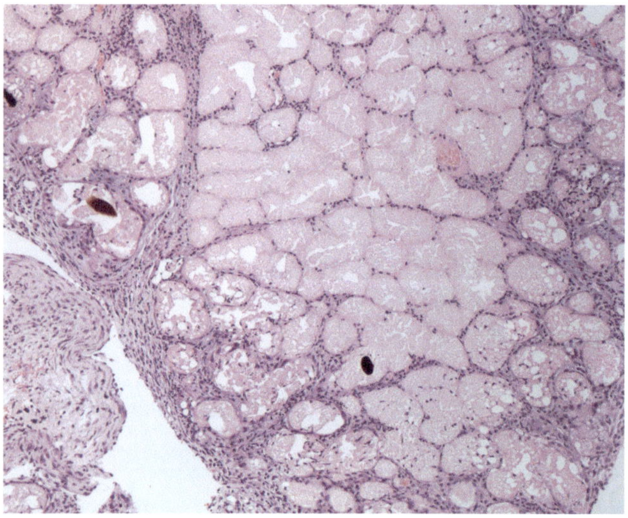

**FIGURE 12-28.** Acinar necrosis, interstitial fibrosis, and inflammation in the harderian gland of a rat. These are spontaneous findings, especially in older animals; they can be associated with orbital bleeding.

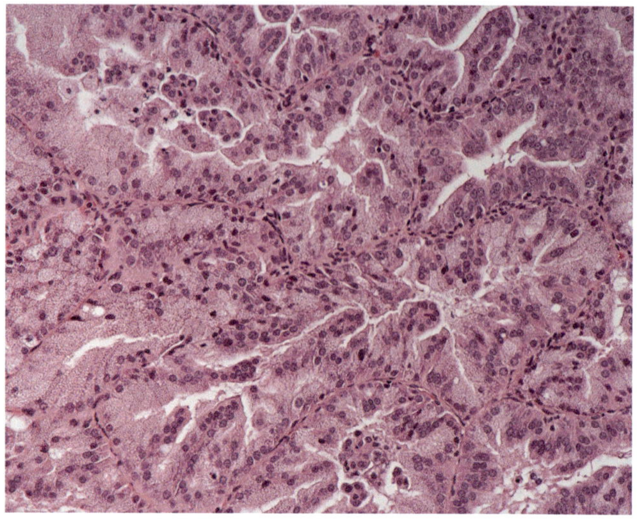

**FIGURE 12-29.** Adenoma in the harderian gland of a rat. The tumour displays papillary proliferation of well-differentiated, vacuolated columnar cells. Benign and malignant harderian gland tumours can be induced by irradiation and a wide range of genotoxic and nongenotoxic compounds. H&E.

## 12.1.6 Lacrimal and Meibomian Glands

A limited number of induced changes are seen in the lacrimal glands. In rodents, focal acinar harderianisation is common in long-term studies as a background change and appears macroscopically as pale foci. The foci reflect lipid accumulation, with the acini closely resembling those of the harderian gland, and their incidence increases in males after 6 months of age (Fig. 12.30). The incidence of this change can be reduced by castration, as it is androgen-dependent.

Several xenobiotics cause reduced secretion of the lacrimal glands, meibomian glands, or both, resulting in secondary changes in the eye. Hypophysectomy induces atrophy of the lacrimal gland in rats; this atrophy can be partially reversed by administration of dihydroxytestosterone and prolactin [63]. Treatment with clonidine induces intracellular oedema and disorganisation of the basal cell layer of the lacrimal gland in rodents. Atrophy of the lacrimal gland appears histologically as reduced size of the acini (Fig. 12.31).

Treatment with a variety of pharmaceuticals, including sulphonamides, anticholinergics, 5-aminosalicylic acid, and β-adrenergic blockers, causes meibomian gland degeneration and atrophy in dogs. The resulting reduction in tear production results in 'dry eye' or keratoconjunctivitis sicca. The affected meibomian glands display acinar degeneration and atrophy, loss of architecture, and mononuclear cell infiltration. Vacuolation of acinar cells and cystic ducts may also be present (Figs. 12.32 and 12.33). Prolonged treatment can result in corneal ulceration and degeneration (Fig. 12.34).

In dogs, spontaneous autoimmune disease associated with circulating autoantibodies occurs in the meibomian glands, with certain breeds being more commonly affected. Histologically, this condition causes degeneration and lymphoid nodules in the gland. A similar condition has been described with use of a β-blocker [14].

Phenazopyridine accumulates in the lacrimal and nictitating glands, as well as the glands of Moll, affecting synthesis of secretory granules and gradually causing destruction of affected cells [64].

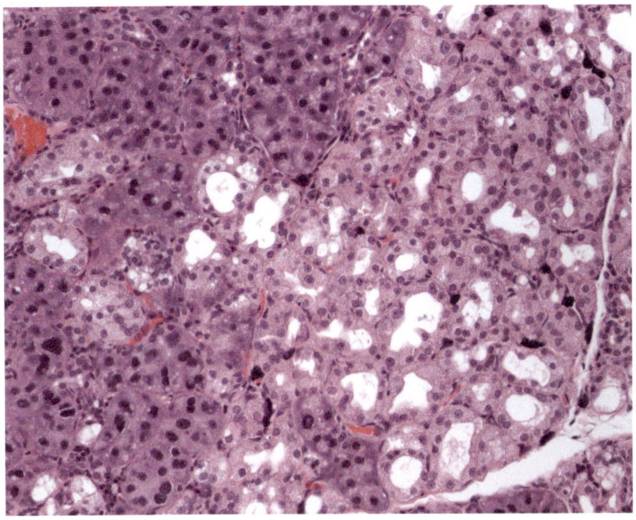

**FIGURE 12-30.** Harderianisation of the lacrimal glands from a rat on a long-term study. This common age-related change is androgen-dependent, so it can be manipulated by castration and hormonal treatment. H&E.

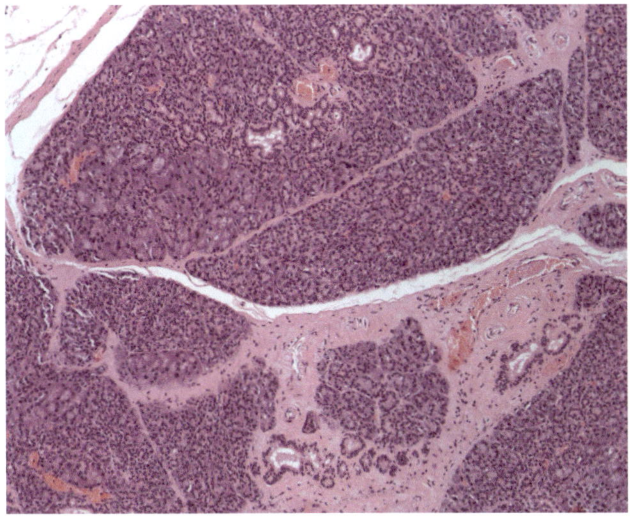

**FIGURE 12-31.** Acinar atrophy of the lacrimal gland in a mouse from a short-term study. Some acini appear normal, but most are small, with loss of cytoplasm and nuclear crowding. This induced change is often mediated through the autonomic nervous system. H&E.

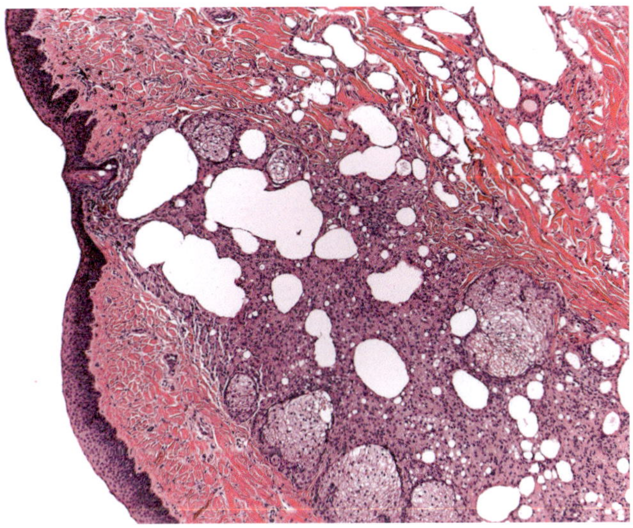

**FIGURE 12-32.** Meibomian gland of a dog with acinar degeneration and atrophy. The acini show loss of architecture with degeneration and vacuolation of the sebaceous cells. Variably sized cystic structures are present, probably representing blocked ducts or acini with subsequent atrophy of the associated acini. H&E.

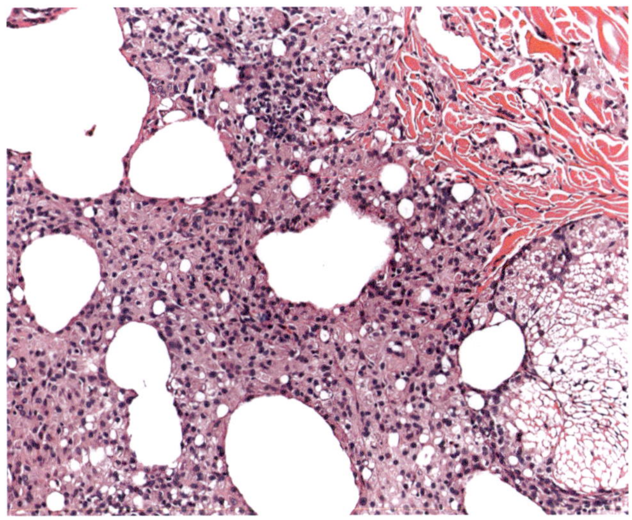

**FIGURE 12-33.** Viewed at greater magnification, the same gland as in Fig. 12.32 shows generalised loss of acinar structure, vacuolation, and degeneration of the acinar cells, with mild lymphohistiocytic infiltration. Among agents that can induce this change are β-adrenergic drugs. H&E.

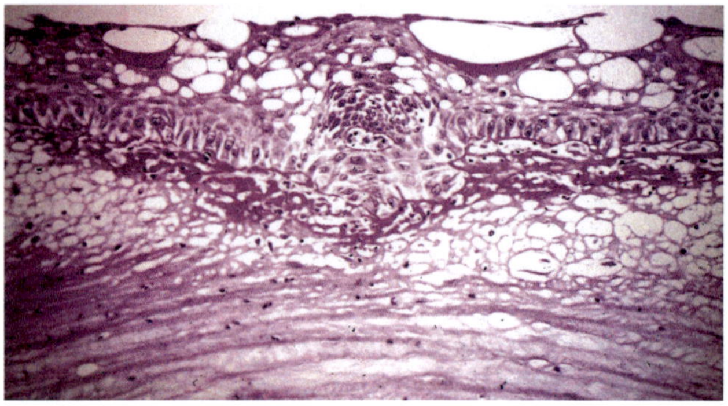

**Figure 12-34.** Cornea of a dog with keratoconjunctivitis sicca induced by a novel antispasmodic compound. The central depressed area probably represents the site of previous ulceration in which the epithelium has repaired, with vesiculation of the superficial epithelial cells and subepithelial swelling and necrosis. H&E (With kind permission from Springer Science+Business Media B.V [14]).

## 12.2 The Ear

The ear is rarely examined histologically in routine safety evaluation studies, at least partially because routine harvesting and histologic examination of the inner ear are made difficult by its location [65]. Also, standard histologic sections give limited information about ototoxicity, the assessment of which requires specialised examination, such as resin or plastic section preparation, or scanning electron microscopy. Electron microscopy is the tool of choice for detecting damage to hair cells in the cochlea. The inner ear is most easily dissected out and examined in the guinea pig, which is the species of choice for ototoxicity testing.

Ototoxicity is induced by a number of mechanisms, with different species being variably affected by xenobiotics. Rats are affected by aromatic solvents such as toluene and styrene and show auditory dysfunction and cochlear pathology, whereas guinea pigs are unaffected. This difference may be due to different metabolic pathways [66]. Age also may influence sensitivity, as older Long-Evans rats have been found to be more resistant than young ones to styrene-induced toxicity [67].

Toxicity is generally due to changes in the inner ear. A number of pharmaceuticals, notably the aminoglycosides and quinine derivatives, have been recognised as ototoxic in humans and laboratory animals. Aminoglycoside antibiotics induce cochlear hair cell degeneration, with degrees of ototoxic potential varying between antibiotics (Fig. 12.35). In rats, kanamycin induces extensive damage to the organ of Corti, with the outer hair cells more severely affected than the inner ones.

Ototoxic compounds affect some areas within the cochlea more often than other areas. Administration of toluene causes loss, primarily of outer hair cells, in the middle and basal turns of the organ of Corti, with corresponding hearing impairment [68]. With many compounds, including toluene and the aminoglycosides, damage continues to progress after exposure ceases [69].

Some compounds induce reversible changes. Loop diuretics, such as furosemide and bumetanide, affect the stria vascularis (which maintains the high potassium content of the endolymph), causing intercellular and intracellular oedema [70]. Salicylate and quinine induce ischaemic damage, which may reverse over time [71].

Some compounds, such as cisplatin, cause permanent damage, possibly through apoptotic mechanisms [72, 73]. Polychlorinated biphenyls induce ototoxicity in juvenile rats, possibly through hypothyroxinaemia, as hypothyroidism is known to affect maturation of the inner ear structures in neonates of some species [74].

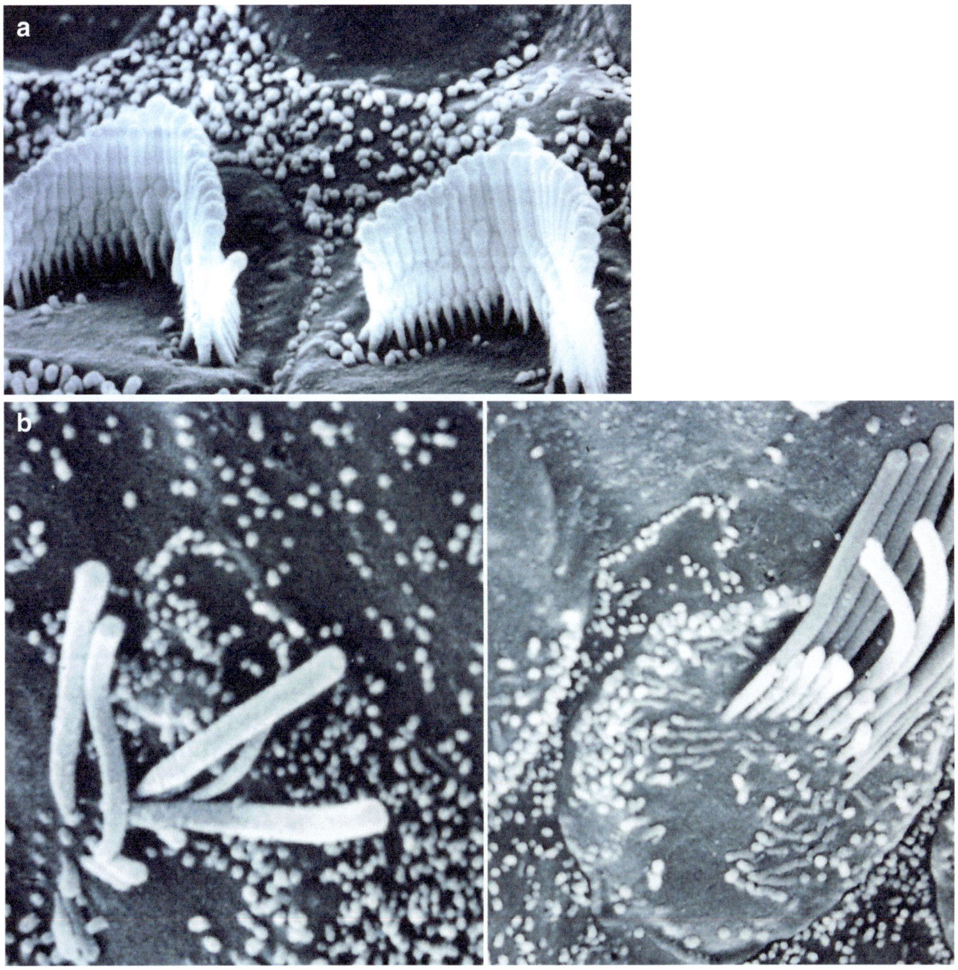


**FIGURE 12-35.** (**a**) Characteristic normal arrangement of the different-length stereocilia of outer hair cells of the guinea pig cochlea. Scanning electron micrograph. (**b**) Normal, collapsed, and damaged stereocilia from the outer hair cells of a gentamicin-treated guinea pig. Scanning electron micrograph (**a**, **b** With kind permission from Springer Science+Business Media B.V [14]).

## 12.2.1 Zymbal's Gland

The Zymbal's gland, a specialised sebaceous gland associated with the ear canal, is specific to rodents. Tumours of this gland occur spontaneously in older rats, forming large masses on the side of the head. A number of genotoxic and nongenotoxic compound classes also induce tumours of this gland, many of them associated with tumours of the skin or preputial or clitoral glands [75, 76]. Tumours of the Zymbal's gland include papillomas, adenomas, and squamous cell carcinomas (Fig. 12.36). Among the many compounds and compound classes that induce tumours of the Zymbal's gland in rats when given orally are nitrosoureas, benzene, and heterocyclic amines [77, 78]. Other substances that induce tumours of the Zymbal's gland include 1–3 butadiene and vinyl chloride given by the inhalation route and 2,3-dibromo-1-propanol applied topically. Early Zymbal's gland changes include ductal squamous hyperplasia and basophilia of the sebaceous acini.

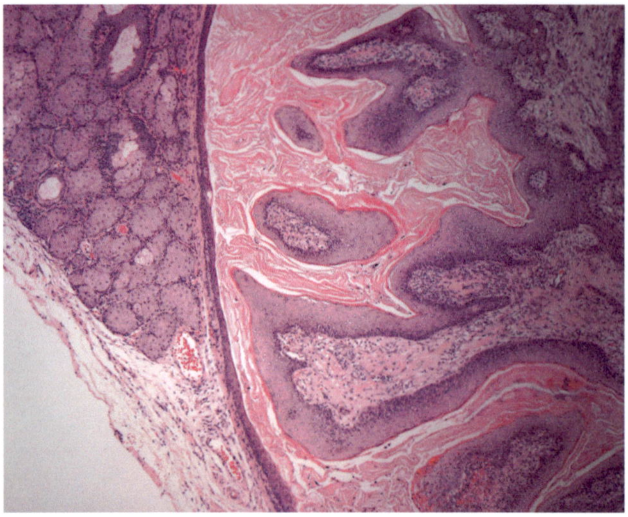

**Figure 12-36.** Squamous cell carcinoma of the Zymbal's gland from a rat. Normal gland is seen on the left. Most of the gland is replaced by a large, cystic tumour consisting of squamous epithelium. The tumour contains abundant keratin; papillary projections are covered by keratinised, hyperplastic squamous epithelium, which is invading the underlying stroma. H&E.

## References


1. Short BG. Safety evaluation of ocular drug delivery formulations: techniques and practical considerations. Toxicol Pathol. 2008;36:49–62.
2. Teixeira L, Dubielzig RR. Eye. In: Haschek WM, Rousseaux CG, Wallig MA, editors. Haschek and Rousseaux's handbook of toxicologic pathology. 3rd ed. Boston: Academic; 2013. p. 2095–185.
3. Galin MA, Nano HD, Hall T. Ocular zinc concentration. Invest Ophthalmol. 1962;1:142–8.
4. Vézina M. Comparative ocular anatomy in commonly used laboratory animals. In: Weir AB, Collins M, editors. Assessing ocular toxicology in laboratory animals. New York: Humana Press; 2013. p. 1–21.
5. Schafer KA, Render JA. Toxicologic pathology of the eye: histologic preparation and alterations of the anterior segment. In: Weir AB, Collins M, editors. Assessing ocular toxicology in laboratory animals. New York: Humana Press; 2013. p. 159–217.
6. Munger RJ, Collins M. Assessment of ocular toxicity potential: basic theory and techniques. In: Weir AB, Collins M, editors. Assessing ocular toxicology in laboratory animals. New York: Humana Press; 2013. p. 23–52.
7. Ver Hoeve JN, Munger RJ, Murphy CJ, Nork TM. Emerging electrophysiological technologies for assessing ocular toxicity in laboratory animals. In: Weir AB, Collins M, editors. Assessing ocular toxicology in laboratory animals. New York: Humana Press; 2013. p. 123–57.
8. Nork TM, Rasmussen CA, Christian BJ, Croft MA, Murphy CJ. Emerging imaging technologies for assessing ocular toxicity in laboratory animals. In: Weir AB, Collins M, editors. Assessing ocular toxicology in laboratory animals. New York: Humana Press; 2013. p. 53–121.
9. Latendresse JR, Warbrittion AR, Jonassen H, Creasy DM. Fixation of testes and eyes using a modified Davidson's fluid: comparison with Bouin's fluid and conventional Davidson's fluid. Toxicol Pathol. 2002;30:524–33.
10. Schafer KA, Render JA. Toxicologic pathology of the eye: alterations of the lens and posterior segment. In: Weir AB, Collins M, editors. Assessing ocular toxicology in laboratory animals. New York: Humana Press; 2013. p. 219–57.
11. Bartlett C. Ocular toxicity regulatory considerations for non-drug Food and Drug Administration (FDA) products and the Environmental Protection Agency (EPA). In: Weir AB, Collins M, editors. Assessing ocular toxicology in laboratory animals. New York: Humana Press; 2013. p. 295–305.
12. Greaves P. Histopathology of preclinical toxicity studies. Eye, in 4th ed. London: Elsevier; 2012, p 822–845.
13. Weir AB, Wilson SD. Nonclinical regulatory aspects for ophthalmic drugs. In: Weir AB, Collins M, editors. Assessing ocular toxicology in laboratory animals. New York: Humana Press; 2013. p. 259–94.
14. Gopinath C, Prentice DE, Lewis DJ. The eye and ear. In: Gopinath C, Prentice D, Lewis DJ, editors. Atlas of experimental toxicologic pathology. Lancaster: MTP Press; 1987. p. 145–55.
15. Garibaldi BA, Goad ME. Lipid keratopathy in the Watanabe (WHHL) rabbit. Vet Pathol. 1988;25:173–4.
16. National Toxicology Program. Toxicology and carcinogenesis studies of malonaldehyde, sodium salt (3-hydroxy-2-propenal, sodium salt) (CAS No. 24382-04-5) in F344/N rats and B6C3F1 mice (gavage studies). Natl Toxicol Program Tech Rep Ser. 1988;331:1–182.
17. Aguirre SA, Huang W, Prasanna G, Jessen B. Corneal neovascularization and ocular irritancy responses in dogs following topical ocular administration of an EP4-prostaglandin E2 agonist. Toxicol Pathol. 2009;37:911–20.
18. Newkirk KM, Chandler HL, Parent AE, Young DC, Colitz CM, Wilkie DA, Kusewitt DF. Ultraviolet radiation-induced corneal degeneration in 129 mice. Toxicol Pathol. 2007;35:819–26.
19. Leure-Dupree AE. Vascularization of the rat cornea after prolonged zinc deficiency. Anat Rec. 1986;216:27–32.
20. Yoshizuka M, McCarthy KJ, Kaye GI, Fujimoto S. Cadmium toxicity to the cornea of pregnant rats: electron microscopy and x-ray microanalysis. Anat Rec. 1990;227:138–43.
21. Reindel JF, Gough AW, Pilcher GD, Bobrowski WF, Sobocinski GP, de la Iglesia FA. Systemic proliferative changes and clinical signs in cynomolgus monkeys administered a recombinant derivative of human epidermal growth factor. Toxicol Pathol. 2001;29:159–73.

22. Pyrah IT, Kalinowski A, Jackson D, Davies W, Davis S, Aldridge A, Greaves P. Toxicologic lesions associated with two related inhibitors of oxidosqualene cyclase in the dog and mouse. Toxicol Pathol. 2001;29:174–9.

23. Kirby TJ. Cataracts produced by triparanol. (MER-29). Trans Am Ophthalmol Soc. 1967;65:494–543.

24. United States Environmental Protection Agency. Pesticide fact sheet: topramezone. 2005. Office of prevention, pesticides and toxic substances (7501C). http://www.epa.gov/opp00001/chem_search/reg_actions/registration/fs_PC-123009_10-Aug-05.pdf.

25. Taradach C, Greaves P. Spontaneous eye lesions in laboratory animals: incidence in relation to age. Crit Rev Toxicol. 1984;12:121–47.

26. Heywood R, Gopinath C. Morphological assessment of visual dysfunction. Toxicol Pathol. 1990;18:204–17.

27. Heng JE, Vorwerk CK, Lessell E, Zurakowski D, Levin LA, Dreyer EB. Ethambutol is toxic to retinal ganglion cells via an excitotoxic pathway. Invest Ophthalmol Vis Sci. 1999;40:190–6.

28. Chung H, Yoon YH, Hwang JJ, Cho KS, Koh JY, Kim JG. Ethambutol-induced toxicity is mediated by zinc and lysosomal membrane permeabilization in cultured retinal cells. Toxicol Appl Pharmacol. 2009;235:163–70.

29. Lucas DR, Newhouse JP. The toxic effect of sodium L-glutamate on the inner layers of the retina. Arch Ophthalmol. 1957;58:193–201.

30. Butler WH, Ford GP, Newberne JW. A study of the effects of vigabatrin on the central nervous system and retina of Sprague Dawley and Lister-Hooded rats. Toxicol Pathol. 1987;15:143–8.

31. Duboc A, Hanoteau N, Simonutti M, Rudolf G, Nehlig A, Sahel JA, Picaud S. Vigabatrin, the GABA-transaminase inhibitor, damages cone photoreceptors in rats. Ann Neurol. 2004;55:695–705.

32. Ford MM, Dubielzig RR, Giuliano EA, Moore CP, Narfstrom KL. Ocular and systemic manifestations after oral administration of a high dose of enrofloxacin in cats. Am J Vet Res. 2007;68:190–202.

33. Wiebe V, Hamilton P. Fluoroquinolone-induced retinal degeneration in cats. J Am Vet Med Assoc. 2002;221:1568–71.

34. Yoshizawa K, Kuro-Kuwata M, Sasaki T, Lai YC, Kanematsu S, Miki H, et al. Retinal degeneration induced in adult mice by a single intraperitoneal injection of N-ethyl-N-nitrosourea. Toxicol Pathol. 2011;39:606–13.

35. Mecklenburg L, Schraermeyer U. An overview on the toxic morphological changes in the retinal pigment epithelium after systemic compound administration. Toxicol Pathol. 2007;35:252–67.

36. Render JA, Carlton WW. Ocular lesions of 6-aminonicotinamide toxicosis in rabbits. Vet Pathol. 1985;22:72–7.

37. Illanes O, Anderson S, Niesman M, Zwick L, Jessen BA. Retinal and peripheral nerve toxicity induced by the administration of a pan-cyclin dependent kinase (cdk) inhibitor in mice. Toxicol Pathol. 2006;34:243–8.

38. Saturno G, Pesenti M, Cavazzoli C, Rossi A, Giusti AM, Gierke B, et al. Expression of serine/threonine protein-kinases and related factors in normal monkey and human retinas: the mechanistic understanding of a CDK2 inhibitor induced retinal toxicity. Toxicol Pathol. 2007;35:972–83.

39. Brown WR, Rubin L, Hite M, Zwickey RE. Experimental papilledema in the dog induced by a salicylanilide. Toxicol Appl Pharmacol. 1972;21:532–41.

40. Parhad IM, Griffin JW, Price DL, Clark AW, Cork LC, Miller NR, Hoffman PN. Intoxication with beta, beta' -iminodipropionitrile: a model of optic disc swelling. Lab Invest. 1982;46:186–95.

41. Smith-Thomas L, Moustafa M, Spada CS, Shi L, Dawson RA, Wagner M, et al. Latanoprost-induced pigmentation in human iridial melanocytes is fibroblast dependent. Exp Eye Res. 2004;78:973–85.

42. Stjernschantz J, Ocklind A, Wentzel P, Lake S, Hu DN. Latanoprost-induced increase of tyrosinase transcription in iridial melanocytes. Acta Ophthalmol Scand. 2000;78:618–22.

43. Yildirim N, Sahin A, Kara S, Baycu C. Latanoprost-induced changes in the iris and trabeculum: an electron-microscopic morphological study. Int Ophthalmol. 2010;30:93–7.

44. Matuk Y, Ghosh M, McCulloch C. Distribution of silver in the eyes and plasma proteins of the albino rat. Can J Ophthalmol. 1981;16:145–50.

45. Bencz Z, Ivan E, Cholnoky E. Analysis of cataract and keratotic damage induced by 4-diethylaminoethoxy-alpha-ethyl-benzhydrol (RGH-6201) in rats. Arch Toxicol Suppl. 1985;8:476–9.

46. Xu GT, Zigler Jr JS, Lou MF. The possible mechanism of naphthalene cataract in rat and its prevention by an aldose reductase inhibitor (ALO1576). Exp Eye Res. 1992;54:63–72.

47. Lou MF, Xu GT, Zigler Jr S, York Jr B. Inhibition of naphthalene cataract in rats by aldose reductase inhibitors. Curr Eye Res. 1996;15:423–32.

48. Yoshizawa K, Oishi Y, Nambu H, Yamamoto D, Yang J, Senzaki H, et al. Cataractogenesis in neonatal Sprague–Dawley rats by N-methyl-N-nitrosourea. Toxicol Pathol. 2000;28:555–64.

49. Miyazono Y, Harada K, Sugiyama K, Ueno M, Torii M, Kato I, et al. Toxicological characterization of N-methyl-N-nitrosourea-induced cataract in rats by LC/MS-based metabonomic analysis. J Appl Toxicol. 2011;31:655–62.

50. Shui YB, Kojima M, Sasaki K. A new steroid-induced cataract model in the rat: long-term prednisolone applications with a minimum of X-irradiation. Ophthalmic Res. 1996;28 Suppl 2:92–101.

51. Shui YB, Vrensen GF, Kojima M. Experimentally induced steroid cataract in the rat: a scanning electron microscopic study. Surv Ophthalmol. 1997;42 Suppl 1:S127–32.

52. Cenedella RJ, Jacob R, Borchman D, Tang D, Neely AR, Samadi A, et al. Direct perturbation of lens membrane structure may contribute to cataracts caused by U18666A, an oxidosqualene cyclase inhibitor. J Lipid Res. 2004;45:1232–41.

53. Gerson RJ, MacDonald JS, Alberts AW, Chen J, Yudkovitz JB, Greenspan MD, et al. On the etiology of subcapsular lenticular opacities produced in dogs receiving HMG-CoA reductase inhibitors. Exp Eye Res. 1990;50:65–78.

54. MacDonald JS, Gerson RJ, Kornbrust DJ, Kloss MW, Prahalada S, Berry PH, et al. Preclinical evaluation of lovastatin. Am J Cardiol. 1988;62:16J–27.

55. von Sallmann L, Grimes P, Collins E. Triparanol-induced cataract in rats. Trans Am Ophthalmol Soc. 1963;61:49–60.

56. Funk J, Landes C. Histopathologic findings after treatment with different oxidosqualene cyclase (OSC) inhibitors in hamsters and dogs. Exp Toxicol Pathol. 2005;57:29–38.

57. Iwai H, Tagawa Y, Hayasaka I, Yanai T, Masegi T. Effects of atropine sulfate on rat harderian glands: correlation between morphological changes and porphyrin levels. J Toxicol Sci. 2000;25:151–9.

58. Westwood FR, Iswaran TJ, Greaves P. Long-term effects of an inotropic phosphodiesterase inhibitor (ICI 153,110) on the rat salivary gland, harderian gland, and intestinal mucosa. Toxicol Pathol. 1991;19.214–23.

59. Breider MA, Bleavins MR, Reindel JF, Gough AW, de la Iglesia FA. Cellular hyperplasia in rats following continuous intravenous infusion of recombinant human epidermal growth factor. Vet Pathol. 1996;33:184–94.

60. Hong HH, Houle CD, Ton TV, Sills RC. K-ras mutations in lung tumors and tumors from other organs are consistent with a common mechanism of ethylene oxide tumorigenesis in the B6C3F1 mouse. Toxicol Pathol. 2007;35:81–5.

61. Kajimura T, Kashimoto Y, Satoh H, Furuhama K. Rapid induction of tumors in the harderian gland of mice receiving urethane after initiation with N-ethyl-N-nitrosourea. J Toxicol Pathol. 2003;16:85–91.

62. Goodrow TL, Nichols WW, Storer RD, Anderson MW, Maronpot RR. Activation of H-*ras* is prevalent in 1,3-butadiene-induced and spontaneously occurring murine Harderian gland tumors. Carcinogenesis. 1994;15:2665–7.

63. Azzarolo AM, Bjerrum K, Maves CA, Becker L, Wood RL, Mircheff AK, Warren DW. Hypophysectomy-induced regression of female rat lacrimal glands: partial restoration and maintenance by dihydrotestosterone and prolactin. Invest Ophthalmol Vis Sci. 1995;36:216–26.

64. Slatter DH, Davis WC. Toxicity of phenazopyridine: electron microscopical studies of canine lacrimal and nictitans glands. Arch Ophthalmol. 1974;91:484–6.

65. Mattsson JL. Ototoxicity: an argument for evaluation of the cochlea in safety testing in animals. Toxicol Pathol. 2000; 28:137–41.

66. Lataye R, Campo P, Pouyatos B, Cossec B, Blachere V, Morel G. Solvent ototoxicity in the rat and guinea pig. Neurotoxicol Teratol. 2003;25:39–50.

67. Campo P, Pouyatos B, Lataye R, Morel G. Is the aged rat ear more susceptible to noise or styrene damage than the young ear? Noise Health. 2003;5:1–18.

68. Johnson AC, Canlon B. Toluene exposure affects the functional activity of the outer hair cells. Hear Res. 1994;72:189–96.

69. Johnson AC, Canlon B. Progressive hair cell loss induced by toluene exposure. Hear Res. 1994;75:201–8.

70. Prepageran N, Scott AR, Rutka JA. Ototoxicity of loop diuretics. In: Roland PS, Rutka JA, editors. Ototoxicity. Hamilton: BC Decker; 2004. p. 42–8.

71. Prepageran N, Rutka JA. Salicylates, nonsteroidal anti-inflammatory drugs, quinine, and heavy metals. In: Roland PS, Rutka JA, editors. Ototoxicity. Hamilton: BC Decker; 2004. p. 28–42.

72. De Freitas MR, Figueiredo AA, Brito GA, Leitao RF, Carvalho Jr JV, Gomes Jr RM, Ribeiro RA. The role of apoptosis in cisplatin-induced ototoxicity in rats. Braz J Otorhinolaryngol. 2009; 75:745–52.

73. Garcia-Berrocal JR, Nevado J, Ramirez-Camacho R, Sanz R, Gonzalez-Garcia JA, Sanchez-Rodriguez C, et al. The anticancer drug cisplatin induces an intrinsic apoptotic pathway inside the inner ear. Br J Pharmacol. 2007;152: 1012–20.

74. Crofton KM, Kodavanti PR, Derr-Yellin EC, Casey AC, Kehn LS. PCBs, thyroid hormones, and ototoxicity in rats: cross-fostering experiments demonstrate the impact of postnatal lactation exposure. Toxicol Sci. 2000;57:131–40.

75. Gold LS, Manley NB, Slone TH, Ward JM. Compendium of chemical carcinogens by target organ: results of chronic bioassays in rats, mice, hamsters, dogs, and monkeys. Toxicol Pathol. 2001;29:639–52.

76. Gold LS, Manley NB, Slone TH, Rohrbach L, Garfinkel GB. Supplement to the Carcinogenic Potency Database (CPDB): results of animal bioassays published in the general literature through 1997 and by the National Toxicology Program in 1997–1998. Toxicol Sci. 2005;85:747–808.

77. Kato T, Migita H, Ohgaki H, Sato S, Takayama S, Sugimura T. Induction of tumors in the Zymbal gland, oral cavity, colon, skin and mammary gland of F344 rats by a mutagenic compound, 2-amino-3, 4-dimethylimidazo[4, 5-f]quinoline. Carcinogenesis. 1989;10:601–3.

78. Kudo M, Ogura T, Esumi H, Sugimura T. Mutational activation of c-Ha-ras gene in squamous cell carcinomas of rat Zymbal gland induced by carcinogenic heterocyclic amines. Mol Carcinog. 1991;4:36–42.

# Index


**A**

Accessory sex glands, 142–145
ACE. *See* Angiotensin-converting enzyme (ACE)
ACTH. *See* Adrenocorticotropic hormone (ACTH)
Adipose tissue
  eosinophilia and inflammation, 249, 250
  focal fat necrosis, 249
  interscapular brown adipose tissue, 248, 249
  lipomas, liposarcomas and angiolipomas, 249
  mesenchymal tumours, 249
  mesenteric white adipose tissue, 249
  sympathomimetic agents, 248
Adrenal glands
  cortex
    cortical adenoma, 175, 176
    cortical atrophy, z. fasciculata, 172, 173
    cortical carcinoma, 175, 176
    cortical hypertrophy, 171
    corticosteroids, 172
    cystic degeneration, 174
    diffuse cortical necrosis, 172
    diffuse hypertrophy, z. glomerulosa, 170
    diffuse necrosis, z. fasciculata, 172, 173
    focal hyperplasia, 175
    focal hypertrophy, z. glomerulosa, 170
    focal lymphoid inflammation, 174, 175
    haemorrhagic cystic degeneration, 174
    hypertrophy/hyperplasia, z. glomerulosa, 170
    induced lesions, 169–170
    intracytoplasmic eosinophilic inclusions, 174
    Na/K ratio, 170
    necrosis, 172
    pigmentation, 174, 175
    steroid synthesis, 170
    vacuolar degeneration, 172, 174
    vacuolation, 172, 173
    xenobiotics, 169
    z. fasciculata and reticularis, 171
  medulla
    agents, 175
    atrophy and fibrosis, 175
    hyperplasia, 175, 177
    necrosis and inflammation, 175
    phaeochromocytoma, 177, 178
Adrenocorticotropic hormone (ACTH), 171
Alimentary system and pancreas
  description, 77
  exocrine pancreas (*see* Pancreas)
  large intestines, 95–99
  oesophagus
    epithelial atrophy, 82
    hyperkeratosis, 82
    impaction, 82
    inflammation and ulceration, 82
    megaoesophagus and dilation, 82
    mucous cells, acinar lumen, 83, 84
    myofibre degeneration, 83
    spontaneous tumours, 83
    transgenic mouse, 82, 83
  oral cavity
    buccal mucosal erosions, 78
    calcium channel blocker, 79
    gingival hyperplasia, 79
    growth factors, 78
    hamster cheek pouch model, 77
    industrial chemicals, 79
    myofibre vacuolation and degeneration, tongue, 78
    papillomas, skin and buccal mucosa, 79
    saliva and squamous epithelium, 77
    skin pigmentation, 77–78
    stomatitis, 78
    sublingual blood sampling, 78
    teeth (*see* Teeth)
    toxicologic changes, 77
  salivary glands
    acinar basophilic foci, 81
    acinar cells, 81, 82
    granular duct, 81
    hyperplasia, 81
    hypertrophy, 81, 82
    novel antineoplastic agent, 81, 82
    sexual dimorphism, 81
    single-cell degeneration and atrophy, serous acini, 81, 82
    types, 81
  small intestines, 90–95
  stomach (*see* Stomach)
Angiotensin-converting enzyme (ACE), 192, 193
Apoptosis, liver
  intracytoplasmic inclusions
    description, 56
    hepatocellular adenomas, 56
    whorl pattern, 56
  nuclear changes
    cytomegaly and karyomegaly, 55
    intranuclear crystalline deposits, 56
    mitotic figures, 55
    multinucleated hepatocytes, 55
    pyridine derivatives, 55
  spheroidal eosinophilic cells, 54
Axonal lesions, 218
Axonopathy
  cervical cord and optic tract, 218, 219
  dorsolateral column, mouse, 218, 220
  eosinophilic bodies/swollen axons, 218, 220
  multifocal, spinal cord, rat, 218, 220
  myelin spheroids and myelinophages, 220, 219
  organophosphates, 218, 219
  tibial nerve, rat, 218, 219



C. Gopinath, V. Mowat, *Atlas of Toxicological Pathology*,
DOI 10.1007/978-1-62703-998-7, © Springer Science+Business Media New York 2014

**B**

Bonchi/bronchioles
  eosinophilic inclusions, 30, 31
  epithelial regeneration, 30
  focal inflammation, 30, 32
  goblet cell hypertrophy/hyperplasia, 30, 31
  inflammation, 30, 32
  mineralisation, bronchiolar epithelium, 30, 31
  neuroendocrine cell hyperplasia, 31, 33
  squamous metaplasia, 30, 33
Bone marrow
  cellularity, 209
  changes, 209
  cytotoxic anticancer agents and antibiotics, 209
  erythroid cellularity, 209, 210
  erythroid/myeloid ratio, 209
  fibro-osseous lesion, 211
  granulocytic cellularity, 209, 210
  histiocytosis, 211
  hypersegmented megakaryocytes, 209, 211
  hypocellularity and megakaryocytes, 209
  immune-mediated thrombocytopenia and megakaryocytosis, 209
  lymphoid follicle, 209, 210
  multifocal histiocytosis, 211
  myelofibrosis and loss, cellularity, 209, 210
  necrosis, haemorrhage and loss of cells, 209, 210
  polychlorinated biphenyls, 209
  resin sections, 209
Bones
  anticonvulsants, 239
  articular cartilage
    rabbit, 238
    rat, 235
  bisphosphonates, 240
  chondroid hyperplasia, 236, 237
  chondromucinous degeneration, 238
  cortical bone, rabbits and rodents, 239
  distal femoral growth, 236, 237
  distal femur, endosteal hyperostosis, 239, 240
  erosion and necrosis, quinolone derivatives, 238
  femoro-tibial joint, 236
  fibro-osseous lesion, mouse, 239
  fluoro-chromelabelling and plastic sections, 235
  growth plate changes, 235
  hedgehog pathway inhibitor, 236
  hyperostosis, 240, 241
  hypertrophic chondrocytes, 235
  hypertrophic growth plate, 235–236
  hypertrophy and mineralisation, 236, 237
  osteoid and formation surfaces, 239
  osteosarcomas, 240
  quinolones and warfarin, 236
  rabbit humerus, 239
  radiation osteopathy, 238
  remodelling, 235
  skeletal system, 235
  teriparatide, 240
  thyromimetics, 238

**C**

Cardiovascular system
  heart (*see* Heart)
  vascular changes
    β-aminopropionitrile causes, 13
    arteriolar hypertrophy, 17
    atherosclerotic plaque, 16, 17
    chronic infusion, 13, 15
    coronary arteries, 16
    drug-induced vascular injury, 13, 14
    fatty streaks, 16
    intimal plaque, 16
    mineralisation and cartilaginous metaplasia, 13, 16
    periarterial connective tissue, 13, 14
    plexiform vasculopathy, 13–15
    thrombosis, 13, 15
    tunica media reveal necrosis, 13, 14
Cataract, 265
CCK. *See* Cholecystokinin (CCK)
Cholangiocarcinomas
  cholangiofibrotic type, 73
  description, 73
  metastasis into lung, 73
Cholecystokinin (CCK), 99, 103, 104
Chronic progressive nephropathy (CPN), 111
Cirrhosis, 71
CL. *See* Corpora lutea (CL)
Cornea
  amphophilic cationic drugs, 254, 255
  cadmium, 256
  cholinesterase-inhibiting effect, 256
  EGFR, 256
  epithelial layer, 254
  focal corneal ulceration, mouse, 255, 256
  4-HPPD, 257
  hyperplasia, 257
  induced changes, 254
  keratitis and dystrophic mineralisation, mouse, 255, 256
  keratoconjunctivitis sicca, 255, 257
  malonaldehyde, 255
  mineralisation, spontaneous finding, 254
  monkey, antineoplastic agent, 255
  multifocal corneal mineralisation and keratitis, 254, 255
  narcotic analgesics/prolonged anaesthesia, 255
  nutritional deficiencies, 256
  vEGF and EGFR inhibitors, 257, 258
Corpora lutea (CL), 150
CPN. *See* Chronic progressive nephropathy (CPN)

**D**

Degeneration
  hyaline and granular, 231
  muscle fibre, 231–232
  myofibre, 230
  seminiferous epithelial, 135
  and spermatids, 136, 137
  tubular dilation, 133
Dogs
  atrophy, 143
  focal hypoplasia, 136
  hyperplasia, 143, 144
  hypertrophy, 143, 144
  sperm granulomas, 140

**E**

EAE. *See* Experimental allergic encephalomyelitis (EAE)
Ear
  aminoglycoside antibiotics, 270
  cisplatin, 270
  description, 270
  furosemide and bumetanide, 270

guinea pig cochlea, 270, 271
ototoxicity and toxicity, 270
Zymbal's gland, 271–272
EGFR inhibitors. *See* Epidermal growth factor receptor (EGFR) inhibitors
Endocrine tumours
adrenal glands (*see* Adrenal glands)
and nonendocrine organs, 169
pancreatic islets (*see* Pancreatic islets)
parathyroid gland (*see* Parathyroid gland)
pituitary gland (*see* Pituitary gland)
thyroid gland (*see* Thyroid gland)
toxic effects, 169
Epidermal growth factor receptor (EGFR) inhibitors, 256, 258
Epididymis
description, 140
endocytic vesicles, 140, 142
epididymal atrophy, 140, 141
epithelial hyperplasia, 141
epithelial inflammation and necrosis, 140, 141
single-cell necrosis, 141, 142
sperm and cell debris, 140, 141
sperm granuloma, 140, 141
toxicity, 140
vacuolation, 140, 142
Erosion
cytotoxic and cytostatic anticancer agents, 78
gastric acids, 93
glandular stomach, 88
impaction, 83
Experimental allergic encephalomyelitis (EAE), 223
Eye
blood-ocular barrier, 253
cornea (*see* Cornea)
Draize test, 254
harderian glands (*see* Harderian glands)
immunoregulatory mechanisms, 253
lacrimal and meibomian glands (*see* Lacrimal and meibomian glands)
lens (*see* Lens)
macular degeneration and glaucoma, 253
ocular drug administration, 253
retina (*see* Retina)
standardised trimming procedures, 254
strains and protocols, 253
surfactants and preservatives, 254
treatment, 254
uveal tract (*see* Uveal tract)
xenobiotic, 254

**F**

Female reproductive cycle
external factors, 149
mammary gland (*see* Mammary gland)
nutritional status and environmental stress, 149
ovaries (*see* Ovaries)
toxicity studies, 149
uterus (*see* Uterus)
vagina and cervix (*see* Vagina and cervix)
Follicle-stimulating hormone (FSH), 190, 193
FSH. *See* Follicle-stimulating hormone (FSH)

**G**

Gall bladder
cholecystitis, 74
cystic mucinous hyperplasia, 74
growth factor inhibitor, 74
ulceration mucosal, 74
GFAP. *See* Glial fibrillary acidic protein (GFAP)
Glial cell changes, 215
Glial fibrillary acidic protein (GFAP), 215, 222, 225
Gliopathies
antiviral agent, 222
cerebral cortex, 222
GFAP, 222
monkey, brain stem, 222, 223
pharmaceutical agent, 222
tellurium and cuprizone, 222
GLP. *See* Glucagon-like peptide (GLP)
Glucagon-like peptide (GLP)
C-cell adenoma, 183, 185
C-cell carcinoma, 183, 185
C-cell hyperplasia, 183, 184

**H**

Harderian glands
acinar necrosis, interstitial fibrosis and inflammation, 267, 268
genotoxic and nongenotoxic compounds, 267, 268
hyperplasia and neoplasia, 267
hyperprolactinaemia, 267
sexual dimorphism, 267
Heart
atrial thrombosis, 11, 12
calcification and cartilaginous metaplasia, 9
cardiomyopathy, 7
cartilaginous metaplasia and fibrosis, 7
catecholamines, 1–2
characterisation, 1
coronary arteritis, 11
degeneration and calcification, 2–4
digitoxin, 9
endocardial inflammation, 4, 5
eosinophilic shrunken myocardial fibres, 2
fat necrosis, 11, 12
glucocorticoids, 9
muramyl peptide, 10
myocardial degeneration, 6
myocardial fibrosis
fibroblast proliferation, 3, 4
pigmentation, 4, 5
myocardial hypertrophy, 10
myocardial necrosis
fibrohistiocytic response, 3
and haemorrhage, 4
necrotic fibres, 8
PTAH, 2
myocardial vacuolation and fibrosis, 8
smooth muscle hyperplasia, 6
spontaneous cardiovascular injury, 1
subendocardial myocardial necrosis and vacuolation, 3
theobromine and digitoxin, 4, 5
tunica media and fibrosis, 6
valvular endocarditis, 11, 13
valvular inflammation, 11, 12
vascular occlusion and recanalisation, 10, 11
vasculitis
and intimal proliferation, 10, 11
myocardial necrosis, 10
Hepatocellular hypertrophy
catalase-positive granules, hepatocytes, 60
centrilobular, 59
cytoplasmic clumping and glycogen lakes, 61

Hepatocellular hypertrophy (*cont.*)
cytoplasmic rarefaction, 61
eosinophilic cells, 59
hepatic enlargement, 61
panlobular, 60
panzonal diffuse hypertrophy, 60
periportal, 60
peroxisome proliferation, 60
smooth endoplasmic reticulum (SER) proliferation, 60–61
Hepatotoxicity, 47, 48
4-Hydroxyphenylpyruvate dioxy-genase (4-HPPD) inhibitors, 257
Hyperplasia
anticonvulsants, 80
bile duct
bile ductules and inflammatory cells, 66
cholangitis, 66
inflammation and fibrosis, 66, 67
periductular fibrosis, 66, 67
cholangiofibrosis
2-acetylaminofluorene (2-AAF) treated rat, 68, 69
description, 68
distended bile duct, 68, 69
diffuse hypertrophy, 86
diffuse nodular
bile salt treated rat, 63
choline-deficient diets, rodents, 63
multifocal regenerative hyperplasia, 63
epididymis, 141
foci of cellular alteration
altered hepatocytes, 64, 65
cystic degeneration, 65
genotoxic carcinogens, 64
granulomas, 65
leucocytosis, sinusoidal and centrilobular, 65
nongenotoxic agents, 64
growth factors, 78
hepatocellular, 62
itocell prominence
carotenoid pigment treated dog, 69, 70
focal sinusoidal dilation, 69, 70
lipid granuloma, 69, 70
peliosis hepatis, 69, 70
serous glandular metaplasia, 59, 70
sinusoidal lining cells, 69, 70
Leydig cells, 137, 138
necrosis, 78
oval cell proliferation, 67
prostatic epithelial hypertrophy, 143
regenerative, 62
spontaneous tumours, 83
squamous cell carcinomas, 79
zonal, 62

**I**

IARC. *See* International Agency for Research on Cancer (IARC)
Induced
acinar atrophy, 100
acinar vacuolation and degeneration, 81
articular cartilage, 238
cadmium, 138
and clitoral glands, 144
corticosteroids, 233
eosinophilic inclusions, 30
erosion/ulceration, 84
exocrine pancreas, 99
gingival hyperplasia, 79
hyperkeratosis, 82, 243
hyperplasia, 81
hyperplastic and neoplastic lesions, 40
hypertrophy, 234
inflammation, 133, 249
kidney and bladder tumours, 126, 127
kidney lesions, 109, 110, 111
lesions in ovary (*See* Ovaries)
lesions of adrenal (*See* Adrenal glands)
lesions of neurons, 217
lesions of thymus, 199
Leydig cell hyperplasia and tumours, 137
lung tumours, 40–41
mineralisation, 86
nasal turbinates, 20, 24
neoplastic and nonneoplastic changes, 19
rhabdomyosarcomas, 234
smooth muscle hypertrophy, 91
stomatitis, 78
6-Sulphanil-aminoindazole, 241
testicular toxicity, 134
toxicity, 37
villous atrophy, 90
vitamin E and selenium deficiency, 231
xanthomas, 245
Induced hepatic tumours
cholangiocarcinoma, 73
hepatocellular tumours, 72
Induced liver lesions
degeneration, 48–49
hyperplasia (*see* Hyperplasia)
hypertrophy, 59–61
inclusions, 56
mineralisation, 59
necrosis, 51–53
pigmentation, 57–58
Induced ovarian and uterine tumours. *See* Ovarian tumours; Uterine tumours
Inflammation
acetylcholine, 256
epidermal/adnexal, 243
fibrosis, 265
granular degeneration, 231
growth hormone, 246
hyperplasia, 257
isolated degenerate muscle fibres, 230
keratitis, 255
lymphocytic infiltration, 264
malonaldehyde, 255
neutrophilic infiltration and corneal hyperplasia, 255
procainamide and D-penicillamine, 234
International Agency for Research on Cancer (IARC), 212
Intestines
large
accumulation enteropathy, foreign-body giant cells, 95, 97
adenomas and adenocarcinomas, 98
caecal adenoma, mouse, 98, 99
caecal hypertrophy, 95, 97
carageenans/dextrans, 95, 98
colonic adenocarcinoma, mouse, 98, 99
description, 95
dextran sodium sulphate, 98
focal ulceration, colonic mucosa, 95, 96
hypertrophy and hyperplasia, 95
inflammation and erosion, 95, 96

iron-containing material, macrophages, 95, 96
mucosal hyperplasia, 98
necrosis and atrophy, 95, 96
role, inflammatory factor, 98
small
Brunner's glands degeneration, 91, 93
Brunner's glands hypertrophy, 91, 92
cysteamine acts, 93
description, 90
erosions and ulceration, 93, 94
focal atypical hyperplasia, 93
glandular epithelial proliferation, 90, 91
lymphangiectasia, 93, 95
mesenteric and serosal lipid granulomas, 93
mucosal hypertrophy and hyperplasia, 90
smooth muscle hypertrophy, 91, 92
storage enteropathies, 93, 94
villous atrophy/stunting, 90, 91
villous hypertrophy, 90, 91
Islet cells
adenoma, 189
atrophy and vacuolation, 188
carcinoma, 189
eosinophilic granularity, 187
hyperplasia, 189
hypertrophy, 189
streptozotocin and alloxan, 187
tumours, 188

**J**
Joints
antigen-antibody complex deposition, 241
arthritis, femoro-tibial joint, 241, 242
intra-articular injections, 241
spontaneous arthritis, 241
synovial hyperplasia, 241
tendon sheath, 241, 242
urate crystals, 241

**K**
Kidney
aminonucleoside, 110
CPN, 111
fibrin thrombi, 111, 112
glomerular injuries, 110, 111
glomerular mineralisation, 111, 112
mesangial storage, 111
morphological changes, 109
nephrons, 109
nephrotoxins, 109
renal changes, 109

**L**
Lacrimal and meibomian glands
acinar atrophy, cytoplasm and nuclear crowding, 268, 269
acinar cells and cystic ducts, 268, 269
corneal ulceration and degeneration, 268, 270
dogs, spontaneous autoimmune disease, 268
harderianisation, androgen-dependent, 268, 269
phenazopyridine accumulates, 268
xenobiotics cause, 268
Large granular lymphocytic (LGL), 212
Larynx
cartilage necrosis and regeneration, 27, 28
epithelium, 27
necrosis, 27
squamous metaplasia, 27
Lens
focal lenticular epithelial hypertrophy and hyperplasia, rat, 265, 266
hyaline bodies, 265, 267
lenticular fibres, 265, 266
morgagnian globules, 265, 266
rat, lenticular epithelial hyperplasia, 265, 266
LGL. *See* Large granular lymphocytic (LGL)
LH. *See* Luteinising hormone (LH)
LHRH. *See* Luteinizing hormone–releasing hormone (LHRH)
Liver
adaptive changes
induced lesions, 48
xenobiotics, 48
apoptosis (*see* Apoptosis, liver)
cholangiocarcinomas, 73
cirrhosis, 71
degeneration, hydropic, 48–49
fatty change (*see* Steatosis)
gall bladder, 74
hepatocellular hypertrophy, 59–61
hepatotoxicity classification, 47
hyperplasia (*see* Hyperplasia)
mineralisation, 59
necrosis, 51–53
neoplasia, 72
pigments
brown granular pigment, 57
cholestatic/obstructive jaundice, 57
copper toxicity, 58
dark brown pigment, Kupffer cells, 58
haematoxylin and eosin (H&E) staining, 58
haemosiderin pigmentation, 57
iron pigmentation, 57
Kupffer cells, antimalarial agent, 58
lipofuscin deposition, 57
porphyrin pigment, 57
vincamine alkaloids, 57
Lungs
alveolar fibrosis, 39
alveolitis, 38
bronchiolar–alveolar adenoma, 40, 42
bronchiolar–alveolar carcinoma, 40, 42
bronchiolar–alveolar hyperplasia, 40, 42
cholesterol clefts, 35, 36
effects, 35
fibrinous pneumonia, 39
fibrosing alveolitis, 41, 44
foamy macrophages, 34, 35
focal pigmented macrophages, 35, 36
focal squamous metaplasia, 41, 43
foreign-body granuloma, 35, 37
granuloma, 35, 36
interstitial inflammation, 39
interstitial pneumonitis and fibrosis, 39
keratin cyst, 41, 43
lipoproteinosis and mineralisation, 35, 38
lymphoid depletion, 39, 40
malignant mesothelioma, 41, 43
metabolic activation, 37
necrotic vasculitis, 40, 41
numerous multilamellar bodies, 35, 37

Lungs (*cont.*)
perivascular/alveolar focus, 35, 37
perivascular lymphocytic infiltration, 40
phospholipidosis, 35, 37
pleural fibrosis, 40, 41
pulmonary artery, 40, 42
pulmonary oedema, 37, 38
squamous cell carcinoma, 41, 43
toxicity, 36
Luteinising hormone (LH), 190
Luteinizing hormone–releasing hormone (LHRH), 192
Lymph nodes
agents, 201
antigenic stimulation and administration, 201
antigen-presenting cells, 201, 203
atypical germinal centre hyperplasia, 201
cellularity in germinal centres, 201, 202
cellularity in paracortex, 201, 202
cystic atrophy, renal lymph node, 201, 202
cystic haemorrhagic degeneration, 201, 202
endothelial venules, 204
erythrophagocytosis, 204, 205
extramedullary haemopoiesis, 204
histiocytosis, 203, 204
inducible changes, 201
mast cell infiltration, 205
necrosis and inflammation, 204, 205
plasmacytosis, 203
reactions, 201
regional nodes, 204
synthetic polysaccharides, 201
vacuolated histiocytes and vacuoles, 203, 204
Lymphoid tumours
agents, 198
bone marrow (*see* Bone marrow)
bronchopneumonia, 198
encephalomyelitis, 198, 199
hypersensitivity, 198
immune stimulation/suppression, 198
immune system's function, 198
immunogenic, 198
interorgan and intercellular homeostatic influences, 197
juvenile immunotoxicity studies, 198
lymph nodes (*see* Lymph nodes)
lymphoproliferative responses, 198
macrophages, 197
monoclonal antibody techniques, 197
neoplasms (*see* Neoplasms)
nutritional deficiencies, 198
organs, 197
spleen (*see* Spleen)
squamous cell papilloma, 198
STP, 198
therapeutics, 198
thymus (*see* Thymus)
toxicity studies, 198
vasculitis, 198, 191

**M**
Male reproductive system
accessory sex glands (*see* Accessory sex glands)
animal studies, 131
epididymis (*see* Epididymis)
fixatives, 131
organ development and fertility, 131
peripu-bertal dogs, 132
testes (*see* Testes)
toxicologic assessment, 131
Mammary gland
acinar dilation and hyperplasia, 163, 164
adenoacanthoma, 163, 166
adenocarcinoma, 163, 166
adenoma, 163, 166
contraceptive steroids, 163
distended, 163, 166
ductular hyperplasia and dilation, 163, 164
feminisation, 163, 165
fibroadenoma, 163, 166
lobular hyperplasia, 163, 164
neuroleptic agents, 163
normal, male rat, 163, 165
oestrous cycle, 163
progestational and oestrogenic compounds, 163
Metabolites
haematogenous transport, 37
toxicity, 20
Muscle
adriamycin causes, 231
atrophy, 232
barring damage, 230
chronic myopathy, 231
colchicine and vincristine, 231
description, 229–230
fatty degeneration, 232
foreign-body reaction, 230
granular degeneration, 231
hyaline generation, 231
hypertrophy, 234
hypolipidaemics,231
isolated degenerate muscle fibre, 230
macrophages and lymphocytes, 234
malignant hyperthermia, 231
myofibre degeneration, cynomolgus monkey, 230
myopathy, 229, 230
nuclei, 229
pathologicchanges, mechanisms, 230
peripheral neuropathy and hind-limb muscle, 233
plasma creatine kinase, 229
PPAR, 231
rhabdomyosarcomas, 234
routine skeletal muscle samples, 229
saline vehicle, myopathy, 234
serotonin, 234
transmission electron microscopy, 260
type I and type II, 229
vitamin E and selenium deficiencies, 231
xenobiotics and pharmaceuticals, 233, 234
Myelinopathy
artefactual vacuolation, rat, 220, 221
basophilic vacuoles, rat, 220, 221
buckthorn toxin and tellurium, 220
cerebellar white matter, rat, 220–221
cerebellum, rat, 220–221
Myocardial lesions, 1, 2, 10

**N**
Nasal turbinates
atrophy, 23
degeneration and ulceration, 23
diffuse olfactory epithelial atrophy, 24
eosinophilic droplets, 21, 23
epithelium and squamous metaplasia, 22

factors, 20
fibrosis, 22
focal epithelial erosion, 20
goblet cell hyperplasia, 20, 21
mild inflammation, 21
necrosis, vomeronasal organ, 23
papilloma, 24, 25
physical and chemical nature, 20
reflux-associated changes, 24, 25
respiratory and squamous metaplasia, 23, 24
ulceration and inflammation, 21

Necrosis
beta cells, 187–188
carbon tetrachloride, 172
centrilobular, 51, 52
cortical, 174
degenerating and necrotic hepatocytes, 53
degeneration, pituitary gland, 190
diffuse, 51, 52
diffuse necrosis, z. fasciculata, 173
distended sinusoidal spaces, blood, 51, 53
fibrosis/inflammation, 51, 52
focal, 51, 53
glycogen loss, 51, 52
haemorrhagic, 174
liquefactive, 193
medulla, 177
midzonal, 51
periportal, 51, 52
reticulin collapse and duplication, 51, 52
single cell, 51
sinusoids, punched-out appearance, 51, 53

Neoplasia
hepatocellular adenoma, 72
hepatocellular carcinoma, 72
Tamoxifen, 72
xenobiotics, 72

Neoplasms
carcinogenicity studies, 212
fischer rat leukaemia, 212
histiocytic sarcoma, 212, 213
immunoblastic lymphoma, 212, 213
immunotyping, 212
lymphoblastic lymphoma, 212
lymphoid tumours, 212
non-lymphoid tumours, 212
plasma cell lymphoma, 212
pleomorphic lymphoma, 212, 213
rodent carcinogenicity bioassays, 212
T-cell lymphoma, 212

Nervous system
adequate fixation and preparation techniques, 215
axonal degeneration and inflammatory cellinfiltration, 223–224
axonopathy (*see* Axonopathy)
blood–brain barrier, 215
choroid plexus vacuolation, 215
CNS tumours, 215, 216
description, 215
EAE, 223
gliopathies (*see* Gliopathies)
multifocal foreign-body granulomata, 223, 224
myelinopathy (*see* Myelinopathy)
neuronopathy (*see* Neuronopathy)
neurotoxic lesions, 215
optic nerve, rats, 223, 224
xenobiotic treatments, 223–224

Neuronopathy
anthracycline antibiotics, 217
cerebellar granular layer, rat, 217
cerebellum, mouse, 217, 218
cytoplasmic vacuolation, 216, 217
dark neurons, cerebrum, mouse, 216
dog, neuronal necrosis and loss, 216
glutamate and kainic acid, 217
neuronal loss and gliosis, 216
phospholipidosis, 217
pigmentation, monkey, 217, 218

## O

Ocular
carcinogenicity studies, 257
teratomas and retinoblastomas, 263

Ovarian tumours
β-adrenergic stimulants, 154
granulosa cell tumour, 154, 155
leiomyoma, 154

Ovaries
agents, 149
atretic follicles, 150
atrophy, 150, 151
corpora lutea, 150, 151
cystic follicles, 150–152
endometriosis, 152, 153
immunohistochemical markers, 150
interstitial gland hyperplasia, 152
ionising radiation and anticancer agents, 150
loss/degeneration, oocytes/follicles, 150
luteinisation, 152, 153
mesothelial proliferation, 152, 153
ovarian tumours (*see* Ovarian tumours)
persistent and enlarged corpus luteum, 150, 151
secondary follicles, 150
sertoliform tubular hyperplasia, 152
smooth muscle hyperplasia, 152, 153
toxicity, 149
tubular hyperplasia, 152

## P

PALS. *See* Periarteriolar lymphoid sheath (PALS)

Pancreas
acinar atrophy, 100
acinar-cell adenomas, rat, 104
acinar-cell carcinomas, 104
acinar-cell vacuolation, 101
acinar hyperplasia, rat, 103, 104
apoptosis, 101
basophilic acinar focus, 101, 103
CCK, 99
chronic pancreatitis, rat, 101, 102
degranulation, 100
diffuse acinar atrophy, 100
eosinophilic foci, 103
eosinophilic, hypertrophic peri-islet acinar cells, rat, 101, 103
fat droplets, 101, 102
fatty changem, cytoplasmic vacuolation, 101, 102
focal acinar atrophy, rat, 100
hepatocyte-like cells, 103, 104
hypertrophy, acinar cells, 101
immunohistochemical staining, insulin, 104, 105
intracytoplasmic lysosomal inclusions, 101, 102
necrotising pancreatitis, 101, 102

Pancreas (*cont.*)
  nesidioblastosis-like lesion, 104, 105
  oral administration, ethanol, 101
  pancreatic acinar unit, 99
  pancreatic hepatocytes, 103
  pancreatic necrosis, 101
  treatment, rats, 103
Pancreatic islets
  angiectasis, 187, 188
  benzothiadiazines and immunomodulators, 187
  cells fibrosis and loss, 188
  eosinophilic granularity, 187
  glucocorticoids, 188
  hepatocyte metaplasia adjacent, 188
  hepatoid metaplasia, 188, 189
  hyalinisation and fibrosis, 188
  hyperplasia, 188
  hypertrophy, 188, 189
  islet cell (*see* Islet cells)
  neuroleptics, 188
  oxine and dithizone, 187
  toxicity studies, 187
  vacuolation, 187
Papilla
  epithelial hyperplasia and inflammation, 122
  intracytoplasmic eosinophilic granular inclusions, 122
  papillary hyperplasia, 122
  pelvic inflammation and hyperplasia, 123
  pyelitis and pelvicdilation, 123
  RPN, 120
  vacuolation, 122
Parathyroid gland
  parathyroiditis, 186
  secondary parathyroid hyperplasia, 186
  toxicity studies, 186
Parynx
  eosinophilic droplets, 25
  epithelium, 25, 26
  lymphoid hyperplasia, 25, 26
PAS. *See* Periodic acid–Schiff (PAS)
PCTs. *See* Proximal convoluted tubules (PCTs)
Periarteriolar lymphoid sheath (PALS), 205–207
Periodic acid–Schiff (PAS), 162
Peroxisome proliferator associated receptor (PPAR)
  mesenchymal tumours, 248
  myofibre degeneration, 231
Phosphotungstic acid haematoxylin (PTAH), 2–4
Pituitary gland
  adenoma, 192, 193
  apoptosis, prolactin-positive cells, 190, 191
  carcinoma, 192, 193
  castration cells, 190, 192
  degeneration and necrosis, 190
  focal hyperplasia, 190, 191
  hypertrophy/hyperplasia, 190
  liquefactive necrosis, 192, 193
  necrosis, 193
  pharmacological effects, 190
  somatotroph, 190, 192
  trophic and inhibitory mechanisms, 190
  undifferentiated and interstitial stellate cells, 190
  vacuolated cells, 190, 191
PPAR. *See* Peroxisome proliferator associated receptor (PPAR)
Proximal convoluted tubules (PCTs)
  lipid deposition, 113
  necrosis and vacuolation, 113
  tubular vacuolation, 112
  vacuolation, 112
PTAH. *See* Phosphotungstic acid haematoxylin (PTAH)

**R**

Rats
  Leydig cell carcinoma, 138, 140
  spermatid retention, 133
  tubular dilation, 133
Renal papillary necrosis (RPN), 120, 121
Respiratory system
  airborne pollutants, inhalation, 19
  bronchi/bronchioles, 30–33
  chemicals and pharmaceuticals, 19
  larynx, 27–28
  lungs (*see* Lungs)
  nasal turbinates (*see* Nasal turbinates)
  pharynx, 26
  terminal bronchioles/alveolar ducts, 33–35
  toxicity, 20
  trachea/tracheal bifurcation, 29–30
Retina
  atrophy, inner nuclear layer, 260, 261
  cationic amphophilic agents, 260
  cell morphology, 259
  cyclin-dependent kinase inhibitors, 261
  degeneration/atrophy, 259
  diets deficiency, 260
  ethambutol and doxorubicin causes, 260
  inner nuclear layer, antineoplastic compound, 260, 262
  nutritional deficiencies and metabolic disorder, 259
  ophthalmoscopy, tapetum lucidum, 259
  outer and inner layers, affected, 260, 262
  outer nuclear and photoreceptor layers, 260
  papilloedema, 263
  photoreceptor cells, 259
  retinoblastoma, rat, 263
  RPE, Bruch's membrane, 261, 262
  subretinal haemorrhage, rat, 261, 262
  swollen, apoptotic and degenerative cells, 260, 261
  tapetum lucidum, dog, 259, 260
  teratoma, rat, 263
  triparanol affects, 263
Retinal pigmented epithelium (RPE)
  cyclin-dependent kinase inhibitors, 261
  lead, naphthalene and oxalates, 261
  photoreceptor layer and choroid, 259
  triparanol affects, 263
Rodent astrocytoma, 225
RPE. *See* Retinal pigmented epithelium (RPE)
RPN. *See* Renal papillary necrosis (RPN)

**S**

Seminal vesicles/prostate
  atrophy, 143
  chronic oestrogenic exposure, 143
  congestion, haemorrhage and inflammation, 144, 145
  focal atypical prostatic hyperplasia, 143, 144
  hyperplasia, 143, 144
  hypertrophy, 143, 144
  organs, changes, 142
  preputial gland, 144
  purulent inflammation, 142, 143
  squamous cell carcinoma, 144, 145

Seminiferous
 epithelial atrophy, 134
 focal hypoplasia, 136
 intratubular fluid, 133
 tubular degeneration, 137
 and vacuolation, 133
Skin
 acanthosis and hyperkeratosis, 245
 anticancerals, 245
 bleomycin causes, 244
 chloracne, rabbit pinna, 245
 cutaneous toxicity, 243
 degeneration and necrosis, 244
 dermal and subcutaneous injections, 247
 diabetic models, 243
 epidermal/adnexa, degenerative changes, 244
 epidermal growth factor and growth hormones, 246
 epidermal hyperplasia, 246
 epidermal pigmentation, 243
 folliculitis and dermal inflammation, 244
 growth hormone injections, 247
 hair follicle growth and atrophy, 245
 hyperkeratosis, 243
 hyperpigmentation, 243
 hyperplasia, 244
 immune-mediated skin toxicity, 244
 inflammation and proliferation, 247
 inflammation, degeneration and hyperplasia, 243
 lymphohistiocytic inflammation, 244
 oxidosqualene cyclase inhibitors, 246
 papilloma, methylnitrosourea, 246
 phototoxicity, 245
 PPAR, 248
 safety assessment studies, 242
 sebaceous gland atrophy, 245
 semiquantitative scoring system, 242
 squamous cell carcinoma, 246
 subcutaneous injection, oil-based vehicles, 247
 tendon sheath, 242
 testing, skin irritancy potential, 242
 thiabendazole, 246
 tumour development, 248
 xanthomas, 245
Society of Toxicologic Pathology (STP), 198, 212
Spleen
 aniline compounds, 208
 antigenic stimulation, 205
 atrophy, white pulp, 205, 206
 capsular fibrosis and inflammation, 208
 cellularity and expansion, marginal zone, 205, 207
 cellularity and prominence, germinal centres, 205, 207
 extramedullary erythroid haemopoiesis, 205, 207
 germinal centre and marginal zone with B cells, 205, 206
 histiocytosis, 205, 207
 indomethacin and aspirin, 205
 long-term treatment, F344 rats, 208
 megakaryocytosis, 208
 metallic tin, 205
 PALS with T cells, 205, 206
 pigs and ruminants, 205
 polymorphonuclear cells, red pulp, 208
 red pulp with macrophages, 205, 206
 stromal cell sarcoma, 208
 T cells loss
  marginal zone, 205, 206
  PALS, 205, 206
Steatosis
 hepatocellular vacuolation
  diffuse, 47, 48
  macrovascular, 49, 50
  microvesicular, 49, 50
 phosphorus, 49
 vacuoles, cytoplasm, 49
Stomach
 enterohepatic circulation, 84
 glandular stomach
  adenoma, 89, 90
  adenomatous hyperplasia, 86
  arteritis, 89
  carcinoid, 89
  chief and parietal cell degeneration, 87
  description, 85
  drugs, 88
  enterochromaffin-like (ECL) cell
   proliferation, 89
  erosion and ulceration, 88
  foveolar hyperplasia, 88
  gastric adenocarcinomas, 89
  globule leucocytes, 86
  intestinal metaplasia, 87
  mechanisms, 88
  mineralisation, 86
  pigment and pigmented macrophages, 86
  protective prostaglandin and gastric acid levels, 88
 rodent forestomach
  dietary deficiency, 84
  drugs, 84
  erosion/ulceration, necrosis, 84, 85
  forestomach hyperplasia and squamous cell
   carcinomas, 84
  gastric squamous cell carcinoma, 84, 85
  hyperplasia and hyperkeratosis, 84, 85
  papilloma, methyl nitrosourea, 84, 85
  pharmaceuticals, 84
STP. *See* Society of Toxicologic Pathology (STP)

**T**

Tachea/tracheal bifurcation
 cilia loss, 29
 inflammation, industrial chemical, 29
 squamous metaplasia, 29, 30
 treatment, 29
Teeth
 ameloblast degeneration, rat, 80
 anticonvulsants, 80
 odontoblast degeneration, rat, 80
 tetracycline and minocycline, 79
 types, 79
 upper and lower incisors, tetracycline
  produces, 79, 80
 vacuolar myopathy, 79, 80
 vincristine and cyclophosphamide, 79
 xenobiotics, 80
Terminal bronchioles/alveolar ducts
 ciliated cuboidal metaplasia, 33, 34
 collagenisation/fibrosis, 33, 35
 factors, 33
 foamy macrophage aggregates, 33, 34
 hyaline membrane formation, 33, 34
 oxidant gases, 33
 squamous metaplasia, 33, 34

Testes
  blood–tubule barrier, 132
  cadmium damages, 133
  cell and stage-specific degeneration, 134
  depletion, elongate spermatids and dividing spermatocytes, 134, 135
  diffuse tubular atrophy, 132, 133
  focal hypoplasia, 136
  heat/immobilisation, 134
  hormonal and metabolic changes, 132
  humans and marmosets, 132
  hypospermatogenesis, 136–137
  hypothalamic–pituitary–gonadal axis, 132
  intratubular fluid, 133
  Leydig cell adenoma, 138, 139
  Leydig cell carcinoma, 138, 140
  Leydig cell hyperplasia, 138, 139
  Leydig cell toxicity, 137, 138
  loss, cell types, 135, 136
  metabolism, 132
  nose-only inhalation studies, 133
  phagocytosis, 133, 134
  seminiferous tubular degeneration, 137, 138
  sertoli and leydig cells, 132
  sertoli cell vacuolation, 137, 138
  spermatid retention, 133, 134
  spermatids, 134, 136, 137
  spermatocoele, 133, 134
  spermatogenic cycle, 132
  toxicity, 132
  tubular degeneration, 135, 136
  tubular dilation, 133
  vacuolation, 134
Thymus
  atrophy in laboratory animals, 199, 200
  glucocorticoids, 199
  immunomodulators, 199
  indistinct cortex/medulla demarcation, 199, 201
  lymphocyte apoptosis, 199, 200
  medullary hyperplasia, 199, 201
  organotin and cyclophosphamide, 199–200
  severe apoptosis and loss, 199, 200
Thyroid gland
  age and iodine content, 178
  agents, 178
  C-cell adenoma, 183, 185
  C-cell area, 183, 184
  C-cell carcinoma, 183, 185
  C-cell hyperplasia, 183, 184
  C-cell tumours, 183
  chronic studies, 180
  chronic thyroiditis, 182, 183
  cystic follicles, 180
  cystic follicular hyperplasia, 180
  dark thyroid, 181–182
  diffuse hyperplasia, 183, 184
  dog treatment, sulfonamide, 179, 180
  focal hyperplasia, 186
  follicular
    adenoma, 181
    atrophy, 181, 182
    carcinoma, 181
    epithelial vacuolation, 182, 183
    hyperplasia, 178, 179
    hypertrophy, 178, 179
    pigmentation, 181–183
    tumours, 181
  goitrogens, 179
  hepatic microsomal enzymes, 180
  long-term studies, 180
  mice, dogs and primates, 179
  monkey treatment, industrial chemical, 180
  morphological effects, 179
  normal thyroid, 178, 179
  rats and humans, species differences, 181
Toxicity
  blood–tubule barrier, 132
  buccal mucosal erosions, 78
  enterohepatic circulation, 84
  fibroplasia, 261
  larynx, 27
  Leydig cells, 137
  lungs, 36
  tapetum lucidum, 253
Tract, 19, 20
Tumours
  lungs, 39
  nasal turbinates, 24
  types, 39

U

Ulceration
  carageenans/dextrans, 95
  epithelial atrophy, 78
  glandular mucosa, 88
Urinary bladder lesions
  angiomatous hyperplasia, 127
  carcinoma, 127
  granulomatous inflammation, 126
  haemangioma, 127
  nodular hyperplasia, 126
  squamous metaplasia, 126
  urothelial carcinoma, 127
  urothelial hyperplasia, 126
Urinary system
  kidney (*see* Kidney)
  papilla, 120–122
  tubular changes
    copper-containing pigment, 114, 116
    cortical tubules, vacuolation, 113
    crystalline nephropathy, 117
    cystic dilation, 117
    cystic hyperplastic tubule, 120, 121
    cytomegaly and karyomegaly, 118, 119
    dilation and casts, 117
    disruption, 113, 114
    distal convolutedtubules, vacuolation, 113
    electron micrograph, 114, 115
    eosinophilia and hypertrophy, 120
    hyaline droplet infiltration, 114, 115
    hyperplasia, 118, 119
    hypertrophy, 114, 116
    interstitial fibrosis/inflammation, 113, 114
    intracytoplasmic eosinophilic inclusions, 114, 115
    intracytoplasmic inclusions, 114, 115
    intranuclear eosinophilic inclusions, 114, 116
    linear cortical scar, 117, 118
    lipid deposition, 111
    $\alpha_2$-microglobulin staining, 114, 115
    mineralisation, 118
    necrosis and vacuolation, 113
    PCT, 112
    pigment deposition, 114

pigmented crystals, 117, 118
vacuolation and crystals, 118
tumours
nephroblastomas, 125
renal tubular adenoma, 125
renal tubular carcinoma, 125
urinary bladder, 126–127
vascular changes
arterial hypertrophy, 123, 124
atherosclerosis, 123
interstitial and peritubular fibrosis, 123
interstitial nephritis, 123
renal cortex, 123
Uterine tumours
cytochrome P450 enzymes, 159
endometrial adenocarcinoma, 159, 160
endometrial polyp, 159, 160
haemangioma, 159, 160
leiomyoma, 159, 160
prolactin inhibition, 159
thick squamous epithelium, hyperkeratosis, 159, 161
Uterus
adenomyosis, 155, 158
angiectasis and angiomatous hyperplasia, 158, 159
atrophy, 158, 159
bromocriptine, 155
decidualisation, 155, 157, 158
decidual plaque, 155, 157
endometrial haemorrhage, 158, 159
endometrial hyperplasia, 155, 156
endometriosis, 155, 158
hypertrophy and vacuolation, 155, 156
mesothelial proliferation, 155, 157
mucometra, 155, 157
multifocal decidualisation, 155, 157
oestrogens, 155
oestrous cycle, 155
papillary projection, 155, 156
pyometra, 155, 157
squamous metaplasia, 155, 156
synthetic growth hormone, 155
uterine tumours (*see* Uterine tumours)
Uveal tract
antiviral agent, 264
blood supply, 264
ciliary bodies and Bruch's membrane, 264
ciliary body, novel anticancer agent, 264, 265
glaucoma, dog, 265
lymphocytic infiltration, 264
melanin synthesis, 264

**V**

Vagina and cervix
atrophy, 161–163
macroscopic changes, 161
mucification, 161, 162
oestrogens and oestrogen receptor modulators, 161
progestogen treatment, 161
thick squamous epithelium, 161
Vascular endothelial growth factor (vEGF) inhibitors, 257, 258
Vascular lesions, 1, 4

**Z**

Zymbal's gland, 271–272

FSC
www.fsc.org
MIX
Papier aus verantwortungsvollen Quellen
Paper from responsible sources
FSC® C105338

If you have any concerns about our products,
you can contact us on
**ProductSafety@springernature.com**

In case Publisher is established outside the EU,
the EU authorized representative is:
**Springer Nature Customer Service Center GmbH**
**Europaplatz 3, 69115 Heidelberg, Germany**

Printed by Libri Plureos GmbH
in Hamburg, Germany